www.medabbrev.com

- Have you used this Internet site?
- You are entitled to a no-cost, one-year, single-user access license.
- See page vii for activation instructions.

Features

- Contains the entire contents of this book
- At no extra cost, add it to your WiFi-enabled devices' home page as an icon, or bookmark it.
- Has a high-speed search engine to find—
  - the meaning(s) of an abbreviation
  - all the abbreviations that contain a particular word
  - trade and generic drug names
- Each week about 20 new entries are added.
- Click any word or drug name and be connected to the Wikipedia definition/monograph.
- You can renew your license each year, see page 417.

MEDICAL ABBREVIATIONS:

32,000 Conveniences at the Expense of Communication and Safety

15th Edition

Neil M Davis, MS, PharmD, FASHP

Professor Emeritus, Temple University
  School of Pharmacy, Philadelphia, PA,
Editor Emeritus, Hospital Pharmacy
President, Safe Medication Practices
  Consulting, Inc.

published by
Neil M Davis Associates
2049 Stout Drive, B-3
Warminster, PA 18974-3861

Phone (215) 442-7430 or (888) 333-1862
  (9 AM-4 PM EST, Mon-Fri)
FAX (215) 442-7432 or (888) 333-4915
E-mail med@neilmdavis.com
Secure Website www.medabbrev.com

Contents

Dedication

This book is dedicated to Julie, my wife, for her support, patience, assistance, and love.

Acknowledgments

The assistance of Evelyn Canizares, Vicki Bell, Gemma Jakeman, Ann Sandt Kishbaugh, Patricia A. Ireland, Allyson Burnett, Sue M. Malone, Matthew Davis, Robin Miller, and Hayley Miller is gratefully acknowledged.

I would like to express my deep appreciation for the many contributions received from readers for their suggested additions and corrections. Please continue to send these to—

Dr. Neil M Davis
2049 Stout Drive, B-3
Warminster, PA 18974

FAX (215) 442-7432 or (888) 333-4915
E-mail   med@neilmdavis.com
Secure Website www.medabbrev.com

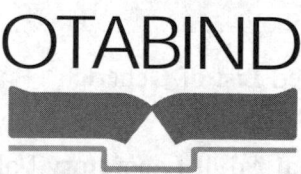

OTABIND

Bound to stay open

The pages in this book open easily and lie flat, a result of the Otabind bookbinding process. Otabind combines advanced adhesive technology and a **free-floating cover** to achieve books that last longer and are bound to stay open.

Preface

The Internet Version: Why Use It and How to Access It

Along with the purchase of each book, the book owner, at no extra cost, is entitled to a single-user license for access to the Internet version of this 15th edition. This license is valid for 12 months from the date of the initial log-in. Internet Explorer 5.0, Firefox 1.0, Safari 3, or Netscape 4.0, or higher can meet the minimum browser requirement. Mobile platforms supported include iPhone®, iPad®, iPod Touch®, DROID™ , Windows® Mobile, BlackBerry®, Palm®, amd other WiFi-enabled devices

Features of the Internet Version

- Updated weekly with about 20 entries (suggestions from users are welcomed and will be incorporated).
- Can instantaneously search for the meanings of abbreviations and acronyms.
- Has a reverse-search feature, for example, looking for all the abbreviations that contain the word "laparoscopic."
- Can search for cross-referenced generic and brand names of drugs.
- Click any word or drug name and be connected to the Wikipedia definition/monograph.
- Can search through the listings of symbols, lists, and normal adult laboratory values.
- Quick access to a "Do Not Use" list of dangerous abbreviations, an explanation as to why they are dangerous, and suggested alternatives to be used. For those facilities that obtain multi-user licenses, they may substitute their own "Do Not Use" list, which they can control and update.
- Can read the full-text of the introductory chapters of the book.
- At no extra cost, add it to your WiFi-enabled device's home page as an icon, or bookmark it.

Instructions for the Initial One-time Log-in

- Access the Website at *www.medabbrev.com*
- Click the **Register** button (on the top-left of the screen)
- You must agree to the Single-User License Agreement which is presented.
- You will be asked for the 8-letter access code that appears on the front inside cover of the book. This will be the only time you are asked for this code.
- At this point just follow the directions.
- Note your sign-in name and your self-assigned password. This name/password will only permit one access at a time, so keep this information confidential to ensure your ready access to the site.

Searching for the Meaning of an Abbreviation on the Internet Version

- Use upper OR lower case letters as the search engine is NOT case sensitive.
- Use normal upper OR lower case letters as the search engine is NOT sensitive to whether the letters are **bold-face** or *italicized.*
- Superscripts and subscripts are to be entered as regular text.
- DO NOT enter periods, commas, hyphens, or spaces (enter afib, not a fib).
- For other details, just follow the simple instructions shown on the Website. The Internet version of the book is essentially the same as the print version except for the fact that it is searchable and is updated weekly with about 20 new entries.

Multi-user Site Licenses are Available

A copy of the Multi-User Site License agreement and its price list is available by clicking the "Submit Suggestions" button on *www.medabbrev.com* where you can type a request to receive it or by calling 888 333 1862 or 215 442 7430. A no-cost, 3-week trial is available.

Extending or Purchasing Internet Access

A 12-month purchase or extension of the Internet version is available. See pricing information on page 417.

Additions, Corrections, and Suggestions are Welcomed

Please send them via any means shown below:

Neil M Davis
2049 Stout Drive, B-3
Warminster PA 18974-3861

FAX 888 333 4915 or 215 442 7432
Email med@neilmdavis.com
Secure website www.medabbrev.com

Thank you for your help in the past.

Have You Used the Internet Version of This Book?

- It is instantaneously searchable for the meanings of abbreviations
- It is reverse searchable (search for all the abbreviations containing a particular word)
- Each week, about 20 new entries are added

See the preface (page vii) for access instructions. A one-year, single-user access is included in the purchase price of the book. Also one-year subscriptions (no book) are available for purchase (see page 417).

WiFi-Enabled Devices

At no extra cost, WiFi-enabled devices can access the Internet version where it can be added as a home-page icon or bookmarked.

computer	iPhone®	iPad®	iPod Touch®	BlackBerry®	DROID™	Windows® Mobile	Palm®

Multi-User Site Licenses are Available

Medical facilities can substitute their own "Do Not Use" list of dangerous abbreviations for the one present. The ability also exists to list abbreviations that are unique to your region and/or organization which would normally not appear in any national list. These lists would be controlled by the facility or company. A no-cost, 3-week trial and pricing information are available by calling 888 333 1862 or 215 442 7430 or via an e-mail request to ev@neilmdavis.com

Chapter 1
Introduction

L isted are current acronyms, symbols, abbreviations, slang and 32,000 of their possible meanings. This list has been compiled to assist individuals in reading and transcribing medical records, medically-related communications, and prescriptions.

WARNING

Abbreviations are a convenience, a time saver, a space saver, a way of fitting a word or phrase into a restricted space on a form or computer, and a way of avoiding the possibility of misspelling words. However, a price can be paid for their use. Abbreviations are sometimes not understood. They can be misread, or are interpreted incorrectly. Their use lengthens the time needed to train individuals in the health fields, wastes the time of healthcare workers in tracking down their meaning, at times delays the patient's care, and occasionally results in patient harm.

The publication of this list of abbreviations is not an endorsement of their legitimacy. It is not a guarantee that the intended meaning has been correctly captured, nor is it an indication that the abbreviation is commonly used. The person who uses an abbreviation must take responsibility for making sure that it is properly interpreted. When an uncommon or ambiguous abbreviation is used and it may not be understood correctly, it should be defined by the writer. Where uncertainty exists, the one who wrote the abbreviation must be contacted for clarification.

There are three types of what are generally termed as abbreviations:
- Acronyms: Lettered abbreviations which are pronounced as a word (e.g., AIDS)
- Initialism: First letter of each word is used and it is *not* pronounced as a word (e.g., HIV)
- Brief Form: A shortened form of a word (e.g., exam)

There are many variations in how an abbreviation can be expressed. Anterior-posterior has been written as AP, A.P., ap, a.p., and A/P. Since there are few standards and those who use abbreviations do not necessarily follow these standards, this book only shows anterior-posterior as AP. This is done to make it easier to find the meaning of an abbreviation as all the meanings of AP are listed together. This elimination of unnecessary duplication also keeps the book at a convenient size, thus enabling it to be sold at a reasonable price.

When an abbreviation is made up of a series of abbreviations, it may not be listed as such. In such instances, the meaning may be determined by looking up each set of abbreviations, as in the example of DTP_a-HIB-PNU-MEN, which means, diphtheria, tetanus toxoids, acellular pertussis; *Haemophilus influenzae* type b conjugate; pneumococcal (*Streptococcus pneumoniae*) conjugate; meningococcal (*Neisseria meningitidis*) conjugate (serogroups unspecified) vaccine.

Lower case letters are used when firm custom dictates as in Ag, Na, mCi, etc. The first letter of brand names are capitalized, whereas nonproprietary names appear in lower case.

The abbreviation ACT is listed as meaning doxorubicin, cyclophosphamide, and paclitaxil. The reason for this apparent disparity is that the official generic names (United States Adopted Names) are shown rather than the brand names Adriamycin and Taxol. In the case of LSD, the official name, lysergide, is given, as well as the chemical name, lysergic acid diethylamide. The Latin derivations for older medical and pharmaceutical abbreviations (*t.i.d.,* *ter in die,* three times daily) may be found in *Remington.*[1]

Some abbreviations which have been encountered or that have been suggested for addition to the book have not been added. Some were obscene or completely insensitive. Slang and drug name abbreviations are shown for informational purposes only and should not be used.

Abbreviations for medical facility names create problems as they are usually not recognized by the readers in other geographic areas. A clue to the fact that one is dealing with such an abbreviation is when it ends with MC, for Medical Center; HS, for Health System; MH, for Memorial Hospital; CH, for Community Hospital; UH, for University Hospital; and H, for Hospital.

The use of abbreviations are not uniform across the country, and usage tends to cluster. Sometimes physicians just make up their own abbreviations. Sometimes a physician-in-training will pick up and use abbreviations used by residents or attendings where they train. Sometimes group practices will start to use certain abbreviations. Sometimes hospitals might have banned certain abbreviations, so you might not see them used at one hospital, while at another hospital they are used. Usage will also vary by specialty.

Form designers and computer programmers should be sensitive to the fact that unrealistic restriction of space for entering data can cause users to create abbreviations which will be unfamiliar to future readers.

As in the medical and other scientific literature, organism and plant names, and non-English words and abbreviations are expressed in *italics* in this book and Internet version, however in the medical transcription field, these are expressed in normal typeface.[2] It also should be noted that in computerized health records, italics, boldface type, superscripts, and subscripts are expressed in normal typeface.

If a meaning for an abbreviation with an ending of an S can not be found, look for that abbreviation without the S. SAEs (serious adverse events) would not be found, but SAE (serious adverse event) is listed.

When an abbreviation cannot be found in this book or when the listed meaning(s) do not make sense, there is a possibility that the abbreviation has been misread. As an example, a reader could not find the meaning of HHTS. On closer examination it really was +HTS, not HHTS. Also EWT could not be identified because it was really ENT.

Some common French and Spanish abbreviations are listed in the book. Because of language structure differences, these abbreviations are often reversed, as in the case of HIV, which in Spanish and French is abbreviated as VIH.

Chapter 5 presents a list of 275 of the most commonly used abbreviations. The purpose of this list is to serve as a primer for whose entering a health-related field.

Chapter 9 contains a cross-referenced list of 3,400 generic and brand drug names. The list contains names of commonly prescribed, new drugs, and recently discontinued drugs. Brand names have their first letter capitalized whereas generic names are in lower case. This list will enable readers to obtain the generic name for brand name products or brand names for generic names. It will also serve as a spelling check.

Coded drug names and abbreviations for drug names are found in the chapter on abbreviations (Chapter 6). Abbreviated drug names should not be used as they pose a safety risk.

Chapter 10 is a table of normal laboratory values. Both the conventional and international values are listed. Each laboratory publishes a list of its normal values. These local lists should be reviewed to see if there are significant differences.

Avoid using abbreviations when naming a diagnosis and/or operative procedures. These are critical points of information, and their meanings must be clear to assure accurate communication for patient care, reimbursement, statistical purposes, and medicolegal documentation.

The Council of Biology Editors (CBE), in their 1983 edition of the *CBE Style Manual* listed about 600 abbreviations gathered from 15 internationally recognized authorities and organizations.[3] The majority of these symbols and abbreviations tend to be more scientifically oriented than those which would appear in medical records. In the few situations where the CBE abbreviations differ from what is presented in this book, the CBE abbreviation has been placed in parentheses after the meaning. As is the practice in the United States, mL has been used rather than ml and the spelling of liter, meter, etc. is used rather than litre and metre, even though ml, litre, and metre are listed in the *CBE Style Manual*. A current edition of the *CBE Style Manual* was published in 2006.[4] Again, in this edition, emphasis is placed on scientific abbreviations.

Only a few of the acronyms and abbreviations for the major cardiologic trials, such as, TIMI- Thrombosis In Myocardial Infarction (trial), have been included in this book. For a list of 4,200 of these acronyms and abbreviations, consult reference number 5.

For a more complete list of abbreviations used for cancer chemotherapy protocols see the appendix of the reference book/web-version, Drug Facts and Comparisons.[6]

The box at the bottom of the front cover is a contrived attention-getter to show how abbreviations are used. The abbreviations are real, just the story is contrived. I would be surprised if most readers could decipher more than half of the abbreviations used since many are not in common use. It reads as follows:

...81 YO WDWNMAM POPTA, BIBA, admitted to CPETU c/o PND & DOE. TBNA in ED last wk for CP relieved by NTG. Prev Adm for PTCA 1995, THR 2005, ICD 2007, IWMI 2010. ATSO Dr Hayley.

Translated as intended, it reads:

...81 **y**ear **o**ld **w**ell-**d**eveloped, **w**ell-**n**ourished, **M**exican-**A**merican **m**ale **p**assed **o**ut **p**rior **t**o **a**rrival. **B**rought **i**n **b**y **a**mbulance, admitted to **c**hest **p**ain **e**valuation and **t**reatment **u**nit, **c**omplained **o**f **p**aroxysmal **n**octurnal **d**yspnea and **d**yspnea **o**n **e**xertion. **T**reated **b**ut **n**ot **a**dmitted in **E**mergency **D**epartment **l**ast **w**eek for **c**hest **p**ain relieved by **n**itroglycerin. **P**revi**o**us **adm**ission for **p**ercutaneous **t**ransluminal **c**oronary **a**ngioplasty 1995, **t**otal **h**ip replacement 2005, **i**mplantable **c**ardioverter **d**efibrillator 2007, **i**nferior **w**all **m**yocardial **i**nfarct 2010. **A**dmit **t**o the **s**ervice **o**f Doctor Hayley.

On the *positive side*, the use of abbreviations in the example—
- Saves time for the writer
- Saves space
- Lessens the possibility of misspellings
- Allows for fitting information into restricted space provided on a form or computer

On the *negative side*, will this uncontrolled use of abbreviations result in—
- Incomplete or erroneous communication with non-emergency room personnel?
- Puzzling documentation?
- An increase in the time necessary to train health personnel?
- Delays in initiating treatment?
- Patient harm?

Over the years certain abbreviations are no longer used because of changes and/or advancements. These obsolete abbreviations are not removed from this book because old records are reviewed for auditing, research, and medicolegal sleuthing. Secondly, some physicians are slow to let go of out-of-date terminology or abbreviations and will likely use early-learned abbreviations out of habit, perhaps for a lifetime. Since the purpose of the book is to help readers decipher whatever it is that they are reading, then there is no logic to restricting abbreviations to only the latest, greatest, and newest of things; the book/web version is needed to help decipher the not-so-new and not-so-great and oldest of abbreviations as well.

An examination of the abbreviations, acronyms, symbols, and their 32,000 meanings is a testimonial to the problems and dangers associated with uncontrolled use of undefined abbreviations.

References

1. Hendrickson R, ed. Remington's The Science and Practice of Pharmacy, 21st ed. Phila., PA: Lippincott Williams and Wilkins, 2006.

2. Sims L. The Book of Style for Medical Transcription, 3rd ed. 2008. Association for Healthcare Documentation Integrity. Modesta, CA.

3. CBE Style Manual, 5th ed. Bethesda, MD: Council of Biology Editors; 1983.

4. Council of Science Editors, Style Manual Committee, Science style and format: the CSE manual for authors, editors, and publishers. 7th ed. Reston (VA): The Council; 2006.

5. Cheng TO, Julian D. Acronyms of cardiologic trials-2002. Int J Cardiol 2003;91:261–351.

6. Facts and Comparisons, St. Louis, Wolters Kluwer Health (factsandcomparisons.com)

Chapter 2

Dangerous, Contradictory, and/or Ambiguous Abbreviations

Many inherent problems associated with abbreviations contribute to or cause errors. Reports of such errors have been published routinely (see Table 1).[1-5]

Healthcare organizations are directed by the Joint Commission to formulate a "Do Not Use" list of dangerous abbreviations which should NOT be used. An example of such a list, which has been adopted from the Institute of Safe Medication Practice Inc. (ISMP) list, is shown as Table 2.

Table 1. Examples of Abbreviations That Have Been Misread or Misinterpreted

---

(1) "HCT250 mg" was intended to mean hydrocortisone 250 mg but was interpreted as hydrochlorothiazide 50 mg (HCTZ50 mg).

(2) Flucytosine was improperly abbreviated as 5 FU, causing it to be read as fluorouracil. Flucytosine is abbreviated 5 FC and fluorouracil is 5 FU.

(3) Floxuridine was improperly abbreviated as 5 FU, causing it to be read as fluorouracil. Floxuridine is abbreviated FUDR and fluorouracil is 5 FU.

(4) MTX was thought to be mechlorethamine. MTX is methotrexate and mechlorethamine is abbreviated HN2.

(5) **The abbreviation "U" for unit is the most dangerous one in the book, having caused numerous ten-fold insulin and heparin overdoses. The word unit should never be abbreviated.** The handwritten U for unit has been mistaken for a zero, causing tenfold errors. The handwritten U has also been read as the number four, six, and as "cc."

(6) OD, meant to signify once daily, has caused Lugol's solution to be given in the right eye.

(7) OJ meant to signify orange juice, looked like OS and caused saturated solution of potassium iodide to be given in the left eye.

(8) IVP, meant to signify intravenous push (Lasix 20 mg IVP), caused a patient to be given an intravenous pyelogram which is the usual meaning of this abbreviation.

(9) Na Warfarin (sodium warfarin) was read as "No Warfarin."

(10) The abbreviation "s̄" for "without" has been thought to mean "with" (c̄).

(11) The order for PT, intended to signify a laboratory test order for prothrombin time, resulted in the ordering of a physical therapy consultation.

(12) The abbreviation "TAB," meant to signify Triple Antibiotic (a coined name for a hospital sterile topical antibiotic mixture), caused patients to have their wounds irrigated with a diet soda. At another facility, with the same set of circumstances, they did not have TAB®, so they used Diet Shasta.®

(13) A slash mark (/) has been mistaken for a one, causing a patient to receive a 100 unit overdose of NPH insulin when the slash was used to separate an order for two insulin doses:

   6 units regular insulin/20 units NPH insulin

(14) Vidarabine, an antiviral agent, was ordered as ara-A; however, ara-C, which is cytarabine, an antineoplastic agent, was given.

(15) On several occasions, pediatric strength diphtheria-tetanus toxoids (DT) have been confused with adult strength tetanus-diphtheria toxoids (Td).

(16) DTP is commonly understood to refer to diphtheria-tetanus-pertussis vaccine, but in some hospitals it is also used as shorthand for a sedative cocktail of Demerol, Thorazine,

5

and Phenergan. Several cases have occurred where a child was vaccinated rather than given the sedative mixture.

(17) What does the abbreviation MR mean? Some will guess measles-rubella vaccine (M-R-Vax II, Merck), while others will assume mumps-rubella vaccine (Biavax II, Merck).

(18) The abbreviation TIW (three times a week) was thought to mean Tuesday and Wednesday when the I was read as a slash mark. Due to confirmation bias (you see what you know), this uncommon abbreviation is seen as the more commonly used TID (three times a day).

(19) PCA, meant to be procainamide, was interpreted as patient-controlled analgesia.

(20) PGE_1 (alprostadil, Caverject) was read as P6 E1 (Alcon's ophthalmic 6% pilocarpine and 1% epinephrine solution).

(21) A nurse transcribed an oral order for the antibiotic aztreonam as AZT, which was subsequently thought to be the antiviral drug zidovudine.

(22) An order for TAC 0.1%, intended to mean triamcinolone cream, was interpreted as tetracaine, Adrenalin, and cocaine solution.

(23) An order for SPA (salt poor albumin) was overlooked because it was not recognized as a drug order.

(24) Therapy was delayed and considerable professional time was wasted when an order for "Bactrim SS q 12 h on S/S" had to be clarified (Bactrim Single Strength every 12 hours on Saturday and Sunday).

(25) A physician wrote an order stating "may take own supply of EPO". The physician meant evening primrose oil, not Epogen (epoetin alfa).

(26) 4-MP was recommended to treat ethylene glycol poisoning. The medical resident mistakenly interpreted this as 6-MP (6-mercaptopurine). 4-MP is fomepizole (4 methylpyrazole) and 6-MP is mercaptopurine (6-mercaptopurine).

(27) An order for lomustine stated it was to be given at "hs". This was misinterpreted as to mean every night. After continuous administration, toxicity resulted in the patient's death. The drug is normally given once every 6 weeks. State complete orders such as "HS $\times$ 1 dose today," "HS nightly," or "HS nightly PRN for sleep."

(28) The directions for an order for Cortisporin Otic Solution indicated "Three drops in ® ear TID." The patient was given the drops in the rear rather than the right ear.

(29) There have been mix-ups between IL-2 and IL-11 when IL-2 is expressed as IL-II (Roman numeral 2). The II has been read as "IL eleven," and vice versa. IL-2 (interleukin 2) is aldesleukin (Proleukin) and IL-11 is oprelvekin (Neumega).

(30) A drug was ordered "Q 10 h." It was read as QID (four times daily). Drugs should not be ordered at unusual hourly intervals such as every 10, 18, or 36 hours, as this has resulted in a host of errors. Standard times are every 2, 3, 4, 6, 8, or 12 hours; once, twice, three, or four times daily; every other day, or Monday, Wednesday, and Friday and once weekly.

(31) 6 IU was read 61 units instead of the intended 6 international units.

(32) A dose of phenytoin was modified and expressed as mg/Kg/d. The d was read as "dose" rather than the intended "day" resulting in 3 extra doses being given.

(33) An order appeared as "If no BM in PM, give MOM in AM p.r.n."

(34) Sometimes ambiguous abbreviations cause financial losses to health providers. For example, an insurance provider may pay less for an office visit for mental retardation than it does for mitral regurgitation. This can happen if the coder is faced with the abbreviation MR.

(35) The abbreviation for "q PM" has been read as 9 PM (a one time dose at 9 PM) rather than every night.

(36) An order was written in a hospital, "Cortisporin 3 drops, AS bid." There was a question about the meaning of AS, but since the patient was scheduled for a colonoscopy it was decided that the meaning was "anal sphincter", so the drug was administered rectally rather than in the left ear as intended. When the patient was asked to roll over for their medicine, I suppose they could have protested that there was nothing wrong with their rectum, but then again, maybe this was part of a complex preparation for their colonoscopy!

(37) A liver transplant patient on readmission had an order handwritten, "MMF 1000 mg PO BID (mycophenolate mofetil)." Mycophenolate mofetil is the immunosuppressive agent CellCept which has been abbreviated MMF. The order was misread as 1000 mg twice

daily MWF (Monday, Wednesday, and Friday). Several doses of this critical drug were omitted before the error was discovered.

(38) A prescription was written for PTU. PTU normally means propylthiouracil, however Purinethol was dispensed in error causing a fatality. Purinethol is never abbreviated PTU. The error probably occurred because both propylthiouracil and Purinethol are available in 50 mg tablets and sit side-by-side on the pharmacy shelf. The prescriber contributed to the error by using nonstandard terminology, an abbreviation.

(39) A nurse mistaken administered Chloral Hydrate Syrup intravenously. This syrup is intended for oral administration only. This was done because the label contained the legend C IV. This was interpreted as intravenous when in fact, C IV stands for a class 4 controlled substance. All controlled substances are indicated as Roman numerals, I, II, III, IV, V. Even though 99.99% of nurses know that drugs in screw-capped bottles, labeled "syrup" are not intended for intravenous administration, it would pay to change C IV to C4 on drug company labels.

(40) After performing spinal surgery a surgeon kept his ICU patients NPO (nothing by mouth), until they had flatus and good **b**owel **s**ounds. His order was: "Strict NPO. Check BS Q2H." The patient had "blood sugar" laboratory tests drawn Q2H!

(41) An order was written for lidocaine 1% s̄ EPINEPHrine. It was misinterpreted as lidocaine 1% with EPINEPHrine. s̄ is a Latin-derived abbreviation for "without" which is rarely used. "Lidocaine 1%" is a safer way to express this order.

(42) There have been mix-ups between DTap and Tdap. DTaP is diphtheria and tetanus toxoids and acellular pertussis vaccine (DAPTACEL and TRIPEDIA, and INFANRIX). It is meant for *active immunization* of pediatric patients 6 weeks through 6 years of age. Tdap is tetanus toxoid, reduced diphtheria toxoid, and acellular pertussis vaccine (BOOSTRIX and ADACEL). It is meant to be used as *booster* shots for older children, adolescents, and adults.

(43) An infant died when she received 5 mg of morphine instead of the handwritten prescribed ".5 mg" dose when the naked decimal point was not seen. This can easily occur if the decimal point happens to fall on a line, or falls on part of a letter from the line above, or when working from poor copies of an original order. Always place a zero in front of a naked decimal (0.5 mg, not .5 mg).

(44) An order was written for Colchicine 1.0 mg IV now. The decimal point was not seen and 10 mg was administered. The patient died. This can easily occur if the decimal point happens to fall on a line, or falls on part of a letter from the line above, or when working from poor copies of an original order. Use 1 mg, not 1.0 mg. A trailing zero can correctly be used where precision is being expressed, such as in reporting a laboratory value, but never in expressing a drug dose or strength.

(45) The pharmacy received an order for a diltiazem drip. No rate of administration was listed, so the pharmacist entered "125 mg UD" in computer rate field. UD is an old-time Latin abbreviation for as directed (*ut dictum*). The nurse did not know the classical meaning of UD and interpreted as meaning unit dose. The nurse then proceeded to give the diltiazem at 125 mg/hr and ran the entire dose over one hour (the rate should have been 5 mg/hr). The nurse then asked for another diltiazem drip and also ran that one over 1 hour. The patient expired. As in many errors, it was not just one thing that caused the error. One of the many factors in causing this error was the use of an ancient abbreviation which should no longer be used.

The author would appreciate receiving other examples of abbreviations that have been misinterpreted causing error or delays so that this section can be expanded. E-mail them to med@neilmdavis.com

---

A prescription could be written with directions as follows: "OD OD OD," to mean one drop in the right eye once daily!

Abbreviations should not be used for drug names as they are particularly dangerous. As previously illustrated, there is the possibility that the writer may, through mental error, confuse two abbreviations and use the wrong one. Similarly, the reader may attribute the wrong meaning to an abbreviation. To further confound the problem, some drug name abbreviations have multiple meanings (see ATR, CPM, CPZ, DXM, FLU, GEM, IBC, KET, NITRO, PIT, PBZ and TMZ in Table 3). The abbreviation AC has been used for three different cancer chemotherapy combinations to mean Adriamycin and either cyclophosphamide, carmustine, or cisplatin.

See chapter 4 which discusses how medical writers, editors, and health professionals can prevent the coining and use of these ambiguous abbreviations. To avoid the introduction of contradictory or ambiguous abbreviations, before coining a new abbreviation, one must do some research. Check this book and Medline to see other possible meanings that already exist for the planned abbreviation. Secondly, rethink if there is really a need to develop an abbreviation for the term.

Beside causing medication errors and incorrect interpretation of medical records, abbreviations can create problems because treatment is delayed while a health professional seeks clarification for the meaning of the abbreviation used. Abbreviations should not be used to designate drugs. The establishment of abbreviations for drug combinations is an ongoing problem and should require facility/organizational approvals.

Certain meanings of abbreviations in the book are followed by a warning, "this is a dangerous abbreviation." This warning could be placed after many abbreviations, but was reserved for situations where errors have been published because these abbreviations were used or where the meaning is critical and not likely to be known. If no alternative abbreviation is suggested, then the term should be spelled out rather than abbreviated. Such warning statements should also appear after every abbreviation for a drug or drug combination.

References

1. Davis NM, Cohen MR. Medication errors: causes and prevention. Warminster, PA: Neil M Davis Associates; 1983.
2. Cohen MR. Medication error reports. Hosp Pharm (appears monthly from 1975 to the present).
3. Cohen MR. Medication errors. Nursing 2011 (appears monthly, starting in Nursing 77, to the present).
4. Davis NM. Med Errors. Am J Nursing (appears monthly from 1994 to 1995).
5. Cohen MR. Medication Errors. American Pharmacists Assoc. Wash. DC, 2011.

Table 2. Dangerous Abbreviations and Dosage Designations

Problem Term	Intended Meaning	Reason for Problem(s)	Suggested Remedy
AU	both ears	Read as OU (both eyes) or not understood	Use "both ears"
cc for expressing liquid measurements	cubic centimeter (same as milliliter [mL])	Read as u (unit) or 00	Use "mL"
D/C	discharge	Interpreted as discontinue medications resulting in premature discontinuance of current medication	Use "discharge"
IN	intranasal	Read as IV or IM or heard as IM	Write "intranasal" "nasally" or use "NAS" if limited by computer space allotted

Table 2. Dangerous Abbreviations and Dosage Designations (*continued*)

Problem Term	Intended Meaning	Reason for Problem(s)	Suggested Remedy
IU	International unit	Misread as IV (intravenous); The I is read as a one (6 IU is read as 61 units)	Use "units" rather than international units, or spell out international units, using a lowercase i
OD	once daily	Interpreted as right eye	Write "once daily"
OJ	Orange juice	Read as OS (left eye) or OD (right eye)	Use "orange juice"
QOD	every other day	Interpreted as meaning "every once a day" or read as q.i.d. (four times daily)	Write "every other day"
QD	once daily	Read or interpreted as q.i.d. (four times daily)	Write "once daily"
q.n.	every night	Read as every hour	Write "once daily at night"
q HS	every night	Read as every hour	Use "once daily at night"
µg	microgram	When handwritten, misread as mg	Use "mcg"
sq or sub q	subcutaneous	The q is read as every	Use "subcut"
ss	sliding scale or 1/2	Read as the numbers 55 and 1/2	Spell out "sliding scale" or "1/2"
T/d (with a dot over the T)	one per day	Interpreted as t.i.d. (three times daily)	Use "one per day"
T1D	type 1 diabetes (melllitus)	Read as TID (three times daily)	Use DM-1
T1DM	type 1 diabetes (mellitus)	Read as TIDM (three times daily with meals)	Use DM-1
TIW	three times a week	Interpreted as T/W (Tuesday & Wednesday); as twice a week; as t.i.d. (three times daily)	Write "three times a week"
U	unit	When handwritten, read as 0, 4, 6, or cc	Use "unit"
Apothecary system of measure (grains, minims, and drams)	Units of measure	Not understood or misunderstood	Use the metric system (mg, g, mL)
Chemical symbols	Drug names or laboratory tests	Not understood or misunderstood	Use full name except for Na, Ca, O_2, K, Cl, KCl and HCl
Such as $MgSO_4$	magnesium sulfate	Not understood or misunderstood, may be read as morphine sulfate	Spell out magnesium sulfate

Table 2. Dangerous Abbreviations and Dosage Designations (*continued*)

Problem Term	Intended Meaning	Reason for Problem(s)	Suggested Remedy
Uncommon Latin words or phrases such as		Not understood or misunderstood	Use
per os	By mouth		by mouth, orally, or PO
ss	1/2		1/2 or one half
UD	As directed		as directed
Lettered abbreviations for drug names or drug protocols	Drug names or drug protocols	Not understood or misunderstood	Use generic and trade name(s); Follow policy for use of protocol names in your facility.
/ (a slash mark)	with, and, or per	Read as one when followed by a number	Use "and", "with" or "per"
Roman numerals	Numbers	Not understood or misunderstood (iv read as intravenous rather than 4; iii, X, L and C, not understood)	Use Arabic numerals (4, 3, 10, 50, 100, etc.)
> and <	"greater than" or "less than"	Not understood or the meaning is reversed	Use "greater than" or "less than"
Drug name and dosage not separated by a space	Inderal 40 mg	Inderal40 mg misread as Inderal 140 mg	Always leave a space between a drug name, dose, and unit of measure
Trailing zeros; 1.0 mg	1 mg	When handwritten decimal point is not seen, read as 10 mg causing a tenfold overdose	Omit the zero, write 1 mg (see note below)
Naked decimal point; .5 mL	0.5 mL	When handwritten decimal point is not seen, read as 5 mL causing a tenfold overdose	Add a zero, 0.5 mL
Abbreviated drug names	A drug name	Misinterpreted or not recognized	Use generic or brand name
Slang	communication	Can be offensive and/or insensitive	Do Not Use slang in verbal or written communications

Note **Exception:** A **trailing zero** may be used where required to demonstrate the level of precision of the value being reported, such as for laboratory results, imaging studies that report size of lesions, or catheter/tube sizes. It should **NOT** be used in medication orders or other medication-related documentation.

Table 3. Examples of Abbreviations That Have Contradictory or Ambiguous Meanings

ABP = ambulatory blood pressure
arterial blood pressure

AC = anticoagulant
anticonvulsant

ACU = acute receiving unit
ambulatory care unit

AMI = amifostine
amitriptyline

APC = advanced pancreatic cancer
advanced prostate cancer

AQoL = Acne Quality of Life
Assessment of Quality of Life
Asthma-related Quality of Life
Australian Quality of Life

ATR = atropine
atracurium

AZT = zidovudine
azathioprine

BC = bladder cancer
breast cancer

BD = behavior disorder
Behçet disease
bipolar disorder
Bowen disease

BM = bone metastases
brain metastases

BNO = bladder neck obstruction
bowels not open

BO = bowel open
bowel obstruction

BR = bright red
brown

BT = bladder tumor
brain tumor
breast tumor

CARBO = Carbocaine
carboplatin (Paraplatin)

CAS = carotid artery stenosis
cerebral arteriosclerosis
coronary artery stenosis

CIA = chemotherapy-induced
amenorrhea
chemotherapy-induced anemia

CLD = chronic liver disease
chronic lung disease

CPM = cyclophosphamide
chlorpheniramine maleate

CPZ = chlorpromazine
Compazine

CRU = cardiac rehabilitation unit
catheterization recovery unit
clinical research unit

DW = dextrose in water
distilled water
deionized water

DXM = dexamethasone
dextromethorphan

ED = eating disorder(s)
elbow disarticulation
emotional disorder
erectile dysfunction

ESLD = end-stage liver disease
end-stage lung disease

FA = folic acid
folinic acid (leucovorin calcium)

FEC = fluorouracil, epirubicin, and
cyclophosphamide
fluorouracil, etoposide, and
cisplatin

FGAs = first generation antihistamines
first generation antipsychotics

FLU = fluconazole (Diflucan)
fludarabine (Fludara)
flunisolide (Aero Bid)
fluoxetine (Prozac)
fluticasone propionate (Flonase)
influenza

FSW = female sex worker
field service worker

GD = Graves disease
Gaucher disease

GEM = gemfibrozil
gemicitabine

HCC = hepatocellular carcinoma
Hürthle cell carcinoma

HD = Hansen disease
Hirschsprung disease
Hodgkin disease
Huntington disease

HO = hand orthosis
hip orthosis

HRF = hypertensive renal failure
hypoxic respiratory failure

HSS = half-strength saline solution
(0.45% sodium chloride
injection)
hypertonic saline solution
(injection), (3, 5, and 7.5%
sodium chloride injection)

ICA = internal carotid artery
intracranial abscess
intracranial aneurysm

IAI = intra-abdominal infection
intra-abdominal injury
intra-amniotic infection

I & D = incision and drainage
irrigation and debridement

IRDM = insulin-required diabetes
mellitus
Insulin resistant diabetes
mellitus

IT = intrathecal
intratracheal
intratumoral
intratympanic

KET = ketamine
ketoconazole

LAM = laminectomy
laparoscopic-assisted
myomectomy
laser-assisted myringotomy

LAPC = locally-advanced pancreatic
cancer
locally-advanced prostatic
cancer

LF = left foot
little finger
long finger

LFD = lactose-free diet
low-fat diet
low-fiber diet

LHSH = long-handled shoe horn
long-handled shower head

LL = left leg
left lung
lower lid
lower limb
lower lip

LNE = lymph node enlargement
lymph node excision

LNU = learned nonuse (splint)
lower and upper (heard as
L & U)

LT = liver transplantation
Lung transplantation

Ltx = liver transplant
lung transplant

LVO = left ventricular opacification
left ventricular output
left ventricular overactivity

MBC = male breast cancer
metastatic breast cancer

Mon = Monday
month

MP = melphalan; prednisone
mitoxantrone; prednisone

MPM = malignant peritoneal mesothelioma
malignant pleural mesothelioma

MS = mental status
milk shake
mitral sound
morning stiffness
morphine sulfate
multiple sclerosis
mitral stenosis
musculoskeletal
medical student
minimal support
muscle strength

MTD = maximum tolerated dose
minimum toxic dose

MTZ = mirtazapine
mitoxantrone

MV = mechanical ventilation
manual ventilation

NABS = no active bowel sounds
normoactive bowel sounds

NAF = Native-American female
Negro-American female
normal adult female

NBM = no bowel movement
normal bowel movement
nothing by mouth

NE = no effect
no enlargement
not evaluated

NITRO = nitroglycerin
sodium nitroprusside

OLB = open-liver biopsy
open-lung biopsy

OPC = operable pancreatic carcinoma
oropharyngeal candidiasis
oropharynx cancer

PBL = primary breast lymphoma
primary brain lymphoma

PBZ = phenylbutazone
pyribenzamine
phenoxybenzamine

PCU = palliative care unit
primary care unit
progressive care unit
protective care unit

PD = Paget disease
panic disorder
Parkinson disease
personality disorder

Pit = Pitocin
Pitressin

PORT = postoperative radiotherapy
postoperative respiratory therapy

PVO = peripheral vascular occlusion
portal vein occlusion
pulmonary venous occlusion

RS = Reiter syndrome
Rett syndrome
Reye syndrome
Raynaud disease (syndrome)
rumination syndrome

RTI = reproductive tract infection
respiratory tract infection

S & S = swish and spit
swish and swallow

SA = suicide alert
suicide attempt

SAD = schizoaffective disorder
social anxiety disorder
seasonal affective disorder

SDBP = seated, standing, or supine
diastolic blood pressure

SGAs = second generation
antihistamines
second generation
antipsychotics

SJS = Schwartz-Jampel syndrome
Stevens-Johnson syndrome
Swyer-James syndrome

SSE = saline solution enema
soapsuds enema

STF = special tube feeding
standard tube feeding

TAC = tetracaine, Adrenalin, and
cocaine solution
triamcinolone cream

3TC = lamivudine (Epivir)
T&C #3 = Tylenol with 30 mg of Codeine

T/E = testosterone to epitestosterone
(ratio)
testosterone to estrogen (ratio)
trunk-to-extremity skinfold
thickness (index)

Table 3. Examples of Abbreviations That Have Contradictory or Ambiguous Meanings (*continued*)

TICU = thoracic intensive care unit
transplant intensive care unit
trauma intensive care unit

TMZ = temazepam
temozolomide

TS = Tay-Sachs (disease)
Tourette syndrome
Turner syndrome

tubal = tubal ligation
tubal pregnancy

Tx = therapist
therapy
traction
transcription
transfer
transfuse
transplant
transplantation
treatment

VAC = etoposide (VePesid), cytarabine
(ara-C, and carboplatin
vincristine, dactinomycin
(actinomycin D), and
cyclophosphamide
vincristine, doxorubicin
(Adriamycin), and
cyclophosphamide

VAD = vincristine, doxorubicin,
(Adriamycin) and
dexamethasone
vincristine, doxorubicin
(Adriamycin) and
dactinomycin

VAP = vincristine, Adriamycin, and
prednisone
vincristine, Adriamycin, and
procarbazine
vincristine, actinomycin D, and
Platinol AQ
vincristine, asparaginase, and
prednisone

WS = Waardenburg syndrome
Werner syndrome
West syndrome
Williams syndrome

Chapter 3
A Healthcare Controlled Vocabulary

Presently there are no standards for abbreviations used in prescribers' orders, consultations, written prescriptions, standing orders, computer order sets, nurse's medication administration records, pharmacy profiles, hospital formularies, etc. Because in the healthcare field everyone does their own thing, there are many variations. These variations in the way abbreviations are expressed are not always understood and at times are misinterpreted. They cause delays in initiating therapy, cause accidents, waste time for everyone in clarifying these documents, lengthen the time it takes to train those working in the healthcare field, lengthen hospital stays, and waste money.

A controlled vocabulary similar to what is used in the aviation industry is needed. Everyone in the aviation industry "follows the book," and uses a controlled vocabulary. All pilots and air traffic controllers say, "alfa", "bravo", "charlie." See Table 1, the phonetic alphabet. They do not go off on their own and say "adam", "beef", "candy!" They say "one three," not thirteen, because thirteen sounds like thirty. Radio transmission in the aviation industry is not easy to decipher, yet because precision is critical, everything possible is done to eliminate error. To prevent errors all radio transmissions are given only in English, every transmission is given in the same order and must be immediately repeated by the receiver to make sure it was heard correctly. Written and oral communication in the medical professions are just as critical and are also not easy to decipher, so establishing a controlled vocabulary is also necessary in this industry.

Listed below are some of the organizations and publications that have ongoing projects related to standardizing medical terminology:

ASTM International (American Society for Testing and Materials International) Committee on Healthcare Informatics (ASTM E31) www.astm.org

HL7 Health Level Seven International (www.hl7.org)

The United States Pharmacopeial Convention, Inc.
12601 Twinbrook Parkway
Rockville, MD, 20852

National Library of Medicine
Unified Medical Language Systems
8600 Rockville Pike
Bethesda, MD, 20894

Council of Science Editors, Style Manual Committee, Science style and format: the CSE manual for authors, editors, and publishers. 7th ed. Reston (VA): The Council; 2006.

American Medical Association, through their *AMA Manual of Style, 10th Edition*. AMA, Chicago, 2008

Computer-Based Patient Record Institute, Inc.
1000 East Woodfield Rd. Suite 102
Schuamburg, IL 60173-5921
http://www.CPRI.org

Association for Healthcare Documentation Integrity through their *The Book of Style for Medical Transcription,* 3rd ed., 2008, Association for Healthcare Documentation Integrity, Modesto, CA

Listed below (Table 2) is the start of a Healthcare Controlled Vocabulary. The basis for this controlled vocabulary is established standard terminology and the result of 43 years of studying medical errors by this author.

It is anticipated that a Healthcare Controlled Vocabulary, with professional organizations' input and backing, will grow and someday evolve into an "official standard." Your suggestions and comments are vital to this growth and eventual recognition. It is always safest to avoid the use of abbreviations unless they are well known in your work environment.

Table 1. Phonetic Alphabet

The International Civil Aviation Organization phonetic alphabet is used by the aviation industry when communications conditions are such that the information cannot be readily received without their use. Health professionals also should use it when it is necessary to orally spell critical information.

Character	Telephony	Phonic	Character	Telephony	Phonic
A	Alfa	(AL-FAH)	S	Sierra	(SEE-AIR-RAH)
B	Bravo	(BRAH-VOH)	T	Tango	(TANG-GO)
C	Charlie	(CHAR-LEE)	U	Uniform	(YOU-NEE-FORM)
		or (SHAR-LEE)			or (OO-NEE-FORM)
D	Delta	(DELL-TA)	V	Victor	(VIK-TAH)
E	Echo	(ECK-OH)	W	Whiskey	(WIS-KEY)
F	Foxtrot	(FOKS-TROT)	X	X-ray	(ECKS-RAY)
G	Golf	(GOLF)	Y	Yankee	(YANG-KEY)
H	Hotel	(HOH-TEL)	Z	Zulu	(ZOO-LOO)
I	India	(IN-DEE-AH)	1	One	(WUN)
J	Juliett	(JEW-LEE-ETT)	2	Two	(TOO)
K	Kilo	(KEY-LOH)	3	Three	(TREE)
L	Lima	(LEE-MAH)	4	Four	(FOW-ER)
M	Mike	(MIKE)	5	Five	(FIFE)
N	November	(NO-VEM-BER)	6	Six	(SIX)
O	Oscar	(OSS-CAH)	7	Seven	(SEV-EN)
P	Papa	(PAH-PAH)	8	Eight	(AIT)
Q	Quebec	(KEH-BECK)	9	Nine	(NIN-ER)
R	Romeo	(ROW-ME-OH)	0	Zero	(ZEE-RO)

Table 2. Examples of a Controlled Vocabulary

Standard	What **not** to use or do	Comments
100 mg (100 space mg)	100mg (100 no space mg)	The USP* standard way of expressing a strength is to leave a space between the number and its units. Leaving this space makes it easier to read the number as can be seen below. 1mg 1 mg 10mg 10 mg 100mg 100 mg
1 mg	1.0 mg	This is a USP standard. When a trailing zero is used, the decimal point is sometimes not seen when working from handwritten copies or when the decimal point falls on a line thus causing a tenfold overdose. These overdoses have caused injury and death. A "trailing zero" may be used only where required to demonstrate the level of precision of the value being reported, such as for laboratory results, imaging studies that report size of lesions, or catheter/tube sizes. It may **NOT** be used in medication orders or other medication-related documentation.
0.1 mL	.1 mL	When the decimal point is not seen, this is read as 1 mL, causing a ten fold overdose.
once daily (Do not abbreviate.)	The abbreviation OD	The classic meaning for OD is right eye. Liquids intended to be given once daily are mistakenly given in the right eye.
	The abbreviation QD	When the q. in q.d. is punctuated too aggressively it looks like Q.I.D. and the medication is given four times daily. When a lower case q is used, the tail of the q has come up between the q and the d to make it look like qid. In the United Kingdom, q.d. means four times daily
unit (Do not abbreviate. Write "unit" using a lower-case u)	The abbreviation U	The handwritten U is mistaken for a zero when poorly written causing a 10 fold overdose (i.e. 6 U regular insulin is read as 60). The poorly written U has also been read as a 4, 6, and cc. Write "unit," leaving a space between the number and the word unit.
mg (lower case mg with no period)	mg,, Mg,, Mg, MG, mgm, mgs	The USP standard expression is the mg
mL (lower case m with a capital L, no period)	mL, ml, ml., mls, mLs, cc	The USP standard expression is the mL for the measurement of liquids

(continued)

17

Table 2. (cont.)

Standard	What **not** to use or do	Comments
Use generic names or brand names	Do not abbreviate drug names or combinations of drugs, such as CPZ, PBZ, NTG, MS, MSO$_4$, 5FC, MTX, 6MP, MOPP, ASA, HCTZ, etc.	Abbreviated drug names and acronyms are not always known to the reader; at times they have more than one possible meaning, or are thought to be another drug.
		When the chemical name "6 mercaptopurine" has been used, six doses of mercaptopurine have been mistakenly administered. The generic name, mercaptopurine, should be used. MgSO$_4$ (magnesium sulfate) has been read as morphine sulfate.
	Do not use shortened names or chemical names in patient-related documents	When an unofficial shortened version of the name norfloxacin, norflox was used, Norflex was mistakenly given.
		An order for Aredia was read as Adriamycin, as some professionals abbreviated the name Adriamycin as "Adria" which looks like Aredia.
The metric system	The apothecary system (grains, drams, minims, ounces, etc.)	The Apothecary system is so rarely used it is not recognized or understood. The symbol for minim (℔) is read as mL; the symbol for one dram (ʒ T) is read as 3 tablespoons, and gr (grain) is read as gram.
Use properly placed commas for numbers above 9999, as in 10,000, or 5,000,000	5000000	Some healthcare workers have difficulty in reading large numbers such as 5000000. The use of commas helps the reader to read these numbers correctly.
600 mg When possible, do not use decimal expressions.	0.6 g	A USP standard. The elimination of decimals lessens the chance for error.
25 mcg	0.025 mg	Mistakes are made when reading numbers less than 1 with decimals.
Use specific concentrations and the time in which intravenous potassium chloride should be administered.	Do not use the term "bolus" in conjunction with the administration of potassium chloride injection.	Some physicians will erroneously indicate that potassium chloride injection should be "bolused" or be given "IV push," vaguely meaning that it should not be dripped in slowly. Many deaths have been reported when prescribers have been taken literally and the potassium chloride was given by bolus or IV push for fluid-restricted patients. Orders should be specific such as, "20 mEq of potassium chloride in 50 mL of 5% dextrose to run over 30 minutes."

Table 2. (cont.)

Standard	What **not** to use or do	Comments
use "and"	Do not use a slash (/) mark or the symbol "&"	A slash mark looks like a one. An order written "6 units regular insulin/20 units NPH insulin," was read as 120 units of NPH insulin. The symbol "&" has been read as a 4.
Orally transmitted medical orders should be read back as heard for verification.	Do not assume that one has spoken or heard correctly.	During oral communications, speakers misspeak and/or transcribers mishear. To minimize these errors, the transmitter must speak clearly and slowly, the transcriber must repeat what was transcribed, and the transmitter must listen attentively when this is being done. Errors are less likely to occur when the prescription is complete. When spelling out words, use the phonetic alphabet shown in Table 1. Oral orders should be avoided whenever possible.
When prescriptions are written or orally transmitted they must be complete. • dosage form must be specified • strength must be specified • directions must be specified • included in the directions must be the purpose or indication.	Incomplete orders	Prescribers on occasion think of one drug and mistakenly order another. Nurses and pharmacists on occasion misread prescriptions because of error, poor handwriting or poor oral communications, or look-alike or sound-alike drugs.[1] When the prescription is complete and the purpose or indication is included, these errors are less likely to occur. Listing the purpose or indication on the prescription label will assist in increasing patient adherence.
Written communications must be legible.	Illegible handwriting	Those who cannot or will not write legibly must print (if this would be legible), type, use a computer, or have an employee write for them and then immediately verify and sign the document. The use of electronic health records will be a great step forward and will solve this problem of poor handwriting.
Prescribe specific doses.	Do not prescribe 2 ampuls or 2 vials	There is often more than one size or concentration of drug available. Failing to be specific will lead to unintended doses being administered.
As required by the Joint Commission, establish a list of dangerous abbreviations which should not be used	Use dangerous abbreviations.	See Chapter 2 of this book "Dangerous, Contradictory, and/or Ambiguous Abbreviations."

Table 2. (cont.)

Standard	What **not** to use or do	Comments
Use h or hr for hour	°	An order written as q 4° has been read as q 40 or the symbol ° has not been understood.
Specify amount of drug to be given in a single dose.[2]	Specify total amount of drug to be administered over a period of time.	Orders such as . . . . 1,600 mg over 4 days have caused death when mistakenly given as a single dose. Order should state . . . 400 mg once daily for four days (2-1-10 to 2-4-10)

*USP = United States Pharmacopeia

1. Davis NM. Look-alike and sound-alike drug names. Hosp Pharm 2010, Supplement Wall-chart (HPJWALLCHARTS.COM)
2. Kohler D. Standardizing the expression & nomenclature of cancer treatment regimens. Am J Health-System Pharm. 1998;55;137–44

Chapter 4

How Medical Writers, Editors, and Health Professionals Can Help Control the Proliferation of Health-Related Abbreviations

I have been collecting medical abbreviations for over 32 years, during which time I co-founded the Institute for Safe Medication Practices and authored 15 editions of the book you are currently reading. The current edition contains 32,000 possible meanings for these health-related abbreviations. If there is such a thing as the world's foremost authority on medical abbreviations, then I am it. What I have learned is that abbreviations are a mixed blessing. They are a convenience, a time saver, a space saver, and a way of avoiding the possibility of misspelling words. However, a price is paid for their use. They can be misread or interpreted incorrectly. Their use lengthens the time needed to train individuals in the health fields, wastes the time of healthcare workers in tracking down their meanings, at times delays patient care, and, more often than people suspect, results in patient harm.

This chapter will discuss:

➢ How and why new abbreviations come into use
➢ The problems created by the use of abbreviations
➢ What medical writers, editors, and health professionals can do to prevent or lessen the problems created by medical abbreviations

The Evolution of Abbreviations

Speaking for myself and, I imagine, the great majority of others, we are used to taking short-cuts in our daily work. When we continually make a written record of a long word or phrase for our personal use, it is only natural to abbreviate it; no one else will see our shortcut and we know what it means. Eventually, we start to use these abbreviations to make it quicker and easier to communicate with the people with whom we work. As time goes on, these abbreviations are used in wider and wider circles.

Abbreviations can also be developed for commercial purposes because it is perceived that abbreviating a word or phrase has appeal to readers and customers. Medical writers and editors may also be the developers of a new abbreviation in order to save space or because they believe this will make for easier reading.

It is instructive to look at an example of how an abbreviation works its way into public use. The abbreviation MRI, for *magnetic resonance imaging,* did not appear in the National Library of Medicine's PubMed until 1983. In 1983 it appeared 13 times. In 2009, it appeared 26,597 times (see table 1). This 1983 date is not quite accurate, as MRI did appear, once in 1977, to mean, *microroughness index.* You would call this a successful abbreviation that has served a useful purpose. New abbreviations appear because of new technology, new equipment, new therapies, new tests, new drug classes, new diseases, new government programs, new insurance programs, new services, because of the need to fit information into restricted space on forms on documents and computers, etc.

The Problem with Abbreviations

There is a learning curve involved with abbreviations. First, learning occurs within a small group of insiders, those within the company that pioneer the development of a product or medical specialists that work on defining a new disease or syndrome. Whether the masses discern that MRI means *microroughness index* or *magnetic resonance imaging* was not a problem; however if your intention is to communicate, HD does not do it; as it could mean *Hansen disease, Hodgkin disease,* or *Huntington disease*. Yes, CHF means *congestive heart failure* 99% of the time, but other times it means *Crimean hemorrhagic fever, chronic heart failure,* and *congenital hepatic fibrosis*. For examples of other ambiguous abbreviations, see page 11. Some abbreviations are contradictory in their various possible meanings, such as BO for bowel *open* or *bowel obstructed* and S & S for *swish and spit* and also for *swish and swallow*.

Some medical abbreviations have proven to be dangerous, and the Joint Commission on Accreditation of Healthcare Organizations (it is obvious why this is abbreviated, JCAHO) has required healthcare facilities to start campaigns to eliminate their use[1,2]. A list of dangerous abbreviations and alternatives is shown on page 8. The JCAHO has changed its name to the Joint Commission. Some of these abbreviations do not appear dangerous in print, but when they are handwritten, as is routinely done in practice, their danger becomes more apparent. Health professionals learn from what they see in print and they will use what they have seen in print when writing by hand in a medical record or a prescription.

What To Do

Avoid using abbreviations

Before using an abbreviation, ask yourself the question: Is it necessary? I have seen long articles where a term is followed by an abbreviation identifying it, and this abbreviation is never used again in the article. Was it really necessary to develop or show this abbreviation?

Before using an abbreviation, authors and editors should determine what is being gained by its use. How much easier will it be to read the article? Will it save a significant amount of space? How cumbersome is the word or phrase being abbreviated? Is it an abbreviation which most of the readers will already be familiar with?

Medical facilities, when formulating their preprinted order sets, protocols, guidelines, etc. should avoid all but the most widely-known abbreviations.

Always avoid using the abbreviations known to be dangerous (see table which appears on page 8).

Test a New Abbreviation Before It Is Introduced

Before a new or unfamiliar abbreviation is coined or used, do some research to see if the abbreviation is also in use with another meaning. If you know that the abbreviation is already commonly in use to mean something else, you should come up with a different abbreviation or not abbreviate the term. I believe the authors and editors of the articles that abbreviated *Crimean hemorrhagic fever and congenital hepatic fibrosis as* CHF, should have known better. One of these problems was resolved when the condition was later referred to in the literature as *Crimean-Congo hemorrhagic fever* (CCHF). The *chronic heart failure* meaning for CHF is more often used outside the United States. The possible meanings of abbreviations can be researched on www.medabbrev.com, www.ncbi.nlm.nih.gov/entrez, and www.google.com. The website www.medabbrev.com (see page vii) is especially useful in that it is updated weekly and it also contains abbreviations which are unique to healthcare facilities that would not be found on other search engines.

Conclusions

There are abbreviations that are dangerous and should not be used (see Chapter 2, Dangerous, Contradictory, and/or Ambiguous Abbreviations, page 5)

There are abbreviations that have ambiguous or contradictory meanings and therefore are not helpful and may be harmful and should not be used. For examples of such abbreviations, see page 11. There are certain abbreviations, which are so rarely used or used only by a select group of specialists that they will not be understood by the average health professional.

It takes experience and the judgment to predict which new abbreviations will make it into the vocabulary of most healthcare professionals. It is best to err on the side of not assigning an abbreviation to a word or group of words, than to assign one.

A price is paid when health professionals use uncommon or multi-definition abbreviations when communicating and sometimes that price is a human life. Medical writers, editors, researchers, hospital administrators, government agencies, health-related industries, etc., can help by following the recommendations presented above. Healthcare professionals must follow this lead.

Table 1. The rate of appearance of the abbreviation MRI
in the National Library of Medicine's PubMed

Year	Number of times MRI appeared
1980–82	0
1983	13
1984	132
1985	471
1986	913
1987	2,002
1989	4,591
2004	15,447
2005	17,404
2006	19,061
2007	22,292
2009	26,597

1. Anon. "National Patient Safety Goals" chapter in Comprehensive Accreditation Manual for Hospitals: The Official Handbook, Refreshed Core, January 2005. The Joint Commission, Oakbrook Terrace, IL. 2005. page NPSG-3

2. www.jointcommission.org (click Prohibited Abbreviations- See goal 2)

Additions, Corrections, and Suggestions are Welcomed

Please send them via any means shown below:

Neil M Davis
2049 Stout Drive, B-3
Warminster PA 18974-3861

FAX 888 333 4915 or 215 442 7432
Email med@neilmdavis.com
Secure website www.medabbrev.com

Thank you for your help in the past.

Have You Used the Internet Version of This Book?

- It is instantaneously searchable for the meanings of abbreviations
- It is reverse searchable (search for all the abbreviations containing a particular word)
- Each week, about 20 new entries are added

See the preface (page vii) for access instructions. A one-year, single-user access is included in the purchase price of the book. Also one-year subscriptions (no book) are available for purchase (see page 417).

WiFi-Enabled Devices

At no extra cost, WiFi-enabled devices can access the Internet version where it can be added as a home-page icon or bookmarked.

computer	iPhone®	iPad®	iPod Touch®	BlackBerry®	DROID™	Windows® Mobile	Palm®

Multi-User Site Licenses are Available

Medical facilities can substitute their own "Do Not Use" list of dangerous abbreviations for the one present. The ability also exists to list abbreviations that are unique to your region and/or organization which would normally not appear in any national list. These lists would be controlled by the facility or company. A no-cost, 3-week trial and pricing information are available by calling 888 333 1862 or 215 442 7430 or via an e-mail request to ev@neilmdavis.com

Chapter 5
Medical Abbreviation Primer

When first entering a medically related field, one must learn the language in order to function. Part of learning this language is to learn the meaning of the abbreviations, acronyms, and symbols in use. This chapter is intended to introduce newcomers to this commonly used medically related shorthand.

The determination of which abbreviations (refers also to acronyms and symbols) are most commonly used is based on the selection by the author with the consultation of experts in various health-related fields. The categorizing of the abbreviations is arbitrary, but is intended to represent the most common use, as the abbreviations could have been placed in many different categories.

This list could have been expanded to include many hundreds-more commonly used abbreviations, but then the list would have been too long to serve as a primer. The absence of an abbreviation from this listing does not mean it is not in common use. Each area of practice and specialty could have added their own commonly used abbreviations.

A few of the abbreviations below have more than one meaning listed. This was done when several meanings are in common use. Many abbreviations have more than one meaning and they must be viewed in their clinical context to arrive at their intended meaning. See Chapter 6 of this book for additional meanings for the abbreviations listed below.

In practice, there are inconsistencies as to how abbreviations are written. They may appear in all capital letters, lower case, or in capital letters and lower case. They may or may not have periods after each letter.

The readers are urged to read Chapter 2, Dangerous, Contradictory, and/or Ambiguous Abbreviations.

Two Hundred and Seventy-Five Commonly Used Medical Abbreviations Arranged by Category—a Primer

Physical Examination, History Portion of the Medical Record, and Discharge Summary

C/O	complains of	ROS	review of systems
CC	chief complaint(s)	SH	social history
CTA	clear to auscultation	Tx	treatment
Dx	diagnosis	CV	cardiovascular
F/U	follow-up	GI	gastrointestinal
FH	family history	GU	genitourinary
H/O	history of	EENT	ears, eyes, nose, and throat
HPI	history of present illness	HEENT	head, ears, eyes, nose, and throat
Hx	history	Ob/Gyn	obstetrics and gynecology
PE	physical examination	Peds	pediatrics
	pelvic examination	UCD	usual childhood diseases
	pulmonary embolism	A & P	auscultation and percussion
PH/SH	personal and social history	ADL	activities of daily living
PI	present illness	CN III	third cranial nerve (there are
PMH	past medical history		CN I to XII)

RCM	right costal margin (there is also a LCM)	o.u.	both eyes
RUQ	right upper quadrant (also there is RLQ, LUQ, and LLQ)	PERRLA	pupils equal, round, reactive to light and accommodation
TM	tympanic membrane	IOP	intraocular pressure
AAO X 3	alert, awake, and oriented to time, place, and person	ROM	range of motion
		VS	vital signs
BM	bowel movement	P	pulse
BP	blood pressure	T	temperature
CVAT	costovertebral angle tenderness	RR	respiratory rate; recovery room
DTR	deep tendon reflex	HR	heart rate
EOMI	extraocular muscles intact	RRR	regular rate and rhythm (heart)
HJR	hepatojugular reflux	WDWNWM	well developed, well nourished, white male (also there are abbreviations for females and other races [WF = white female; AAF = African-American female]
JVD	jugular venous distention		
IBW	ideal body weight		
LBW	lean body weight		
BSA	body surface area		
LMP	last menstrual period	YO	year old
NAD	no apparent distress no apparent disease	DOB	date of birth
		+	positive; present; plus
NC/AT	normocephalic, atraumatic	−	negative; absent; minus
NKA	no known allergies	c̄	with
NKDA	no known drug allergies	ō	negative; without
o.d.	right eye	W/O	without
o.s.	left eye		

Diseases and Symptoms

AD	Alzheimer disease	SOB	shortness of breath
AIDS	acquired immunodeficiency syndrome	URI	upper respiratory infection
		TB	tuberculosis
HIV	human immuno-deficiency virus	CVA	cerebrovascular accident; costovertebral angle
AMI	acute myocardial infarction		
MI	myocardial infarction	DVT	deep vein thrombosis
CHF	congestive heart failure	NV	nausea and vomiting
ACS	acute coronary syndrome	NVD	nausea, vomiting, and diarrhea
HT	hypertension (also HTN) height		neck vein distention
		PONV	postoperative nausea and vomiting
DM	diabetes mellitus		
AODM	adult onset diabetes mellitus	PUD	peptic ulcer disease
IDDM	insulin dependent diabetes mellitus	GERD	gastroesophageal reflux disease
		RA	rheumatoid arthritis
NIDDM	noninsulin-dependent diabetes mellitus	OA	osteoarthritis
		SLE	systemic lupus erythematosus
PD	Parkinson disease	TIA	transient ischemic attack
AOM	acute otitis media	HA	headache
Ca	cancer	BPH	benign prostatic hypertrophy (hyperplasia)
COAD	chronic obstructive airway disease		
COPD	chronic obstructive pulmonary disease	UTI	urinary tract infection
		STD	sexually transmitted disease
DOE	dyspnea on exertion	MVA	motor vehicle accident

Clinical Laboratory

ANA	antinuclear antibody	AST	aspartate aminotransferase
Alb	albumin	BG	blood glucose; blood gases
ALT	alanine aminotransferase	BS	blood sugar bowel sounds breath sounds
LFT	liver function test		
aPTT	activated partial thromboplastin time	BUN	blood urea nitrogen

CK-MB	creatine kinase, MB fraction		Mg	Magnesium (also Mg^{++})
CO_2	carbon dioxide		Na	Sodium (also Na^+)
CPK	creatinine phosphokinase		OGTT	oral glucose tolerance test
CrCl	creatinine clearance		PSA	prostate-specific antigen
SCr	serum creatinine		UA	urinalysis
C & S	culture and sensitivity		VDRL	Venereal Disease Research
ESR	erythrocyte sedimentation rate			Laboratory (test for syphilis)
Gluc	glucose		CBC	complete blood count
FBS	fasting blood sugar		Diff	differential (blood count)
HbA_{1c}	glycosylated hemoglobin		Eos	eosinophil
CHOL	cholesterol		Fe	iron
HDL	high-density lipoprotein		Hct	hematocrit
LDL	low-density lipoprotein		Hgb	hemoglobin
LDH	lactic dehydrogenase		H&H	hemoglobin and hematocrit
Trig	triglycerides		Plt	platelets
INR	international normalized ratio		MCV	mean corpuscular volume
DB	direct bilirubin		RBC	red blood cell (count)
TB	total bilirubin		Segs	segmented neutrophils
TP	total protein		WBC	white blood cell (count)
Ca	Calcium (also Ca^{++})		ABG	arterial blood gases
Cl	Chloride (also Cl^-)		WNL	within normal limits
K	Potassium (also K^+)			

Other Diagnostic Tests, Procedures, and Treatments

ECG	electrocardiogram		CT	computer tomography
EEG	electroencephalogram		IVP	intravenous pyelogram
FEV_1	forced expiratory volume in one second		MRI	magnetic resonance imaging
			PET	positron emission tomography
IPPB	intermittent positive-pressure breathing		US	ultrasound
			CABG	coronary artery bypass graft
PFT	pulmonary function tests		PCTA	percutaneous transluminal
PEEP	positive end-expiratory pressure			coronary angioplasty
MUGA	multigated (radionuclide) angiogram		PT	physical therapy
			D & C	dilatation and curettage

Physicians' Orders and Prescriptions

ASAP	as soon as possible		tab	tablet
OOB	out of bed		inj	injection
BRP	bathroom privileges		i	one
CPR	cardiopulmonary resuscitation		ii	two
DNR	do not resuscitate		*q*	*every (as in q 6 hours)*
DAW	dispense as written		h	hour(s)
DC or D/C	discharge		*b.i.d.*	*twice daily*
	discontinue		*t.i.d.*	*three times daily*
I/O	intake and output		*q.i.d.*	*four times daily*
LD	loading dose		*q.a.m.*	every morning
NAS	no salt added		*q.p.m.*	every evening
n.p.o.	nothing by mouth		*a.c.*	*before meals*
p.o.	by mouth; postoperative		*p.c.*	*after meals*
IM	intramuscular		*h.s.*	*bedtime*
IV	intravenous		n.r.	no refills (prescriptions)
SC	subcutaneous		*p.r.n.*	*as required; whenever necessary*
SQ	subcutaneous (subcut preferred)			
PICC	percutaneous indwelling central catheter		MRx1	may repeat one time
			Rx	*prescription*
				pharmacy
IVPB	intravenous piggyback		OTC	over-the-counter (no prescription
NGT	nasogastric tube			required)
cap	capsule			

| Stat | immediately | | TO | telephone order |
| TKO | to keep (vein) open | | VO | verbal order |

Drug Names
(Presented for informational purposes only; they should *not* be used)

APAP	acetaminophen		$MgSO_4$	magnesium sulfate
ASA	aspirin		MOM	milk of magnesia
5D/W	dextrose 5% injection (in water)		NaCl	sodium chloride
Dig	digoxin		NS	normal saline (0.9% sodium
ETOH	alcohol (ethyl alcohol)			chloride; same as NSS)
$FeSO_4$	ferrous sulfate		NSS	normal saline solution (0.9%
H_2O	water			sodium chloride)
H_2O_2	hydrogen peroxide		O_2	oxygen
HCl	hydrochloride (when following a		PCN	penicillin
	drug name, as in thiamine HCl		tPA	tissue plasminogen activator
	[thiamine hydrochloride])		IVF	intravenous fluids
	hydrochloric acid (when it appears		TPN	total parenteral nutrition
	separately [not as part of a drug		lytes	electrolytes (sodium, potassium,
	name])			chloride, etc.)
KCl	potassium chloride			

Drug Classes

ABX	antibiotic(s)		OC	oral contraceptive
COX-2 I	cyclooxygenase-2 inhibitor		PPI	proton pump inhibitor
MAOI	monoamine oxidase inhibitor		SSRI	selective serotonin reuptake
NSAID	nonsteroidal anti-inflammatory			inhibitor
	drug		TCA	tricyclic antidepressant

Units of Measure

cm	centimeter (2.54 cm = 1 inch)		mEq	milliequivalent
g	gram (28.35 g = 1 ounce)		mg	milligram (1,000 mg = 1 gram [g])
kg	kilogram (1 kg = 2.2 pounds)		mL	milliliter (1,000 mL = 1 liter [L])
L	liter (l L = 1,000 mL = 1 quart		mmHg	millimeters of mercury
	plus about 2 ounces)		°C	degrees Centigrade (Celsius)
lb	pound (1 lb = 0.454 Kg)		°F	degrees Fahrenheit
mcg	microgram (1,000 mcg			
	= 1 milligram [mg])			

Hospital Locations

CCU	cardiac care unit		OB	obstetrics
DR	delivery room		OR	operating room
ED	emergency department		PACU	postanesthesia care unit
ER	emergency room (same as ED)		PICU	pediatric intensive care unit
ICU	intensive care unit			pulmonary intensive care unit
L & D	labor and delivery		RD	radiology department
LDR	labor, delivery, and recovery		SICU	surgical intensive care
MICU	medical intensive care unit			unit
NICU	neonatal intensive care unit			

Miscellaneous

APRN	Advanced Practice Registered		MAR	medication administration
	Nurse			record
ARNP	Advanced Registered Nurse		MD	Doctor of Medicine
	Practitioner		PA	Physician Assistant
CNS	Clinical Nurse Specialist		PharmD	Doctor of Pharmacy
DO	Doctor of Osteopathy		RPh	Registered Pharmacist
LPN	Licensed Practical Nurse		RN	Registered Nurse
MA	Medical Assistant			

Chapter 6

Lettered and Numbered Abbreviations, Acronyms, and Slang

This chapter starts with numbers, abbreviations which start with a number or numbers, and Roman numerals. It is followed by lettered abbreviations and acronyms.

The letter-by-letter (dictionary) system of alphabetizing is used ("*ad lib*" is listed under ADL).

When an abbreviation ending with an S can not be found, check for the abbreviation without the S as it may be the plural form of one that is listed.

Brand names (proprietary names) have their first letter capitalized, whereas nonproprietary (generic) names are in lower-case letters.

Although shown for informational purposes, drug names should not be abbreviated as the meaning may not be known to the reader or interpreted as intended.

Slang is presented for informational purposes only and should not be used.

The listing of symbols and Greek letters can be found in Chapter 7.

Some of the meanings shown are very specialized or new and will not be understood by the majority of health professionals. These very specialized abbreviations are presented for informational purposes and their use in healthcare documentation should be done with assurance that they will be understood. See WARNING in chapter 1.

Number(s) or Begins with Number(s)

½ and ½	half Dakin solution and half glycerin
½ NSS	sodium chloride 0.45% (½ normal saline solution)
1°	first degree
	primary
1:1	one-to-one (individual session with staff)
100	one hundred (1×10^2)
1,000	one thousand (1×10^3)
1,500	fifteen hundred
	Health Insurance Claim Form
	HCFA 1500
10,000	ten thousand (1×10^4)
100,000	one hundred thousand (1×10^5)
1,000,000	one million (1×10^6)
10,000,000	ten million (1×10^7)
100,000,000	one hundred million (1×10^8)
1,000,000,000	one billion (1×10^9)
17K	17-ketosteroids
$_1O_2$	singlet oxygen
1-TU	1 tuberculin unit
2°	second degree
	secondary
2/2	secondary to

222	aspirin, caffeine, and codeine (8 mg) tablets (Canada)
24°	twenty-four hours (24 hr is safer as the ° is seen as zero)
25(OH)D	25-hydroxyvitamin D
282	aspirin, caffeine, codeine, and meprobamate (Canada)
2-CDA	cladribine (Leustatin; chlorodeoxyadenosine)
2D	two-dimensional
2X2	gauze dressing folded 2″ by 2″
24/7	24 hours a day, 7 days a week
3°	tertiary
	third degree
356h	Application to Market a New Drug, Biologic or an Antibiotic Drug for Human Use (FDA form number)
3D	three-dimensional
3D-CT	3-dimensional computed tomography
3MP	Magnetic Mini-Mover Procedure
3TC	lamivudine (Epivir)
3V	3-vessel
3X	three times
4	for (as in TI4 "therapeutic interchange for. . .")
	four
420	Marijuana
4-AP	4-aminopyridine (Ampyra)
4D-CT	four-dimensional computed tomography
4WW	four-wheel walker
4X4	gauze dressing folded 4″ by 4″
5 + 2	5 days of cytarabine and 2 days of daunorubicin, leukemia therapy
5-ASA	mesalamine (Asacol; Rowasa)
5FU	fluorouracil
5S's	Sort, Set-In-Order, Shine, Standardize and Sustain (steps to make the work environment Lean)
5-TU	5 tuberculin units
5YSR	5-year survival rate(s)
642	propoxyphene tablets (Canada)
6MP	mercaptopurine (Purinenthol)
7/24	7 days a week, 24 hours a day
7 + 3	7 days of cytarabine and 3 days of daunorubicin, leukemia therapy
7's	Serial 7's; a mental status examination (starting with 100, count backward by 7's)
777	Ortho Novum 777® (a triphasic oral contraceptive)

Roman Numerals (should not be used because they are not universally understood)

i	one
ii	two
iii	three
iv	four (a dangerous expression as it is read as intravenous, use 4; for additional meanings see the letters IV)
v	five (for additional meaning see the letter V)
vi	six
vii	seven
viii	eight
ix	nine
x	ten (for additional meanings see the letter X)
xi	eleven
xii	twelve
xx	twenty
XL	forty (for additional meanings see the letters XL)
L	fifty (for additional meaning see the letter L)
C	hundred (for additional meanings see the letter C)
M	thousand (for additional meanings see the letter M)

A

A	accommodation
	Acinetobacter
	acute
	adenosine (also referred to as Ado)
	age
	alive
	ambulatory
	angioplasty
	anterior
	anxiety
	apical
	arterial
	artery
	Asian
	assessment
	assistance
	auscultation
A+	blood type A positive (A positive is preferred)
A−	blood type A negative (A negative is preferred)
A′	ankle
@	at
Ⓐ	assist
(a)	axillary temperature
ā	anterior
	before
A₁	aortic first heart sound
A₂	aortic second sound
A250	5% albumin 250 mL
A1000	5% albumin 1000 mL
A II	angiotensin II
AA	accelerated approval (FDA)
	acetic acid
	achievement age
	active assistive
	acute asthma
	affected area
	affirmative action
	African American
	Alcoholics Anonymous
	alcohol abuse
	alopecia areata
	alveolar-arterial gradient
	amino acid
	anaplastic astrocytoma
	androgenetic alopecia
	anesthesiologist assistant
	anti-aerobic
	antiarrhythmic agent
	aortic aneurysm
	aplastic anemia
	arachidonic acid
	arm ankle (pulse ratio)

	ascending aorta
	ascorbic acid (vitamin C)
	audiologic assessment
	Australia antigen
	authorized absence
	automobile accident
	cytarabine (ara-C) and doxorubicin (Adriamycin)
aa	of each
A&A	aid and attendance
	albuterol and ipratropium bromide (Atrovent) (this combination is available as Combivent Aerosol and DuoNab inhalation solution)
	arthroscopy and arthrotomy
	awake and aware
A-a	alveolar arterial (gradient)
a/A	arterial-alveolar (gradient)
AIIA	Angiotensin II antagonist
AAA	abdominal aortic aneurysmectomy (aneurysm)
	acute anxiety attack
	apply to affected area
	Area Agencies on Aging
	aromatic amino acids
	arterio-arterial anastomosis
A&AA	active and active assistive
AAAASF	American Association for Accreditation of Ambulatory Surgery Facilities
AAAE	amino acid activating enzyme
AAAHC	Accreditation Association of Ambulatory Health Care
AABB	American Association of Blood Banks
AABR	automated auditory brainstem response
AAC	Adrenalin, atropine, and cocaine
	advanced adrenocortical cancer
	antimicrobial agent-associated colitis
	augmentative and alternative communication
AACD	aging-associated cognitive decline
AACG	acute-angle closure glaucoma
AACLR	arthroscopic anterior cruciate ligament reconstruction
AACVPR	American Association of Cardiovascular and Pulmonary Rehabilitation (guidelines)
AAD	acid-ash diet
	antibiotic-associated diarrhea
A₁AD	alpha₁-antitrypsin deficiency
AADA	Abbreviated Antibiotic Drug Application
AADC	aromatic L-amino acid decarboxylase

[A-a]Do$_2$	alveolar-arterial oxygen tension gradient	alkylating agent score
AAE	active assistance exercise	allergic Aspergillus sinusitis
	acute allergic encephalitis	androgenic-anabolic steroid
AAECS	amino acid enriched cardioplegic solution	Ann Arbor stage (Hodgkin disease staging system)
A/AEX	active assistive exercise	aortic arch syndrome
AAF	African-American female	Associate's Degree, Applied Science
	altered auditory feedback	atlantoaxis subluxation
AAFB	alcohol acid-fast bacilli	atomic absorption spectroscopy
AAFO	active ankle-foot orthoses	atypical absence seizure
AAG	alpha-1-acid glycoprotein	

AASCRN	amino acid screen
AAH	acute alcoholic hepatitis	AASH	adrenal androgen-stimulating hormone
	atypical adenomatous hyperplasia	
AAI	acute alcohol intoxication	AASLD	American Association for the Study of Liver Disease (Practice Guidelines)
	arm-ankle index	
	atlantoaxial instability	
	atrial demand-inhibited (pacemaker)	AASM	American Academy of Sleep Medicine (practice parameters)
AAK	atlantoaxial kyphosis	AAST	American Association for the Surgery of Trauma (trauma grading)
AAL	anterior axillary line	
AALNC	Legal Nurse Consultant (American Association of Legal Nurse Consultants)	AAST-OIS	American Association for the Surgery of Trauma—Organ Injury Scale
AAM	African-American male	AASV	antibody-associated systemic vasculitis
	amino acid mixture	
AAMI	age-associated memory impairment	AAT	activity as tolerated
AAMS	acute aseptic meningitis syndrome		alpha-antitrypsin
AAMT	American Association for Medical Transcription (now ADHI)		androgen ablation therapy
		at all times
AAN	AIDS-associated neutropenia		atrial demand-triggered (pacemaker)
	analgesic abuse nephropathy	
	analgesic-associated nephropathy		atypical antibody titer
	attending's admission notes		automatic atrial tachycardia
AANA	American Association of Nurse Anesthetists	A$_1$AT	alpha$_1$-antitrypsin
AAO	alert, awake, & oriented	A$_1$AT-P$_i$	alpha$_1$-antitrypsin (phenotyping)
AAO × 3	alert, awake and oriented to time, place, and person	AAU	acute anterior uveitis
		AAV	adeno-associated vector
AAOC	antacid of choice		adeno-associated virus
AAP	acute anterior poliomyelitis	AAV-GAD	glutamic acid decarboxylase (gene viral transfer with the) adeno-associated virus
	American Academy of Pediatrics (guidelines)	
	assessment adjustment pass	AAVV	accumulated alveolar ventilatory volume
AAPC	antibiotic-associated pseudomembranous colitis	
AAPMC	antibiotic-associated pseudomembranous colitis	AAWD	antiandrogen withdrawal
		AB	abortion
a/ApO$_2$	arterial-alveolar oxygen tension ratio		Ace® bandage
			antibiotic
AAPSA	age-adjusted prostate-specific antigen		antibody
			Aphasia Battery
AAR	antigen-antiglobulin reaction		apical beat
	automated anesthesia record		armboard
AARF	atlantoaxial rotatory fixation (subluxation; dislocation)		attentional blink
			products meeting bioequivalence requirements for generic pharmaceuticals
AAROM	active-assistive range of motion	
AAS	acute abdominal series	Aβ	beta-amyloid peptide

A/B	acid-base ratio	ABCs	A_{1c} level (glycosylate hemoglobin
	apnea/bradycardia		A_{1c}), Blood pressure, and
A > B	air greater than bone (conduction)		Cholesterol level (ABCs of
A & B	apnea and bradycardia		diabetes care)
	assault and battery		abstinence, fidelity ("being
AB+	AB positive blood type		faithful"), or condom use (ABCs
	(AB positive preferred)		of HIV prevention)
AB−	AB negative blood type		airway, breathing, and circulation
	(AB negative preferred)		stabilization (ABCs of
ABA	applied behavioral analysis		resuscitation)
ABBI	Advanced Breast Biopsy		aneurysmal bone cysts
	Instrumentation	ABD	after bronchodilator
abbr MDRD	abbreviated Modification of Diet in		automated border detection
	Renal Disease		detection
ABC	abacavir (Ziagen)		type of plain gauze dressing
	abbreviated blood count	Abd	abdomen
	Aberrant Behavior Checklist		abdominal
	absolute band counts		abductor
	absolute basophil count	ABDCT	atrial bolus dynamic computer
	activity-based costing		tomography
	advanced breast cancer	AC followed	doxorubicin (Adriamycin) and
	airway, breathing, and circulation	by D	cyclophosphamide followed by
	all but code (resuscitation order)		docetaxel
	aneurysmal bone cyst	ABD GR	abdominal girth
	antigen-binding capacity	ABD PB	abductor pollicis brevis
	apnea, bradycardia, and cyanosis	Abd/pel	abdomen/pelvis
	applesauce, bananas, and cereal	ABD PL	abductor pollicis longus
	(diet)	ABE	acute bacteria endocarditis
	argon-beam coagulator		adult basic education
	Aristotle Basic Complexity		average bioequivalence
	(Score)		botulism equine trivalent antitoxin
	aspiration, biopsy and cytology	ABECB	acute bacterial exacerbations of
	artificial beta cells		chronic bronchitis
	automated blood count	ABEP	auditory brain stem-evoked
	(no differential)		potentials
	automatic brightness control		aortic blood flow
	(radiology)	ABER	abduction and external rotation
	avidin-biotin complex	Abeta	amyloid beta
ABCD	age, blood pressure, clinical	A-beta42	beta-amyloid 42
	features, and duration of	ABF	aortobifemoral (bypass)
	symptoms (prognostic score for		aortobronchial fistula
	short term risk of stroke after	ABG	air/bone gap
	transient ischemic attack)		aortoiliac bypass graft
	amphotericin B cholesteryl		arterial blood gases
	sulfate complex (Amphotec;		axiobuccogingival
	amphotericin B colloid	ABH	abnormal bile hybrid
	dispersion)		Ativan, Benadryl, and Haldol
	asymmetry, border irregularity,	ABI	ankle brachial index (ankle-to-arm
	color variation, and diameter		systolic blood pressure ratio)
	more than 6 mm (melanoma		atherothrombotic brain infarction
	warning signs in a mole)		auditory brainstem implant
	automated blood count (differential	ABID	antibody identification
	done manually)	A Big	atrial bigeminy
ABCDE	botulism toxoid pentavalent	ABK	aphakic bullous keratopathy
ABCS	Active Bacterial Core Surveillance	ABL	abetalipoproteinemia
	(CDC)		acute blood loss
	automated blood count, STKR		allograft bound lymphocytes
	(differential done by machine)		axiobuccolingual

ABLA	acute blood loss anemia
ABLB	alternate binaural loudness balance
ABLC	amphotericin B lipid complex (Abelcet)
ABLV	Australian bat lyssavirus
A/B Mods	apnea/bradycardia moderate stimulation
ABMS	acute bacterial maxillary sinusitis
	autologous bone marrow support
A/B MS	apnea/bradycardia mild stimulation
ABMT	autologous bone marrow transplantation
ABN	abnormality(ies)
	Advance Beneficiary Notice
abnl bld	abnormal bleeding
ABNM	American Board of Nuclear Medicine
abnor.	abnormal
ABO	absent bed occupant
	blood group system (A, AB, B, and O)
ABP	ambulatory blood pressure
	androgen-binding protein
	arterial blood pressure
ABPA	allergic bronchopulmonary aspergillosis
ABPB	axillary brachial plexus block
ABPI	Association of the British Pharmaceutical Industry
ABPM	axillary brachial plexus block
ABPM	allergic bronchopulmonary mycosis
	ambulatory blood pressure monitoring
ABQAURP	American Board of Quality Assurance and Utilization Review Physicians
ABR	absolute bed rest
	auditory brain-stem response
ABRS	acute bacterial rhinosinusitis
ABS	absent
	absorbed
	absorption
	Accu-Check® (blood glucose)
	acute brain syndrome
	admitting blood sugar
	Alterman-Bishop stent
	amniotic band syndrome
	antibody screen
	at bedside
ABSA	adjusted body surface area
ABSH	asymmetrical basal septal hypertrophy
ABSS	Anderson Behavioral State Scale
A/B SS	apnea/bradycardia self-stimulation
ABT	aminopyrine breath test
	antibiotic therapy
	autologous blood therapy

ABVD	doxorubicin (Adriamycin)®, bleomycin, vinblastine, and dacarbazine (DTIC)
ABW	actual body weight
	adjusted body weight
ABx	antibiotics
AC	abdominal circumference
	acceleration capacity (heart)
	acetate
	acromioclavicular
	activated charcoal
	acute
	African Caribbean
	air conditioned
	air conduction
	anchored catheter
	antecubital
	anticoagulant
	anticonvulsant
	arm circumference
	assist control
	autologous cell
	axillary crutches
	before meals
	doxorubicin (Adriamycin) and cyclophosphamide
a.c.	before meals
A-C	Astler-Coller (stages of colorectal cancer)
A/C	anterior chamber of the eye
	assist/control
A & C	alert and cooperative
A₁C	glycosylated hemoglobin A_{1C}
5-AC	azacitidine (Vidaza)
9AC	rubitecan (9-aminocamptothecin; Orathecin)
ACA	acrodermatitis chronica atrophicans
	acyclovir
	adenocarcinoma
	against clinical advice
	aminocaproic acid (Amicar)
	annual clothing allowance
	anterior cerebral artery
	anterior communicating artery
	anticanalicular antibodies
AC/A	accommodation convergence– accommodation (ratio)
ACABS	acute community-acquired bacterial sinusitis
ACAD	anterior circulation arterial dissection
ACAS	acute community-acquired sinusitis
	asymptomatic carotid artery study
ACAT	acyl coenzyme A: cholesterol acyltransferase
ACB	alveolar-capillary block
	antibody-coated bacteria
	aortocoronary bypass

	before breakfast	ACDFs	adult children from dysfunctional families
AcB	assist with bath	ACDK	acquired cystic disease of the kidney
AC & BC	air and bone conduction		
ACBE	air contrast barium enema	ACDs	anticonvulsant drugs
ACBG	aortocoronary bypass graft	ACE	acute care of the elderly (nursing unit)
AC-BPPV	anterior canal benign paroxysmal positional vertigo		adrenocortical extract
ACBT	active cycle of breathing techniques		adverse clinical event
			aerosol-cloud enhancer
ACC	acalculous cholecystitis		angiotensin-converting enzyme
	accident		antegrade colonic enema
	accommodation		antegrade continence enema
	acinar cell carcinoma		doxorubicin (Adriamycin), cyclophosphamide, and etoposide
	adenoid cystic carcinomas		
	administrative control center		
	advanced colorectal cancer	ACEI	angiotensin-converting enzyme inhibitor
	ambulatory care center		
	American College of Cardiology (guidelines)	ACET	air-conduction estimated from tympanometry
	amylase creatinine clearance		antepartum continuous epidural therapy
	anterior cingulate cortex		
	anterior corticcal cataract	ACF	aberrant crypt focus
	automated cell count		accessory clinical findings
ACCE	Academic Clinical Coordinator Educator		acute care facility
			anterior cervical fusion
ACC-NCDR	American College of Cardiology-National Cardiovascular Data Registry	ACG	accelerography
			adjusted clinical groups
			angiocardiography
AcCoA	acetyl-coenzyme A	ACGME	Accreditation Council for Graduate Medical Education
ACCP	American College of Chest Physicians		
		ACH	adrenal cortical hormone
ACCR	amylase creatinine clearance ratio		aftercoming head
ACCU	acute coronary care unit		arm girth, chest depth, and hip width
ACCU✔	Accucheck® (blood glucose monitoring)		
		ACh	acetylcholine
ACD	absolute cardiac dullness	ACHA	air-conduction hearing aid
	absorbent cover dressing	AChE	acetylcholinesterase
	acid-citrate-dextrose	AChEIs	acetylcholinesterase inhibitors
	advanced cervical dilation	ACHES	abdominal pain, chest pain, headache, eye problems, and severe leg pains (early danger signs of oral contraceptive adverse effects)
	allergic contact dermatitis		
	alveolar capillary dysplasia		
	anemia of chronic disease		
	anterior cervical diskectomy		
	anterior chamber depth		
	anterior chamber diameter	AC & HS	before meals and at bedtime
	anterior chest diameter	ACI	acceleration index
	average cost per day		adrenal cortical insufficiency
	before dinner		aftercare instructions
	dactinomycin (actinomycin D; Cosmegen)		anabolic-catabolic index
			anemia of chronic illness
ACDC	antibody complement-dependent cytolysis		autologous chondrocyte implantation
		ACIOL	anterior chamber intraocular lens
AC-DC	bisexual (homo- and heterosexual)	ACIP	Advisory Committee on Immunization Practices (of the Centers for Disease Control and Prevention)
ACDDS	Alcoholism/Chemical Dependency Detoxification Service		
ACDF	anterior cervical diskectomy and fusion		
		ACIS	automated cellular imaging system

35

ACJ	acromioclavicular joint	ACPP	adrenocorticopolypeptide
A/CK	Accu-Check® (blood glucose)	ACPPD	average cost per patient day
ACL	accessory collateral ligament (hand)	ACPP PF	acid phosphatase prostatic fluid
	Allen Cognitive Level	ACPS	anterior cervical plate stabilization
	American cutaneous leishmaniasis	ACQ	acquired
	anterior cruciate ligament (knee)		Areas of Change Questionnaire
aCL	anticardiolipin (antibody)	ACQ-5	asthma control questionnaire (5-item
ACLA	aclarubicin		symptom and activity version)
ACLF	adult congregate living facility	ACR	acute cellular rejection
ACLR	anterior cruciate ligament repair		adenomatosis of the colon and
ACLS	advanced cardiac (cardiopulmonary) life support		rectum
			albumin to creatinine ratio
	Allen Cognitive Level Screen		American College of Radiology
ACLs	atypical cribriform lesions		American College of
ACM	alternative/complementary medicine		Rheumatology
			anterior chamber reformation
	Arnold-Chiari malformation		anticonstipation regimen
ACME	arginine catabolic mobile element	ACR20	American College of
	aphakic cystoid macular edema		Rheumatology
	Automated Classification of Medical Entities		rating scale (20% or more improvement)
ACMT	advanced combined modality therapy	ACRC	advanced colorectal cancer
		ACRD	acquired cystic renal disease
ACMV	assist-controlled mechanical ventilation	ACRES	amplification created restriction enzyme site
ACN	acetonitrile	ACRN	AIDS-Certified Registered Nurse
	acute conditioned neurosis	ACS	abdominal compartment syndrome
ACNP	Acute Care Nurse Practitioner		anterior compartment syndrome
ACNU	nimustine HCl (Nidran; Acnu)		acute confusional state
ACO	Accountable Care Organization (established by the Patient Protection and Affordable Care Act. 2010)		acute coronary syndromes
			American Cancer Society
			anodal-closing sound
			automated corneal shaper
	anterior capsular opacification		before supper
ACOA	Adult Children of Alcoholics	ACSF	anterior cervical spine fixation
ACOG	American College of Obstetricians and Gynecologists		artificial cerebrospinal fluid
		ACSL	automatic computerized solvent
A COMM A	anterior communicating artery		litholysis
ACOPIA	inability to cope	ACSM	American College for Sports Medicine
ACOS-OG	American College of Surgeons Oncology Group		
		ACSVBG	aortocoronary saphenous vein bypass graft
ACP	accessory conduction pathway		
	acid phosphatase	ACSW	Academy of Certified Social Workers
	adamantinomatous craniopharyngioma		
		ACT	activated clotting time
	adenocarcinoma of the prostate		aggressive comfort treatment
	advance care planning		allergen challenge test
	ambulatory care program		anticoagulant therapy
	anesthesia-care provider		artemisinin-based combination therapy
	anterior cervical plate		
	antrochoanal polyp		assertive community treatment (program)
ACPA	anticytoplasmic antibodies		
AC-PC line	anterior commissure-posterior commissure line		doxorubicin (adriamycin), cyclophosphamide, and paclitaxel (Taxol)
AC-PH	acid phosphatase		
ACPO	acute colonic pseudo-obstruction	ACT-D	dactinomycin (Cosmegen)

Act Ex	active exercise
ACTG	AIDS Clinical Trial Group
ACTH	corticotropin (adrenocorticotropic hormone)
ACT-Post	activated clotting time post-filter
ACT-Pre	activated clotting time pre-filter
ACTSEB	anterior chamber tube shunt encircling band
ACU	ambulatory care unit
ACUP	adenocarcinoma of unknown primary (origin)
ACUV	air-contrast ultrasound venography
ACV	acyclovir (Zovirax)
	amifostine, cisplatin, and vinblastine
	assist control ventilation
	atrial/carotid/ventricular
A-C-V	A wave, C wave, and V wave
ACVBP	doxorubicin (Adriamycin), cyclophosphamide, vindesine, bleomycin, and prednisone
ACVD	acute cardiovascular disease
ACVP	doxorubicin (Adriamycin), cyclophosphamide, vincristine, and prednisone
ACW	anterior chest wall
	apply to chest wall
acyl-CoA	acyl coenzyme A
AD	accident dispensary
	admitting diagnosis
	advanced dementia
	advance directive (living will)
	air dyne
	alcohol dependence
	alternating days (this is a dangerous abbreviation)
	Alzheimer disease
	androgen deprivation
	antidepressant
	assistive device
	atopic dermatitis
	autistic disorder
	axillary dissection
	axis deviation
	right ear
A&D	admission and discharge
	alcohol and drug
	ascending and descending
	vitamins A and D
ADA	adenosine deaminase
	American Dental Association
	American Diabetes Association
	Americans with Disabilities Act
	anterior descending artery
	awareness during anesthesia
ADAM	adjustment disorder with anxious mood

ADaM	Analysis Data Model
ADAMs	a disintegrin and metallo-proteinases (a family of multidomain transmembrane and secreted proteins)
ADAS	Alzheimer Disease Assessment Scale
ADAS-COG	Alzheimer Disease Assessment Scale-Cognitive Subscale
ADAT	advance diet as tolerated
ADAU	adolescent drug abuse unit
ADB	amorous disinhibited behavior
ADC	Aid to Dependent Children
	AIDS (acquired immune deficiency syndrome) dementia complex
	analog-to-digital converter (radiology)
	anxiety disorder clinic
	apparent diffusion coefficient (radiology)
	average daily census
	average daily consumption
ADCA	autosomal dominant cerebellar ataxia
ADCC	antibody-dependent cellular cytotoxicity
A.D.C. VAAN DIML	mnemonic for formatting physician orders: Admit, Diagnosis, Condition, Vitals, Activity, Allergies, Nursing procedures, Diet, Ins and outs, Medication, Labs
ADD	adduction
	annual disability density
	arrest in dilation/descent
	attention-deficit disorder
	average daily dose
ADDH	attention-deficit disorder with hyperactivity
ADDL	additional
ADDLs	amyloid-derived diffusible ligands
ADDM	adjustment disorder with depressed mood
ADDP	adductor pollicis
ADDs	AIDS (acquired immune deficiency syndrome)-defining diseases
ADDU	alcohol and drug dependence unit
ADE	acute disseminated encephalitis
	adverse drug event
ADEM	acute disseminating encephalomyelitis
ADEN	adenoids
ADE-NOCA	adenocarcinoma
ADEPT	antibody-directed enzyme prodrug therapy

ADFT	atrial defibrillation threshold		alternative dispute resolution
ADFU	agar diffusion for fungus		doxorubicin (Adriamycin)
ADG	atrial diastolic gallop	ADRB2	beta-2 adrenergic receptor
	axiodistogingival	ADRD	Alzheimer disease and related
ADH	antidiuretic hormone		disorders
	atypical ductal hyperplasia	ADRIA	doxorubicin (Adriamycin)
ADHD	attention-deficit hyperactivity	ADRV	adult diarrhea rotavirus
	disorder	ADS	admission day surgery
ADHF	acute decompensated heart failure		anatomical dead space
ADI	acceptable daily intake		anonymous donor's sperm
	acute diaphragmatic injury		antibody deficiency syndrome
	AIDS (acquired immunodeficiency	ADs	advance directives (living wills)
	symdrome) defining illness	ADSD	autosomal-dominant striatal
	allowable (acceptable) daily intake		degeneration
	axiodistoincisal	AdSD	adductor spasmodic dysphonia
A-DIC	doxorubicin (Adriamycin) and	ADSU	ambulatory diagnostic surgery
	dacarbazine		unit
ADJ	adjusted	ADT	admission, discharge, and transfer
Adj Dis	adjustment disorder		alternate-day therapy
Adj D/O	adjustment disorder		androgen deprivation treatment
ADL	activities of daily living		(therapy)
ADLD	autosomal dominant		antiarrhythmic drug therapy
	leukodystrophy		anticipate discharge tomorrow
ADLG	average duration of life gained		any damn thing (a placebo)
ad lib	as desired		Auditory Discrimination Test
	at liberty	ADTP	Adolescent Day Treatment
ADM	abductor digiti minimi (muscle)		Program
	acceptance of disability modified		Alcohol-Dependence Treatment
	acellular dermal matrix		Program
	administered (dose)	ADTR	Academy of Dance Therapists,
	admission		Registered
	adrenomedullin	ADU	automated dispensing unit
	doxorubicin (Adriamycin)	ADV	adenovirus vaccine, not otherwise
ADMA	asymmetrical dimethyl arginine		specified
ADME	absorption, distribution,	adv	adventitious sounds (wheezes and
	metabolism, and excretion		rhonchi)
ADNFLE	autosomal dominant nocturnal	ADV$_4$	adenovirus vaccine, type 4, live,
	frontal lobe epilepsy		oral
ADO	adenosine (also referred to as A)	ADV$_7$	adenovirus vaccine, type 7, live,
	axiodisto-occlusal		oral
ADOA	autosomal-dominant optic atrophy	A5D5W	alcohol 5%, dextrose 5% in water
Ad-OAP	doxorubicin (Adriamycin),		for injection
	vincristine, (Oncovin)	ADX	audiological diagnostic
	cytarabine, (Ara C) and	ADx™	urine drug screen for six drugs of
	prednisone		abuse
ADOL	adolescent	AE	above elbow (amputation)
ADON	Assistant Director of Nursing		accident and emergency
ADP	arterial demand pacing		(department)
	adenosine diphosphate		acute exacerbation
ADPC	active distance to palmar crease		adaptive equipment
ADPKD	autosomal dominant polycystic		adverse event
	kidney disease		air entry
ADPV	anomaly of drainage of pulmonary		androgen excess
	vein		anoxic encephalopathy
ADQ	abductor digiti quinti		antiembolitic
	adequate		arm ergometer
ADR	acute dystonic reaction		aryepiglottic (fold)
	adverse drug reaction	A/E	adaptive equipment

A&E	accident and emergency (department)	AES	adult emergency service anti-embolic stockings
AEA	above-elbow amputation anti-endomysium antibody	AEs	adverse events
		AET	alternating esotropia atrial ectopic tachycardia
AEB	as evidenced by atrial ectopic beat	AF	acid-fast acoustical feedback afebrile
AEC	absolute (blood) eosinophil count at earliest convenience automatic exposure control (radiology)		amniotic fluid anterior fontanel antifibrinogen aortofemoral ascitic fluid atrial fibrillation
AECB	acute exacerbations of chronic bronchitis		
AECG	ambulatory electrocardiogram	AF-AFl	atrial fibrillation and atrial flutter
AECOPD	acute exacerbation of chronic obstructive pulmonary disease	AFB	acid-fast bacilli aorto-femoral bypass aspirated foreign body
AED	antiepileptic drug automated (automatic) external defibrillator	AFB_1	aflatoxin B_1
		AFBG	aortofemoral bypass graft
AEDD	anterior extradural defects	AFBY	aortofemoral bypass (graft)
AEDF	absent end-diastolic flow (umbilical-artery Doppler ultrasonography)	AFC	adult foster care air filled cushions alveolar fluid clearance
AEDH	acute epidural hematoma	AFDC	Aid to Families with Dependent Children
AEDP	assisted end-diastolic pressure automated external defibrillator pacemaker	AFE	amniotic fluid embolization autofluorescence endoscopy
AEE	asthma-exacerbation episodes	AFEB	afebrile
aEEG	amplitude-integrated electroencephalography	AFEU	ante partum fetal evaluation unit
		AF/FL	atrial fibrillation/atrial flutter
AEEU	admission entrance and evaluation unit	aFGF	acidic fibroblast growth factor
		AFH	adult family home angiomatoid fibrous histiocytoma anterior facial height
AEF	aortoesophageal fistula		
AEFI	adverse events following immunization	AFI	acute febrile illness amniotic fluid index
AEG	air encephalogram Alcohol Education Group	A fib	atrial fibrillation
AEIOU TIPS	mnemonic for the diagnosis of coma: Alcohol, Encephalopathy, Insulin, Opiates, Uremia, Trauma, Infection, Psychiatric, and Syncope	AFIP	Armed Forces Institute of Pathology
		AFKO	ankle-foot-knee orthosis
		AFL	air/fluid level atrial flutter
AELBM	after each loose bowel movement	AFLP	acute fatty liver of pregnancy amplified fragment length polymorphism
AEM	active electrode monitor ambulatory electrogram monitor antiepileptic medication		
		A Flu	atrial flutter
AEP	auditory evoked potential	AFM	active fetal movement acute *Plasmodium falciparum* malaria aerosol face mask atomic force microscopy doxorubicin (Adriamycin), fluorouracil, and methotrexate
AEq	age equivalent		
AER	acoustic evoked response albumin excretion rate auditory evoked response		
AERD	aspirin-exacerbated respiratory disease		
Aer. M.	aerosol mask	AFM×2	double-aerosol face mask
AERS	adverse event reporting system	AFO	ankle-fixation orthotic ankle-foot orthosis
AERs	adverse event reports		
Aer. T.	aerosol tent		

AFOF	anterior fontanelle and open and flat	AGECAT	automatic geriatric examination for computer-assisted taxonomy
AFOSF	anterior fontanelle open, soft, and flat	AGF	angle of greatest flexion
AFP	acute flaccid paralysis	AGG	agammaglobulinemia
	alpha-fetoprotein	aggl.	agglutination
	anterior faucial pillar	AGHD	adult growth hormone deficiency
	ascending frontal parietal	AGI	alpha-glucosidase inhibitor
AFQT	Armed Forces Qualification Test	AGIB	acute gastrointestinal bleeding
AFRD	acute febrile respiratory disease	AGL	acute granulocytic leukemia
AFRIMS	Armed Forces Research Institute of Medical Sciences	A GLAC-TO-LK	alpha galactoside leukocytes
AFRRI	Armed Forces Radiological Research Institute	AGMA	anion-gap metabolic acidosis
		AGN	acute glomerulonephritis
AFRS	allergic fungal rhinosinusitis	AGNB	aerobic gram-negative bacilli
AFS	allergic fungal sinusitis	$AgNO_3$	silver nitrate
	amputation-free survival	AgNORs	argyrophilic nucleolar organizer regions (staining)
	atomic fluorescence spectrometry	α_1-AGP	alpha$_1$-acid glycoprotein
AFT	arrived to find	AGPT	agar-gel precipitation test
Aft/Dis	aftercare/discharge	AGS	adrenogenital syndrome
AFTN	autonomously functioning thyroid nodule		Alagille syndrome
			American Geriatric Society (guidelines)
AFV	amniotic fluid volume		
AFVSS	afebrile, vital signs stable	AG SYND	adrenogenital syndrome
AFX	air-fluid exchange	AGT	alanine-glyoxylate aminotransferase
AFx	atypical fibroxanthoma		
AG	abdominal girth		angiotensinogen
	adrenogenital	AGTT	abnormal glucose tolerance test
	aminoglycoside	AGU	aspartylglycosaminuria
	Amsler grid	AGUS	atypical glandular cells of uncertain significance
	anaplastic glioma		
	anion gap	AGV	Ahmed glaucoma valve
	antigen	AGVHD	acute graft-versus-host disease
	antigravity	AGVI	Ahmed glaucoma valve implantation
	atrial gallop		
Ag	silver	AH	abdominal hysterectomy
A/G	albumin to globulin ratio		amenorrhea and hirsutism
AGA	accelerated growth area		amenorrhea-hyperprolactinemia
	acute gonococcal arthritis		antihyaluronidase
	androgenetic alopecia		auditory hallucinations
	antigliadin antibody	A&H	accident and health (insurance)
	appropriate for gestational age	AHA	acetohydroxamic acid (Lithostat®)
	average gestational age		acquired hemolytic anemia
AGAS	accelerated graft atherosclerosis		American Health Association (guidelines)
AG/BL	aminoglycoside/beta-lactam		
AGC	absolute granulocyte count		autoimmune hemolytic anemia
	advanced gastric cancer	AHAs	alpha hydroxy acids
	atypical glandular cells	AHase	antihyaluronidase
	automatic gain control (radiology)	AHB_c	hepatitis B core antibody
AGCUS	atypical glandular cells of undetermined significance	AHC	acute hemorrhagic conjunctivitis
			acute hemorrhagic cystitis
AGD	agar gel diffusion		Adolescent Health Center
AGE	acute gastroenteritis		alternating hemiplegia of childhood
	advanced glycation end product(s)		avoidable hospitalization conditions
	angle of greatest extension		
	anterior gastroenterostomy	AHCA	Agency for Healthcare Administration
	arterial gas embolism		

American Healthcare Association
AHCPR   Agency for Health Care
    Policy and Research
AHCs   academic health centers
AHD   alien-hand syndrome
    antecedent hematological disorder
    arteriosclerotic heart disease
    autoimmune hemolytic disease
AHDI   Association for Healthcare
    Documentation Integrity
AHE   acute hemorrhagic
    encephalomyelitis
    amygdalo-hippocampectomy
AHEC   Area Health Education Center
AHF   antihemophilic factor
    Argentine hemorrhagic fever
    (Junin virus) vaccine
AHF-M   antihemophilic factor (human),
    method M, (monoclonal
    purified)
AHFS   acute heart failure syndrome(s)
    American Hospital Formulary
    Service
AHG   antihemophilic globulin
AHGS   acute herpetic gingival stomatitis
AHHD   arteriosclerotic hypertensive heart
    disease
AHI   apnea-hypopnea index
AHJ   artificial hip joint
AHL   apparent half-life
AHM   ambulatory Holter monitoring
AHMO   anterior horizontal mandibular
    osteotomy
AHN   adenomatous hyperplastic nodule
    Assistant Head Nurse
AHO   a history of
    Albright hereditary osteodystrophy
AHP   acute hemorrhagic pancreatitis
    acute hepatic panel (see page 356)
    American Herbal Pharmacopeia
    and Therapeutic Compendium
AHPB   adjusted historic payment base
AhpF   alkyl hydroperoxide reductase,
    F isomer
AHR   acute humoral rejection
    adjusted hazard ratios
    airway hyperresponsiveness
AHRE   atrial high-rate event
AHRF   acute hypoxemic respiratory failure
AHRQ   Agency for Healthcare Research
    and Quality
AHS   adaptive hand skills
    allopurinol hypersensitivity
    syndrome
    Alpers-Huttenlocher syndrome
    anticonvulsant hypersensitivity
    syndrome

AHSA   Assistant Health Services
    Administrator
AHSCT   autologous hemopoietic stem-cell
    transplantation
AHSG   fetuin-A (alpha2-Heremans Schmid
    glycoprotein
AHSP   alpha hemoglobin stabilizing
    protein
AHST   autologous hematopoietic stem cell
    transplantation
AHT   alternating hypertropia
    antihyaluronidase titer
    autoantibodies to human
    thyroglobulin
AHTG   antihuman thymocyte globulin
AI   accidentally incurred
    accommodative insufficiency
    allelic imbalance
    American Indian
    allergy index
    aortic insufficiency
    apical impulse
    apnea index
    artificial insemination
    artificial intelligence
A & I   Allergy and Immunology
    (department)
    auscultation and inspection
AIA   Accommodation Independence
    Assessment
    allergen-induced asthma
    allyl isopropyl acetamide
    anti-insulin antibody
    aspirin-induced asthma
AIAA   aromatase inhibitor-associated
    arthralgia
AI-Ab   anti-insulin antibody
AIAN   American Indian and Alaska
    Native
AIBF   anterior interbody fusion
AIC   amount in controversy
AICA   anterior inferior cerebellar artery
    anterior inferior communicating
    artery
AICBG   anterior interbody cervical bone
    graft
AICD   activation-induced cell death
    automatic implantable cardioverter/
    defibrillator
AICM   anti-inflammatory controller
    medication
AICS   acute ischemic coronary syndromes
AID   absolute iron deficiency
    acute infectious disease
    aortoiliac disease
    artificial insemination donor
    automated infusion device

	automatic implantable defibrillator		acute insulin response
AIDH	artificial insemination donor husband	AIRE	autoimmune regulator (gene)
AIDKS	acquired immune deficiency syndrome with Kaposi sarcoma	AIRR	acute infusion-related reaction
AIDP	acute inflammatory demyelinating polyradiculoneuropathy	AIS	Abbreviated Injury Score acute ischemic stroke adolescent idiopathic scoliosis anti-insulin serum
AIDS	acquired immunodeficiency syndrome	AISA	acquired idiopathic sideroblastic anemia
AIE	acute inclusion body encephalitis	AIS/ISS	Abbreviated Injury Scale/ Injury Severity Score
AIED	autoimmune inner-ear Disease		
AIEOP	Italian Association of Pediatric Hematology and Oncology (cancer study group)	AIT	adoptive immunotherapy Advanced Individual Training (Army) amiodarone-induced thyrotoxicosis auditory integration therapy
AIF	aortic-iliac-femoral		
AIGHL	anterior band of the inferior glenohumeral ligament	AITD	autoimmune thyroid disease autoimmune thyroiditis
AIH	artificial insemination with husband's sperm asymptomatic incidentally hyperprolactinemia autoimmune hepatitis	AITN	acute interstitial tubular nephritis
		AITP	autoimmune thrombocytopenia purpura
		AIU	absolute iodine uptake adolescent inpatient unit
AIHA	autoimmune hemolytic anemia		
AIHD	acquired immune hemolytic disease	AIVC	absence of the inferior vena cava
AIIRs	airborne infection isolation rooms	AIVR	accelerated idioventricular rhythm
AIIS	anterior inferior iliac spine	AJ	ankle jerk
AILD	angioimmunoblastic lymphadenopathy with dysproteinemia	AJFAT	Ankle Joint Functional Assessment Tool
		AJCC	American Joint Committee on Cancer
AILT	angioimmunoblastic T-cell lymphoma	AJO	apple juice only
AIM	anti-inflammatory medication	AJR	abnormal jugular reflex
AIMS	Abnormal Involuntary Movement Scale Arthritis Impact Measurement Scales	AK	above-knee (amputation) actinic keratosis artificial kidney
		AKA	above-knee amputation alcoholic ketoacidosis all known allergies also known as
AIN	acute interstitial nephritis anal intraepithelial neoplasia anterior interosseous nerve		
AINS	anti-inflammatory non-steroidal	a.k.a.	also known as
AIO	all-in-one (lipid emulsion, protein, carbohydrate, and electrolytes combined total parenteral nutrition)	AKC	atopic keratoconjunctivitis
		AKI	acute kidney injury acute kidney insufficiency
		AKP	anterior knee pain
AIOD	aortoiliac occlusive disease	AKS	alcoholic Korsakoff syndrome arthroscopic knee surgery
AION	anterior ischemic optic neuropathy		
AIP	acute infectious polyneuritis acute intermittent porphyria acute interstitial pneumonia asymptomatic inflammatory prostatitis autoimmune pancreatitis	AKU	artificial kidney unit
		AL	acute leukemia argon laser artemether-lumefantrine (antimalarial drug combination [Riamet; Coarten]) arterial line assisted living attachment level (dental) axial length left ear
AIPC	androgen-independent prostate cancer		
AIPH	acute idiopathic pulmomary hemorrhage		
AIR	accelerated idioventricular rhythm acetylcholine-induced relaxation		

Al	aluminum		anaplastic lymphoma kinase
ALA	adrenalin (epinephrine), lidocaine, and amethocaine (tetracaine)		anterior lamellar keratoplasty
			automated lamellar keratoplasy
	alpha-linolenic acid (α-linolenic acid)	ALK Ø	alkaline phosphatase
		ALK ISO	alkaline phosphatase isoenzymes
	alpha-lipoic acid	ALK-P	alkaline phosphatase
	amebic liver abscess	ALK PHOS ISO	alkaline phosphatase isoenzyme
	aminolevulinic acid (Levulan)		
	antileukotriene agent	ALL	acute lymphoblastic leukemia
	antilymphocyte antibody		acute lymphocytic leukemia
	as long as		allergy
ALAC	antibiotic-loaded acrylic cement	ALLD	arthroscopic lumbar laser diskectomy
ALAD	abnormal left axis deviation		
ALA-GLN	alanyl-glutamine	ALLO	allogeneic
ALARA	as low as reasonably achievable	Allo-BMT	allogeneic bone marrow transplantation
ALAT	alanine aminotransferase (also ALT; SGPT)		
		Allo-HCT	allogenic hematopoietic cell transplant
ALAX	apical long axis		
ALB	albumin	Allo-HSCT	allogeneic hematopoietic stem cell transplantation
	albuterol		
	anterior lenticular bevel	allo-SCT	allogeneic stem cell transplantation
ALBUMS	aldehyde linker-based ultrasensitive mismatch scanning	ALM	acral lentiginous melanoma
			alveolar lining material
ALC	acetyl-L-carnitine (Alcar)		autoclave-killed *Leishmania major*
	acute lethal catatonia		
	alcohol	ALMI	anterolateral myocardial infarction
	alcoholic liver cirrhosis	ALN	anterior lower neck
	allogeneic lymphocyte cytotoxicity		anterior lymph node
	alternate level of care		axillary lymph nodes
	Alternate Lifestyle Checklist	ALND	axillary lymph node dissection
	axiolinguocervical	ALNM	axillary lymph node metastasis
ALCA	anomalous left coronary artery	ALO	apraxia of eyelid opening
ALCL	anaplastic large-cell lymphoma		axiolinguo-occlusal
ALC R	alcohol rub	ALOC	altered level of consciousness
ALD	adrenoleukodystrophy	Al(OH)₃	aluminum hydroxide
	alcoholic liver disease	ALOS	average length of stay
	aldolase	ALP	alkaline phosphatase
ALDH	aldehyde dehydrogenase		argon laser photocoagulation
ALDO	aldosterone		Alupent
ALDOST	aldosterone	Alpha1 (M)	Alpha 1 microglobulin
ALF	acute liver failure	Alpha-syn	alpha-synuclein
	arterial line filter	ALPS	autoimmune lymphoproliferative syndrome
	assisted living facility		
ALFT	abnormal liver function tests	ALPSA	anterior labroligamentous periosteal sleeve avulsion
ALG	antilymphoblast globulin		
	antilymphocyte globulin	ALPZ	alprazolam (Xanax)
ALGB	adjustable laparoscopic gastric banding	ALR	adductor leg raise
		ALRI	acute lower-respiratory-tract infection
ALH	atypical lobular hyperplasia		
ALHE	angiolymphoid hyperplasia with eosinophilia		anterolateral rotary instability
		ALS	acid-labile subunit
ALI	Abbott Laboratories, Inc.		acute lateral sclerosis
	acute lung injury		advanced life support
	argon laser iridotomy		amyotrophic lateral sclerosis
ALIF	anterior lumbar interbody fusion		antilymphocyte serum
A-line	arterial catheter	ALSG	Australian Leukemia Study Group
ALJ	administrative law judge	ALSOB	alcohol-like substance on breath
ALK	alkaline	ALT	alanine aminotransferase(SGPT)

	anterolateral thigh		Arm Motor Ability Test
	antibiotic lock technique (catheter infection prevention)	A-MAT	amorphous material
		AMAT S/E	Arm Motor Ability Test for shoulder/elbow
	argon laser trabeculoplasty		
	autolymphocyte therapy	AMAT W/H	Arm Motor Ability Test for wrist/hand
2 *alt*	every other day (this is a dangerous abbreviation)	AMB	ambulate
ALTB	acute laryngotracheobronchitis		ambulatory
ALTE	acute (aberrant, apparent) life threatening event		amphotericin B (Fungizone)
			as manifested by
ALTF	anterolateral thigh flap	AMBDs	autoimmune mucocutaneous blistering diseases
alt hor	every other hour (this is a dangerous abbreviation)	AMBER	advanced multiple beam equalization radiography
ALTP	argon laser trabeculoplasty		
ALUP	Alupent	AMBS	ambulates
ALv	attachment level (dental)	Ambu	artificial-respiration device consisting of a bag that is squeezed by hand
ALVAD	abdominal left ventricular assist device		
ALVAL	aseptic lymphocytic vasculitis-associated lesion(s)	AMC	arm muscle circumference
			arthrogryposis multiplex congenita
ALWMI	anterolateral wall myocardial infarct	AMCD	Aerospacel Medical Certification Division (of the Federal Aviation Administration)
ALZ	Alzheimer disease		
AM	adult male		
	aerosol mask	aMCI	amnestic mild cognitive impairment
	amalgam		
	anovulatory menstruation	AM/CR	amylase to creatinine ratio
	anterior midpapillary	AMD	age-related macular degeneration
	morning (a.m.)		arthroscopic microdiskectomy
	myopic astigmatism		axiomesiodistal
AMA	advanced maternal age		dactinomycin (actinomycin D; Cosmegen)
	against medical advice (This implies the patient was seen and his/her discharge is being addressed by a care provider and the patient signs a form that he/she is leaving against medical advice. Check to see if this conforms to your facility's definition.) (see LWBS LWBT)		methyldopa (alpha methyldopa)
		AMDR	acceptable macronutrient distribution range
		AME-	acute metabolic encephalopathy
			adenomyoepithelioma
			agreed medical examination
			anthrax meningoencephalitis
			apparent mineralocorticoid excess (syndrome)
	American Medical Association		Aviation Medical Examiner
	antimitochondrial antibody	AMegL	acute megakaryoblastic leukemia
AMAC	adults molested as children	AMES-LAN	American sign language
AMAD	activity median aerodynamic diameter		
		AMF	aerobic metabolism facilitator
AMBI	acute multiple brain infarcts		amifostine (Ethyol)
AM Care	brushing teeth, washing face and hands		amonafide
			autocrine motility factor
AMAD	morning admission	AMFYOYO	adios, my friend, you're on your own (polite form) (slang)
AM/ADM	morning admission		
AMAG	adrenal medullary autograft	AMG	acoustic myography
AMAL	amalgam		aminoglycoside
AMAN	acute motor axonal neuropathy		axiomesiogingival
AMAP	American Medical Accreditation Program		Federal Republic of Germany's equivalent to United States Food, Drug, and Cosmetic Act
	as much as possible		
Amask	aerosol mask	AMGA	American Medical Group Association
AMAT	anti-malignant antibody test		

AMI	acute myocardial infarction	AMSAN	acute motor sensory axonal
	amifostine (Ethyol)		neuropathy
	amitriptyline	AMSIT	portion of the mental status
	axiomesioincisal		examination:
AMKL	acute megakaryocytic leukemia		A—appearance,
AML	acute myelogenous leukemia		M—mood,
	angiomyolipoma		S—sensorium,
	anterior mitral leaflet		I—intelligence,
AMLOS	arithmetic mean length of stay		T—thought process
AMLR	auditory midlatency response	AMT	abbreviated mental test
	Marketing Authorization		Adolph's Meat Tenderizer
	Application (French)		allogeneic (bone) marrow
AMM	agnogenic myeloid metaplasia		transplant
AMML	acute myelomonocytic leukemia		alpha-methyltryptamine
AMMOL	acute myelomonoblastic		aminopterin
	leukemia		amniotic membrane transplantation
AMN	adrenomyeloneuropathy		amount
amnio	amniocentesis	AM&T	adenoidectomy with myringotomy
AMN SC	amniotic fluid scan		and tympanostomy tube insertion
AMOL	acute monoblastic leukemia	AMTS	Abbreviated Mental Test Score
AMOVA	analysis of molecular variance	AMU	accessory-muscle use
AMP	adenosine monophosphate		atomic mass units (radiology)
	ampere	AMV	alveolar minute ventilation
	ampicillin		assisted mechanical ventilation
	ampul	AMY	amylase
	amputation	AMY/CR	amylase/creatinine ratio
	antipressure mattress	AN	acoustic neuromas
AMPA	alpha-amino-3-hydroxy-5-methyl-		Alaska Native
	4-isoxazoleproprionic acid		amyl nitrate
	(subtype of glutamate receptors)		anorexia nervosa
AMPLE	allergies, medications, past medical		anticipatory nausea
	history, last meal, events leading		Associate Nurse
	to admission (used for history		avascular necrosis
	and physical examination)	ANA	American Nurses Association
AMPPE	acute multifocal placoid pigment		anastrozole (Arimidex)
	epitheliopathy		antinuclear antibody
A-M pr	Austin-Moore prosthesis	ANAD	anorexia nervosa and associated
AMPS	Assessment of Motor and Process		disorders
	Skills	ANADA	Abbreviated New Animal Drug
AMPT	metyrosine (alphamethylpara		Application
	tyrosine)	ANAG	acute narrow angle glaucoma
AMR	acoustic muscle reflex	ANA	anaerobic swab
	alternating motion rates	SWAB	
	amrubicin	ANC	absolute neutrophil count
AMRI	anterior medial rotary instability		antenatal care
AMS	absorbable metal stent(s)		antenatal course
	accelerator mass spectrometry	ANCA	antineutrophil cytoplasmic
	acute maxillary sinusitis		antibody
	acute mountain sickness	anch	anchored
	adult male sling (for male urinary	ANCN	absolute neutrophil count nadir
	incontinence)	ANCOVA	analysis of covariance
	aggravated in military service	AND	allow natural death
	altered mental status		anterior nasal discharge
	amylase		Associate's Degree in Nursing
	aseptic meningitis syndrome		axillary node dissection
	atypical mole syndrome	ANDA	Abbreviated New Drug Application
	auditory memory span	anes	anesthesia
m-AMSA	amsacrine (acridinyl anisidide)	ANF	antinuclear factor

atrial natriuretic factor
ANG   angiogram
     angiotensin
Ang-2   angiopoietin-2
ANG II   angiotensin II
ANGIO   angiogram
ANH   acute normovolemic hemodilution
     artificial nutrition and hydration
     assisted nutrition and hydration
ANISO   anisocytosis
ANK   ankle
     appointment not kept
ANL   acceptable noise level
ANLL   acute nonlymphoblastic leukemia
ANM   Assistant Nurse Manager
ANMAT   Argentina Regulatory Agency
     (Administratión Nacional de
     Medicamentos, Alimentos y
     Tecnologia Médica)
ANN   artificial neural network(s)
     axillary node-negative
ANNA   artificial neural network analysis
ANOVA   analysis of variance
ANP   Adult Nurse Practitioner
     atrial natriuretic peptide (anaritide
     acetate)
     axillary node–positive
ANPR   advanced notice of proposed rule
     making
ANS   answer
     autonomic nervous system
ANSER   Aggregate Neurobehavioral
     Student Health and Education
     Review
ANSI   American National Standards
     Institute
ANT   anterior
     anthrax vaccine, not otherwise
     specified
     enpheptin (2-amino-5-nitrothiazol)
ANT_a anthrax vaccine, absorbed
ante   before
ANTI   anti–blood group A antiglobulin
   A:AGT   test
Anti bx   antibiotic
anti-D   anti-D immune globulin
anti-GAD   antibodies to glutamic acid
     decarboxylase
anti-HBc   antibody to hepatitis B core
     antigen (HBcAg)
anti-HBe   antibody to hepatitis B e antigen
     (HBeAg)
anti-HBs   antibody to hepatitis B surface
     antigen (HBsAg)
anti-Sm   anti-*Schistosoma mansoni*
     (antibody)
ant sag D   anterior sagittal diameter
ANTU   alpha naphthylthiourea

ANUG   acute necrotizing ulcerative
     gingivitis
ANV   acute nausea and vomiting
ANVISA   National Health Surveillance
     Agency (Brazil)
ANX   anxiety
     anxious
ANZDATA   Australia and New Zealand
     Dialysis and Transplant
     Registry
AO   abdominal obesity
     acridine orange (stain)
     Agent Orange
     Alveolar osteitis (also known as
     dry socket)
     anaplastic oligodendrogliomas
     anterior oblique
     aorta
     aortic opening
     aortography
     axio-occlusal
     plate, screw (orthopedics)
     right ear
A-O   atlanto-occipital (joint)
A/O   alert and oriented
A & O   alert and oriented
A&O × 1   alert and oriented to person
A&O × 2   alert and oriented to person and
     place
A&O × 3   awake and oriented to person,
     place, and time
A&O × 4   awake and oriented to person,
     place, time, and object
AOA   American Osteopathic Association
     anaplastic oligoastrocytoma
AOAA   aminooxoacetic acid
AOAP   as often as possible
AOAs   adult offspring of alcoholics
AOB   alcohol on breath
AOBC   aortic occlusion balloon catheter
AOBL   anemia of blood loss
AOBS   acute organic brain syndrome
AOC   abridged ocular chart
     advanced ovarian cancer
     amoxicillin, omeprazole, and
     clarithromycin
     anode opening contraction
     antacid of choice
     area of concern
AOCD   anemia of chronic disease
AOCL   anodal opening clonus
AOCN   Advanced Oncology Certified
     Nurse
AOD   adult-onset diabetes
     alcohol and (and/or) other drugs
     alleged onset date
     anaplastic oligodendroglioma
     arterial occlusive disease

	Assistant-Officer-of-the-Day
AODA	alcohol and other drug abuse
AODM	adult-onset diabetes mellitus
AOE	acute otitis externa
A of 1	assistance of one
A of 2	assistance of two
AOFAS	American Orthopaedic Foot and Ankle Society (clinical rating scale)
AOI	apnea of infancy
	area of induration
ao-il	aorta-iliac
AOIVM	angiographically occult intracranial vascular malformation
AOL	augmentation of labor
AOLC	acridine-orange leukocyte cytospin
AOLD	automated open lumbar diskectomy
AOM	acute otitis media
	alternatives of management
AONAD	alert, oriented, and no acute distress
AOO	anodal opening odor
	continuous arterial asynchronous pacing
AO/OTA	Association for Osteosynthesis/ Orthopaedic Trauma Association (fracture classification)
AOP	anemia of prematurity
	anodal opening picture
	aortic pressure
	apnea of prematurity
AOR	adjusted odds ratio
	Alvarado Orthopedic Research
	at own risk
	auditory oculogyric reflex
AORC	arthritis and other rheumatic conditions
AORT REGURG	aortic regurgitation
AORT STEN	aortic stenosis
AOS	ambulatory outpatient surgery
	anode opening sound
	antibiotic order sheet
	aortic ostial stenoses
	arrived on scene
AOSC	acute obstructive suppurative cholangiotomy
AOSD	adult-onset Still disease
AOTB	alcohol on the breath
AOTe	anodal opening tetanus
AOX	antioxidant(s)
AP	abdominal pain
	abdominoperineal
	acute pancreatitis
	aerosol pentamidine
	alkaline phosphatase
	angina pectoris

	antepartum
	anterior-posterior (x-ray)
	antibiotic prophylaxis
	aortopulmonary
	apical periodontitis
	apical pulse
	appendectomy
	appendicitis
	arterial pressure
	arthritis panel (see page 356)
	atrial pacing
	attending physician
	doxorubicin (Adriamycin); cisplatin (Platinol)
A&P	active and present
	anterior and posterior
	assessment and plans
	auscultation and percussion
A/P	accounts payable
	ascites/plasma ratio
$A_2 > P_2$	second aortic sound greater than second pulmonic sound
4-AP	4-aminopyridine (Ampyra)
APA	aldosterone-producing adenoma
	American Psychiatric Association
	anticipatory postural adjustment
	antiphospholipid antibody
APAA	anterior parietal artery aneurysm
APAC	acute primary angle closure
APACHE	Acute Physiology and Chronic Health Evaluation
APAD	anterior-posterior abdominal diameter
APAG	antipseudomonal aminoglycosidic
APAP	acetaminophen (N acetylpara-aminophenol; Tylenol; paracetamol)
APB	abductor pollicis brevis
	atrial premature beat
APBI	accelerated partial breast irradiation
APBSCT	autologous peripheral blood stem cell transplantation
APC	absolute phagocyte count
	activated protein C
	acute pharyngoconjunctiivitis (fever)
	adenoidal-pharyngeal-conjunctival
	adenomatous polyposis of the colon and rectum
	advanced pancreatic cancer
	Advance Practice Clinician
	advanced prostate cancer
	Ambulatory Payment Classification
	annual percentage change
	antigen-presenting cell
	argon plasma coagulator
	aspirin, phenacetin, and caffeine (no longer marketed in the US)

	asymptomatic prostate cancer
	atrial premature contraction
	autologous packed cells
APCD	adult polycystic disease
APCE	affinity probe capillary electrophoresis
APCIs	atrial peptide clearance inhibitors
APCKD	adult polycystic kidney disease
AP-CT	abdominal and pelvic computer tomography
APD	acid peptic disease
	action potential duration
	afferent pupillary defect
	anterior-posterior diameter
	atrial premature depolarization
	automated peritoneal dialysis
	pamidronate disodium (aminohydroxypropylidene diphosphate)
APDC	Anxiety and Panic Disorder Clinic
AP-DRGs	all-patient diagnosis-related groups
APDT	acellular pertussis vaccine with diphtheria and tetanus toxoids
APE	absolute prediction error
	acute psychotic episode
	acute pulmonary edema
	anterior pituitary extract
	doxorubicin (Adriamycin), cisplatin (Platinol-AQ), and etoposide
APECED	autoimmune polyendocrinopathy-candidiasis ectodermal dystrophy
ApEn	approximate entropy
APER	abdominoperineal excision of the rectum
aPFC	anterior pre-frontal cortex
APG	ambulatory patient group
	Apgar (score)
Apgar	appearance (color), pulse (heart rate), grimace (reflex irritability), activity (muscle tone), and respiration (score reflecting condition of newborn)
APH	adult psychiatric hospital
	alcohol-positive history
	antepartum hemorrhage
APhA	American Pharmacists Association
APHIS	Animal and Plant Health Inspection Service
API	active pharmaceutical ingredients
	Asian-Pacific Islander
APIS	Acute Pain Intensity Scale
APIVR	artificial pacemaker-induced ventricular rhythm
APKD	adult polycystic kidney disease
	adult-onset polycystic kidney disease
APL	abductor pollicis longus

	accelerated painless labor
	acute promyelocytic leukemia
	anterior pituitary-like (hormone)
	chorionic gonadotropin
AP & L	anteroposterior and lateral
APLA	antiphospholipid antibody
APLD	automated percutaneous lumbar diskectomy
APLS	antiphospholipid syndrome
APME	acute postinfectious measles encephalitis
APML	acute promyelocytic leukemia
APMPPE	acute posterior multifocal placoid pigment epitheliopathy
APMS	acute pain management service
APN	acquired pendular nystagmus
	acute panautonomic neuropathy
	acute pyelonephritis
	Advanced Practice Nurse
APO	adverse patient occurrence
	apolipoprotein A-1
	doxorubicin (Adriamycin), prednisone, and vincristine (Oncovin)
APO(a)	apolipoprotein (A)
APO B	apolipoprotein B
APOE	apolipoprotein E
APOE-4	apolipoprotein-E (gene)
APOLT	auxiliary partial orthotopic liver transplantation
APOPPS	adjustable postoperative protective prosthetic socket
APP	alternating pressure pad
	amyloid precursor protein
	appetite
	assume pain present
APPG	aqueous procaine penicillin G (dangerous terminology; since it is for intramuscular use only; write as penicillin G procaine)
APPLA	another planned permanent living arrangement
appr	approximate
approx	approximate
appt	appointment
APPY	appendectomy
APR	abdominoperineal resection
	acute radiation proctitis
	anatomical programmed radiography
	average payment rate
AP & R	apical and radial (pulses)
APR-DRGs	all-patient refined diagnosis-related groups
APRT	abdominopelvic radiotherapy
APRV	airway pressure release ventilation
APS	acute pain service

	Acute Physiology Scoring (system)		aural rehabilitation
	adult protective services		autorefractor
	Adult Psychiatric Service		axial rotation
	antiphospholipid syndrome	Ar	argon
APSAC	anistreplase (anisoylated plasminogen streptokinase activator complex)	A&R	adenoidectomy with radium advised and released
		A-R	apical-radial (pulses)
APSD	Alzheimer presenile dementia	A/R	accounts receivable
APSP	assisted peak systolic pressure	ARA	Action Research Arm (test)
APSS	Associated Professional Sleep Societies		adenosine regulating agent
		Ara	arabinose
APT	antiplaletelet therapy	ara-A	vidarabine (Vira-A)
	apartment	ara-AC	fazarabine
aPTT	activated partial thromboplastin time	ara-C	cytarabine (Cytosar-U)
		ARAD	abnormal right axis deviation
APU	ambulatory procedure unit antepartum unit	ARAS	ascending reticular activating system
APUD	amine precursor uptake and decarboxylation		atherosclerotic renal-artery stenosis
APV	amprenavir (Agenerase)	ARB	angiotensin II receptor blocker
	approximate priming volume (amount of fluid needed to prime an IV access device)		antibiotic-resistant bacteria
			any reliable brand
		ARBOR	arthropod-borne virus
APVC	partial anomalous pulmonary venous connection	ARBOW	artificial rupture of bag of water
		ARC	abnormal retinal correspondence
APVR	aortic pulmonary valve replacement		adult residential care
			AIDS-related complex
APVT	advanced portal vein thrombosis		Alcohol Rehabilitation Center
APW	aortopulmonary window		anomalous retinal correspondence
AQ	amodiaquine		American Red Cross
aq	water		autologous red cells
AQ	accomplishment quotient	ARCBS	American Red Cross Blood Services
AQoL	Assessment of Quality of Life	ARCC	autosomal recessive congenital cataract
	Asthma-related Quality of Life		
	Australian Quality of Life	ARCOS	Automation of Reports and Consolidated Orders System (for controlled substances)
AQP4	aquaporin-4		
aq dest	distilled water		
AQLQ-J	Asthma Quality of Life Questionnaire—Juniper	ARD	acute respiratory disease
			adult respiratory distress
AQLQ-M	Asthma Quality of Life Questionnaire—Marks		antibiotic removal device
			antibiotic retrieval device
AQOL	acne quality of life		aphakic retinal detachment
AQR	ain't quite right (slang)	ARDMS	American Registry of Diagnostic Medical Sonographers
A quad	atrial quadrageminy		
AR	Achilles reflex	ARDS	adult respiratory distress syndrome
	acoustic reflex	ARE	active-resistive exercises
	active resistance	ARF	acute renal failure
	airway resistance		acute respiratory failure
	alcohol related		acute rheumatic fever
	allergic rhinitis		amylase-rich food (flour)
	androgen receptor	ARFF	at risk for falling
	ankle reflex	ARFI	acoustic radiation force impulse (imaging)
	aortic regurgitation		
	apoptotic rate	ARG	alkaline reflux gastritis
	Argyll Robertson (pupil)		arginine
	assisted respiration	ARGNB	antibiotic-resistant gram-negative bacilli
	at risk		

ARH	autosomal recessive hypercholesterolemia
ARHL	age-related hearing loss
ARHNC	advanced resected head and neck cancer
ARI	acute renal insufficiency
	acute respiratory infection
	acute respiratory illness
	aldose reductase inhibitor
	arousal index
ARIF	arthroscopic reduction and internal fixation
ARIMA	autoregressive integrated moving average (model)
ARJP	autosomal recessive juvenile parkinsonism
ARL	acquired immunodeficiency syndrome (AIDS)-related lymphoma
	average remaining lifetime
ARLD	alcohol-related liver disease
ARM	anxiety reaction, mild
	artificial rupture of membranes
ARMD	age-related macular degeneration
ARMS	alveolar rhabdomyosarcoma
	amplification refractory mutation system
	at-risk mental state
ARN	acute retinal necrosis
ARNA	American Radiological Nurses Association
ARND	alcohol-related neurodevelopmental disorder
ARNP	Advanced Registered Nurse Practitioner
AROM	active range of motion
	artifical rupture of membranes
ARP	absolute refractory period
	acute radiation proctitis
	alcohol rehabilitation program
	asparagine-rich protein
ARPC	androgen-resistant prostate cancer
ARPE	amylase-rich pleural effusion
ARPF	anterior release posterior fusion
ARPKS	autosomal recessive polycystic kidney disease
ARPN	Advanced Practice Registered Nurse
ARPT	acid reflux provocation test
ARR	absolute risk reduction
	Academy of Radiology Research
	anterior rectal resection
	arrive
aRR	adjusted rate ratio
ARROM	active resistive range of motion
ARRS	American Roentgen Ray Society
ARRT	American Registry of Radiologic Technologists

ARS	acute radiation sickness
	antirabies serum
ART	Accredited Record Technician (for newer title, see RHIT)
	Achilles (tendon) reflex test
	acoustic reflex threshold(s)
	adjuvant radiation therapy
	androgen replacement therapy
	anesthesia release time (patient-on-table until release for surgical preparation)
	antiretroviral therapy
	arterial
	assessment, review, and treatment
	assisted reproductive technology
	automated reagin test (for syphilis)
ARTIC	articulation
Art T	art therapy
ARU	acute receiving unit
	alcohol rehabilitation unit
ARV	AIDS-related virus
	antiretroviral
ARVC	arrhythmogenic right ventricular cardiomyopathy
ARVD	arrhythmogenic right ventricular dysplasia
	atherosclerotic renovascular disease
ARVMB	anomalous right ventricular muscle bundles
ARVs	antiretroviral drugs
ARW	Accredited Rehabilitation Worker
ARWY	airway
AS	activated sleep
	active surveillance
	alpha-synuclein
	American Samoa
	anabolic steroid
	anal sphincter
	androgen suppression
	Angelman syndromes
	ankylosing spondylitis
	anterior synechia
	anxiety sensitivity
	aortic stenosis
	artesunate (an antimalarial agent)
	Asperger syndrome
	atherosclerosis
	atropine sulfate
	AutoSuture®
	doctor called through answering service
	left ear
ASA	American Society of Anesthesiologists
	American Statistical Association
	angiosarcoma
	argininosuccinate
	aspirin (acetylsalicylic acid)

as soon as

atrial septal aneurysm

ASA I   **American Society of Anesthesiologists' classification** Healthy patient with localized pathological process. Emergency operations are designated by "E" after the classification.)

ASA II   A patient with mild to moderate systemic disease

ASA III   A patient with severe systemic disease limiting activity but not incapacitating

ASA IV   A patient with incapacitating systemic disease

ASA V   Moribund patient not expected to live without the operation

ASA VI   A patient declared brain-dead whose organs are being removed for donor purposes

5-ASA   mesalamine (5-aminosalicylic acid; Asacol; Rowasa) (this is a dangerous abbreviation as it is mistaken for five aspirin tablets)

ASAA   acquired severe aplastic anemia

ASACL   American Society of Anesthesiologists Classification (see ASA I)

ASAD   arthroscopic subacromial decompression

ASA+ERDP   aspirin and extended-release dipyridamole (Aggrenox)

aSAH   aneurysmal subarachnoid hemorrhage

AS/AI   aortic stenosis/aortic insufficiency

ASAM PPC-2   Patient Placement Criteria published by the American Society of Addiction Medicine, Second Edition

ASAP   Alcohol and Substance Abuse Program

as soon as possible

atypical small acinar proliferation

ASAT   abdomminal subcutaneous adipose tissue

aspartate aminotransferase (also AST; SGOT)

ASB   anesthesia standby

anterior skull base

asymptomatic bacteriuria

ASBMS   American Society for Metabolic & Bariatric Surgery

ASBO   adhesive small-bowel obstruction

ASBs   artificially sweetened beverages

A's & B's   apnea and bradycardia

ASC   active symptom control

adult stem cell

altered state of consciousness

ambulatory surgery (surgical) center

anterior subcapsular cataract

antimony sulfur colloid

apocrine skin carcinoma

ascorbic acid (vitamin C)

ASCA   antisaccharomyces cerevisiae

ASCAD   atherosclerotic coronary artery disease

ASCCC   advanced squamous cell cervical carcinoma

ASCCHN   advanced squamous cell carcinoma of the head and neck

ASCI   acute spinal cord injury

ASCO   American Society of Clinical Oncology

ASCR   autologous stem cell rescue

ASCS   autologous stem cell support

ASCs   adipose-derived stem cells

ASCT   allogeneic stem cell transplantation

autologous stem cell transplantation

ASCUS   atypical squamous cell of undetermined significance

ASCVD   arteriosclerotic cardiovascular disease

ASCVR   arteriosclerotic cardiovascular renal disease

ASD   acute stress disorder

adjacent segment disease

air-space disease

aldosterone secretion defect

androstenedione

annual summary dose (ionizing radiation)

atrial septal defect

autism spectrum disorder(s)

ASD I   atrial septal defect, primum

ASD II   atrial septal defect, secundum

ASDA   American Sleep Disorders Association (criteria)

ASDC   Association of Sleep Disorders Centers

ASDH   acute subdural hematoma

ASDPs   antisocial personality disorders

ASE   abstinence symptom evaluation

acute stress erosion

a-Se   amorphous selenium

ASES   American Shoulder and Elbow Score

ASEX   Arizona Sexual Experiences (sexual dysfunction scale)

ASF   anterior spinal fusion

asymmetric screen film (radiology)

auditory spatial facilitation

ASFA   Adoption and Safe Families Act

ASFR   age-specific fertility rate

ASG	atrial septal graft	ASOTP	Affiliate Sex Offender Treatment Provider
ASH	American Society of Hematology (guidelines)	ASP	acute suppurative parotitis
	asymmetric septal hypertrophy		acute symmetric polyarthritis
AsH	hypermetropic astigmatism		antisocial personality
ASHD	arteriosclerotic heart disease		application service provider
ASI	active specific immunotherapy		asparaginase
	Addiction Severity Index		aspartic acid
	Anxiety Status Inventory	ASPD	antisocial personality disorder
	Arterial Stiffness Index	ASPDV	anterior superior pancreaticoduodenal vein
aSi	amorphous silicon		
ASIA	**American Spinal Injury Association (Score)**	ASPVD	arteriosclerotic peripheral vascular disease
	A-Complete—No preservation of any motor and/or sensory function below the zone of injury	ASQ	Ages and Stages Questionnaire
		ASQ:SE	Ages and Stages Questionnaire—Social Emotional
		ASR	aldosterone secretion rate
	B-Incomplete—Preserved sensation		articular surface replacement
	C-Incomplete—Preserved motor (nonfunctional)		automatic speech recognition
		ASRA	Alcohol Severity Rating Scale
	D-Incomplete—Preserved motor (functional)	ASRM	American Society for Reproductive Medicine (Infertility with endometriosis score/staging)
	E-Complete Recovery		
ASIH	absent, sick in hospital	ASS	anterior superior supine
ASIMC	absent, sick in medical center		aspirin (some European countries)
ASIS	anterior superior iliac spine		assessment
ASK	antistreptokinase	ASSRs	auditory steady-state responses
ASK™	Applied Semantic Knowledgebase	ASST	autologous serum skin test
ASKase	antistreptokinase	asst	assistant
ASL	American Sign Language	AST	allergy skin test
	antistreptolysin (titer)		androgen suppression therapy
ASLO	antistreptolysin-O		Aphasia Screening Test
ASLV	avian sarcoma and leukosis virus (Rous virus)		aspartate aminotransferase (same as SGOT)
ASM	atrial systolic murmur		astemizole (Hismanal)
AsM	myopic astigmatism		astigmatism
ASMA	antismooth-muscle antibody	AstdVe	assisted ventilation
ASMI	anteroseptal myocardial infarction	ASTH	asthenopia
ASN	Associate's of Science in Nursing	ASTI	acute soft tissue injury
ASO	accessory sinus ostia	AS TOL	as tolerated
	administrative services only (contract)	ASTIG	astigmatism
		ASTM	American Society for Testing and Materials
	AIDS (acquired immunodeficiency syndrome) service organization(s)	ASTRO	American Society for Therapeutic Radiation and Oncology
	aldicarb sulfoxide		astrocytoma
	allele-specific oligodeoxy-nucleotide (probes)	ASTZ	antistreptozyme test
		ASU	acute stroke unit
	Amplatzer Septal Occluder		ambulatory surgical unit
	antisense oligonucleotides	ASV	antisnake venom
	antistreptolysin-O titer	ASVD	arteriosclerotic vessel disease
	arterial switch operation	ASYM	asymmetric(al)
	arteriosclerosis obliterans	ASX	asymptomatic
	automatic stop order	AT	abdominothoracic
As$_2$O$_3$	arsenic trioxide (Trisenox)		activity therapy (therapist)
ASOC	advanced-stage ovarian cancer		Addiction Therapist
ASOT	antistreptolysin-O titer		anaerobic threshold

	antithrombin
	applanation tonometry
	ataxia-telangiectasia
	atraumatic
	atrial tachycardia
AT1	angiotensin II type 1
AT 10	dihydrotachysterol (Hytakerol; DHT®)
ATA	atmosphere absolute
	authority to administer
ATB	antibiotic
	aquatic therapy bar
	atypical tuberculosis
ATBF	African tick-bite fever
ATC	acute toxic class
	aerosol treatment chamber
	alcoholism therapy classes
	all-terrain cycle
	anaplastic thyroid carcinoma
	antituberculous chemoprophylaxis
	around-the-clock
	Arthritis Treatment Center
	Athletic Trainer, Certified
ATCC	American Type Culture Collection
ATCCS	acute traumatic central cord syndrome
ATD	antithyroid drug(s)
	anticipated time of discharge
	aqueous tear deficiency
	asphyxiating thoracic dystrophy
	autoimmune thyroid disease
ATE	adipose tissue extraction
AT-EI	assistive technology and environmental interventions
ATEM	analytical transmission electron microscopy
ATEs	arterial thromboembolic events
ATF	Alcohol, Tobacco, and Firearms (Bureau)
	arrived to find
At Fib	atrial fibrillation
ATFL	anterior talofibular ligament
AT III FUN	antithrombin III functional
ATG	antithymocyte globulin
ATHR	angina threshold heart rate
ATI	Abdominal Trauma Index
	acute traumatic ischemia
ATL	Achilles tendon lengthening
	adult T-cell leukemia
	anterior temporal lobectomy
	anterior tricuspid leaflet
	antitension line
	atypical lymphocytes
ATLL	adult T-cell leukemia/lymphoma
ATLP	anterior thoracolumbar locking (implant) plate
ATLS	acute tumor lysis syndrome

	advanced trauma life support
ATM	acute transverse myelitis
	ataxia telangiectasia mutated (gene)
	atmosphere
At ma	atrial milliamp
ATN	acute tubular necrosis
ATNC	atraumatic normocephalic
aTNM	autopsy staging of cancer
ATNR	asymmetrical tonic neck reflex
ATO	arsenic trioxide (Trisenox)
ATOD-C	Alcohol, Tobacco and Drugs, Certified
ATP	ability to pay
	according-to-protocol
	addiction treatment program
	adenosine triphosphate
	anterior tonsillar pillar
	antitachycardia pacing
	autoimmune thrombocytopenia purpura
ATP III	Adult Treatment Panel III
ATPase	adenosine triphosphatase
ATPS	ambient temperature & pressure, saturated with water vapor
ATR	Achilles tendon reflex
	anterior temporal-lobe resection
	atracurium (Tracrium)
	atrial
	atropine
ATRA	all-*trans* retinoic acid (tretinoin-Vesanoid)
atr fib	atrial fibrillation
ATRO	atropine
ATRX	acute transfusion reaction
ATSDR	Agency for Toxic Substances and Disease Registry
ATTN	attending
	attention
ATU	alcohol treatment unit
ATUE	abbreviated therapeutic use exemption
ATV	all-terrain vehicle
ATS	American Thoracic Society (guidelines)
	antimony trisulfide
	antitetanic serum (tetanus antitoxin)
	anxiety tension state
ATSO	admit to (the) service of
ATSO4	atropine sulfate
ATSP	asked to see patient
ATT	alternating triple therapy
	antitetanus toxoid
	arginine tolerance test
ATTN	attending
	attention

ATTR	amyloid transtyretin
at. wt	atomic weight
ATX	atelectasis
ATZ	anal transitional zone
AU	allergenic (allergy) units
	arbitrary units
	both ears (this is a dangerous abbreviation, as it may be seen as OU [both eyes])
Au	gold
A/U	at umbilicus
198Au	radioactive gold
AUA score	American Urological Association— pertains to benign prostatic hypertrophy symptoms
AUB	abnormal uterine bleeding
AuBMT	autologous bone marrow transplant
AUC	analytical ultracentrifugation
	area under the curve
AUCt	area under the curve to last time point
AUD	alcohol use disorder
	amplifiable units of DNA (deoxyribonucleic acid)
	arthritis of unknown diagnosis
	auditory
AUD COMP	auditory comprehension
aud hallu	auditory hallucinations
AUDIT	Alcohol Use Disorders Identification Test
AUG	acute ulcerative gingivitis
AUGIB	acute upper gastrointestinal bleeding
AUIC	area under the inhibitory curve
AUL	acute undifferentiated leukemia
AuNPs	gold nanoparticles
AUR	acute urinary retention
AUS	acute urethral syndrome
	artificial urinary sphincter
	auscultation
AuSCT	autologous stem cell transplantation
AutD	autistic disorder
AUTO	autologous
AUTO SP	automatic speech
AV	anteverted
	anticipatory vomiting
	arteriovenous
	atrioventricular
	auditory visual
	auriculoventricular
A:V	arterial-venous (ratio in fundi)
AVA	anthrax vaccine, adsorbed
	aortic valve area
	aortic valve atresia
	arteriovenous anastomosis

AVA-EE	aortic valve area epicardial echocardiography
AVB	atrioventricular block
	Aventis Behring
AVC	acrylic veneer crown
	aortic valve classification
	atrioventricular conduction
AVD	aortic valve disease
	apparent volume of distribution
	arteriosclerotic vascular disease
	atrioventricular delay
	cerebrovascular accident (French, Spanish)
AVDP	asparaginase, vincristine, daunorubicin, and prednisone
	avoirdupois
AVDO2	arteriovenous oxygen difference
AVE	aortic valve echocardiogram
	atrioventricular extrasystole
AVED	ataxia with isolated vitamin E deficiency
AVF	arteriovenous fistula
	augmented unipolar foot (left leg)
avg	average
AVGS	autologous vein graft stent
AVGs	ambulatory visit groups
AVH	acute viral hepatitis
AVHB	atrioventricular heart block
AVHs	auditory verbal hallucinations
	auditory and visual hallu cinations
AVJA	atrioventricular junction ablation
AVJR	atrioventricular junctional rhythm
AVL	American visceral leishmaniasis
	augmented unipolar left (left arm, electrocardiogram lead)
AVLT	auditory verbal learning test
AVM	arteriovenous malformation
AVN	arteriovenous nicking
	atrioventricular node
	avascular necrosis
AVNB	atrioventricular nodal block
AVNERP	atrioventricular node effective refractory period
AVNR	atrioventricular nodal re-entry
AVNRT	atrioventricular node recovery time
	atrioventricular nodal re-entry tachycardia
A-VO2	arteriovenous oxygen difference
AVOC	avocation
AVP	arginine vasopressin
	Aventis Pasteur
AVPU	alert, (responds to) verbal (stimuli), (responds to) painful (stimuli), unresponsive (mnemonic used by EMTs to judge patients' level of consciousness)

AVR	aortic valve replacement	AzdU	azidouridine
	augmented unipolar right (right arm electrocardiogram lead)	AZE	azelastine hydrochloride (Astelin)
AVRP	atrioventricular refractory period	AZM	acquisition zoom magnification
AVRT	atrioventricular reciprocating tachycardia		azithromycin (Zithromaz; Z-Pak)
AVS	aortic valve sclerosis	AZOOR	acute zonal occult outer retinopathy
	atriovenous shunt		
AVSD	atrioventricular septal defect	AZQ	diaziquone
AVSS	afebrile, vital signs stable	AZT	zidovudine
AVT	atrioventricular tachycardia		(azidothymidine; Retrovir)
	atypical ventricular tachycardia	A-Z test	Aschheim-Zondek test
AvWS	acquired von Willebrand syndrome		(diagnostic test for pregnancy)
AW	abdominal wall		
	abnormal wave		
	airway		
A/W	able to work		
A&W	alive and well		
AWA	alcohol withdrawal assessment		
	as well as		
A waves	atrial contraction wave		
AWB	autologous whole blood		
AWC	approach with care		
AWD	alcohol withdrawal delirium		
	alive with disease		
AWDW	assault with a deadly weapon		
AWE	acetowhite epithelium		
AWI	anterior wall infarct		
AWMI	anterior wall myocardial infarction		
AWO	airway obstruction		
AWOL	absent without leave		
AWP	airway pressure		
	average wholesale price		
AWRU	active wrist rotation unit		
AWS	alcohol withdrawal seizures (syndrome)		
	Axillary Web syndrme		
AWSA	Alcohol Withdrawal Severity Assessment (scale)		
AWU	alcohol withdrawal unit		
ax	axillary		
AX	axis		
AXB	axillary block		
AXC	aortic cross clamp		
ax-fem.fem.	axilla-femoral-femoral (graft)		
AXFR	axillofemoral reconstruction		
AXND	axillary node dissection		
AXR	abdomen x-ray		
AxSYM®	immunodiagnostic testing equipment		
AXT	alternating exotropia		
AY	acrocyanotic (infant color)		
AYA	adolescents and young adults		
AZA	azathioprine (Imuran)		
5 AZA-CdR	5-Aza-2'-deoxycitidine (decitabine; Dacogen)		
5-AZC	azacitidine (Vidaza)		

B

B	bacillus
	bands
	bilateral
	black
	bloody
	bolus
	both
	botulism (Vaccine B is botulism toxoid)
	brother
	buccal
	See "Plan B"
Ⓑ	both
B+	blood type B positive (B positive is preferred)
B−	blood type B negative (B negative is preferred)
B_1	thiamine HCl
B I	Billroth I (gastric surgery)
B II	Billroth II (gastric surgery)
B_2	riboflavin
B_3	nicotinic acid
b/4	before
B_5	pantothenic acid
B_6	pyridoxine HCl
B_7	biotin
B_8	adenosine phosphate
B_9	benign
B_{12}	cyanocobalamin
B19	parvovirus B19
B52	combined 5 mg of lorazepam (Haldol) IV and 2 mg of haloperidol (Ativan) IV (slang)
BA	backache
	Baker Act (Florida mental health act enabling involuntary commitment)
	Baptist
	benzyl alcohol
	bile acid
	biliary atresia
	bioavailability
	blood agar
	blood alcohol
	Boehler angel
	bone age
	Bourns assist
	branchial artery
	broken appointment
	bronchial asthma
	buccoaxial
	butyric acid
Ba	barium
B > A	bone greater than air

B < A	bone less than air
B & A	brisk and active
BAA	beta-adrenergic agonist
BAAM	Beck airway airflow monitor
Bab	Babinski
BAC	Bacterial Artficial Chromosome
	benzalkonium chloride
	blood-alcohol concentration
	breast arterial calcification
	bronchioloalveolar carcinoma
	buccoaxiocervical
BACCA	basal cell cancer
BACE	beta-site APP (amyloid precursor protein)-cleaving enzyme
BACI	bovine anti-cryptosporidium immunoglobulin
BACM	blocking agent corticosteroid myopathy
BACON	bleomycin, doxorubicin, lomustine, vincristine, and mechlorethamine
BACOP	bleomycin, doxorubicin (Adriamycin), cyclophosphamide, vincristine, and prednisone
BACPAC	Bulk Activities Post Approval Change
BACs	bacterial artificial chromosomes
BACT	bacteria
	base-activated clotting time
BAD	Benadryl, Ativan, and Decadron
	bipolar affective disorder
	blunt aortic disruption
BADL	basic activities of daily living
BADLS	Bristol Activities of Daily Living Scale
BaE	barium enema
BAE	bronchial artery embolization
BAEDP	balloon aortic end diastolic pressure
BAEP	brain stem auditory evoked potential
BAERs	brain stem auditory evoked responses
BaEV	baboon endogenous virus
BAG	buccoaxiogingival
BAHA	bone-anchored hearing aids
BAI	blunt abdominal injury
	breath-actuated inhalers
	Brief Assessment Interview
BAIQ	below average intelligence quotient
BAK cage	an interbody fusion system used to stabilize the spine
BAL	balance
	blood-alcohol level
	British antilewisite (dimercaprol)
	bronchoalveolar lavage
BALB	binaural alternate loudness balance
BALF	bronchoalveolar lavage fluid

B-ALL	B cell acute lymphoblastic leukemia	
BALP	baseline bone alkaline phosphatase	
BALT	bronchus-associated lymphoid tissue	
BAM	bony acetabular morphology Brain Acoustic Monitor	
BaM	barium meal	
BAMC	Brooke Army Medical Center	
BAMS	bioaerosol mass spectrometry	
BAN	breath activated nebulizer British Approved Name	
Banana Bag	a yellow colored intravenous infusion containing a multivitamin product, folic acid, thiamine hydrochloride, and possibly magnesium sulfate in 5% dextrose or 0.9% sodium chloride. Contents can vary. Used for alcoholic patients. (slang)	
BAND	band neutrophil (stab)	
BANS	back, arm, neck and scalp	
BAO	basal acid output	
BAoV	bicuspid aortic valve	
BAP	balloon angioplasty blood agar plate	
BAPS	balance activation proprioceptive system biomechanical ankle platform system	
BAPT	Baptist	
baPWV	brachial-ankle pulse wave velocity	
BAR	biofragmentable anastomotic ring	
Barb	barbiturate	
BARN	bilateral acute retinal necrosis	
BAR Troche	Benadryl, Ativan, and Reglan troche	
BAS	balloon atrial septostomy Barnes Akathisia Scale behavioral activation system bile acid sequestrants boric acid solution bronchial asthma (in) status	
BaS	barium swallow	
BASA	baby aspirin (81 mg chewable tablets of aspirin)	
BASC	Behavior Assessment System for Children	
BASIS	Basic Achievement Skills Individual Screener	
BASK	basket cells	
BASMI	Bath Ankylosing Spondylitis Metrology Index	
baso.	basophil	
BASO STIP	basophilic stippling	
BAT	Behavioral Avoidance Test best available therapy	

	blunt abdominal trauma	
	borreliacidal-antibody test	
	brightness acuity tester	
BATF	Bureau of Alcohol, Tobacco and Firearms	
BATO	boronic acid adduct of technetium oxime	
batt	battery	
BAVP	balloon aortic valvuloplasty	
BAU	bioequivalent allergy units	
BAV	bicuspid aortic valve	
BAVMs	brain arteriovenous malformations	
BAW	bronchoalveolar washing	
BB	baby boy backboard back to back bad breath bed bath bed board beta-blocker blanket bath blood bank blow bottle blue bloaters body belts both bones breakthrough bleeding breast biopsy bronchial brushing brush biopsy buffer base bulging bag (amniotic sac is found to be protruding from the cervix during a pelvic or speculum examination)	
B&B	bismuth and bourbon bowel and bladder	
B/B	backward bending	
BBA	born before arrival	
BBAS	blade and balloon atrial septostomy	
BBB	baseball bat beating blood-brain barrier bundle branch block	
BBBB	bilateral bundle branch block	
BBC	bilateral breast cancer Brown-Buerger cystoscope	
BBCS	bumps, bruises, cuts and scrapes (that is no serious injuries) (slang)	
BBD	baby born dead before bronchodilator benign breast disease	
BBE	biofield breast examination	
BBFA	both bones forearm	
BBFF	both bone foreman fracture	
BBFP	blood and body fluid precautions	
BBH	blood-bank hold	

BBI	Bowman Birk inhibitor	BCB	Brilliant cresyl blue (stain)
BBIC	Bowman Birk inhibitor concentrate	BCBR	bilateral carotid body resection
BBL	bottle blood loss	BC/BS	Blue Cross/Blue Shield
BBM	banked breast milk	BCC	basal cell carcinoma
BBOW	bulging bag of water		birth control clinic
BBP	blood-borne pathogen	BCCa	basal cell carcinoma
	butyl benzyl phthalate	BCD	basal cell dysplasia
BBR	bibasilar rales		bleomycin, cyclophosphamide, and
BBS	Bardet-Biedl syndrome		dactinomycin
	Berg Balance Scale		borderline of cardial dullness
	bilateral breath sounds	BCDCSW	Board Certified Diplomate in
BBSE	bilateral breath sounds equal		Clinical Social Work
BBSI	Brigance Basic Skills Inventory	BCDH	bilateral congenital dislocated hip
BBT	basal body temperature	BCE	basal cell epithelioma
	Buteyko breathing technique		beneficial clinical event
BB to MM	belly button to medial malleolus		bilateral cervical exploration
B Bx	breast biopsy	BCEDP	breast cancer early detection
BC	back care		program
	base curve	B cell	B lymphocyte
	basket catheter	BCETS	Board Certified Expert in
	battered child		Traumatic Stress
	bed and chair	BCF	basic conditioning factor
	beta carotene		Baylor core formula
	bicycle	BCG	bacille Calmette-Guérin vaccine
	birth control		bicolor guaiac
	bladder cancer	BCH	benign cephalic histiocytosis
	blood culture		benign coital headache
	Blue Cross	BCHA	bone-conduction hearing aid
	Board Certified	BChE	butyrylcholinesterase
	bone conduction	BCI	blunt carotid injury
	Bourn control	BCIE	bullous congenital ichthyosiform
	breast cancer		erythroderma
	buccocervical	BCIR	Barnett continent intestinal
	buffalo cap (cap for intravenous		reservoir
	line)	BCL	basic cycle length
B/C	because		bio-chemoluminescence
	blood urea nitrogen/creatinine ratio	B/C/L	BUN, (blood urea nitrogen),
B&C	bed and chair		creatinine, lytes (electrolytes)
	biopsy and curettage	B-CLL	B-cell chronic lymphocytic
	board and care		leukemia
	breathed and cried	BCLP	bilateral cleft lip and palate
BCA	balloon catheter angioplasty	BCLS	basic cardiac life support
	basal cell atypia	BCM	below costal margin
	bichloracetic acid		birth control medication
	bicinchoninic acid		birth control method
	brachiocephalic artery		body cell mass
BCa	breast cancer	BCMA	bar-code medication administration
BCAA	branched-chain amino acids	BCME	bis (chloromethyl) ether
BC < AC	bone conduction less than air	BCNP	Board Certified Nuclear Pharmacist
	conduction	BCNSP	Board Certified Nutrition Support
BC > AC	bone conduction greater than air		Pharmacist
	conduction	BCNU	bacteria-controlled nursing unit
BCAO	bilateral carotid artery occlusion		carmustine (BiCNU; Gliadel)
B. cat	*Branhamella catarrhalis*	BCOC	bowel care of choice
B-CAVe	bleomycin, lomustine (CCNU),		bowel cathartic of choice
	doxorubicin (Adriamycin), and	BCOP	Board Certified Oncology
	vinblastine (Velban)		Pharmacist

BCP	biochemical profile	1,4-butanediol
	birth control pills	twice daily (in the United
	blood cell profile	Kingdom, Australia, and
	carmustine, cyclophosphamide, and	elsewhere)
	prednisone	bd twice daily (in the United
BCPAP	Broun continuous positive airway	Kingdom, Australia, and
	pressure	elsewhere)
BCPP	Board Certified Psychiatric	B-D Becton Dickinson and Company
	Pharmacist	BDAE Boston Diagnostic Aphasia
BCPNN	Bayesian Confidence Propagation	Examination
	Neural Network	BDAS balloon dilation atrial septostomy
BCPS	Board Certified Pharmacotherapy	BDBS Bonnet-Dechaume-Blanc syndrome
	Specialist	BDC burn-dressing change
BCQ	breast central quadrantectomy	BDCM bromodichloromethane
BCR	bicaudate ratio	BDD body dysmorphic disorder
	breakpoint cluster region (gene)	bronchodilator drugs
	bulbocavernosus reflex	BDE bile duct exploration
BCRE	black cohosh root extract	boron dose enhancer
BCRS	Brief Cognitive Rate Scale	BDF bilateral distal femoral
BCRT	breast-conservation followed by	black divorced female
	radiation therapy	BDI Beck Depression Inventory
BCS	battered child syndrome	bile duct incision
	breast-conserving surgery	bile duct injury
	Budd-Chiari syndrome	BDI SF Beck Depression Inventory-Short
BCSC	breast cancer stem cells	Form
BCSF	bone cell stimulating factor	BDL below detectable limits
BCSS	bone cell stimulating substance	bile duct ligation
BCT	Bag Carrying Test	B-DLCL diffuse large B-cell lymphoma
	breast-conserving therapy	BDM black divorced male
	broad complex tachycardias	BDNF brain-derived neurotrophic factor
BCTP	bi-component triton tri-n-butyl	BDOD brain-dead organ donor
	phosphate	B-DOPA bleomycin, dacarbazine, vincristine
BCU	burn care unit	(Oncovin), prednisone, and
BCUG	bilateral cystourethrogram	doxorubicin (Adriamycin)
BCVA	best corrected visual acuity	BDP beclomethasone dipropionate
BCVI	blunt cerebrovascular injury	(Beconase AQ; QVAR)
BCX	blood culture	best demonstrated practice
B&D	bathing and dressing	BDR background diabetic retinopathy
BD	band neutrophil	bile duct reconstruction
	base deficit	black dot ringworm
	base down	bronchodilator response
	behavior disorder	bulk dose regimen
	Behçet disease	BDS bile duct stone(s)
	bile duct	BDSM bondage and discipline, dominance
	biotinidase deficiency	and submission,
	bipolar disorder(s)	(sadomasochism)
	birth date	BDUs battle dress uniforms
	birth defect	BDV Borna disease virus
	blood donor	BE bacterial endocarditis
	bortezomib and dexamethasone	barium enema
	Bowen disease	Barrett esophagus
	brain dead	base excess
	Breslow depth	below elbow
	bronchial drainage	binge eating
	bronchodilator	bioequivalence
	buccodistal	bread equivalent
	Buerger disease	breast examination

Be	beryllium	BFA	baby for adoption
B ↑ E	both upper extremities		basilic forearm
B ↓ E	both lower extremities		bifemoral arteriogram
B & E	brisk and equal	BFB	biofeedback
BEA	below-elbow amputation	BFC	benign febrile convulsion
BEAC	carmustine (BiCNU), etoposide, cytarabine (ara-C), and cyclophosphamide	BFD	blackfoot disease
		BFEC	benign focal epilepsy of childhood
		bFGF	basic fibroblast growth factor
BEACOPP	bleomycin, etoposide, doxorubicin (Adriamycin), cyclophosphamide, vincristine (Oncovin), procarbazine, and prednisone	BFI	Brief Fatigue Inventory
		BFL	breast firm and lactating
		B-FLY	butterfly
		BFM	Berlin-Frankfurt-Munster(cancer study group)
BEAM	brain electrical activity mapping		black married female
	carmustine (BCNU), etoposide, cytarabine (ara-C), and methotrexate		body fat mass
			bright field microscope
		BFNC	benign familial neonatal convulsions
BEAR	Bourn electronic adult respirator		
BEP	benign essential blepharospasm	BFP	biologic false positive
BEC	bacterial endocarditis		blue fluorescent protein
BECs	bronchial epithelial cells	BFR	Backward Functional Reach (test)
BECT	barium enema computed tomography		blood filtration rate
			blood flow rate
BED	binge-eating disorder	B. frag	Bacillus fragilis
	biochemical evidence of disease	BFs	breast-feeds
	biological effective dose	BFT	bentonite flocculation test
	biological equivalent dose		biofeedback training
BEE	basal energy expenditure	BFU$_e$	erythroid burst-forming unit
BEF	bilateral endothelial fistula	BG	baby girl
	bronchoesophageal fistula		basal ganglia
BEGA	best estimate of gestational age		blood glucose
BEH	behavior		bone graft
	benign essential hypertension	B-G	Bender-Gestalt (test)
Beh Sp	behavior specialist	BGA	Bundesgesundheitsamt (German drug regulatory agency)
BEI	bioelectric impedance		
	butanol-extractable iodine	B-GA-	beta galactosidase
BEL	blood ethanol level	LACTO	
BEP	bleomycin, etoposide, and cisplatin (Platinol)	BGC	basal-ganglion calcification
		BGCT	benign glandular cell tumor
	brain stem evoked potentials	BGDC	Bartholin gland duct cyst
BE-PEG	balanced electrolyte with polyethylene glycol	BGDR	background diabetic retinopathy
		BGL	blood glucose level
BESS	bilateral endoscopic sinus surgery	BGM	blood glucose monitoring
		bGS	biopsy Gleason score
BEST	bio-electrical stimulation therapy	BGT	Bender-Gestalt test
BET	bacterial endotoxins test		blood glucose testing
BEV	beams-eye view	BGTT	borderline glucose tolerance test
	billion electron volts	BH	bowel habits
	bleeding esophageal varices		Braxton Hicks (contractions)
BF	biofeedback		breath holding
	black female	BHA	butylated hydroxyanisole
	bone fragment	BHBC	bicyclist hit by car
	boyfriend	BHC	benzene hexachloride
	breakfast fed		Braxton Hicks contractions
	breast-fed	bHCG	beta human chorionic gonadotropin
B/F	bound-to-free ratio	BHD	carmustine, hydroxyurea, and dacarbazine
B & F	back and forth		
%BF	percentage of body fat	BHDS	Birt-Hogg-Dube syndrome

B-HEXOS- A-LK	beta hexosaminidase A leukocytes	BIG-IV	botulism immune globulin intravenous (human)
BHGI	The Breast Health Global Initiative	BIH	benign intracranial hypertension
BHI	biosynthetic human insulin brain-heart infusion		bilateral inguinal hernia
		BIID	body integrity identity disorder
BHL	bilateral hilar lymphadenopathy	BIL	bilateral
BHMCO	behavioral health managed care organization		brother-in-law
		BILAT SLC	bilateral short leg case
BHN	bridging hepatic necrosis	BILAT SXO	bilateral salpingo-oophorectomy
BHP	boarding home placement	Bili	bilirubin
	British Herbal Pharmacopeia	BILI-C	conjugated bilirubin
BHR	Birmingham hip resurfacing	BIL MRY	bilateral myringotomy
	bronchial hyperresponsiveness (hyperactivity)	BIMA	bilateral internal mammary arteries
		BIN	twice a night (this is a dangerous abbreviation)
BHRT	bioidentical-hormone replacement therapy		
		BIND	Biological Investigational New Drug
BHS	Beck Hopelessness Scale		
	Behavioral Health Services	BIO	binocular indirect ophthalmoscopy
	beta-hemolytic streptococci	BIOF	biofeedback
	breath-holding spell	BIP	bipolar affective disorder
BHT	borderline hypertensive		bleomycin, ifosfamide, and cisplatin (Platinol)
	breath hydrogen test		
	butylated hydroxytoluene		bleomycin-induced pneumonitis
BHWU	Bair Hugger warming unit		brain injury program
BI	Barthel Index	BIPA	Benefits Improvement and Protection Act
	base in		
	bleeding index (dental)	BiPAP	bilevel (biphasic) positive airway pressure
	Boehringer Ingelheim Pharmaceuticals, Inc.		
		BiPD	biparietal diameter
	bowel impaction	BIPP	bismuth iodoform paraffin paste
	brain injury	BIR	back internal rotation
Bi	bismuth	BI-RADS	Breast Imaging Reporting and Data System (American College of Radiology)
BIA	bioelectrical impedance analysis		
	biospecific interaction analysis		
BIB	brought in by	BIRB	Biomedical Institutional Review Board
BIBA	brought in by ambulance		
BIC	brain injury center	BIS	behavioral inhibition system
BICAP	bipolar electrocoagulation therapy		Bispectral Index
bicarb	bicarbonate	Bi-SLT	bilateral, sequential single lung transplantation
BiCNU®	carmustine		
BICR	blinded independent central review	bisp	bispinous diameter
BICROS	bilateral contralateral routing of signals	BIT	behavioral inattention test
			burp in transit (gas seen in the stomach on an abdominal film) (slang)
BICU	burn intensive care unit		
BID	brought in dead		
BID	twice daily (b.i.d. preferred)	BITA	bilateral internal thoracic artery
b.i.d.	twice daily	BITC	benzyl isothiocyanate
BIDA	amonafide	BiV	biventricular pacing
BiDil®	hydralazine and isosorbide dinitrate	BIVAD	bilateral ventricular (biventricular) assist device
BIDS	bedtime insulin, daytime sulfonylurea	BIW	twice a week (this is a dangerous abbreviation)
BIF	bifocal	BIZ-PLT	bizarre platelets
BiFC	bimolecular fluorescence complementation (assay)	BJ	Bence Jones (protein)
			biceps jerk
BIG	botulism immune globulin		body jacket
	Breast International Group		bone and joint
BIGEM	bigeminal	BJE	bone and joint examination

	bones, joints, and extremities
BJI	bone and joint infection
BJLO	Benton Judgment Line Orientation (test)
BJM	bones, joints, and muscles
BJOA	basal joint osteoarthritis
BJP	Bence Jones protein
BJR	Bezold-Jarisch reflex
BK	below knee (amputation)
	bradykinin
	bullous keratopathy
BKA	below-knee-amputation
BKC	blepharokeratoconjunctivitis
bkft	breakfast
Bkg	background
BKTT	below-knee to toe (cast)
BKV	BK polyomavirus
BKVAN	BK virus (polyomavirus)-associated nephropathy
BKWC	below-knee walking cast
BKWP	below-knee walking plaster (cast)
BL	balloon laryngoplasty
	baseline (fetal heart rate)
	bioluminescence
	bland
	blast cells
	blood level
	blood loss
	blue
	bronchial lavage
	Burkitt lymphoma
B/L	brother-in-law
BLA	Biological License Application
	blood-loss anemia
BLB	Boothby-Lovelace-Bulbulian (oxygen mask)
	bronchoscopic lung biopsy
BLBK	blood bank
BLBS	bilateral breath sounds
BL = BS	bilateral equal breath sounds
BlCa	blader cancer
bl cult	blood culture
B-L-D	breakfast, lunch, and dinner
bldg	bleeding
bld tm	bleeding time
BLE	both lower extremities
BLEED	ongoing *b*leeding, *l*ow blood pressure, *e*levated prothrombin time, *e*rratic mental status, and unstable comorbid *d*isease (risk factors for continued gastrointestinal bleeding)
BLEO	bleomycin sulfate
BLESS	bath, laxative, enema, shampoo, and shower
BLG	bovine beta-lactoglobulin
BLI	blast lung injury

BLIC	beta-lactamase inhibitor combination
BLIP	beta-lactamase inhibiting protein
BLL	bilateral lower lobe
	blood lead level
	brows, lids, and lashes
BLLS	bilateral leg strength
BLM	bleomycin sulfate
BLN	bronchial lymph nodes
BLOB	backward loss of balance
BLOBS	bladder obstruction
BLOC	brief loss of consciousness
BLOKS	Boston Leeds Osteoarthritis Knee Score
BLP	blastomycosis-like pyoderma (also known as pyoderma vegetans)
BLPB	beta-lactamase-producing bacteria
BLPO	beta-lactamase-producing organism
BLQ	below the limit of quantification
	both lower quadrants
BLR	blood flow rate
BLS	basic life support
	Bureau of Labor Statistics
BLT	bilateral lung transplantation
	blood-clot lysis time
	brow left transverse
B.L. unit	Bessey-Lowry units
BLV	bovine leukemia virus
BM	bacterial meningitis
	black male
	bone marrow
	bone metastases
	bowel movement
	brain metastases
	breast milk
	budget manager
	bullous myringitis
BMA	biomedical application
	bismuth subsalicylate, metronidazole, and amoxicillin
	bone marrow aspirate
	British Medical Association
BMAT	basic motor ability test(s)
BMB	bone marrow biopsy
BMBF	German Ministry of Education and Research
BMC	bone marrow cells
	bone marrow culture
	bone mineral content
BMCS	balloon-mounted coronary stents
BMD	Becker muscular dystrophy
	benchmark dose
	bipolar manic depressive
	bipolar mood disorder
	bone marrow depression
	bone mineral density
	broth microdilution
BMDC	bone marrow-derived (stem) cells

BME	basal medium Eagle (diploid cell culture)		bladder neck
			bulimia nervosa
	biomedical engineering	BNBAS	Brazelton Neonatal Behavioral
	bone marrow edema		Assessment
	brief maximal effort	BNC	binasal cannula
BMET	basic metabolic panel (see page 356)		bladder neck contracture
		BNCT	boron neutron capture therapy
BMF	between meal feedings	BND	bloody, near dead (slang)
	black married female	BNE	but not exceeding
BMFDS	Burke-Marsden-Fahn dystonia rating scale	BNF	British National Formulary
		BNI	blind nasal intubation
BMG	benign monoclonal gammopathy	BNL	below normal limits
BMGF	Bill & Melinda Gates Foundation		breast needle localization
BMH	bone marrow harvest	Bn M	bone marrow
BMI	body mass index	B-NHL	B-cell non-Hodgkin lymphoma
BMJ	bones, muscles, joints	BNO	bladder neck obstruction
BMK	birthmark		bowels not open
BML	bone marrow lesion	BNP	brain natriuretic peptide
BMM	black married male		B-type natriuretic peptide
	bone marrow metastases		(nesiritide [Natrecor])
	bone marrow micrometastases	BNPA	binasal pharyngeal airway
BMMC	bone marrow mononuclear T cells	BNR	bladder neck retraction
BMMM	bone marrow micrometastases	BNS	benign nephrosclerosis
BMMNC	bone marrow mononuclear cell	BNT	back to normal
B-MODE	brightness modulation		behavioral naltrexone therapy
BMP	basic metabolic profile (panel) (see page 356)		Boston Naming Test
		BO	base out
	behavior management plan		because of
	bone morphogenetic protein		behavior objective
BMPC	bone marrow plasmacytosis		body odor
BMPs	bone-morphogenic proteins		bowel obstruction
BMQ	Beliefs about Medicines Questionnaire		bowel open
			bucco-occlusal
BMR	basal metabolic rate	B & O	belladonna & opium
	best motor response		(suppositories)
BMRM	bilateral modified radical mastectomy	BOA	behavioral observation audiometry
			born on arrival
BMS	bare-metal stents		born out of asepsis
	Bristol-Myers Squibb Company	BOB	ball-on-back
	burning mouth syndrome	BOC	beats of clonus
BMSC	bone marrow-derived stem cells	BOCF	baseline observation carried forward
BMT	bilateral myringotomy and tubes		
	bismuth subsalicylate, metronidazole, and tetracycline	BOD	bilateral orbital decompression
			Board of Drugs (Sweden)
	bone marrow transplant		burden of disease
BMTH	bismuth, metronidazole, tetracycline, and a histamine H_2-receptor antagonist	BODE	body mass index, airflow obstruction, dyspnea, and exercise capacity (index)
BMTN	bone marrow transplant neutropenia	Bod Units	Bodansky units
		BOE	bilateral otitis externa
BMTT	bilateral myringotomy with tympanic tubes	BOH	Board of Health
			bundle of His
BMTU	bone marrow transplant unit	BOLD	bleomycin, vincristine (Oncovin), lomustine, and dacarbazine
BMTx	bone marrow transplant		
BMU	basic multicellular unit		blood oxygenation level-dependent
BMY	Bristol-Myers Squibb	BOM	benign ovarian mass
BMZ	betamethasone (Celestone)		bilateral otitis media
BN	battalions	BOMA	bilateral otitis media, acute

BOME	bilateral otitis media with effusion		borderline personality disorder
BOMH	Board of Mental Health		bronchopulmonary dysplasia
BOMP	bleomycin, vincristine (Oncovin),	BPd	diastolic blood pressure
	mitomycin, and cisplatin	BPD/DS	biliopancreatic diversion with a
	(Platinol)		duodenal switch (surgery for
BoNTA	botulinum toxin type A		obesity)
BOO	bladder outlet obstruction	BPE	benign enlargement of the prostate
BOOP	bronchitis obliterans-organized	BPF	Brazilian purpuric fever
	pneumonia		bronchopleural fistula
BOP	bleeding on probing	BPH	benign prostatic hypertrophy
BOR	bortezomib (Velcade)		bronchopulmonary hygiene
	bowels open regularly	BPG	bypass graft
	bronchio-oto-renal (syndrome)		penicillin G benzathine (Bicillin L-
BORN	State Board of Registration in		A; Permapen) for IM use only
	Nursing	BPI	bactericidal/permeability increasing
BORospA	borreliosis (Lyme disease, *Borrelia*		(protein)
	sp.) vaccine, outer surface		Brief Pain Inventory
	protein A	BPIG	bacterial polysaccharide immune
BORR	best overall response rate		globulin
BOS	base of support	BPL	benzylpenicilloylpolylysine
	bronchiolitis obliterans syndrome		bone probing length (dental)
BOSS	Becker orthopedic spinal system	BPLA	blood pressure, left arm
BOT	base of tongue	BPLND	bilateral pelvic lymph node
	borderline ovarian tumors		dissection
BOU	burning on urination	BPM	beats per minute
BOUGIE	bougienage		breaths per minute
BOVR	Bureau of Vocational	BPN	bacitracin, polymyxin B, and
	Rehabilitation		neomycin sulfate
BOW	bag of water	BPO	benign prostatic obstruction
BOW-I	bag of water–intact		benzoyl peroxide
BOW-R	bag of water–ruptured		bilateral partial oophorectomy
BP	bathroom privileges	BPOC	barcode point-of-care
	bed pan	BPOP	bizarre parosteal
	bench press		osteochondromatous
	benzoyl peroxide		proliferation (Nora's Lesion)
	biological parent(s)	BPP	biophysical profile
	bipolar	BPPP	bilateral pedal pulses present
	birthplace	BP,P,R,T,	blood pressure, pulse, respiration,
	blood pressure		and temperature
	bodily pain	BPPV	benign paroxysmal positional
	body powder		vertigo
	British Pharmacopeia	BPR	beeper
	bullous pemphigoid		blood per rectum
	bypass		blood pressure recorder
bp	base pair(s) (genetics)		body position retraining (sleep
BP-200	Bourn Infant Pressure Ventilator		medicine)
BPA	birch pollen allergy	BPRS	Brief Psychiatric Rating Scale
	bisphenol A	BPS	bilateral partial salpingectomy
BPAD	bipolar affective disorder		blood pump speed
BPAP	bilevel positive airway pressure	BPs	systolic blood pressure
BPAR	biopsy-proven actue rejection	BPSD	behavioral and psychological
BPb	whole blood lead concentration		symptoms of dementia
BPC	British Pharmaceutical Codex		bronchopulmonary segmental
BPCF	bronchopleural cutaneous fistula		drainage
BPI	bipolar disorder, Type I	BPSO	bilateral prophylactic salpingo-
BPII	bipolar type II disorder		oophorectomy
BPD	benzoporphyrin derivative	BPT	BioPort Corporation
	biparietal diameter	BPTB	bone-patellar tendon-bone (graft)

BPV	benign paroxysmal vertigo	BRN	brown
	benign positional vertigo	BRO	brother
	bovine papilloma virus	BROM	back range of motion
BPW	bilateral pick-up walker	BRONJ	bisphosphonate-related
Bq	becquerel		osteonecrosis of the jaw
BQL	below quantifiable levels	BRONK	bronchoscopy
BQR	brequinar sodium	BRP	bathroom privileges
BR	bathroom	BRR	Bannayan-Riley-Ruvalcaba
	bedrest		(syndrome)
	Benzing retrograde	BR RAO	branch retinal artery occlusion
	birthing room	BRRB	bright red rectal bleeding
	blink rate	BRRS	Bannayan-Riley-Ruvalcaba
	blink reflex		syndrome
	bowel rest	BR RVO	branch retinal vein occlusion
	brachioradialis	BRS	baroreceptor reflex sensitivity
	breast		brain reward system
	breast reconstruction	BrS	breath sounds
	breech	BRSV	bovine respiratory syncytial virus
	bridge	BRU	basic remodeling unit (osteon)
	bright red		brucellosis (*Brucella melitensis*)
	brown		vaccine
Br	bromide	BRVO	branch retinal vein occlusion
	bromine	BS	barium swallow
BRA	bananas, rice (rice cereal), and		bedside
	applesauce		before sleep
	brain		Behçet syndrome
BrAC	breath alcohol content		Bennett seal
BRADY	bradycardia		blind spot
BRAF	v-raf murine sarcoma viral		blood sugar
	oncogene homolog B1		Blue Shield
BRANCH	branch chain amino acids		bone scan
BRAO	branch retinal artery occlusion		bowel sounds
BRAS	bilateral renal artery stenosis		breath sounds
BRAT	bananas, rice (rice cereal),	B & S	Bartholin and Skene (glands)
	applesauce, and toast		bending and stooping
	Baylor rapid autologous transfuser		Brown and Sharp (suture sizes)
	blunt thoracic abdominal trauma	BS×4	bowel sounds in all four
BRATT	bananas, rice (rice cereal),		quadrants
	applesauce, tea, and toast	BSA	body surface area
BRB	blood-retinal barrier		bowel sounds active
	bright red blood		Brief Scale of Anxiety
BRBR	bright red blood per rectum	BSAB	Balthazar Scales of Adaptive
BRBPR	bright red blood per rectum		Behavior
BRC	bladder reconstruction	BSAb	broad-spectrum antibiotics
BrCa	breast cancer	bsAbs	bispecific antibodies
BRCA1	breast cancer gene 1	BSAP	bone-specific alkaline phosphatase
BRCA2	breast cancer gene 2	BSB	bedside bag
BRCM	below right costal margin		body surface burned
BrdU	bromodeoxyuridine	BSC	basosquamous (cell) carcinoma
BRET	bioluminescence resonance energy		bedside care
	transfer		bedside commode
BRex	breathing exercise		best supportive care
Br Fdg	breast-feeding		biological safety cabinet
BRFS	biochemical relapse-free survival		Biomedical Science Corps
BRFSS	Behavioral Risk Factor		burn scar contracture
	Surveillance System (CDC)	BSCC	bedside commode chair
BRJ	brachial radialis jerk		Bjork-Shiley convexo-concave
BRM	biological response modifiers		(valves)

BSCVA	best spectacle-corrected visual acuity	BSSO	bilateral sagittal split osteotomy
BSD	baby soft diet	BSSRO	bilateral sagittal split-ramus osteotomy
	bedside drainage	BSSS	benign sporadic sleep spikes
	brain stem death	BSST	breast self-stimulation test
BSE	bovine spongiform encephalopathy	BST	bedside testing
	breast self-examination		bovine somatotropin
	broccoli sprout extracts		brain-stem tumors
BSEC	bedside easy chair		brief stimulus therapy
BSepF	black separated female	bst	boost
BSepM	black separated male	BSU	Bartholin, Skene, urethra (glands)
BSER	brain stem evoked responses		behavioral science unit
BSF	black single female	BSu	blood sugar
	busulfan (Myleran)	BSUTD	baby shots up to date
BSG	Bagolini striated glasses		Base Service Unit
	brain stem gliomas	BSW	Bachelor of Social Work
BSGA	beta streptococcus group A		bedscale weight
BSGI	breast-specific gamma imaging	BSX	bypass surgery
BSI	bloodstream infection	BT	bedtime
	body substance isolation		behavioral therapy
	brain stem injury		bituberous
	Brief Symptom Inventory		bladder tumor
BSL	baseline		Blalock-Taussig (shunt)
	Biological Safety Level		bleeding time
	blood sugar level		blood transfusion
BSL-1	Biosafety Level 1		blood type
BS L base	breath sounds diminished, left base		blue tongue
			blunt trauma
BSM	black single male		bowel tones
	blood safety module		brachytherapy
	body surface mapping		brain tumor
BSN	Bachelor of Science in Nursing		breast tumor
	bowel sounds normal		bronchial thermoplasty
BSNA	bowel sounds normal and active	Bt	*Bacillus thuringiensis*
BSNMT	Bachelor of Science in Nuclear Medicine Technology	B-T	Blalock-Taussig (shunt)
		B/T	between
BSNT	breast soft and nontender	Bt#	bottle number
BSNUTD	baby shots not up to date	BTA	below the ankle
BSO	bilateral salpingo-oophorectomy		bladder tumor antigen
	l-buthionine sulfoximine		bladder tumor-associated analytes
bSOD	bovine superoxide dismutase		botulinum toxic type A (Botox)
BSOM	bilateral serous otitis media	BTA-A	botulinum toxin type A (Botox)
BSP	body substance precautions	BTAI	blunt traumatic aortic injury
	bone sialoprotein	BTB	back to bed
	Bromsulphalein®		beat-to-beat (variability)
BSPA	bowel sounds present and active		breakthrough bleeding
BSPM	body surface potential mapping	BTBV	beat-to-beat variability
BSR	body stereotactic radiosurgery	BTC	behind-the-counter (drugs)
	bowels sounds regular		bilateral tubal cautery
BSRI	Bem Sex Role Inventory		biliary tract cancer
BSRT (R)	Bachelor of Science in Radiologic Technology (Registered)		bladder tumor check
			by the clock
BSS	Baltimore Sepsis Scale	BTCP	breakthrough cancer pain
	bedside scale	BTD	bortezomib, thalidomide, and dexamethasone
	bismuth subsalicylate		
	black silk sutures		bridge to decision (refers to heart transplantation)
BSS®	balanced salt solution		
BSSG	sitogluside	BTE	Baltimore Therapeutic Equipment

	behind-the-ear (hearing aid)	BUS	Bartholin, urethral, and Skene
	bisected, totally embedded		glands
BTF	blenderized tube feeding		bladder ultrasound
BTFS	breast tumor frozen section		bulbourethral sling
BTG	beta thromboglobulin	BUSV	Bartholin urethral Skeins vagina
B-Thal	beta thalassemia	BUT	biopsy urease test
BTHOOM	beats the hell out of me (better		break up time
	stated as "differed diagnosis")	Butt Paste	16% Zinc Oxide ointment.
BTI	biliary tract infection		Contents and strength can vary.
	bitubal interruption		(slang and a commercial
BTKA	bilateral total knee arthroplasty		product)
BTL	bilateral tubal ligation	BV	bacterial vaginitis
BTM	bilateral tympanic membranes		bevacizumab (Avastin)
	bismuth subcitrate, tetracycline,		biological value
	and metronidazole		blood volume
BTMEAL	between meals	BVAD	biventricular assist device
BTO	bilateral tubal occlusion	BVAS	Birmingham Vasculitis Activity
BTP	bismuth tribromophenate		Score
	breakthrough pain	BVD	bovine viral diarrhea
	β-trace protein	BVDU	bromovinlydeoxyuridine (brivudin)
BTPABA	bentiromide	BVE	blood volume expander
BTPS	body temperature pressure	BVF	bulboventricular foramen
	saturated	BVH	biventricular hypertrophy
BTR	bladder tumor recheck	BVL	bilateral vas ligation
BTS	Blalock-Taussig shunt	BVM	bag valve mask
BTSH	bovine thyrotropin	BVMG	Bender Visual-Motor Gestalt (test)
BTT	bridge to (heart) transplantation	BVO	branch vein occlusion
BTU	behavior therapy unit	BVP	blood volume processed
BTW	back to work		(hemodialysis)
	between	BVR	Bureau of Vocational
	by-the-way		Rehabilitation
BTW M	between meals	BVRO	bilateral vertical ramus osteotomy
BTX	Botulinum toxin type A (Botox)	BVRT	Benton Visual Retention Test
BtxA	botulinum toxin type A (Botox)	BVT	basilica vein transposition
BTZ	bortezomib (Velcade)		bilateral ventilation tubes
BU	base up (prism)	BVZ	bevacizumab (Avastin)
	below umbilicus	BW	bandwidth (radiology)
	Bethesda units (hematology)		birth weight
	Bodansky units		bite-wing (radiograph)
	burn unit		body water
	busulfan (Myleran)		body weight
BUA	broadband ultrasound attenuation	B & W	Black and White (milk of magnesia
BUCAT	busulfan, carboplatin, and thiotepa		& aromatic cascara fluidextract)
BuCy	busulfan and cyclophosphamide	BWA	bed-wetter admission
BUD	budesonide (Rhinocort)	BWC	bladder-wash cytology
BUdR	bromodeoxyuridine	BWCO	baby won't come out (needs
BUE	both upper extremities		Caesarian) (slang)
BUFA	baby up for adoption	BWCS	bagged white cell study
BULB	bilateral upper lid blepharoplasty	BWF	Blackwater fever
BUN	blood urea nitrogen	BWFI	bacteriostatic water for injection
	bunion	BWidF	black widowed female
BUO	bleeding of undetermined origin	BWidM	black widowed male
BUPE	buprenorphine and naloxone	BWS	battered woman syndrome
	(Suboxone) (slang)		Beckwith-Wiedemann syndrome
Bupi	bupivacaine (Marcaine,	BWs	bite-wing (x-rays)
	Sensorcaine)	BWSE	black widow spider envenomation
BUR	back-up rate (ventilator)	BWSTT	body weight-supported treadmill
Burd	Burdick suction		training

BWT	bowel wall thickness
BWX	bite-wing x-ray
Bx	behavior
	biopsy
B × B	back-to-back
BX BS	Blue Cross and Blue Shield
BXM	B-cell crossmatch
BXO	balanitis xerotica obliterans
ΦBZ	phenylbutazone
BZD	benzodiazepine
BZDZ	benzodiazepine
BZP	benzyl piperazine (known as 1-benzylpiperazine, A2, Frenzy, Nemesis, Lovely and Lovelies)

C

C	ascorbic acid (Vitamin C)
	carbohydrate
	Catholic
	Caucasian
	Celsius
	centigrade
	Chlamydia
	clubbing
	conjunctiva
	constricted
	cyanosis
	cytidine (also referred to as Cyd)
	hundred
$\bar{c}$	with
C′	cervical spine
C+	with contrast
C−	without contrast
C 1	cyclopentolate 1% ophthalmic solution (Cyclogyl)
C0-C2	occipitocervical spine junction
C_1–C_7	cervical vertebra 1 through 7
C_1–C_8	cervical nerves 1 through 8
C_1–C_9	precursor molecules of the complement system
C_1–C_{12}	cranial nerves 1 to 12
C3-C6	subaxial spine junction
C3	complement C3
C4	complement C4
CI-CV	Drug Enforcement Agency scheduled substances class one through five
C_{II}	second cranial nerve
CA	cancelled appointment
	cancer
	cancer antigen
	Candida albicans
	carcinoma
	cardiac arrest
	carotid artery
	celiac artery
	cellulose acetate (filter)
	Certified Acupuncturist
	chronologic age
	competent authority
	Cocaine Anonymous
	community-acquired
	compressed air
	continuous aerosol
	coracoacromial (ligament)
	coronary angioplasty
	coronary artery
Ca	calcium
	cancer

C/A	conscious, alert	CADD®	Computerized Ambulatory Drug Delivery (pump)
C+A	children and adolescents	CADL	communication activities of daily living (speech/ cognitive test)
Ca++	calcification		
	calcium		
CA 125	cancer antigen 125	CADP	computer-assisted design of prosthesis
C&A	Clinitest® and Acetest®		
CAA	cerebral amyloid angiopathy	CADRF	coronary artery disease risk factors
	coloanal anastamosis	CADXPL	cadaver transplant
	crystalline amino acids	CAE	cellulose acetate electrophoresis
CAAP-1	Certified Associate Addiction Professional Level 1		coronary artery endarterectomy
			cyclophosphamide, doxorubicin
CAB	catheter-associated bacteriuria		(Adriamycin), and etoposide
	cellulose acetate butyrate	CAEC	cardiac arrhythmia evaluation center
	combined androgen blockade		
	complete abortion		Cook airway exchange catheter
	complete atrioventricular block	CaEDTA	calcium disodium edetate
	Consumer Affairs Branch (FDA)	CAERS	CFSAN (Center for Food Safety and Applied Nutrition) Adverse Events Reporting System (FDA)
	coronary artery bypass		
CAB-BAGE	coronary artery bypass graft (CABG)		
		CAEV	caprine arthritis encephalitis virus
CABG	coronary artery bypass graft	CAF	chronic atrial fibrillation
CaBI	calcium bone index		controlled atrial flutter/fibrillation
CaBP	calcium-binding protein		coronary artery fistula
CABS	coronary artery bypass surgery		cyclophosphamide, doxorubicin (Adriamycin), and fluorouracil
CAC	cardioacceleratory center		
	carotid artery calcification (calcium)	CAFF	controlled atrial fibrillation/flutter
	Certified Alcohol Counselor	CAFSA	cerebellar ataxia with free sialic acid (syndrom)
	Community Action Center		
	computer-assisted coding	CAFT	Clinitron® air fluidized therapy
	computerized autocoding	CAG	chronic atrophic gastritis
	coronary artery calcification		closed angle glaucoma
CACB	chronic angle closure glaucoma		continuous ambulatory gamma globin (infusion)
CACD	central areolar choroidal dystrophy		
CA-ChEIs	centrally acting cholinesterase inhibitors		coronary arteriography
			critical angle of Gissane
CACI	computer-assisted continuous infusion	CaG	calcium gluconate
		CAGE	a questionnaire for alcoholism evaluation C Have you ever felt the need to cut down on your drinking? A Have you ever felt annoyed by criticism of your drinking? G Have you ever felt guilty about your drinking? E Have you ever taken a drink (eye opener) first thing in the morning?
CaCl₂	calcium chloride		
CaCO₃	calcium carbonate		
CACP	cisplatin		
CACS	cancer-related anorexia/cachexia		
	coronary artery calcium score		
CAD	cadaver (kidney donor)		
	calcium alginate dressing		
	cervical artery dissection		
	computer-aided detection		
	computer-aided diagnosis	CAH	chronic active hepatitis
	computer-aided dispatch		chronic aggressive hepatitis
	coronary atherosclerotic disease		congenital adrenal hyperplasia
	coronary artery disease	CAHB	chronic active hepatitis B
CaD	calcium and vitamin D (fortified milk)	CAI	carbonic anhydrase inhibitors
			carboxyamide aminoimidazoles
CADAC	Certified Alcohol and Drug Abuse Counselor		carotid artery injury
			chronic ankle instability
CADASIL	cerebral autosomal dominant arteriopathy with subcortical infarcts and leukoencephalopathy		computer-assisted instructions
		'caid	Medicaid
		CAIRO	CApecitabine, IRinotecan, and Oxaliplatin

CAIV cold-adapted influenza virus vaccine

CAL callus
calories (cal)
chronic airflow limitation
clinical attachment level (dental)
computer-assisted learning

C_{alb} albumin clearance

calc calculation

cal ct calorie count

CALD chronic active liver disease

CALGB Cancer and Leukemia Group B

CALI chromophore-assisted laser inactivation

CALLA common acute lymphoblastic leukemia antigen

CAM campylobacter vaccine
Caucasian adult male
cell adhesion molecules
child abuse management
complementary and alternative medicine
confusion assessment method
controlled ankle motion
cystic adenomatoid malformation

CAMA Chronic and Acute Medical Assistance
corrected-arm-muscle area

CAMCOG Cambridge Cognitive Examination

CAMD Coalition Againsst Major Diseases
computer-aided molecular design

CAMF cyclophosphamide, Adriamycin, methotrexate, and fluorouracil

CAMP cyclophosphamide, doxorubicin (Adriamycin), methotrexate, and procarbazine

cAMP cyclic adenosine monophosphate

CA-MRSA community-associated methicillin-resistant *Staphylococcus aureus*

CAMs cell adhesion molecules

CA-MSSA community-acquired methicillin-susceptible *Staphylococcus aureus*

CAMT congenital amegakaryocytic thrombocytopenia

CAN cardiovascular autonomic neuropathy
Certified Nurse Assistant
chronic allograft nephropathy
contrast-associated nephropathy
cord around neck

CA/N child abuse and neglect

CAN-A Certified Nursing Assistant-Advanced

CANC cancelled

c-ANCA antineutrophil cytoplasmic antibody

CANDA computer-assisted new drug application

CAN-KLB *Candida albicans, Klebsiella pneumoniae* vaccine

CANP Certified Adult Nurse Practitioner

CANS complaints of the arm, neck and/or shoulders

CAO chronic airway (airflow) obstruction
coronary artery occlusion

CaO_2 arterial oxygen concentration

$Ca(OH)_2$ calcium hydroxide

CAOS computer-assisted orthopedic surgery

CaOx calcium oxalate

CAP cancer of the prostate
capsule
cellulose acetate phthalate
Certified Addiction Professional
cervical acid phosphatase
chaotic atrial tachycardia
chemistry admission profile
chloramphenicol
College of American Pathologists (cancer checklist)
community-acquired pneumonia
compound action potentials
cyclophosphamide, doxorubicin (Adriamycin), and cisplatin

CaP cancer of the prostate

Ca/P calcium to phosphorus ratio

CA4P combretastatin A4 prodrug

CAPA Certified Ambulatory Perianesthesia Nurse
Corrective and Preventive Action (related to FDA)

CAPB central auditory processing battery

CAPD central auditory processing disorder
continuous ambulatory peritoneal dialysis

CAPLA computer-assisted product license application

CAPP Child Abuse Prevention Program

CaPPS calcium pentosan polysulfate

CAPS aspects of **c**ognition, **a**ffective state, **p**hysical condition, and **s**ocial factors (patient assessment; parameters)
caffeine, alcohol, pepper, and spicy food (dietary restrictions)
cryopyrin-associated periodic syndromes

CAPS-SX Clinical Administered PTSD (Post-traumatic Stress Disorder) Scale–One Week Symptom Version

CAPWA computerized arterial pulse waveform analysis

CAR	cancer-associated retinopathy	CAST®	color allergy screening test
	cardiac ambulation routine	CASWCM	Certified Advanced Social Work
	carotid artery repair		Case Manager
	carotid artery rupture	CAT	Cardiac Arrest Team
	coronary artery revascularization		carnitine acetyl transferase
	Coxsackie adenovirus receptor		catalase
CA-RA	common adductor-rectus abdominis		cataract
CARB	carbohydrate		category
CARBO	Carbocaine		Children's Apperception Test
	carboplatin (Paraplatin)		coital alignment technique
CARD	Cardiac Automatic Resuscitative		complementary and alternative
	Device		therapy
CARES	Cancer Rehabilitation Evaluation		computed axial tomography
	System		methcatinone
CARF	Commission on Accreditation of	CAT/	Cognitive Adaptive Test/Clinical
	Rehabilitation Facilities	CLAMS	Linguistic and Auditory
CARM	Centre for Adverse Reactions		Milestone Scale
	Monitoring (New Zealand)	CAT DQ	Cognitive Adaptive Test
	Classification Association Rule		Development Quotient
	Mining	CATH	catheter
C-arm	fluoroscopy image intensifier		catheterization
CARN	Certified Addiction Registered		Catholic
	Nurse	CATS	catecholamines
CARN-AP	Certified Addictions Registered	CATSHL	camptodactyly, tall stature, and
	Nurse - Advanced Practice		hearing loss (syndrome)
CARS	Childhood Autism Rating Scale	CATT	card agglutination test with stained
	coherent anti-Stokes Raman		trypanosomes
	scattering	CAU	caudal
CART	classification and regression tree		Caucasian
	combination antiretroviral therapy	cAu	colloidal gold
CARTI	community-acquired respiratory	CAUTI	catheter-associated urinary tract
	tract infection(s)		infection
CAS	carotid angioplasty and stenting	CAV	cardiac allograft vasculopathy
	carotid artery stenosis (stenting)		computer-aided ventilation
	cerebral arteriosclerosis		congenital absence of vagina
	Chemical Abstracts Service		cyclophosphamide, doxorubicin
	Clinical Asthma Score		(Adriamycin), and vincristine
	collision avoidance system	CAV-1	canine adenovirus type 1
	combined androgen suppression	CAVB	complete atrioventricular block
	computer-assisted surgery	CAVC	common artrioventricular canal
	coronary artery stenosis		complete atrioventricular canal
CASA	cancer-associated serum antigen	CAVE	Content Analysis of Verbatim
	Center on Addiction and Substance		Explanation
	Abuse		cyclophosphamide, doxorubicin,
	computer-assisted semen analysis		(Adriamycin) vincristine, and
	court appointed special advocate		etoposide
CaSC	carcinoma of the sigmoid colon	CAVH	continuous arteriovenous
CASH	chemotherapy-associated		hemofiltration
	steatohepatitis	CAVHD	continuous arteriovenous
CASHD	coronary arteriosclerotic heart		hemodialysis
	disease	CAVM	cerebral arteriovenous
CA-SAI	community-acquired		malformation
	Staphylococcus aureus	CAV-P-VP	cyclophosphamide, doxorubicin
	infections		(Adriamycin), vincristine,
CASL	continuous arterial spin labeled		cisplatin, and etoposide
	(magnetic resonance imaging)	CAVR	continuous arteriovenous
CASP	Child Analytic Study Program		rewarming
CASS	computer-aided sleep system	CAVS	calcific valve stenosis

CAVSD   complete atrioventricular septal defect

CAVU   continuous arteriovenous ultrafiltration

CAW   carbonaceous-activated water (Willard Water)

CAX   central axis

Ca x P   calcium times phosphorus product

CB   cerebellopontine
cesarean birth
chronic bronchitis
code blue
concha (conchae) bullosa
conjugated bilirubin (direct)
(umbilical) cord blood

c/b   complicated by

C & B   chair and bed
crown and bridge

CB1   cannabinoid receptor, type 1

CBA   chronic bronchitis and asthma
cost-benefit analysis
County Board of Assistance

CBAPF   Certified Board of Addiction Professionals

CBASP   Cognitive Behavioral Analysis System of Psychotherapy

CBAVD   congenital bilateral absence of the vas deferens

CBB   cord blood bank
criterion-based benchmark

CBBS   clear, bilateral, breath sounds

CBBs   cell-based biosensors

CBC   carbenicillin
complete blood count
contralateral breast cancer

CBCC   cisplatin-based combination chemotherapy

CBCDA   carboplatin

CBCL   Child Behavior Checklist

CBCT   community based clinical trials
cone-beam computed tomography

CBD   closed bladder drainage
common bile duct
corticobasal degeneration

CBDE   common bile duct exploration

CBDI   common bile duct injury

CBDS   common bile duct stone(s)

CBDT   cisplatin, carmustine, dacarbazine, and tamoxifen

CBE   Changes Being Effected (FDA regulatory term)
charting by exception
child birth education
clinical breast examination

CBEFM   Clear-blue Easy Fertility Monitor

CBER   Center for Biologics Evaluation and Research (FDA)

CBF   cerebral blood flow

CBFS   cerebral blood flow studies

CBFV   cerebral blood flow velocity

CBG   capillary blood glucose

CBGM   capillary blood glucose monitor

CBH   collimated beam handpiece (for laser)

CBI   Caregiver Burden Index
continuous bladder irrigation

CBLI   cumulative blood lead index

CBM   cryopreserved bone marrow

CBMC   cord blood mononuclear cell

CBN   chronic benign neutropenia
collected by nurse

CBO   cerebral blood oxygenation

CBP   chronic benign pain
copper-binding protein

CBPP   contagious bovine pleuropneumonia

CBPS   Community Based Prevention Services
congenital bilateral perisylvian syndrome
coronary bypass surgery

CBR   carotid bodies resected
chronic bedrest
clinical benefit rate
clinical benefit responders
complete bedrest

CB1R   cannabinoid-1 receptor

CBRAM   controlled partial rebreathing-anesthesia method

CBRN   chemical, biological, radiological, or nuclear (agents)

CB RRR s M/R/G   cardiac beat, regular rhythm and rate without murmurs, rubs, or gallops

CBrS   clear breath sounds

CBS   capillary blood sugar (see CBG)
Caregiver Burden Screen
Charles Bonnet syndrome
chronic brain syndrome
coarse breath sounds
corticobasal syndrome
Cruveilhier-Baumgarten syndrome

CBSE   clinical bedside swallow evaluation

CBT   cognitive behavioral therapy
cord blood transplant

CBTC   Canadian Brain Tumor Consortium

CBU   cumulative breath units

CBV   central blood volume
cyclophosphamide, carmustine (BiCNu), and etoposide (VePesid)

CBW   corrected body weight
cotton bollworm
current body weight

CBZ   carbamazepine (Tegretol)

CBZE   carbamazepine epoxide

CC	cardiac catheterization	CCB	calcium channel blocker(s)
	Care Coordinator		Community Care Board
	Catholic		corn, callus, and bunion
	cerebral concussion	CCBT	Certified Cognitive Behavioral
	cervical cancer		Therapist
	chart check (as in 24 hour CC)	CCC	Cancer Care Center
	chief complaint		central corneal clouding (Grade 0+
	choriocarcinoma		to 4+)
	chronic complainer		Certificate of Clinical Competency
	chronic constitpation		child care clinic
	circulatory collapse		cholangiocellular carcinoma
	clean catch (urine)		circulating cancer cells
	Clinical Coordinator		closed chest compressions
	clomiphene citrate (Clomid)		Comprehensive Cancer Center
	comfort care		concordance correlation coefficient
	complications and comorbidity		continuous curvilinear
	coracoclavicular		capsulorrhexis
	cord compression		Coricidin Cough and Cold (slang)
	corpus callosum	C/cc	colonies per cubic centimeter
	creatinine clearance	CC & C	colony count and culture
	critical care	CCC-A	Certificate of Clinical Competence
	critical condition		in Audiology
	cubic centimeter (cc); Note, mL is	CCCE	Clinical Center Coordinator
	the standard designation for		Educator
	expressing liquid measurements.	CCCN	Certified Continence Care Nurse
	It is preferred as a poorly written	CCC-SP	Certificate of Clinical Competence
	cc looks like the dangerous		in Speech-Language Pathology
	abbreviation for unit "u" or 00	CCD	central core disease
	with correction (with glasses)		charged-coupled device (radiology)
C_c	concentration of drug in the central		childhood celiac disease
	compartment		chin-chest distance
C/C	cholecystectomy and operative		clinical cardiovascular disease
	cholangiogram		colpocystodefecography
	complete upper and lower dentures		Continuity of Care Document
	counseling and coordination	CCDC	Certified Chemical Dependency
	(of care)		Counselor
CCII	Clinical Clerk–2nd year	CCDC-1	Certified Chemical Dependency
C & C	cold and clammy		Counselor, Level One
CCA	calcium-channel antagonist	CCDS	color-coded duplex sonography
	Certified Coding Associate	CCE	clubbing, cyanosis, and edema
	cholangiocarcinoma		colon capsule endoscopy
	circumflex coronary artery		countercurrent electrophoresis
	common carotid artery	CC-EMG	corpus cavernosum
	concentrated care area		electromyography
	continuous cool aerosol	CCF	cephalin cholesterol flocculation
	countercurrent chromatography		Cleveland Clinic Foundation
	critical care area		compound comminuted fracture
CCa	colon cancer		congestive cardiac failure
CCAM	congenital cystic adenomatoid		crystal-induced chemotactic factor
	malformation (of the lung)	CCFA	cycloserine cefoxitin fructose agar
CCAP	capsule cartilage articular	CCFE	cyclophosphamide, cisplatin,
	preservation		fluorouracil, and estramustine
CCAT	common carotid artery thrombosis	CCFs	chronic-care facilities
C-CATODSW	Certified Clinical Alcohol,	CCG	Children's Cancer Group
	Tobacco and Other Drugs Social	CCgR	complete cytogenetic response
	Worker	CCH	chronic community care home
CCAVC	complete common atrioventricular		Cook County Hospital
	canal		cluster headache

CCHB	congenital complete heart block	CCR	California Cancer Registry
CCHD	complex congenital heart disease		cardiac catheterization recovery
	cyanotic congenital heart disease		cardiocerebral resuscitation
CCHF	Congo-Crimean		complete cytogenetic remission
	hemorrhagic fever		conventional care regimens
CCHO	consistent carbohydrate		Continuity of Care Record
CCHS	congenital central hypoventilation		continuous complete remission
	syndrome		counterclockwise rotation
CCI	chronic coronary insufficiency	C_{cr}	creatinine clearance
	Correct Coding Initiative	cCR	complete clinical remission
	corrected count increment	CCRC	Certified Clinical Research
CCJAP	Certified Criminal Justice		Coordinator
	Addiction Professional		continuing care residential
CCJAS	Certified Criminal Justice		community
	Addiction Specialist	CC-RCC	clear-cell renal-cell carcinoma
CCK	cholecystokinin	CCRN	Certified Critical Care Registered
CCK-OP	cholecystokinin octapeptide		Nurse
CCK-PZ	cholecystokinin pancreozymin	CCRT	combined chemoradiotherapy
CCL	cardiac catheterization laboratory		concurrent chemoradiotherapy
	critical condition list	CCRU	critical care recovery unit
CCl_4	carbon tetrachloride	CCS	California Children's Services
CCLE	chronic cutaneous lupus		cell cycle-specific
	erythematosus		certified coding specialist
CCM	calcium citrate malate		color contrast sensitivity
	cerebral cavernous malformation	CC & S	cornea, conjunctiva, and sclera
	Certified Case Manager	CCSA	Canadian Cardiovascular Society
	cervical compression myelopathy		Angina (score)
	children's case management	CCSE	Cognitive Capacity Screening
	corneal confocal microscopy		Examination
	country coordinating mechanism	CCSK	clear cell sarcoma of the kidney
	Critical Care Medicine	CCSP	Certified Chiropractic Sports
	cyclophosphamide, lomustine		Physician
	(CCNU; CeeNU), and		Clara cell secretory protein
	methotrexate	CCS-P	Certified Coding Specialist,
CCMHC	Certified Clinical Mental Health		Physician-Based
	Counselor	CCSS	Childhood Cancer Survivor Study
CCMS	capture compound mass	CCSV	cell-cultured smallpox vaccine
	spectrometry	CCSVI	chronic cerebrospinal venous
CCMSU	clean catch midstream urine		insufficiency
CCMU	critical care medicine unit	CCT	calcitriol
CCN	continuing care nursery		carotid compression tomography
	cyr61, ctfg, nov (family of		central corneal thickness
	proteins)		Certified Cardiographic Technician
CCNS	cell cycle-nonspecific		closed cerebral trauma
	Certified Clinical Nurse Specialist		closed cranial trauma
CCNU	lomustine (CeeNu)		collision cell technology
CCO	continuous cardiac output		congenitally corrected transposition
	Corporate Compliance Officer		(of the great vessels)
CCOHTA	Canadian Coordinating Office for		Critical Care Technician
	Health Technology Assessment		crude coal tar
C-collar	cervical collar	CCTA	coronary computed tomographic
CCoV	canine coronavirus		angiography
CCP	crystalloid cardioplegia	CCTGA	congenitally corrected transposition
	cyclic citrullinated peptide		of the great arteries
CCPD	continuous cycling (cyclical)	CCT in PET	crude coal tar in petroleum
	peritoneal dialysis	CCTV	closed circuit television
CCPs	Corporate Compliance Programs	CCU	coronary care unit
CCQ	California Child Q-set		critical care unit

CCUA	clean catch urinalysis	
CCUP	colpocystourethropexy	
CCV	Critical Care Ventilator (Ohio)	
	critical closing volume	

CCUA   clean catch urinalysis
CCUP   colpocystourethropexy
CCV   Critical Care Ventilator (Ohio)
   critical closing volume
CCW   childcare worker
   counterclockwise
CCWR   counterclockwise rotation
CCX   complications
CCY   cholecystectomy
CD   cadaver donor
   candela
   Castleman disease
   celiac disease
   cervical dystonia
   cesarean delivery
   character disorder
   chemical dependency
   childhood disease
   chlorproguanil-dapsone (Lapdap)
   chronic dialysis
   circular dichroism
   closed drainage
   Clostridium difficile
   clusters of differentiation
   common duct
   communication disorders
   compact disc
   complementarity-determining
   complicated delivery
   conduct disorder
   conjugate diameter
   contact dermatitis
   continuous drainage
   conventional denture
   convulsive disorder
   cortical dysplasia
   Crohn disease
   cumulative doses
   cycle day, referring to cycle day
      number of the menstrual cycle;
      e.g.: CD#1, first day of
      menstrual cycle
   cyclodextran
   cytarabine and daunorubicin
Cd   cadmium
   concentration of drug
C/D   cigarettes per day
   cup-to-disc ratio
CD4   antigenic marker on helper/inducer
      T cells (also called OKT 4, T4,
      and Leu3)
CD8   antigenic marker on suppressor/
      cytotoxic T cells (also called
      OKT 8, T8, and Leu 8)
C&D   curettage and desiccation
   cystectomy and diversion
   cytoscopy and dilatation
CDA   Certified Dental Assistant

C

   chenodeoxycholic acid (chenodiol)
   Clinical Document Architecture
   congenital dyserythropoietic
      anemia
2-CDA   cladribine (Leustatin;
      chlorodeoxyadenosine)
CDA4CDT   Clinical Documentation
      Architecture for Common
      Document Types (project)
CDAD   *Clostridium difficile*-associated
      diarrhea
CDAI   Crohn Disease Activity Index
CDAK   Cordis Dow Artificial Kidney
CDAP   continuous distended airway
      pressure
CDASH   Clinical Data Acquisition Standards
      Harmonization
CDB   cough and deep breath
CDC   calculated day of confinement
   cancer detection center
   carboplatin, doxorubicin, and
      cyclophosphamide
   Centers for Disease Control and
      Prevention
   Certified Drug Counselor
   chenodeoxycholic acid (chenodiol)
   Clostridium difficile colitis
CDCA   chenodeoxycholic acid (chenodiol)
CDCC   complement-dependent cellular
      cytotoxicity
CDCP   Centers for Disease Control and
      Prevention (CDC is official
      abbreviation)
CDCR   conjunctivodacryocystorhinostomy
CdCS   Cri du Chat syndrome
CDD   Certificate of Disability for
      Discharge
   Clostridium difficile disease
   cytidine deaminase
CDDN   Certified Developmental
      Disabilities Nurse
CDDP   cisplatin (Platinol)
CDE   canine distemper encephalitis
   Certified Diabetes Educator
   common data element
   common duct exploration
CDER   Center for Drug Evaluation and
      Research (FDA)
CDFI   color Doppler flow imaging
CDG   carbohydrate-deficient glycoprotein
   congenital disorders of
      glycosylation
CDGE   constant denaturant gel
      electrophoresis
CDGP   constitutional delay of growth and
      puberty
CDGS   carbohydrate-deficient glycoprotein
      syndrome

CDH	chronic daily headache	CDRs	complementary determining regions
	congenital diaphragmatic hernia		
	congenital dislocation of hip	CDRS	Children's Depression Rating Scale
	congenital dysplasia of the hip	CDR(V)	cup-to-disc ratio vertical
CDHP	5-chloro-2 4-dihydroxypyridine	CDS	Chemical Dependency Specialist
CDI	Children's Depression Inventory		Chronic Disease Score
	clean, dry, and intact		closed-door seclusion
	Clostridium difficile infection		cognitive dysfunction syndrome (veterinary)
	color Doppler imaging		
	conformation-dependent immunoassay		color Doppler sonography
			continuous dopamine stimulation
	Cotrel Duobosset Instrumentation	CDSC	Communicable Disease Surveillance Centre (United Kingdom)
CDIC	*Clostridium difficile*-induced colitis		
C Dif	*Clostridium difficile*	CDSPIES	congestive heart failure, drugs, spasm, pneumothorax, infection, embolism, and secretions (differential diagnosis mnemonic)
C Diff	*Clostridium difficile*		
CDISC	Clinical Data Interchange Standards Consortium		
CDJ	choledochojejunostomy		
CDK	climatic droplet keratopathy	CDSR	Cochrane Database of Systematic Reviews
	cyclin-dependent kinase		
CDKI	cyclin-dependent kinase inhibitor	CDSS	Cervical Dystonia Severity Scale
CDK2	cyclin-depenent kinases 2	CDSSs	clinical decision support systems
CDLC	continuous double-loop closure	CDT	carbohydrate-deficient transferrin
CDLE	chronic discoid lupus erythematosus		catheter-directed thrombolysis
			Chemical Dependency Technician
CdLS	Cornelia de Lange syndrome		clinical development team
CDM	charge description master		Clock-Drawing Test
	clinical data management		*Clostridium difficile* toxin
	clinical development monitor		complete decongestive therapy (for lymphedema)
CDMS	Certified Disability Management Specialist		
			connecting discourse tracking (measure of speech perception)
	clinically-definite multiple sclerosis		
CDO	cartilage disorder		cystic dysplasia of the testis
CDONA/ LTC	Certified Director of Nursing Administration in Long-Term Care		current dental terminology
			cytolethal distending toxin
		CDTA	cyclohexane-1,2-diaminetetraacetic acid
CDP	cancer detection program		
	chemical dependence profile	CDTM	collaborative drug therapy management
	Chemical Dependency Professional		
	Child Development Program	CDTS	Composite Drug Toxicity Score
	clinical development plan	CDU	chemical dependency unit
	complete decongestive physiotherapy		color-coded duplex ultrasonography
	crystalline degradation product	CDV	canine distemper virus
	cytidine diphosphate		cardiovascular
CDQ	corrected development quotient		cyclophosphamide, doxorubicin, and vincristine
CDR	cancer detection rate		
	Cause of Death Registry	CDX	chlordiazepoxide (Librim)
	clinical data repository	cDXA	central dual-energy X-ray absorptiometry
	Clinical Dementia Rating		
	cognitive dietary restraint	cdyn	dynamic compliance
	commonly deleted region	CE	California encephalitis
	continuing disability review		capillary electrophoresis
	recordable compact disc		capsule endoscopy
CDRH	Center for Devices and Radiological Health		carboplatin and etoposide
			cardiac enlargement
CDR(H)	cup-to-disc ratio horizontal		cardiac enzymes

	cardioesophageal	CEFOX	cefoxitin (Mefoxtin)
	Carpentier-Edwards (heart-valve	CEFTAZ	ceftazidime
	prosthesis)	CEFUR	cefuroxime
	cataract extraction	CEI	continuous extravascular infusion
	central episiotomy		converting enzyme inhibitor
	chemoembolization	CEJ	cementoenamel junction (dental)
	chest expansion		cervical-enamel junction (dental)
	cholesterol ester	CEL	cardiac exercise laboratory
	community education	CELIP	Claims Expansion Line-item
	Conformité Européne (an		Processing
	indication of compliance to all	CELP	chronic erosive lichen planus
	EU directives)	CELs	contrast-enhancing lesions
	conjugated estrogens	CEM	Clinical Event Manager
	consultative examination		confocal endo microscopy
	continuing education	CEMD	consultative examination by
	contrast echocardiology		physician
	cystic echinococcosis	CE-MRA	contrast-enhanced magnetic
C&E	consultation and examination		resonance angiography
	cough and exercise	ceMRI	contrast-enhanced magnetic
	curettage and electrodesiccation		resonance imaging
CEA	carcinoembryonic antigen	CEN	Certified Emergency Nurse
	carotid endarterectomy		European Committee for
	continuous epidural anesthesia		Standardization
	cost-effectiveness analysis	CENOG	computerized electroneuro-
CEB	calcium entry blocker		ophthalmogram
	carboplatin, etoposide, and	CEO	chief executive officer
	bleomycin	CEOT	calcifying epithelial odontogenic
CEBV	chronic Epstein-Barr virus		tumor
CEC	capillary electrochromatography	CEP	cardiac enzyme panel
	Cardiac Evaluation Center		Certified Emergency Paramedic
	Council for Exceptional Children		chronic eosinophilic pneumonia
CECA	Childhood Experience of Care and		cognitive evoked potential
	Abuse (interview)		congenital erythropoietic porphyria
CECD	congenital endothelial corneal		countercurrent electrophoresis
	dystrophy		cyclophosphamide, etoposide, and
CEc̄/IOL	cataract extraction with intraocular		cisplatin (Platinol AQ)
	lens	CEPE	cataract extraction by
CECS	chronic exertional compartment		phacoemulsification
	syndrome	CEPH	cephalic
	Courtauld Emotional Control Scale		cephalosporin
CECT	contrast-enhanced computed	CEPH	cephalin flocculation
	tomography	FLOC	
CED	Camurati-Engelmann disease	CEPP (B)	cyclophosphamide, etopside,
	cavity evaluation device		procarbazine, prednisone, and
	clinically effective dose		bleomycin
	convection-enhanced delivery	CER	comparative effectiveness research
	cystoscopy-endoscopy dilation		conditioned emotional response
CEDS	Certified Eating Disorders	CE&R	central episiotomy and repair
	Specialist	CERA	continuous erythropoiesis receptor
CEE	Central European encephalitis		activator (methoxy polyethylene
	conjugated equine estrogen		glycol-epoetin beta [MICERA])
	(Premarin; conjugated estrogen)		cortical evoked response
CEF	chick embryo fibroblast		audiometry
	cyclophosphamide, epirubicin, and	CERAD	Consortium to Establish a Registry
	fluorouracil		for Alzheimer Disease
CEFM	continuous external fetal	CERC	Crisis Emergency and Risk
	monitoring		Communication (training)
CEFOT	cefotaxime (Claforan)	CERD	chronic end-stage renal disease

CERT	Centers for Education and Research on Therapeutics	CFCs	chlorofluorocarbons
	Comprehensive Error Rate Testing	CFD	color-flow Doppler
	Community Emergency Response Teams		computational fluid dynamics
	Computer Emergency Response Team	CFDS	color flow Doppler sonography
CERULO	ceruloplasmin	CFEOM	congenital fibrosis of the extraocular muscles
CERV	cervical	CFF	critical fusion (flicker) frequency
CES	cauda equina syndrome	CFFT	critical flicker fusion threshold
	central excitatory state	CFG	comfort function goal (guideline for pain tolerance)
	cognitive environmental stimulation		convergent functional genomics
	estrogen, conjugated (conjugated estrogen substance)	CFH	chemical fume hood
CESB	chronic electrical stimulation of the brain		complement factor H
CES-D	Center for Epidemiologic Studies – Depression	CFI	Center for the Intrepid
			chemotherapy-free intervals
			confrontation fields intact
CESI	cervical epidural steroid injection	CFIDS	chronic fatigue immune dysfunction syndrome
CET	common extensor tendon	CFL	cadaveric fascia lata
CETC	circulating epithelial tumor cells		calcaneofibular ligament
CETN	Certified Enterostomal Therapy Nurse		cisplatin, fluorouracil, and leucovorin calcium
CETP	cholesteryl ester transfer protein	CFLX	ciprofloxacin (Cipro)
CEU	Utah residents with ancestry from northern and western European ancestry (populations included in HapMap - see HapMap)		circumflex
		CFM	cerebral function monitor
			close fitting mask
			craniofacial microsomia
			cyclophosphamide, fluorouracil, and mitoxantrone
CEUS	contrast-enhanced ultrasonography	CFNS	chills, fever, and night sweats
CEV	cyclophosphamide, etoposide, and vincristine		craniofrontonasal syndrome
CE w/IOL	cataract extraction with intraocular lens	CFOI	Census of Fatal Occupational Injuries (US Bureau of Labor Statistics report)
CF	calcium leucovorin (citrovorum factor)	CFP	cystic fibrosis protein
	cancer-free	CFPT	cyclophosphamide, fluorouracil, prednisone, and tamoxifen
	cardiac failure	CFR	case-fatality rates
	Caucasian female		*Code of Federal Regulations*
	Christmas factor		coronary flow reserve
	cisplatin and fluorouracil	CFRB	critical findings read back
	complement fixation	CFRD	cystic fibrosis-related diabetes
	contractile force	CFRDM	cystic fibrosis-related diabetes mellitus
	correction factor		
	count fingers	CFRN	Certified Flight Registered Nurse
	cystic fibrosis	CFRP	carbon-fiber reinforced polymer
C3F8	perfluoropropane	CFS	cancer family syndrome
C&F	cell and flare		Child and Family Service
	chills and fever		childhood febrile seizures
	condoms and foam		chronic fatigue syndrome
CFA	common femoral artery		congenital fibrosarcoma
	complete Freund adjuvant		craniofacial surgery
	cryptogenic fibrosing alveolitis	CFSAN	Center for Food Safety and Applied Nutrition (FDA)
	cystic fibrosis anthropathy	CFT	capillary filling time
CFAC	complement-fixing antibody consumption		chronic follicular tonsillitis
C-factor	cleverness factor		chronic food toxicity (obesity) (slang)
CFCF	carbon fiber composite frame cage		

	complement fixation test	C-GRD	coffee-ground
CFTR	cystic fibrosis transmembrane (conductance) regulator	CGRN	Certified Gastroenterology Registered Nurse
	cystic fibrosis transmembrane receptor	CGRP	calcitonin gene-related peptide
CFU	colony-forming units	CGS	cardiogenic shock
	criteria for use		catgut suture
CFU-E	colony-forming unit–erythroid		centimeter-gram-second system
CFU-G	colony-forming unit–granulocyte	CGTT	cortisol glucose tolerance test
CFU-G/M	colony-forming unit– granulocyte/macrophage	cGVHD	chronic graft-versus-host disease
CFU-M	colony-forming unit–macrophage	cGy	centigray
CFU-Mk	colony-forming unit– megakaryocyte	CH	Caribbean Hispanic
			chest
CFU-S	colony-forming unit–spleen		chief
CFV	common femoral vein		child (children)
CFVR	coronary flow velocity reserve		chronic
CFX	circumflex artery		cluster headache
CG	cardiogreen (dye)		concentric hypertrophy
	caregiver		congenital hypothyroidism
	cholecystogram		convalescent hospital
	Cockcroft-Gault (formula for estimating creatinine clearance)		crown-heal
		C_h	hepatic clearance
	contact guard (physical therapy)	ch^1	Christ Church chromosone
	contact guarding	CH_{50}	total hemolytic complement
	contralateral groin	C&H	cocaine and heroin
CGA	clonal group A	CHA	compound hypermetropic astigmatism
	comprehensive geriatric assessment		congenital hypoplastic anemia
	contact guard assist	CHAD	cyclophosphamide, altretamine, (hexamethylmelamine), doxorubicin (Adriamycin), and cisplatin (DDP)
	corrected gestation age		
CGB	chronic gastrointestinal (tract) bleeding		
CGCG	central giant-cell granuloma	CHADS	an index that quantifies baseline risk of stroke for individuals with atrial fibrillation (congestive heart failure, hypertension, age greater than 75, diabetic, and history of stroke)
CGCR	Clinical Global Consensus Rating		
CGD	chronic glycogen deficit		
	chronic granulomatous disease		
	cobalt gray equivalent		
CGF	continuous gavage feeding (infant feeding)	CHAI	Commission for Healthcare Audit and Inspection (United Kingdom)
cGFR	calculated glomerular filtration rate		
CGI	Clinical Global Impressions (scale)		continuous hepatic artery infusion
CGIC	Clinical Global Impression of Change	CHAID	Chi Square Automatic Interaction Detection
CGI-S	Clinical Global Impressions, Severity of Illness	CHAM-OCA	cyclophosphamide, hydroxyurea, dactinomycin, methotrexate, vincristine, leucovorin, and doxorubicin
CGL	chronic granulocytic leukemia		
	with correction/with glasses		
CGM	continuous glucose monitoring		
	cortical gray matter	CHAM-PUS	Civilian Health and Medical Program of the Uniformed Services
CGMP	Current Good Manufacturing Practices		
cGMP	cyclic guanosine monophosphate	CHAMPVA	Civilian Health and Medical Program-Veterans Administration
CGMS	continuous glucose monitoring systems		
CGN	Certified Gastroenterology Nurse	Chandelier sign	used to describe a patient who experiences extreme pain during a physical examination (slang)
	chronic glomerulonephritis		
cGN	crescentic glomerulonephritis		
CGP	certification in Geriatric Pharmacy	CHAP	child health associate practitioner

	cyclophosphamide, altretamine, (hexamethylmelamine), doxorubicin (Adriamycin), and cisplatin (Platinol)	CHEMO	chemotherapy
		ChemoRx	chemotherapy
		chemo/XRT	chemotherapy with radiation therapy
CHAQ	childhood health assessment questionnaire	CHEOPS	Children's Hospital of Eastern Ontario Pain Scale
CHARGE	coloboma (of eyes), hearing deficit, choanal atresia, retardation of growth, genital defects (males only), and endocardial cushion defect	CHEP	Canadian Hypertension Education Program
			cricohyoidoepiglottopexy
		CHESS	chemical shift suppression
CHART	complaint, history, assessment, Rx (treatment), transport	CHF	chronic heart failure
			congestive heart failure
			Crimean hemorrhagic fever
	continuous hyperfractionated accelerated radiotherapy	CHFV	combined high-frequency of ventilation
	Craig Handicap Assessment and Reporting Technique	CHG	change
			chlorhexidine gluconate
CHB	chronic hepatitis B	CHI	chikungunya virus vaccine
	complete heart block		closed head injury
	congenital heart block		Consolidated Health Informatics
	Han Chinese from Beijing (populations included in HapMap - see HapMap)		contrast harmonic imaging
			creatinine-height index
			crushing head injury (injuries)
CHBHA	congenital Heinz body hemolytic anemia	CHIBLOC	closed head injury, brief loss of consciousness
CHC	community health center	CHID	Combined Health Information Database
	concentric hypertrophic cardiomyopathy		
		CHIK	Chikungunya (virus)
CH_3- CCNU	semustine	CHIKV	Chikungunya virus
		CHILD	congenital hemidysplasia with ichthyosiform nevus and limb defects (syndrome)
CHCT	caffeine-halothane contracture test		
cHct	central hematocrit		
CHD	canine hip dysplasia	CHIN	community health information network
	center hemodialysis		
	changed diaper	CHIP	Children's Health Insurance Program
	childhood diseases		
	chronic hemodialysis		comprehensive health insurance plan
	common hepatic duct		
	congenital heart defect		iproplatin
	congenital heart disease	ChIP	chromatin immunoprecipitation
	coordinate home care	CHIR	Chiron Corporation
	coronary heart disease	Chix	chickenpox
CHE	chronic hepatic encephalopathy	CHL	conductive hearing loss
	comprehensive health examination	CHLC	Cooperative Human Linkage Center
CHEDDAR	Chief Compliant; History: social and physical as well as contributing factors; Examination; Details of problems and complaints; Drugs and dosage—list current meds; Assessment, diagnostic process, total impression; Return visit information or referral (format of documentation)		
		ChloMP	chlorambucil, mitoxantrone, and prednisolone
		ChlVPP	chlorambucil, vinblastine, procarbazine, and prednisone
		CHM	complete hydatidiform mole
		CHMP	Committee for Medicinal Products for Human Use (EMEA)
		CHN	central hemorrhagic necrosis
CHEF	clamped homogeneous electric field		Certified Hemodialysis Nurse
			Chinese herb nephropathy
ChEI	cholinesterase inhibitor		Community Health Nurse
			community nursing home
CHEM 7	see page 356	CHO	carbohydrate

	Chemical Hygiene Officer	CHUC	Certified Health Unit Coordinator
	Chinese hamster ovary	CHVP	cyclophosphamide, doxorubicin
–CHO	aldehyde		(hydroxydaunorubicin),
C_{H_2O}	free-water clearance		teniposide (VM26), and
CHO_a	cholera vaccine, attenuated live		prednisone
	(oral)	CHW	community health workers
CHOC	chocolate	CHWG	chewing gum
CHO_{cn}-	cholera vaccine,	CHX	chlorhexidine (Peridex; Periogard)
LPS	lipopolysaccharide-toxin	CI	cardiac index
	conjugate		cerebral infarction
$C_2 H_5 OH$	alcohol (ethyl alcohol)		cesium implant
CHO_{i-w}	cholera vaccine, inactivated whole		Clinical Instructor
	cell		cochlear implant
CHO_{i-w-BS}	cholera vaccine, inactivated whole		cognitively impaired
	cell, B subunit		colon inertia
chol	cholesterol		commercial insurance
c̄ hold	withhold		complete iridectomy
Chole	cholecystectomy		confidence interval
CHO_o	cholera, oral vaccine		continuous infusion
CHOP	cyclophosphamide, doxorubicin		contraindications
	(hydroxy-daunorubicin),		convergence insufficiency
	vincristine (Oncovin),		core imprint (cytology)
	prednisone		coronary insufficiency
CHOP-	cyclophosphamide,	μCi	microcurie
Bleo	doxorubicin	Ci	curie(s)
	(hydroxydaunorubicin),	CI30	cumulative incidence at 30 years
	vincristine (Oncovin),	CIA	calcaneal insufficiency avulsion
	prednisone, and bleomycin		chemotherapy-induced amenorrhea
CHO_{tox}	cholera toxin/toxoid vaccine		chemotherapy-induced anemia
CHP	Certification in Healthcare Privacy		chronic idiopathic anhidrosis
CHPB	Canadian Health Protection Branch		collagen-induced arthritis
	(the equivalent of the U.S. Food		common line artery
	and Drug Administration)	CIAA	competitive insulin autoantibodies
CHPN	Certified Hospice and Palliative	CIACS	cocaine-induced acute coronary
	Nurse		syndrome
CHPV	Codman Hakim programmable	CIAED	collagen-induced autoimmune ear
	valve		disease
CHPX	chickenpox	cIAI	complicated intraabdominal
CHR	Cercaria-Hullen reaction		infections
	chronic	CIB	Carnation Instant Breakfast®
	complete hematological response		crying-induced bronchospasm
ChronoHAI	circadian-based hepatic artery		cytomegalic inclusion bodies
	infusion	CIBD	chronic inflammatory bowel
CHRN	Certified Hyperbaric Registered		disease
	Nurse	CIBI	Clinician Interview-Based
CHRPE	congenital hypertrophy of the		Impression (of change)
	retinal pigment epithelium	CIBIC	Clinician Interview-Based
CHRS	congenital hereditary retinoschisis		Impression of Change
CHS	Chediak-Higashi syndrome	CIBIC-	Clinician Interview-
	contact hypersensitivity	plus	Based Impression of Change
CHT	Certified Hand Therapist		with Caregiver Input
	Certified Hyperbaric Technician	CIBP	chronic intractable benign pain
	Certified Hypnotherapist	C-IBS	constipated predominant irritable
	chemotherapy		bowel syndrome
	closed head trauma	CIC	cardioinhibitory center
ChT	chemotherapy		Certified in Infection Control
CHTN	chronic hypertension		circulating immune complexes
CHU	closed head unit		clean intermittent catheterization

C

completely in-the-canal (hearing aid)

coronary intensive care

CICE   combined intracapsular cataract extraction

CICI   chemotherapy-induced cognitive impairment

CICU   cardiac intensive care unit

CICVC   centrally inserted central venous catheter

CID   Center for Infectious Diseases (CDC)

Central Institute for the Deaf

cervical immobilization device

chemotherapy-induced diarrhea

clinically important difference

collision-induced dissociation

combined immunodeficiency

cytomegalic inclusion disease

CIDP   chronic inflammatory demyelinating polyradiculoneuropathy (polyneuropathy)

CIDS   cellular immunodeficiency syndrome

continuous insulin delivery system

CIDs   clinically important differences

CIE   capillary immunoelectrophoresis

chemotherapy-induced emesis

congenital ichthyosiform erythroderma

counterimmunoelectrophoresis

crossed immunoelectrophoresis

CIEA   continuous infusion epidural analgesia

CIEF   capillary isoelectric focusing

CIEP   counterimmunoelectrophoresis

crossed immunoelectrophoresis

CIFN   chemotherapy-induced fever and neutropenia

CI 5-FU   continuous infusion of fluorouracil

CIG   cigarettes

CIH   Certified in Industrial Health

continuous infusion haloperidol

CIHD   chronic ischemic heart disease

CIHI   Canadian Institute for Health Information

CIHR   Canadian Institutes of Health Research

CII   continuous insulin infusion

CIIA   common internal iliac artery

CIL   carbamazepine-induced lupus

CIM   change in menses

chemotherapy-induced mucositis

constraint-inducedmovement

convective interaction media

corticosteroid-induced myopathy

critical illness myopathy

CIMCU   cardiac intermediate care unit

CIMT   carotid (artery) intimamedia thickness

constraint-induced movement therapy

CIN   cervical intraepithelial neoplasia

chemotherapy-induced neutropenia

chromosomal (chromosome) instability

chronic interstitial nephritis

contrast-induced nephropathy

C_{IN} insulin clearance

CIN3+   cervical intraepithelial neoplasia grade 3 or worse

CINAHL   Cumulative Index to Nursing and Allied Health

CINCA   chronic infantile neurologic cutaneous arthropathy

CIND   cognitive impairment, no dementia

CINE   chemotherapy-induced nausea and emesis

cineangiogram

CINV   chemotherapy-induced nausea and vomiting

CIO   corticosteroid-induced osteoporosis

CIOMS   The Council for International Organization of Medical Sciences

CIP   Cardiac Injury Panel

Certified IRB (Institutional Review Board) Professional

critical illness polyneuropathy

CIPD   chronic intermittent peritoneal dialysis

CIPN   chemotherapy-induced peripheral neuropathy

CipRGC   ciprofloxacin-resistant *Neisseria gonorrhoeae*

CIR   continent intestinal reservoir

CIRB   central institutional review board

Circ   circulation

circumcision

circumference

circumflex

circ. & sen.   circulation and sensation

CIRF   cocaine-induced respiratory failure

CIRM   California Institute of Regenerative Medicine

CIRS-G   Cumulative Illness Rating Scale-Geriatric

CIRT   carbon ion radiotherapy

CIS   Cancer Information Service (National Cancer Institute)

carcinoma in situ

clinically isolated syndrome

Commonwealth of Independent States

	continuous interleaved sampling
CI&S	conjunctival irritation and swelling
CISC	clean intermittent self-catheterization
CISCA	cisplatin, cyclophosphamide, and doxorubicin (Adriamycin)
CISCOM	The Centralized Information Service for Complementary Medicine
CISD	critical incident stress debriefing (used by EMTs)
Cis-DDP	cisplatin (Platinol)
CISH	chromogen in situ hybridization
CISM	critical incident stress management (debriefing used by EMTs)
CIS-R	Clinical Interview Schedule, Revised
CISS	constructive interface in steady state (imaging)
CI-Stim	cochlear implant stimulation
CIT	chemotherapy-induced toxicities
	cold ischemia time
	constraint-induced therapy (protocol)
	conventional immunosuppressive therapy
	conventional insulin therapy
CIT IDS	citation identifiers (National Library of Medicine)
CITP	capillary isotachophoresis
CITR	Collaborative Islet Transplant Registry
CIU	chronic idiopathic urticaria
	crisis intervention unit
CIV	common iliac vein
	continuous intravenous (infusion)
CIVD	cold-induced vasodilatation
CIVI	continuous intravenous infusion
CIXU	constant infusion excretory urogram
CIWA-Ar	Clinical Institute Withdrawal Assessment for Alcohol–revised
CJD	Creutzfeldt-Jakob disease
cJET	congenital junctional ectopic tachycardia
CJR	centric jaw relation
CJS	chronic joint symptoms
	Criminal Justice System
CK	check
	conductive keratoplasty
	creatine kinase
CK-BB	creatine kinase BB band (primarily in brain)
CKC	cold-knife conization
CKD	chronic kidney disease
CKD-MBD	chronic kidney disease with mineral and bone disorders
C/kg	coulomb per kilogram (radiology)
CK-ISO	creatine kinase isoenzyme
CK-MB	creatine kinase MB fraction (primarily in cardiac muscle)
CK MM	creatine kinase MM fraction (primarily in skeletal muscle)
CKW	clockwise
Cl	chloride (Cl^-)
CL	central line
	chemoluminescence
	clear liquid
	cleft lip
	cloudy
	confidence limits
	contact lens
	critical list
	cutaneous leishmaniasis
	cycle length
	lung compliance
C_L	compliance of the lungs
C-L	consultation-liaison
CLA	community living arrangements
	congenital lactic acidosis
	congenital laryngeal atresia
	conjugated linoleic acid
CLABSI	central line-associated bloodstream infection
C lam	cervical laminectomy
CLAMS DQ	Clinical Linguistic and Auditory Milestone Scale Development Quotient
CLAMSS	cleavage- and ligation-associated mutation-specific sequencing
CLAP	contact laser ablation of prostate
CLARE	contact lens-associated acute red eye
CLAS	Cancer Linear Analogue Scale
	congenital localized absence of skin
CLASS	computer laser-assisted surgical system
CLASS I	congestive heart failure with no limitation with ordinary activity (New York Heart Association Classification)
CLASS II	congestive heart failure with slight limitation of physical activity
CLASS III	congestive heart failure with marked limitation of physical activity
CLASS IV	congestive heart failure with inability to engage in any physical activity without symptoms
Clav	clavicle
CLB	chlorambucil (Leukeran)
	coccidian-like body
CLB_{atx}	*Clostridium botulinum* antitoxin
CLBBB	complete left bundle branch block

CLBD	cortical Lewy body disease
CLBP	chronic low back pain
CLB$_{tox}$	*Clostridium botulinum* toxoid vaccine
CLC	Community Living Center
	cork leather and celastic (orthotic)
CL/CP	cleft lip and cleft palate
CLD	central lung distance
	chronic liver disease
	chronic lung disease
	Clostridium difficile vaccine
Cl$_d$	dialysis clearance
CLDP	chronic lung disease of prematurity
CLE	centrilobular emphysema
	congenital lobar emphysema
	constant-load exercise
	continuous lumbar epidural (anesthetic)
	cutaneous lupus erythematosus
CLED	cysteine lactose electrolyte-deficient (agar)
CLEIA	chemiluminescent enzyme immunoassay
CLEP	college level examination program
CLF	cholesterol-lecithin flocculation
CLG	clorgyline
CLH	chronic lobular hepatitis
C$_h$	hepatic clearance
CLI	central lymphatic irradiation
	clomipramine (Anafranil)
	critical leg (limb) ischemia
CLIA	chemiluminescent immunoassay
	Clinical Laboratory Improvement Act
CLINDA	clindamycin (Cleocin)
ClinROs	clinician-reported outcomes
Cl$_{int}$	intrinsic clearance
CLL	chronic lymphocytic leukemia
CLLE	columnar-lined lower esophagus
cl liq	clear liquid
CLM	colorectal liver metastases
	cutaneous larva migrans
CLN	centrolobular necrosis
CLNC	Certified Legal Nurse Consultant
Cl$_{nr}$	nonrenal clearance
CLO	Campylobacter-like organism
	close
	cod liver oil
CLOX	clock-drawing task (cognitive impairment test)
CL & P	cleft lip and palate
CL PSY	closed psychiatry
CLPU	contact lens-induced peripheral ulceration
Cl$_r$	renal clearance
CLRB	clinical laboratory (results) read back
Cl Red	closed reduction

CLRO	community leave for reorientation
CLS	capillary leak syndrome
	community living skills
CLSE	calf-lung surfactant extract (Infasurf)
CLSI	Clinical and Laboratory Standards Institute
CLSM	confocal laser scanning microscopy
CLT	chronic lymphocytic thyroiditis
	complex lymphedema therapy
	cool lace tent
Cl$_T$	total body clearance
CLV	cuff-leak volume
	cutaneous leukocytoclastic vasculitis
CL VOID	clean voided specimen
CLW$_c$	*Clostridium welchii* type C (Pigbel) toxoid vaccine
clysis	hypodermoclysis
CLZ	clozapine (Clozaril)
cm	centimeter (2.54 cm = 1 inch)
CM	capreomycin (Capastat)
	CarboMedics (heart valve prosthesis)
	cardiac monitor
	cardiomegaly
	cardiomyopathy
	care manager
	care management
	case management
	case manager
	Caucasian male
	centimeter (cm) (2.54 cm = 1 inch)
	cerebral malaria
	Chiari malformation
	chondromalacia
	chronic migraine (headache)
	cochlear microphonics
	common migraine
	continuous microwave
	continuous murmur
	contrast media
	costal margin
	cow's milk
	culture media
	cutaneous melanoma
	cystic mesothelioma
	tomorrow morning (this is a dangerous abbreviation)
cm	centimeter (2.54 cm = 1 inch)
cM	centimorgan (one one-hundredth of a morgan; the unit of distance on a linkage map)
CM-I	Chiari malformation Type I
cm1	circumflex marginal 1
cm2	circumflex marginal 2
cm^2	square centimeters
cm^3	cubic centimeter

CMA	Certified Medical Assistant		Community Mental Health Center
	Certified Movement Analyst		Community Migrant Health Center
	chromosomal microarray analysis	CMHN	Community Mental Health Nurse
	compound myopic astigmatism	CMI	case mix index
	cost-minimization analysis		cell-mediated immunity
	cow's milk allergy		clomipramine (Anafranil)
CMAF	centrifuged microaggregate filter		collagen meniscus implant
CMAI	Cohen-Mansfield Agitation inventory		Consumer Medicine Information (Australia)
CMAJ	*Journal of the Canadian Medical Association*		Cornell Medical Index
		CMID	cytomegalic inclusion disease
CMAP	compound muscle action potential	C_{min}	minimum concentration of drug
CMAPs	compound muscle action potentials	CMIR	cell-mediated immune response
C_{max}	maximum concentration of drug	CMJ	carpometacarpal joint
CMB	carbolic methylene blue		cervicomedullary junction
CMBBT	cervical mucous basal body temperature	CMK	congenital multicystic kidney
		CML	cell-mediated lympholysis
CMC	carboxymethylcellulose		chronic myelogenous leukemia
	carpal metacarpal (joint)		chronic myeloid leukemia
	Chemistry, Manufacturing, and Controls (section)	CML5	lower second premolar
		CML-BP	blastic phase chronic myeloid leukemia
	chloramphenicol		
	chronic mucocutaneous candidiasis	CML-CP	chronic myeloid leukemia in chronic phase
	clinically meaningful change		
	closed mitral commissurotomy	CMM	Comprehensive Major Medical (insurance)
CMCD	carboxymethylcellulose dressing		
CMCN	Certified Managed Care Nurse		continuous metabolic monitor
CMD	congenital muscular dystrophy		cutaneous malignant melanoma
	corrected mass defect	CMME	chloromethyl methyl ether
	cytomegalic disease	CMML	chronic myelomacrocytic leukemia
CMDRH	Center for Medical Devices and Radiological Health (of the Food and Drug Administration)	CMMS	Columbia Mental Maturity Scale
		CMN	Certificate of Medical Necessity
			congenital melanocytic nevi
CME	cervicomediastinal exploration (examination)		congenital mesoblastic nephroma
		CMO	cardiac minute output
	continuing medical education		cetyl myristoleate
	cystoid macular edema		Chief Medical Officer
CMER	current medical evidence of record		comfort measures only (resuscitation order)
CMF	chondromyxoid fibroma		
	cyclophosphamide, methotrexate and fluorouracil		consult made out
		CMO 1	corticosterone methyl oxidase type 1
CMFP	cyclophosphamide, methotrexate, fluorouracil, and prednisone	CMOP	cardiomyopathy
		C-MOPP	cyclophosphamide, mechloreth- amine, vincristine (Oncovin), procarbazine, and prednisone
CMFT	cyclophosphamide, methotrexate, fluorouracil, and tamoxifen		
CMFVP	cyclophosphamide, methotrexate, fluorouracil, vincristine, and prednisone	CMP	cardiomyopathy
			chondromalacia patellae
			comprehensive (complete) metabolic profile (see page 356)
CMG	Case-Mix Group		
	cystometrogram		cushion mouthpiece
CMGM	chronic megakaryocytic granulocytic myelosis	CMPA	cow's milk protein allergy
		CMPF	centromedian-parafascicular
CMGN	chronic membranous glomerulonephritis		cow's milk, protein-free
		CMPS	chronic myofascial pain syndrome
CMGs	case-mix groups	CMPT	cervical mucous penetration test
CMH	Cochran Mantel Haenszel	CMR	cardiometabolic risk
	current medical history		cardiovascular magnetic resonance
CMHC	Certified Mental Health Counselor		cerebral metabolic rate

C

chief medical resident
child (1-4 years) mortality rates
chloroform-methanol residue
crude mortality rate

CMRI   cardiac magnetic resonance imaging

CMRIT   combined modality radioimmunotherapy

CMRNG   chromosomally mediated resistant *Neisseria gonorrhoeae*

CMRO   chronic multifocal recurrent osteomyelitis

$CMRO_2$ cerebral metabolic rate for oxygen

cMRSA   community-associated methicilllin-resistant *Staphylococcus aureus*

CMS   cardiometabolic syndrome
Centers for Medicare and Medicaid Services (replaces Health Care Financing Administration [HCFA])
children's medical services
circulation motion sensation
chocolate milkshake
constant moderate suction
continuous motion syndrome

CMSC   Certified Medical Staff Coordinator

CMSUA   clean midstream urinalysis

CMT   carpometatarsal (joint)
Certified Massage Therapist
Certified Medication Technician
Certified Medical Transcriptionist
Certified Music Therapist
cervical motion tenderness
Charot-Marie-Tooth (phenotype) (disease)
Chiropractic manipulative treatment
choline magnesium trisalicylate (Trilisate)
combined modality therapy
continuing medication and treatment
cutis marmorata telangiectasia

CMT2C   type 2C Charcot-Marie-Tooth disease

CMTS   color, motion, temperature, and sensation

CMTX   chemotherapy treatment

CMUA   continuous motor unit activity

CMV   cisplatin, methotrexate, and vinblastine
controlled mechanical ventilation
conventional mechanical ventilation
cool mist vaporizer
cytomegalovirus
cytomegalovirus vaccine

CMVIG   cytomegalovirus immune globulin

CMVS   culture midvoid specimen

cmWP   centimeters of water pressure

CN   charge nurse
congenital nystagmus
cranial nerve
tomorrow night (this is a dangerous abbreviation)

Cn   cyanide

C/N   contrast-to-noise ratio

CN II–XII   cranial nerves 2 through 12

CNA   Certified in Nursing Administration
Certified Nursing Assistant
chart not available

C_{Na} sodium clearance

CNAA   Certified in Nursing Administration, Advanced

CNAG   chronic narrow angle glaucoma

CNAP   continuous negative airway pressure

CNB   core-needle biopsy

CNC   clinical nurse coordinator
Community Nursing Center
Consonant-Vowel Nucleus-Consonant (Maryland CNC word list)

CNCbl   cyanocobalamin (vitamin B_{12})

CNCH   chondrodermatitis nodularis chronica helicis

CND   canned
cannot determine
chronic nausea and dyspepsia

CNDC   chronic nonspecific diarrhea of childhood

CNDM2   cerebral neuropathology of type 2 diabetes mellitus

CNE   Chief Nurse Executive
chronic nervous exhaustion
continuing nursing education
could not establish
culture-negative endocarditis

CNEP   continuous negative extrathoracic pressure

C-NES   conversion nonepileptic seizures

CNF   cyclophosphamide, mitoxantrone (Novatantrone), and fluorouracil

CNG   complete, no growth

CNH   central neurogenic hypernea
contract nursing home

CNHC   chronodermatitis nodularis helicis chronicus
community nursing home care

CNI   calcineurin inhibitors

CNL   chemonucleolysis
chronic neutrophilic leukemia
Connaught Laboratories

CNLCP   Certified Nurse Life Care Planner

CNLD   chronic neonatal lung disease

CNLSD	condensation nucleation light scattering detection		complained of
			complaints
CNM	certified nurse midwife		under care of
CNMP	chronic nonmalignant pain	^{60}Co	radioactive isotope of cobalt
CNMT	Certified Nuclear Medicine Technologist	CO_2	carbon dioxide
		CO_3	carbonate
CNN	Certified in Nephrology Nursing	COA	children of alcoholic
	congenital nevocytic nevus		chronic obstructive asthma
CNNP	Certified Neonatal Nurse Practitioner		coenzyme A
			condition on admission
CNO	Chief Nursing Officer	CoA	coarctation of the aorta
	community nursing organization	COAD	chronic obstructive airway disease
CNOP	cyclophosphamide, mitoxantrone (Novantrone), vincristine (Oncovin), and prednisone		chronic obstructive arterial disease
		COAG	chronic open angle glaucoma
		COAGSC	coagulation screen
CNOR	Certified Nurse, Operating Room	COAP	cyclophosphamide, vincristine (Oncovin), cytarabine (ara-C), and prednisone
CNP	capillary nonprofusion		
CNPB	continuous negative pressure breathing		
		COAR	coarctation
CNPI	Checklist for Nonverbal Pain Indicators	COARCT	coarctation
		COB	chronic obstructive bronchitis
CNPS	cardiac nuclear probe scan		cisplatin, vincristine (Oncovin), and bleomycin
CNR	contrast-to-noise ratio (radiology)		
CNRN	Certified Neurosurgical Registered Nurse		coordination of benefits
		COBE	chronic obstructive bullous emphysema
CNS	central nervous system		
	Certified Nutrition Specialist	COBRA	Consolidated Omnibus Budget Reconciliation Act of 1985
	Clinical Nurse Specialist		
	coagulase-negative staphylococci	COBS	chronic organic brain syndrome
	Crigler-Najjar syndrome	COBT	chronic obstruction of biliary tract
CNSC	Certified Nutrition Support Clinician		
		COC	calcifying odontogenic cyst
CNSD	Certified Nutrition Support Dietitian		chain of custody
			combination oral contraceptive
CNSHA	congenital nonspherocytic hemolytic anemia		continuity of care
		COCCIO	coccidioidomycosis
CNSN	Certified Nutrition Support Nurse	COCM	congestive cardiomyopathy
CNT	could not tell	COCN	Certified Ostomy Care Nurse
	could not test	CoCr	cobalt-chromium alloy
CNTA	combined neurosurgical and transfacial approach	COD	carotid occlusive disease
			cataract, right eye
CNTF	ciliary neurotrophic factor		cause of death
CNV	choroidal neovascularization		chronic oxygen dependency
	contingent negative variation		codeine
	copy number variations		coefficient of oxygen delivery
CNVM	choroidal neovascular membrane		condition on discharge
		CODAS	chronotherapeutic oral drug absorption system
CO	carbon monoxide		
	cardiac output	Code	**Meanings can vary from region to region**
	castor oil		
	centric occlusion		Code Blue – Medical emergency – adult
	Certified Orthoptist		
	cervical orthosis		Code Brown – a patient's bed containing feces (slang)
	corneal opacity		
	corn oil		Code Gray – Combative person
	court order		Code Orange – Hazardous material spill/release
Co	cobalt		
C/O	check out		Code Pink – Infant abduction

	Code Purple – Child abduction
	Code Red – Fire
	Code Silver – Person with a weapon and/or a hostage situation
	Code Triage External – An external disaster
	Code Triage Internal – An internal disaster
	Code White – Medical emergency – pediatric
	Code Yellow – Bomb threat a patient's bed containing urine (slang)
	Code 99 – patient in cardiac or respiratory arrest
CODES	Crash Outcome Data Evaluation System (National Highway Traffic Safety Administration-sponsored)
COD-MD	cerebro-oculardysplasia muscular dystrophy
CODO	codocytes
COE	Centers of Excellence court-ordered examination
COEPS	cortically originating extrapyramidal symptoms
COER-24	24-hour controlled-onset, extended-release (dosage form)
COFS	cerebro-oculo-facioskeletal
COG	center of gravity Central Oncology Group Children's Oncology Group cognitive function tests
COGN	cognition
COGTT	cortisone-primed oral glucose tolerance test
COH	carbohydrate controlled ovarian hyperstimulation
COHb	carboxyhemoglobin
COHN	Certified Occupational Health Nurse
COHN/CM	Certified Occupational Health Nurse/Case Manager
COHN-S	Certified Occupational Health Nurse - Specialist
COHN-S/CM	Certified Occupational Health Nurse - Specialist Case Manager
COI	conflict of interest
Coke	Coca-Cola® cocaine
COL	colonoscopy
COLD	chronic obstructive lung disease Computer Output to Laser Disk
COLD A	cold agglutin titer
Collyr	eye wash
col/mL	colonies per milliliter

colp	colporrhaphy
COLPO	colposcopy
COLTRU	*colletotrichum truncatum*
COM	calcium oxalate monohydrate center of mass chronic otitis media citrate of magnesia
COMBO	combination ultrasound with electrical stimulation
COME	chronic otitis media with effusion
COMF	comfortable
COMLA	cyclophosphamide, vincristine (Oncovin), methotrexate, calcium leucovorin, and cytarabine (ara-C)
COMM E	Committee E, a German Federal Health Agency committee for the evaluation of herbal remedies
COMP	Committee on Orphan Medicinal Products (EMEA) compensation complications composite compound compress cyclophosphamide, vincristine (Oncovin), methotrexate, and prednisone
CompSAS	complex sleep apnea syndrome
CO-MRSA	community-onset methicillin-resistant *Staphylococcus aureus*
COMS	clinical outcomes management system
COMT	catechol-*O*-methyl-transferase Certified Ophthalmic Medical Technologist
COMTA	Commission on Message Therapy Accreditation
CON	catheter over a needle certificate of need conservatorship
CON A	concanavalin A
conc.	concentrated
CONEP	National Commission for Ethics in Research (Brazil)
CONG	congenital gallon
CONJ	conjunctiva
CONPA-DRI I	cyclophosphamide, vincristine, doxorubicin, and melphalan
CONPA-DRI II	conpadri I plus high-dose methotrexate
CONPA-DRI III	conpadri I plus intensified doxorubicin
CONS	consultation

CoNS	coagulase-negative staphylococci	COR P	cor pulmonale
CONT	continuous	CORT	Certified Operating Room
	contusions		Technician
CON-TRAL	contralateral	COS	cataract, left eye
			change of shift
CONTU	contusion		Chief of Staff
CONV	conversation		childhood-onset schizophrenia
Conv. ex.	convergence excess		clinically observed seizure
ConvRX	conventional therapy		controlled ovarian stimulation
–COOH	carboxylic acid		course of treatment
CO-Ox	Co-oximetry		Crisis Outpatient Services
COP	center of pressure	C_{osm}	osmolal clearance
	change of plaster	COSTART	Coding symbols for a thesaurus of
	cicatricial ocular pemphigoid		adverse reaction terms
	Colibacilosis porcina vaccine	COT	content of thought
	colloid osmotic pressure		court-ordered treatment
	complaint of pain	COTA	Certified Occupational Therapy
	cryptogenic organizing		Assistant
	pneumonia	COTE	comprehensive occupational
	cycophosphamide, vincristine		therapy evaluation
	(Oncovin), and prednisone	COTT CH	cottage cheese
CoP	Communities of Practice	COTX	cast-off, to x-ray
	Conditions of Participation	COU	cardiac observation unit
COP 1	copolymer 1		cataracts, both eyes
COPA	cuffed oropharyngeal airway	COV	coefficient of variation
COPAdM	cyclophosphamide, vincristine	COW	circle of Willis
	(Oncovin), prednisone,	COWA	controlled oral word association
	doxorubicin (Adriamycin) and	COWAT	Controlled Oral Word Association
	methotrexate		Test
COP-BLAM	cyclophosphamide, vincristine (Oncovin), prednisone, bleomycin, doxorubicin (Adriamycin), and procarbazine (Matulane)	COWS	Clinical Opioid Withdrawal Scale
			cold to the opposite and warm to
			the same
		COX	Coxsackie virus
			cyclo-oxygenase
			cytochrome C oxidase
COPD	chronic obstructive pulmonary disease	COX-2	cyclo-oxygenase-2
		CP	calculation point
COPE	chronic obstructive pulmonary emphysema		centric position
			cerebellopontine (angles)
COPP	cyclophosphamide, vincristine, procarbazine, and prednisone		cerebral palsy
			Certified Paramedic
COPS	community outpatient service		chemical peel
COPT	circumoval precipitin test		chemistry profiles
CoQ10	coenzyme Q_{10}		chest pain
COR	coefficient of reproducibility		chloroquine-primaquine
	complete oral rehabilitation		chondromalacia patella
	conditioned orientation response		chronic pain
	coronary		chronic pancreatitis
CoR	custodian of records		cleft palate
cOR	crude odds ratio		clinical pathway
CORA	conditioned orientation reflex audiometry		Clinical Psychologist
			closing pressure
CORBA	Common-Object Request Broker Architecture		cold pack
			constrictive pericarditis
CORE	cardiac or respiratory emergency		convenience package
CORF	Comprehensive Outpatient Rehabilitation Facility		cor pulmonale
			creatine phosphokinase
CORLN	Certified Otorhinolaryngology and Head/Neck Nurse		cricopharyngeal

cyclophosphamide and cisplatin (Platinol)

cystopanendoscopy

process capability

C_p concentration of drug plasma

phosphate clearance

Cp *Chlamydia pneumoniae*

C/P carbohydrate-to-protein ratio

C&P compensation and pension

complete and pain-free (range of motion)

complete and pushing

cystoscopy and pyelography

CPA cardiopulmonary arrest

carotid photoangiography

cerebellar pontile angle

chest pain alert

child protection agency

color power angiography

conditioned play audiometry

congenital primary aphakia

costophrenic angle

cyclophosphamide (Cytoxan)

cyproterone acetate (Androcur)

CPAF chlorpropamide-alcohol flush

C_{PAH} para-amino hippurate clearance

CPAN Certified Postanesthesia Nurse

CPAP continuous positive airway pressure

CPB cardiopulmonary bypass

cisplatin, cyclophosphamide, and carmustine (BiCNU)

competitive protein binding

CPBA competitive protein-binding assay

CPBP cardiopulmonary bypass

CPC cancer prevention clinic

cerebral palsy clinic

Certified Professional Coder

cetylpyridinium chloride

chronic passive congestion

clinicopathologic conference

coil planet centrifuge

continue plan of care

CPC 1 Cerebral Performance Category 1 (There are also Categories 2 to 5)

CPC-H Certified Procedural Coder, Hospital-Based

CP-CML chronic phase chronic myeloid leukemia

CP/CPPS chronic prostatitis/chronic pelvic pain syndrome

CPCR cardiopulmonary-cerebral resuscitation

CPCS clinical pharmacokinetics consulting service

CPCs calcium phosphate cements

CPD cephalopelvic disproportion

chorioretinopathy and pituitary dysfunction

chronic peritoneal dialysis

citrate-phosphate-dextrose

cPd colloidal palladium

CPDA-1 citrate-phosphate-dextrose-adenine-one

CPDA-2 citrate-phosphate-dextrose-adenine-two

CPDD calcium pyrophosphate deposition disease

CPDG2 carboxypeptidase-G2

CPDN Certified Peritoneal Dialysis Nurse

CPDR Center for Prostate Disease Research (Department of Defense)

CPE cardiogenic pulmonary edema

chronic pulmonary emphysema

Clinical Pastoral Education

Clostridium perfringens enterotoxin

clubbing, pitting, or edema

complete physical examination

continuing professional education

cytopathic effect

CPEB cytoplasmic polyadenylation element binding (protein)

CPE-C cyclopentenylcytosine

CPEFM Clear-Plan Easy Fertility Monitor

CPEO chronic progressive external ophthalmoplegia

CPER chest pain emergency room

CPET cardiopulmonary exercise testing

CPETU chest pain evaluation and treatment unit

CPEx cardioipulmonary exercise (testing)

CPF cerebral perfusion pressure

chlorpyrifos (an insecticide)

CPFT Certified Pulmonary Function Technologist

CPFX ciprofloxacin (Cipro)

CPG clinical practice guidelines

CPG2 carboxypeptidase G2

CPGN chronic progressive glomerulonephritis

CPH chronic paroxysmal hemicrania

chronic persistent hepatitis

CPHQ Certified Professional in Healthcare Quality

CPhT Certified Pharmacy Technician

CPI chronic public inebriate

constitutionally psychopathia inferior

CPID chronic pelvic inflammatory disease

CPIP chronic pulmonary insufficiency of prematurity

CPK creatine phosphokinase (BB, MB, MM are isoenzymes)

CPK-1 creatine phosphokinase MM fraction

CPK-2	creatine phosphokinase MB fraction
CPK-BB	creatine phosphokinase BB fraction
CPKD	childhood polycystic kidney disease
CPK-MB	creatine phosphokinase of muscle band
CPL	criminal procedure law
CPM	cancer pain management
	central pontine myelinolysis
	chlorpheniramine maleate
	chronic progressive myelopathy
	Clinical Practice Model
	continue present management
	continuous passive motion
	counts per minute
	cycles per minute
	cyclophosphamide (Cytoxan)
CPmax	peak serum concentration
CPMDI	computerized pharmacokinetic model-driven drug infusion
CPmin	trough serum concentration
CPMM	constant passive motion machine
CPMP	Committee for Proprietary Medicinal Products (of the European Union)
CPN	central parenteral nutrition
	Certified Pediatric Nurse
	chronic pyelonephritis
	common peroneal nerve
	complete parenteral nutrition
CPNA	Certified Pediatric Nurse Associate
CPNB	continuous peripheral nerve block
CPNI	common peroneal nerve injury
CPO	chief privacy officer
	continue present orders
	curved periacetabular osteotomy
CPOE	computerized physician (prescriber) order entry
CPOM	continuous pulse oximeter monitoring
CPON	Certified Pediatric Oncology Nurse
CPOX	chicken pox
CPP	central precocious puberty
	cerebral perfusion pressure
	chronic pelvic pain
	coronary perfusion pressure
	cryo-poor plasma
CPPB	continuous positive pressure breathing
CPPD	calcium pyrophosphate dihydrate
	cisplatin
CP & PD	chest percussion and postural drainage
CPPS	chronic pelvice pain syndrome
CPPV	continuous positive pressure ventilation
CPQ	Conner Parent Questionnaire

CPR	cardiopulmonary resuscitation
	computer-based patient records
	computerized patient record
	customary, prevailing and reasonable (charge payment method)
	tablet (French)
CPR-1	all measures except cardiopulmonary resuscitation
CPR-2	no extraordinary measures (to resuscitate)
CPR-3	comfort measures only
CPRAM	controlled partial rebreathing anesthesia method
CP/ROMI	chest pain, rule out myocardial infarction
CPRS	Categorical Pain Relief Scale
	computerized patient record system
CPRS-OCS	Comprehensive Psychiatric Rating Scale, Obsessive-Compulsive Subscale
CPRU	cardiac procedure recovery unit
CPS	carbamyl phosphate synthetase
	cardiopulmonary support
	Center for Prevention Services (CDC)
	cervical pedicle screw
	chest pain syndrome
	child protective services
	Chinese paralytic syndrome
	chloroquine-pyrimethamine sulfadoxine
	chronic paranoid schizophrenia
	clinical performance score
	clinical pharmacokinetic service
	CoaguChek® Plus System
	coagulase-positive staphylococci
	Cognitive Performance Scale
	complex partial seizures
	counts per second
	cumulative probability of success
CPs	clinical pathways
CPS I	carbamyl phosphate synthetase I
cPSA	complexed prostate-specific antigen
CPSC	Consumer Product Safety Commission
CPSI	Chronic Prostatitis Symptom Index
CPSN	Certified Plastic Surgical Nurse
CPSP	central post-stroke pain
CPT	camptothecin
	carnitine palmitoyl transferase
	chest physiotherapy
	child protection team
	chromo-perturbation
	chronic paranoid type
	cold pressor test

	Continuous Performance Test		Clinical Research Associate
	corticosteroid pulse treatment		colorectal anastomosis
	current perception threshold		Contract Research Assistant
	Current Procedural Terminology (coding system)		corticosteroid-resistant asthma cranial
CPT-2011	Current Procedural Terminology, 2011 Edition	CRAB	carbapenem-resistant *Acinetobacter baumannii*
CPT-11	irinotecan hydrochloride (Camptosar)	CRABP	cellular retinoic acid binding protein
CPTA	Certified Physical Therapy Assistant	CRAbs	chelating recombinant antibodies
CPT/C	current perception threshold, computerized	CRADA	Cooperative Research and Development Agreement (with NIH)
CPTH	chronic post-traumatic headache	CRAFFT	car, relax, alone, friends, forget, trouble (questionnaire to assess teenage risk of substance abuse)
CPU	children's psychiatric unit clinical pharmacology unit		
CPUE	chest pain of unknown etiology	CRAG	cerebral radionuclide angiography
CPUM	Certified Professional in Utilization Management	CrAg	cryptococcal antigen
CPV	canine parvovirus cowpox virus	CRAMS	circulation, respiration, abdomen, motor, and speech
CPX	complete physical examination	CRAN	craniotomy
CPZ	Compazine® or chlorpromazine (CPZ is a dangerous abbreviation as it could be either)	CRAO	central retinal artery occlusion
		CRAX	crackers
		CRB	Clinical Review Board correct retinal boundaries
CQ	chloroquine	CRBBB	complete right bundle branch block
CQDS	cumulative quality disruption score	CRBIs	catheter-related bloodstream infections
CQI	continuous quality improvement		
CR	caloric restrictions	CRBP	cellular retinol-binding protein
	capillary refill	CRBSI	catheter-related bloodstream infections
	cardiac rehabilitation		
	cardiorespiratory	CRC	case review committee
	case reports		child-resistant container
	chief resident		clinical research center
	chorioretinal		Clinical Research Coordinator
	clockwise rotation		colorectal cancer
	closed reduction	CR & C	closed reduction and cast
	colon resection	CrCl	creatinine clearance
	complete remission	CrCl₃	chromic chloride
	computed radiography	CRCLM	colorectal cancer liver metastases
	contact record	CRCS	colorectal cancer screening
	controlled release	CRD	childhood rheumatic disease
	cosmetic rhinoplasty		chronic renal disease
	creamed		chronic respiratory disease
	credentialing		colorectal distension
	crutches		cone-rod dystrophy
	cycloplegia retinoscopy		congenital rubella deafness
Cr	caloric restrictions		crown-rump distance
	chromium	CRE	cumulative radiation effect
	creatinine	CREAT	serum creatinine
C/R	conscious, rational	CREC	ciprofloxacin-resistant *Escherichia coli*
C & R	convalescence and rehabilitation cystoscopy and retrograde		
		CREF	cycloplegic refraction
CR₁	first cranial nerve	CRELM	screening tests for Congo-Crimean, Rift Valley, Ebola, Lassa, and Marburg fevers
CRA	central retinal artery		
	chronic rheumatoid arthritis		
	cis-retinoic acid (isotretinion, Accutane®)		
		CREP	crepitation

CREST	calcinosis, Raynaud disease, esophageal dysmotility, sclerodactyly, and telangiectasia	CRO	cathode ray oscilloscope contract research organization(s)
CRF	cancer-related fatigue cardiac risk factors case report form chronic renal failure corticotrophin-releasing factor	CROACC	cannot rule out anything, correlate clinically (slang)
		CROM	cervical range of motion chronic refractory osteomyelitis
CRFs	clinical risk factors	CROMY	chronic refractory osteomyelitis
CRG-L2	Cancer related gene-Liver 2	Crook-U	a prison ward in a hospital (slang)
CRH	corticotropic-releasing hormone	CROS	contralateral routing of signals
CRFZ	closed reduction of fractured zygoma	CRP	canalith repositioning procedure chronic relapsing pancreatitis coronary rehabilitation program C-reactive protein
CRH	corticotropin-releasing hormone		
CRHCa	cancer-related hypercalcemia	C&RP	curettage and root planning
CRI	Cardiac Risk Index catheter-related infection chronic renal insufficiency	CRPA	C-reactive protein agglutinins
		CRPC	castration-refractory prostate cancer
CRIB	Clinical Risk Index for Babies	CRPD	chronic restrictive pulmonary disease
CRIE	crossed radioimmunoelectrophoresis		
CRIF	closed reduction and internal fixation	CRPF	chloroquine-resistant *Plasmodium falciparum*
CRIM	cross-reacting immunologic material	CRPP	closed reduction and percutaneous pinning
CRIMF	closed reduction/intermaxillary fixation	CRPS	complex regional pain syndromes
		CRPS I	complex regional pain syndrome type I
CRIS	controlled-release infusion system	CRQ	Chronic Respiratory (Disease) Questionnaire
crit	hematocrit		
CRKL	crackles	CRR	community rehabilitation residence
CRL	crown rump length	CRRN	Certified Rehabilitation Registered Nurse
CRLM	colorectal liver metastases		
CRM	circumferential resection margins continual reassessment method cream cross-reacting mutant	CRRN-A	Certified Rehabilitation Registered Nurse - Advanced
		CRRT	continuous renal replacement therapy
CRM +	cross-reacting material positive	CRS	care record summary Carroll Self-Rating Scale catheter-related sepsis Center for Scientific Review (NIH) Chemical Reference Substances child restraint system(s) Chinese restaurant syndrome chronic rhinosinusitis cocaine-related seizure(s) colon-rectal surgery congenital rubella syndrome continuous running suture cryoreductive surgery cytokine-release syndrome
CRMD	children with retarded mental development		
CRMO	chronic recurrent multifocal osteomyelitis		
CRMPC	castration-resistant metastatic prostate cancer		
CRN	Certified Radiologic Nurse crown		
CRNA	Certified Registered Nurse Anesthetist		
CRNFA	Certified Registered Nurse, First Assistant		
CRNH	Certified Registered Nurse in Hospice	CRSD	circadian rhythm sleep disorder
CRNI	Certified Registered Nurse Intravenous	CRST	calcification, Raynaud phenomenom, scleroderma, and telangiectasia
CRNL	Certified Registered Nurse - Long-Term Care		
CRNO	Certified Registered Nurse in Ophthalmology	CRT	cadaver renal transplant capillary refill time Cardiac Rescue Technician cardiac resynchronization therapy cartilage roof triangle
CRNP	Certified Registered Nurse Practitioner		

C

	cathode ray tube		Cushing syndrome
	central reaction time		cycloserine
	Certified Rehabilitation Therapist		o-chlorobenzylidene malononitrile
	chemoradiotherapy	C&S	conjunctiva and sclera
	choice reaction time		cough and sneeze
	circuit resistance training		culture and sensitivity
	copper reduction test	C/S	cesarean section
	cranial radiation therapy		consultation
CRT-D	cardiac resynchronization therapy defibrillator		culture and sensitivity
		CSA	central sleep apnea
Cr Tr	crutch training		childhood sexual abuse
CRTs	case report tabulations		compressed spectral activity
CRTT	Certified Respiratory Therapy Technician		Controlled Substances Act
CRTX	cast removed take x-ray		controlled substance analogue
CRTx	chemoradiotherapy		corticosteroid-sensitive asthma
CRU	cardiac rehabilitation unit		cryosurgical ablation
	catheterization recovery unit	CsA	cyclosporine (cyclosporin A)
	clinical research unit	CsA-ME	cyclosporine microemulsion (Neoral)
CRV	central retinal vein		
CRVF	congestive right ventricular failure	CSAP	cryosurgical ablation of the prostate
CRVO	central retinal vein occlusion		
CRx	chemotherapy	CSB	caffeine sodium benzoate
CIIRx	Century II Bicarbonate Dialysis Machine		Cheyne-Stokes breathing
			Children's Services Board
CRYO	cryoablation	CSBF	coronary sinus blood flow
	cryosurgery	CSBM	complete spontaneous bowel movements
CRYST	crystals		
CS	cardiogenic shock	CSBO	complete small bowel obstruction
	cardioplegia solution	CSC	central serous chorioretinopathy
	cat scratch		cornea, sclera, and conjunctiva
	cervical spine		cryogen spray cooling
	cesarean section		cryopreserved stem cells
	Chemstrip	CSCC	cutaneous squamous cell carcinoma
	chest strap	CSCI	continuous subcutaneous infusion
	cholesterol stone	CsCl	cesium chloride
	chlorobenzylidene malononitrile	CSCR	central serous chorioretinopathy
	cigarette smoker	CSCS	Certified Strength and Conditioning Specialist
	clinically significant		
	Clinical Specialist	CSCs	cancer stem cells
	clinical stage	CSD	cat scratch disease
	close supervision		celiac sprue disease
	conditionally susceptible		conduction system disorder (disease)
	congenital syphilis		
	conjunctiva-sclera		congenital sensorineural deafness
	consciousness		cortical spreading depression
	conscious sedation	C S&D	cleaned, sutured, and dressed
	consultation	CSDD	Center for the Study of Drug Development
	consultation service		
	controlled substances (manufacture, importation, possession, use and distribution of certain drugs of potential abuse that are regulated by US government)	CSDH	chronic subdural hematoma
			combined systolic and diastolic hypertension
		CSE	combined spinal/epidurals
			cross-section echocardiography
	coronary sinus	CSEA	combined spinal-epidural anesthesia
	corticosteroid(s)		
	cranial setting	C sect.	cesarean section

CSEP	core-stabilization exercise programs		cervical spine pain
			chiral stationary phase
CSF	cerebrospinal fluid		cutaneous silent period
	colony-stimulating factors	C-SPI	Certified Specialist in Poison Information
CSFELP	cerebrospinal fluid electrophoresis		
CSFP	cerebrospinal fluid pressure	C-spine	cervical spine
CSGIT	continuous-suture graft-inclusion technique	CSR	central supply room
			Cheyne-Stokes respiration
C-Sh	chair shower		clinical statistical report
CSH	carotid sinus hypersensitivity		combat stress reaction
	chronic subdural hematoma		corrected sedimentation rate
	combat surgical hospital(s)		corrective septorhinoplasty
CSHQ	Children's Sleep Habits Questionnaire	C-S RT	craniospinal radiotherapy
		CSS	Canadian Stroke Scale (score)
CSI	chemical shift imaging		carotid sinus stimulation
	Computerized Severity Index		Central Sterile Services
	continuous subcutaneous infusion		chemical sensitivity syndrome
	coronary stent implantation		chewing, sucking, and swallowing
	corticosteroid injection		child safety seats
	craniospinal irradiation		Churg-Strauss syndrome
CsI	cesium iodide	C_{SS}	concentration of drug at steady-state
CSICU	cardiac surgery intensive care unit		
		CSSD	closed system sterile drainage
CSID	congenital sucrase-isomaitase deficiency	C-SSRS	Columbia Suicide Severity Rating Scale
CSII	continuous subcutaneous insulin infusion	CSSS	coronary subclavian steal syndrome
		CSSSIs	complicated skin and skin-structure infections
CSIO	continuous subcutaneous infusion of opiates		
		CSSU	cardiac short-stay unit
CS IV	clinical stage 4	CST	cardiac stress test
CSL	chemical safety level		castration
CSLO	confocal scanning laser ophthalmoscopy		central sensory conducting time
			cerebroside sulfotransferase
CSLU	chronic status leg ulcer		Certified Surgical Technologist
CSM	carotid sinus massage		cesarean section prior to labor at term
	cerebrospinal meningitis		
	cervical spondylotic myelopathy		contraction stress test
	circulation, sensation, and movement		convulsive shock therapy
			cosyntropin stimulation test
	Committee on Safety of Medicines (United Kingdom)		static compliance
		C_{STAT}	static lung compliance
CSMC	Cedars-Sinai Medical Center (Los Angeles, CA)	CSTD	closed-system (drug) transfer device
CSME	cotton-spot macular edema	CSTE	Council of State and Territorial Epidemiologists
CSMN	chronic sensorimotor neuropathy		
CSN	Certified School Nurse	CSTO	cat smarter than owner (Veterinary slang)
	cystic suppurative necrosis		
CSNB	congenital stationary night blindness	CSU	cardiac surgery unit
			cardiac surveillance unit
CSNRT	corrected sinus node recovery time		cardiovascular surgery unit
CSNS	carotid sinus nerve stimulation		casualty staging unit
CSO	Chief Security Officer		catheter specimen of urine
	Consumer Safety Officer (FDA)	CSVD	cerebral small-vessel disease
	copied standing orders	CSVT	cerebral sinovenous thrombosis
CSOM	chronic serous otitis media	CSW	cerebral salt-wasting (syndrome)
	chronic suppurative otitis media		Clinical Social Worker
CSP	cellulose sodium phosphate		commercial sex worker

C

CSWCM	Certified Social Work Case Manager		cyclophosphamide, thiotepa, and carboplatin
CSWD	conservative sharp wound debridement	CTCAE v3.0	Common Terminology Criteria for Adverse Events, version 3.0
	corticosteroid withdrawal		(National Cancer Institute
CSWs	commercial sex workers		grading system for treatment-
CSWSS	continuous spike-waves during slow sleep		related toxicities; grade 1 = mild, grade 2 = moderate,
CSX	cardiac syndrome X		grade 3 = severe, grade 4 =
CT	calcitonin		life-threatening or disabling,
	calf tenderness		grade 5 = death related to
	cardiothoracic		adverse event)
	carpal tunnel	CTCL	cutaneous T-cell lymphoma
	cellulose triacetate (filter)		(mycosis fungoides)
	cervical traction	CTCOFR	Composite Time to Complete
	chemotherapy		Organ Failure Resolution
	chest tube	CT & DB	cough, turn & deep breath
	Chlamydia trachomatis	CTD	carboxy-terminal domain
	circulation time		carpal tunnel decompression
	client		chest tube drainage
	clinical trial		Common Technical Document
	clotting time		connective tissue disease
	coagulation time		corneal thickness depth
	coated tablet		cumulative trauma disorder
	compressed tablet	CTDI	computed tomography dose index
	computed tomography	CTDW	continues to do well
	Coomb test	CTE	chronic traumatic encephalopathy
	corneal thickness	CTEP	Cancer Therapy Evaluation
	corneal transplant		Program
	corrective therapy		Center for Therapy Evaluation
	cytarabine and thioguanine		Programs (National Cancer
	cytoxic drug		Institute)
C_t	concentration of drug in tissue	CTEPH	chronic thromboembolic
C/T	compared to		pulmonary hypertension
C7-T2	cervicothoracic spine junction	CTF	clanging tuning fork (test)
CTA	catamenia (menses)		Colorado tick fever
	clear to auscultation		continuous tube feeding
	composite tissue allograft	CTG	cardiotocography
	computed tomographic angiography	C/TG	cholesterol to triglyceride ratio
		CTGA	complete transposition of the great
CTAB	clear to auscultation, bilaterally		arteries
C-TAB	cyanide tablet		corrected transposition of the great
CTAP	clear to auscultation and percussion		arteries
	computed tomography during	CTGF	connective tissue growth factor
	arterial portography	CTH	clot to hold
CTB	ceased to breathe	CTHA	computed tomography hepatic
	cholera toxin B		arteriography
CTC	Cancer Treatment Center	CTI	cavotricuspid isthmus
	circular tear capsulotomy		certification of terminal illness
	circulating tumor cells	cTI	cardiac troponin I
	Clinical Trial Certificate (United Kingdom's equivalent to the Investigational New Drug Application)	CTIBL	cancer treatment-induced bone loss
		CTICU	cardiothoracic intensive care unit
		CTID	chemotherapy-induced diarrhea
	Common Toxicity Criteria	CTJ	cervicothoracic junction
	computed tomographic colonography	CTL	cervical, thoracic, and lumbar
			chronic tonsillitis

	control (subjects)
	cytotoxic T-lymphocytes
CTLG	computed tomographic lymphography
CTLM	computed tomography-laser mammography
CTLSO	cervicothoracic-lumbosacral orthosis
CTM	Chlor-Trimeton
	clinical trials materials
	computed tomographic myelography
CT/MPR	computed tomography with multiplanar reconstructions
CTMS	clinical trial management systems
CTN	calcitonin
	Certified Transcultural Nurse
C & T N, BLE	color and temperature normal, both lower extremities
cTnC	cardiac troponin C
cTnI	cardiac troponin I
cTNM	clinical-diagnostic staging of cancer
CTnT	cardiac troponin T
CTO	chronic total (coronary) occlusion
CTP	comprehensive treatment plan
CTPA	clear to percussion and auscultation
	computed tomographic pulmonary angiography
CTPN	central total parenteral nutrition
CTQ	Childhood Trauma Questionnaire
CTR	capsular tension ring
	carpal tunnel release
	carpal tunnel repair
	Certified Tumor Registrar
	cosmetic transdermal reconstruction
CTRB	Clinical Trial Review Board
	critical tests read back
CTRS	Certified Therapeutic Recreation Specialist
	Conners Teachers Rating Scale
CT-RT	chemo-radiotherapy
CTS	cardiothoracic surgeon
	carpal tunnel syndrome
	closed-tube sampling
CTSIB	Clinical Test Sensory Interaction Balance
CTSP	called to see patient
CTT	congenital trigger thumb
	cotton-thread test
CTTH	chronic tension-type headache
CTU	computed tomographic urography
CTV	clinical target volumes (radiation therapy)
	clinical tumor volume
CTVT	canine transmissible venereal tumor

CTW	central terminal of Wilson
CTX	cerebrotendinous xanthomatosis
	cervical traction
	chemotherapy
	Clinical Trial Exemption
	cyclophosphamide (Cytoxan)
CTX-1	C-telopeptide type 1
CTXN	contraction
CTZ	chemoreceptor trigger zone
	co-trimoxazole (sulfamethoxazole and trimethoprin)
CU	cause undetermined
	cause unknown
	chronic undifferentiated
	clinical units
	color unit
	communicates understanding
	convalescent unit
	Cuprophan (filter)
Cu	copper
C_u	urea clear clearance
C/U	checkup
	creatinine/urea ratio
CUA	Certified Urologic Associate
	clean urinalysis
	cost-utility analysis
CUC	chronic ulcerative colitis
	Clinical Unit Clerk
CUCNS	Certified Urologic Clinical Nurse Specialist
CUD	cause undetermined
	controlled unsterile delivery
CUFCM	Century Ultrafiltration Control Machine
CUG	cystourethrogram
Cu-IUD	copper intrauterine device
CUNP	Certified Urologic Nurse Practitioner
CUOG	Canadian Urologic Oncology Group
CUP	carcinoma of unknown primary (site)
CUPS	carcinoma of unknown primary site
CUR	curettage
	cystourethrorectocele
CURN	Certified Urologic Registered Nurse
CUS	carotid ultrasound
	chronic undifferentiated schizophrenia
	compression ultrasonography
	contact urticaria syndrome
CUSA	Cavitron ultrasonic suction aspirator
CUT	chronic undifferentiated type (schizophrenia)
CUTA	congenital urinary tract anomaly

CV   cardiovascular
     cell volume
     cisplatin and etoposide (VePesid)
     coefficient of variation
     color vision
     common ventricle
     consonant vowel
     contrast venography
     curriculum vitae
C/V   cervical/vaginal
CVA   cerebrovascular accident
     costovertebral angle
     cough-variant asthma
CVAAS   cold vapor atomic absorption
     spectrometry
CVAD   central venous access device
CVAH   congenital virilizing adrenal
     hyperplasia
CVAT   costovertebral angle tenderness
CVB   chronic villi biopsy
     group B coxsackievirus
CVB3   coxsackievirus B3
CVC   central venous catheter
     chief visual complaint
     consonant-vowel-consonant
CVD   cardiovascular disease
     cisplatin, vinblastine, and
       decarbazine
     collagen vascular disease
CVDU   chronic ventilator-dependent unit
CVEB   cisplatin, vinblastine, etoposide,
     and bleomycin
CVENT   controlled ventilation
CVEs   cerebrovascular events
CVF   cardiovascular failure
     cardiovascular fitness
     central visual field
     cervicovaginal fluid
     cobra venom factor
     colovesical fistula
     confrontational visual fields
CVG   cochleovestibular ganglion
     coronary vein graft
     cutis verticis gyrata
CVHC   Cardiovascular Health Clinic
CVHD   chronic valvular heart disease
CVI   carboplatin, etoposide, ifosfamide,
     and mesna uroprotection
     cerebrovascular insufficiency
     chronic venous insufficiency
     common variable
       immunodeficiency (disease)
     continuous venous infusion
CVICU   cardiovascular intensive care unit
CVID   common variable immune
     deficiency
CVINT   cardiovascular intermediate
CVL   central venous line

     cervicovaginal lavage
     clinical vascular laboratory
CVLP   chimeric virus-like particles
CVLT   California Verbal Learning Test
CVM   Center for Veterinary Medicine
     (NIH)
CVMP   Committee for Medicinal Products
     for Veterinary Use (EMEA)
CVMT   cervical-vaginal, motion tenderness
CVN   central venous nutrient
     Certified Vascular Nurse
CVNSR   cardiovascular normal sinus rhythm
CVO   central vein occlusion
     conjugate diameter of pelvic inlet
CvO_2 mixed venous oxygen content
CVOD   cerebrovascular obstructive disease
CVOR   cardiovascular operating room
CVP   central venous pressure
     cyclophosphamide, vincristine, and
       prednisone
CVPP   lomustine, vinblastine,
     procarbazine, and prednisone
CVR   cerebral vascular resistance
     cerebrovascular resuscitation
     coronary vascular reserve
CVRI   coronary vascular resistance
     index
CVRS   Cardiovascular-Respiratory Score
CVS   cardiovascular surgery
     cardiovascular system
     challenge virus standard
     chorionic villi sampling
     clean voided specimen
     continuing vegetative state
CVSCU   cardiovascular special care unit
CVSD   congenital ventricular septal
     defect
CVST   cardiovascular stress test
     cerebral venous sinus
       thrombosis
CVSU   cardiovascular specialty unit
CVT   calf vein thrombosis
     cephalic vein transposition
     cerebral venous thrombosis
CVTC   central venous tunneled catheter
CVU   chronic venous ulceration
     clean voided urine
CVUG   cysto-void urethrogram
CVVH   continuous venovenous
     hemofiltration
CVVHDF   continuous venovenous
     hemodiafiltration
Cvx   cervix
CW   careful watch
     case worker
     chest wall
     clockwise
     compare with

C

C/W	consistent with crutch walking	CYP3A4	cytochrome P450 enzyme 3A4 (there are many cytochrome
CWA	chemical warfare agents		P450 enzymes, such as CYP2E1,
CWAF	Chemical Withdrawal Assessment		CYP1A1, CYP2D6, etc.)
	Flowsheet	CYP450	cytochrome P450 system
CWAP	continuous wave arthroscopy pump	CYRO	cryoprecipitate
CWCN	Certified Wound Care Nurse	CysC	cystatin C
CWD	canal-wall down	CYSTA	cystathionine
	cell-wall defective	CYSTO	cystogram
	change wet dressing		cystoscopy
	chronic wasting disease	CYT	cyclophosphamide
CWE	cotton-wool exudates	Cyt	cytosine
CWL	Caldwell-Luc	CYTA	cytotoxic agent
CWM	comprehensive weight management	CYVA DIC	cyclophosphamide,
CWMS	color, warmth, movement, and		vincristine, Adriamycin, and
	sensation		dacarbazine (DTIC)
CWOCN	Certified Wound, Ostomy and	CZ	central zone (prostate needle
	Continence Nurse		biopsy location)
CWP	centimeters of water pressure	CZE	capillary zone electrophoresis
	childbirth without pain	CZI	crystalline zinc insulin (regular
	chronic widespread pain		insulin)
	coal worker's pneumoconiosis	CZP	clonazepam (Klonopin)
	cold wet packs	CZT	cadmium zinc telluride
cWPW	concealed Wolff-Parkinson-White		
	syndrome		
CWR	clockwise rotation		
CWS	Certified Wound Care Specialist		
	comfortable walking speed		
	cotton-wool spots		
CWT	compensated work training		
CWV	closed wound vacuum		
CX	cancel		
	cervix		
	chronic		
	circumflex		
	circumflex artery		
	culture		
	cylinder axis		
	cystectomy		
Cx	consultation		
CXA	circumflex artery		
CxBx	cervical biopsy		
CxMT	cervical motion tenderness		
CXR	chest x-ray		
CXTX	cervical traction		
CY	calendar year		
	cyclophosphamide (Cytoxan)		
C&Y	Children with Youth (program)		
CYA	cover your ass		
CyA	cyclosporine		
CyADIC	cyclophosphamide, doxorubicin		
	(Adriamycin), and dacarbazine		
CYC	cyclophosphamide		
Cyclo C	cyclocytidine HCl		
Cyd	cytidine (also referred to as C)		
CYF	Children, Youth and Families		
CYL	cylinder		
CYP	cytochrome P-450 system		

C

D

D	daughter		Dental Assistant
	day		diagnostic arthroscopy
	dead		diastolic augmentation
	decay		direct admission
	dependent		direct agglutination
	depression		disc area
	dextrose	Da	diversional activity
	dextro		dopamine
	diarrhea		drug addict
	diastole		drug aerosol
	dictated	Da	daltons
	dilated	D/A	discharge and advise
	diminished	D & A	drug & alcohol
	Dinamap (blood pressure monitor)	DAA	dead after arrival
	diopter		dissection aortic aneurysm
	distal	DA/A	drug/alcohol addiction
	distance	DAB	days after birth
	divorced		diamino benzidine
	dream		Deutsche Arzneibuch (German Pharmacopeia)
D+	note has been dictated/look for report	DABA	Diplomate of the American Board of Anesthesiology
D−	note not dictated, save chart for doctor	DAC	day activity center
$D_{0(2/7/07)}$	Day zero (the day treatment begins, February 7th, 2007)		decitabine
			disabled adult child
			Division of Ambulatory Care
D_1	day one (first day of treatment)	DACi	deacetylase inhibitor
	first diagonal branch (coronary artery)	DACL	Depression Adjective Checklists
		DACS	density-adjusted cell sorting
D-1	dorsal vertebrae 1 to 12	DACT	dactinomycin (Cosmegen)
D-12	dorsal nerves 1-12	DAD	diffuse alveolar damage
D_2	second diagonal branch (coronary artery)		diode array detector
			Disability Assessment of Dementia
	ergocalciferol		dispense as directed
			drug administration device
2/d	twice a day (this is a dangerous abbreviation)		father
		DADS	distal acquired demyelinating symmetrical (neuropathy)
2-D	two-dimensional	DAE	diving air embolism
3-D	three-dimensional	DAEC	diffuse-adherence *Entamoeba coli*
D_3	cholecalciferol		
D-3+7	cytarabine and daunorubicin	DAF	decay-accelerating factor
4D	4 prism diopters		delayed auditory feedback
4-D	four-dimensional	DAFE	Dial-A-Flow Extension®
D5	dextrose 5% injection	DAFM	double-aerosol face mask
5xD	five times a day (this is a dangerous abbreviation)	DAFNE	dose adjustment for normal eating
		DAG	diacylglycerol
D-15	Farnsworth panel D-15 color vision test		dianhydrogalactitol
		DAH	diffuse alveolar hemorrhage
D50	50% dextrose injection		disordered action of the heart
$D_{5/.45}$	dextrose 5% in 0.45% sodium chloride injection	DAI	diffuse axonal injury
		DAIDS	Division of AIDS (of the National Institute of Allergy and Infectious Diseases, NIH)
DA	darbepoetin alfa (Aranesp)		
	dark adaptation (test)	DAL	diffuse aggressive lymphomas
	Debtors Anonymous		drug analysis laboratory
	degenerative arthritis	DALE	disability-adjusted life expectancy
	delivery awareness	DALK	deep anterior lamellar keratoplasty

DALM	dysplasia-associated lesion or mass		direct antiglobulin test
DALY	disability-adjusted life year(s)	DAU	daughter
DAM	diacetylmonoxine		drug abuse urine
DAMA	discharged against medical advice	DAUNO	daunorubicin
DAMP	deficits in attention, motor control, and perception	DAVA	vindesine sulfate (Eldisine; desacetyl vinblastine amide sulfate)
DAN	diabetic autonomic neuropathy	DAVE	The Data Assessment and
DANA	drug-induced antinuclear antibodies		Verification program
DAo	descending aorta	DAVM	dural arteriovenous malformation
DAOM	depressor anguli oris muscle	DAV SEP	deviated septum
DAP	dapsone	DAW	dispense as written
	diabetes-associated peptide	DAWN	Drug Abuse Warning Network
	diastolic augmentation pressure	dB	decibel
	distending airway pressure	DB	database
	dose area product (radiology)		date of birth
	Draw-A-Person		Decision Board
DAPT	Draw-A-Person Test		deep breathe
DAR	daily affective rhythm		demonstration bath
	data, action, response		dermabrasion
DARB	darbepoetin alfa (Aranesp)		diaphragmatic breathing
DARE	data, action, response, and evaluation		difficulty breathing
			direct bilirubin
DARP	drug abuse rehabilitation program		double blind
	drug abuse reporting program	D2B	door-to-balloon (time)
DARPA	Defense Advanced Research Projects Agency (US Department of Defense)	DBA	Diamond-Blackfan anemia
		dBA	decibel, weighted according to the A scale
DARQ	diarylquinoline	DB & C	deep breathing and coughing
DART	developmental and reproductive toxicology (protocols)	DBD	milolactol (dibromodulicitol)
		DBDS	Dementia Behavior Disturbance Scale
D/ART	depression/awareness, recognition and treatment		
		DBE	deep breathing exercise
DAS	data acquisition system (radiology)		double-balloon enteroscopy
	day of admission surgery		double-balloon endoscopy
	developmental apraxia of speech	DBED	penicillin G benzathine (for IM use only; Bicillin L-A)
	died at scene		
	disease activity score	dBEMCL	decibel effective masking contralateral
	distractive auditory stimuli		
	dynamometer anchoring station	D₅BES	dextrose in balanced electrolyte solution
DAs	daily activities		
DASE	dobutamine-atropine stress echocardiography	DBG	dabigatran etexilate (Pradaxa)
		DBH	double-bundle hamstring (tendon graft)
DASH	Dietary Approaches to Stop Hypertension (diet)		
		DBI	documented by initials
	Disabilities of the Arm, Shoulder and Hand (questionnaire/rating)	DBI®	phenformin HCl
		DBIL	direct bilirubin
DASI	Duke Activity Status Index	DBKT	Diabetes: Basic Knowledge Test
DAST	Drug Abuse Screening Test	DBL	double beta-lactam
DAT	daunorubicin, cytarabine, (ara-C), and thioguanine	DBM	dibenzoylmethane
			donor breast milk
	definitely abnormal tracing (electrocardiogram)	DBMT	displacement bone marrow transplantation
	dementia of the Alzheimer type	DBP	D-binding protein
	diet as tolerated		diastolic blood pressure
	diphtheria antitoxin		dibutyl phthalate
	direct agglutination test	DBPCFC	double-blind, placebo-controlled food challenge
	direct amplification test		

DBPT	dacarbazine (DTIC), carmustine (BCNU), cisplatin (Platinol), and tamoxifen	DCCV	direct current cardioversion
		DCD	developmental coordination disorder
DBQ	debrisoquin		donation after cardiac death
DBS	deep brain stimulation	DC'd	discontinued
	desirable body weight	DCE	delayed contrast-enhancement
	diminished breath sounds		designated compensable event
	dorsal blocking splint		detection-controlled estimation
	dried blood stain		distal clavicle excision
DBSs	dietary botanical supplements	D&C&E	dilation, curettage, and evacuation
DBT	dialectical behavior therapy	DCE-MRI	dynamic contrast enhanced magnetic resonance imaging
	drug benefit threshold		
DBW	dry body weight	DCF	data collection form
DBZ	dibenzamine		Denomination Commune Francaise (French-approved nonproprietary name)
DC	daunorubicin and cytarabine		
	daycare		
	deceleration capacity (heart)		docetaxel, cisplatin, and fluorouracil
	decrease		
	dendritic cells		pentostatin (Nipent; 2′ deoxycoformycin)
	dextrocardia		
	diagonal conjugate	DCFS	Department of Children and Family Services
	direct Coombs (test)		
	direct current	DCG	diagnostic cardiogram
	discharge (This is a dangerous abbreviation as it is read as discontinue)	DCH	delayed cutaneous hypersensitivity
		DCI	decompression illness
		DCIA	deep circumflex iliac artery (flap)
	discomfort	DCIS	ductal carcinoma *in situ*
	displacement chromatography	DCL	diffuse cutaneous leishmaniasis
	Doctor of Chiropractic	DC-LAMP	dendritic cell-lysosomal-associated membrane protein
	dorsal compartment		
D&C	dilatation and curettage	DCLHb	diaspirin cross-linked hemoglobin
	direct and consensual	DCM	dementia care mapping
D/C	disconnect		dilated cardiomyopathy
	discontinue	DCMP	dilated cardiomyopathy
DCA	deoxycholic acid	DCMXT	dichloromethotrexate
	dichloroacetate	DCN®	Darvocet N
	directional coronary atherectomy	DCNU	chlorozotocin
	disk/condyle adhesion	DCO	damage control orthopedics
	double-cup arthroplasty		death certificates only (cases known only from death certificates)
	sodium dichloroacetate		
DCAG	double-coronary artery graft		
DCAP-BTLS	deformities, contusions, abrasions, and punctures/penetrations, burns, tenderness, lacerations, and swelling (an assessment mnemonic used by EMTs)		diffusing capacity of carbon monoxide
		DCP	discharge planner (plan)
			dynamic compression plate
		DCP®	calcium phosphate, dibasic
DC-ART	disease controlling anti-rheumatic therapy	DCPM	daunorubicin, cytarabine, prednisolone, and mercaptopurine
DC&B	dilation, currettage, and biopsy		
DCBE	double-contrast barium enema	DCPN	direction-changing positional nystagmus
DCC	day care center(s)		
	diabetes care clinic	DCR	dacryocystorhinostomy
	direct current cardioversion		delayed cutaneous reaction
DCCF	dural carotid-cavernous fistula		digital contact radiography
DCCs	day care centers		disease control rate
DCCT	Diabetes Control and Complications Trial (questionnaire)		distal clavicle resection
		DCRC	disseminated colorectal cancer
		DCRF	data case report forms

3DCRT	three-dimensional conformal radiation therapy		diarrhea and dehydration
			divorced and desperate (middle aged female who visits doctor
DCS	damage-control surgery		weekly just for male attention)
	decompression sickness		(slang)
	dorsal column stimulator		drilling and drainage
DCSA	double-contrast shoulder	DDA	dideoxyadenosine
	arthrography	DDAH	dimethylarginine
DCSAD	Diagnostic Classification of Sleep		dimethylaminohydrolase
	and Arousal Disorders	DDAVP®	desmopressin acetate
dcSSc	diffuse cutaneous systemic	DDC	dose-dense chemotherapy
	sclerosis		zalcitabine (dideoxy-cytidine;
DCSW	Diplomate in Clinical Social Work		Hivid)
DCT	daunorubicin, cytarabine, and	DDCI	dopadecarboxylase inhibitor
	thioguanine	DDD	defined daily doses
	decisional conflict theory		degenerative disk disease
	deep chest therapy		dense deposit disease
	direct (antiglobulin) Coombs test		fully automatic pacing
	dynamic contour tonometry	DDDR	pacemaker code (D = chamber
3D-CT	three-dimensional computed		paced-**d**ual, D = chamber
	tomography		sensed-**d**ual, D = response to
4D-CT	four-dimensional computed		sensing-**d**ual, R =
	tomography		programmability-**r**ate
DCTM	delay computer tomographic		modulation)
	myelography	DDDR-70	dual-chamber rate responsive
DCU	day care unit		pacing at 70/minute
DCUS	duplex-color ultrasonography	DDE	dichlorodiphenylethylene
DCVC	dual-channel virus counter	DDEB	dystrophic epidermolysis bullosa
DCW	direct care worker	DDFS	distant disease free survival
DCYS	Department of Children and Youth	DDGB	double-dose gallbladder (test)
	Services	DDH	developmental dysplasia of the hip
DD	D-dimer	DDHT	double-dissociated hypertropia
	delayed diarrhea	DDI	didanosine (dideoxyinosine; Videx)
	delivery date		dressing dry, intact
	denileukin diftitox (Ontak)	DDIs	drug-drug interactions
	dependent drainage	DDis	developmental disorder
	Descemet detachment	DDiv	Doctor of Divinity
	detrusor dyssynergia	DDLS	dedifferentiated liposarcoma
	developmentally delayed	DDMAC	Division of Drug Marketing,
	developmental disabilities		Advertising and
	developmental dyslexia		Communications (FDA)
	developmentally disabled	DDMC	diabetes disease management
	dialysis dementia		clinic
	died of the disease	DDNS	digestive disease and nutrition
	differential diagnosis		service
	disc diameter	DDP	cisplatin (Platinol)
	discharge diagnosis	DDPS	Detailed Descriptions of
	Doctor of Divinity		Pharmacovigilance Systems
	dose-dense	DDR	direct digital radiography
	double dose (used by Radiology)	DDRA	dead despite resuscitation attempt
	down drain	DDRE	Division of Drug Risk Evaluation
	dry dressing		(FDA)
	dual disorder	DDRUL	dorsal distal radioulnar ligament
	Duchenne dystrophy	DDS	Denys-Drash Syndrome
	due date		dialysis disequilibrium syndrome
	dysthymic disorder		Doctor of Dental Surgery
D/D	diarrhea/dehydration		dopamine dysregulation syndrome
D → D	discharge to duty		double-decidual sac (sign)
D & D	debridement and dressing		

	4, 4-diaminodiphenyl-sulfone (dapsone)	DEFIB	defibrillate
D & Ds	death and doughnuts (morbidity and mortality conferences) (slang)	DEFT	defendant
			driven equilibrium Fourier transform (technique)
DDST	Denver Development Screening Test	DEG	diethylene glycol
		degen	degenerative
DDT	chlorophenothane	DEHP	diethylhexyl phthalate
DDTP	drug dependence treatment program	DEJ	dentin-enamel junction
		DEL	delivered
DDx	differential diagnosis		delivery
DE	dermal epidermal (junction)		deltoid
	digitalis effect	DELM	digital epiluminescence microscopy
	diminished emotionality	DEM	drug evaluation matrix
D_5E_{48}	5% Dextrose and Electrolyte 48	demo	demonstration
D_5E_{75}	5% Dextrose and Electrolyte 75	DEMRI	dynamic enhanced magnetic resonance imaging
2-DE	two-dimensional echocardiography		
	two-dimentional gel electrophoresis		delayed-enhancement magnetic resonance imaging
3-DE	three-dimensional echocardiography	Denver II	Denver Developmental Screening Test - second edition
D&E	dilation and evacuation	DENV	dengue virus
DEA	diethylamine	DEP	dependent
DEA#	Drug Enforcement Administration number (physician's federal narcotic number)	DEPs	diesel exhaust particles
		DEP ST SEG	depressed ST segment
DEAE	diethylaminoethyl	DER	disulfiram-ethanol reaction
DEB	diepoxybutane (test)	DERM	dermatology
	drug eluting bead	DES	desflurane (Supreme)
	dystrophic epidermolysis bullosa		diethylstilbestrol
DEC	deciduous (primary teeth)		diffuse esophageal spasm
	decrease		disequilibrium syndrome
	diethylcarbamazine (Hetrazan)		Dissociative Experience Scale
	Drug Evaluation and Classification (a standardized curriculum to train police officers)		drug-eluting stent
			dry-eye syndrome
			dysfunctional elimination syndrome (urology)
DECA	nandrolone decanoate (Deca-Durabolin)	DESAT	desaturation
DECAFS	Department of Children and Family Services	DESF	desflurane (Suprane)
		DESI	Drug Efficacy Study Implementation
DECEL	deceleration		
DEcIDE	Developing Evidence to Inform Decisions about Effectiveness (centers)	DESS	double-echo steady state (magnetic resonance imaging)
		DET	diethyltryptamine
DECT	dual-energy computed tomography		Dionne Egress Test
decub	decubitus		dipyridamole echocardiography test
DED	diabetic eye disease	DETOX	detoxification
	died in emergency department	DEV	deviation
	dry eye disease		duck embryo vaccine
DEEDS	drugs, exercise, education, diet, and self-monitoring	DEVR	dominant exudative vitreoretinopathy
DEEG	depth electroencephalogram	DEX	dexamethasone
	deteriorating electroencephalogram		dexrazoxane (Zinecard)
DEET	diethyltoluamide		dexter (right)
DEF	decayed, extracted, or filled		dexverapamil
	defecation	DEXA	dual-energy x-ray absorptiometry
	deficiency	DF	day frequency (of voiding)
2-DEF	two-dimensional echo-derived ejection fraction		decayed and filled
			deferred

defibrotide
degree of freedom
dengue fever
dexfenfluramine
diabetic father
diagnostic findings
diastolic filling
dietary fiber
dorsiflexion
drug-free
dye-free

DFA   delayed feedback audiometry
diet for age
difficulty falling asleep
direct fluorescent antibody
distal forearm

DFCI   Dana-Farber Cancer Institute

DFD   defined formula diets
degenerative facet disease

DFE   dilated fundus examination
distal femoral epiphysis

DFG   direct forward gaze

DFI   disease-free interval
diabetic foot infection
Druggan-Forsythe-Iversen (agar)

DFLE   disability-free life expectancy

DFM   decreased fetal movement
deep finger massage
deep friction massage

DFMC   daily fetal movement count

DFMR   daily fetal movement record

DFO   deferoxamine (Desferal)

DFOM   deferoxamine (Desferal)

DFP   diastolic filling period
isoflurophate (diisopropyl
flurophosphate)

DFR   diabetic floor routine
dialysate flow rate (hemodialysis)

DFRC   deglycerolized frozen red cells

DFS   disease-free survival
Division of Family Services
Doppler flow studies

DFSP   dermatofibrosarcoma protuberans

DFT   defibrillation threshold (testing)

DFTD   Tasmanian devil facial tumor
disease

DFU   dead fetus in uterus
diabetic foot ulcer

DFV   D'Aoust Fineman virus
dengue fever vaccine
diarrhea, fever, and vomiting

DFW   Dexide face wash

DFWO   dorsiflexory wedge osteotomy

DFYS   Division of Family and Youth
Services (government agency)

DFX   deferasirox (Exjade)

DG   diagnosis
dorsal glides

---

downward gaze
Duarte galactosemia

DGA   DiGeorge anomaly
disseminated granuloma annulare

DGC   dystrophin-glycoprotein complex

DGE   delayed gastric emptying

DGF   delayed graft function

DGGE   denaturing gradient gel
electrophoresis

DGI   disseminated gonococcal infection

DGL   deglycyrrhizinated licorice

DGR   duodenogastric reflux

DGM   ductal glandular mastectomy

DGS   DiGeorge syndrome

DGs   documentation guidelines

DGT   daughter
decaffeinated green tea

DH   delayed hypersensitivity
Dental Hygienist
Department of Health
dermatitis herpetiformis
developmental history
diaphragmatic hernia

D+H   delusions and hallucinations

D-H   Dimon-Hughston (intertrochanteric
osteotomy technique)

DHA   dihydroxyacetone
docosahexaenoic acid

DHAC   dihydro-5-azacytidine

DHAD   mitoxanthrone HCl (Novantrone)

DHANP   Diplomate of the Homeopathic
Academy of Naturopathic
Physicians

DHAP   dexamethasone, high-dose
cytarabine, (ara-A) cisplatin
(Platinol)
docosahexaenoic acid-paclitaxel

DHA-TP   dihydroartemisinin, trimethoprim,
and piperaquine

DHBV   duck hepatitis B virus

DHCA   deep hypothermia circulatory arrest

DHCC   dihydroxycholecalciferol

DHD   daily hemodialysis
desire for hastened death
dissociated horizontal deviation

DHE   dental health education

DHE 45®   dihydroergotamine mesylate

DHEA   dehydroepiandrosterone

DHEAS   dehydroepiandrosterone sulfate

DHF   dengue hemorrhagic fever
diastolic heart failure

DHFR   dihydrofolate reductase

DHHS   Department of Health and Human
Services

DHI   Dizziness Handicap Inventory
dynamic hyperinflation

DHIC   detrusor hyperactivity with
impaired contractility

D

DHL	diffuse histocytic lymphoma
DHP	dental hygiene program
	dihydropyridine
DHP-1	dehydropeptidase-1
DHPG	ganciclovir
DHPLC	denaturing high-performance liquid chromatography
DHPR	dihydropteridine reductase
DHPS	dihydopteroate synthase
DHR	delayed hypersensitivity reaction
DHS	deoxyhypusine synthase
	Department of Human Services
	duration of hospital stay
	dynamic hip screw
DHST	delayed hypersensitivity test
DHT	dihydrotachysterol (Hytakeral; DHT®)
	dihydrotestosterone
	dissociated hypertropia
	Dobhoff tube
DHTF	Dobhoff tube feeding
DI	(Beck) Depression Inventory
	date of injury
	Debrix Index
	detrusor instability
	diabetes insipidus
	diagnostic imaging
	Disability Index
	dorsal interossei
	drug interactions
D&I	debridement and irrigation
	dry and intact
DIA	diameter
	drug-induced agranulocytosis
	drug-induced amenorrhea
	Drug Information Association
diag.	diagnosis
DIAM	drug-induced aseptic meningitis
DIAP-PERS	(causes of transient incontinence) delirium/confusion, infection, (urinary), atrophic urethritis/vaginitis, pharmaceuticals, psychological, excessive excretion (e.g., CHF, hyperglycemia) restricted mobility, and stool impaction
DIAS	diastolic
DIAS BP	diastolic blood pressure
Diath SW	diathermy short wave
DIAZ	diazepam (Valium)
DIB	disability insurance benefits
DIBC	drug-induced blood cytopenias
DIBD	drug-induced behavioral disinhibition
DIB-R	Diagnostic Interview for Borderlines (personality disorders)-Revised

DIBS	dead-in-bed syndrome
D-IBS	diarrhea-predominant irritable bowel syndrome
DIC	dacarbazine (DTIC-Dome)
	diagnostic imaging center
	differential interference contrast
	disseminated intravascular coagulation
	drug information center
DICC	dynamic infusion cavernosometry and cavernosography
DICE	dexamethasone, ifosfamide, cisplatin, and etopside, with mesna
DICLOX	dicloxacillin (Dynapen)
DICOM	Digital Imaging and Communication in Medicine
DICP	demyelinated inflammatory chronic polyneuropathy
DICT	dose-intensive chemotherapy
DID	death(s) from intercurrent disease
	delayed ischemia deficit
	dissociative identity disorder
	drug-induced disease
di,di	dichorionic, diamniotic
DIE	died in emergency department
	drug-induced esophagitis
DIEA	deep inferior epigastric artery (flap)
DIED	died in emergency department
DIEP	deep inferior epigastric perforator
DIF	differentiation-inducing factor
DIFF	differential blood count
DIFFC	dropped in for friendly chat (no medical problem) (slang)
DIG	digoxin (this is a dangerous abbreviation)
DIH	died in hospital
DIHS	Division of Immigration Health Services
	drug-induced hypersensitivity syndrome
DIJOA	dominantly inherited juvenile optic atrophy
DIL	daughter-in-law
	dilute
	drug-induced lupus
	drug information leaflet
DILC	dose-intensity limiting criterium
DILD	diffuse infiltrative lung disease
	drug-induced liver disease
DILE	drug-induced lupus erythematosus
DILI	drug-induced liver injury
DILS	diffuse infiltrative lymphocytosis syndrome
	drug-induced lupus syndrome
DIM	diindolylmethane

	diminish
D₅IMB	Ionosol MB with 5% dextrose injection
DIMD	drug-induced movement disorders
DIMOAD	diabetes insipidus, diabetes mellitus, optic atrophy, and deafness
DIMS	disorders of initiating and maintaining sleep
DIN	disease impact number
	ductal intraepithelial neoplasia
DIND	delayed ischemic neurologic deficit
DINK	a patient who did not keep (appointment)
DIO	diet-induced obesity
	dorsal interosseus
DIOS	distal ileal obstruction syndrome
	distal intestinal obstruction syndrome
DIP	desquamative interstitial pneumonia
	diphtheria toxoid vaccine
	diplopia
	distal interphalangeal
	drip infusion pyelogram
	drug-induced parkinsonism
	urinalysis dipstick (slang)
DIP$_{ant}$	diphtheria antitoxin
DIPC	dynamic infusion pharmacocavemosometry
DIPJ	distal interphalangeal joint
DIR	directions
DIRD	drug-induced renal disease
DIS	daily interruption of sedation
	Diagnostic Interview Schedule (questionnaire)
	digital imaging spectrophotometer
	dislocation
DISA	disseminated autonomy
DiSA	*Dirofilaria immitis* (heartworm) somatic antigen(s)
DISC	discharge
	disabled infectious single cycle (virus)
	dynamic integrated stabilization chair
DISC-IV	Diagnostic Interview Schedule for Children-Version 4
disch.	discharge
DISCUS	Dyskinesia Indentification System Condensed User Scale
DISH	diffuse idiopathic skeletal hyperostosis
DISI	dorsal intercalated segmental (segment) instability
DISIDA	diisopropyl iminodiacetic acid
D₅ISOM	5% Dextrose and Isolyte M

D₅ISOP	5% Dextrose and Isolyte P
DISR	drug-induced skin reactions
DIST	distal
	distilled
DIT	diiodotyrosine
	drug-induced thrombocytopenia
DIU	death in utero
	diuretic(s)
DIV	double-inlet ventricle
DIVA	digital intravenous angiography
Div ex	divergence excess
DIVP	dilute intravenous Pitocin
DJD	degenerative joint disease
DK	dark
	diabetic ketoacidosis
	diseased kidney
	don't know
DKA	diabetic ketoacidosis
	didn't keep appointment
DKB	deep knee bends
DKC	double knee to chest
	dyskeratosis congenita
DKD	diabetic kidney disease
D-K-S	Damus-Kaye-Stansel (operation/procedure)
DKTC	double-knee to chest (stretch)
DL	danger list
	deciliter (dL; 100 mL)
	diagnostic laparoscopy
	direct laryngoscopy
	drug level
	dual lumen
	ductal lavage
dL	deciliter (100 mL)
D$_L$	maximal diffusing capacity
DLAR	direct low-anterior resection
DLB	dementia with Lewy bodies
	direct laryngoscopy and bronchoscopy
DLBCL	diffuse large B-cell lymphoma
DLBD	diffuse Lewy body disease
DLB&E	direct laryngoscopy, bronchoscopy and esophagoscopy
DLBL	diffuse large B-cell lymphoma
DLC	double-lumen catheter
DLCL	diffuse large cell lymphoma
DLCO sb	diffusion capacity of carbon monoxide, single breath
DLD	date of last drink
	deterministic lateral displacement
DLE	decrement-load exercise
	discoid lupus erythematosus
	disseminated lupus erythematosis
DLEK	deep lamellar endothelial keratoplasty
DLF	digitalis-like factor
	ductal lavage fluid

DLI	donor leukocyte infusions	DMAS	Drug Management and Authorization Section
DLIF	digoxin-like immunoreactive factors	DMAs	data mining algorithms
	direct lumbar interbody fusion	DMAT	disaster medical assistance team
DLIS	digoxin-like immunoreactive substance	dmax	depth of maximum dose
		DMB	data monitoring board
DLMP	date of last menstrual period	DMBA	dimethylbenzanthracene
DLNG	dl-norgestrel	DMC	dactinomycin, methotrexate, and cyclophosphamide
DLNMP	date of last normal menstrual period		data monitoring committee
DLNs	distant lymph nodes		diabetes management center
DLP	dislocation of patella	DMCS	Dyggve-Melchior-Clausen syndrome
	dose-length product (radiology)		
	double-limb progression	DMD	Descemet membrane detachment
DLPD	diffuse lymphocytic poorly differentiated		disciform macular degeneration
			Doctor of Dental Medicine
DLPFC	dorsolateral prefrontal cortex		drowsiness monitoring device
DLQI	Dermatology Life Quality Index		Duchenne muscular dystrophy
D5LR	dextrose 5% in lactated Ringer injection	DMD w/ SRNM	disciform macular degeneration with subretinal neovascular membrane
DLROW	a test used in mental status examinations (patient is asked to spell WORLD backwards)	DME	diabetic macular edema
			Director of Medical Education
DLRT	dogleg radiotherapy		durable medical equipment
DLS	daily living skills	DMEC	data-monitoring and ethics committee
	digitalis-like substances		
	dynamic light scattering	DMEM	Dulbecco Modified Eagle Medium
DLSC	double-lumen subclavian catheter		
DLST	drug-induced lymphocyte stimulation test	DMEPA	Division of Medication Error Prevention and Analysis (FDA)
DLT	dose-limiting toxicity	DMEPOS	durable medical equipment, prosthetics, orthotics, and supplies
	double-lung transplant		
DLTT	dosing least toxic time		
DLU	diffused lung uptake	DMERC	Durable Medical Equipment Regional Carrier
DLV	delavirdine (Rescriptor)		
DLW	doubly labeled water	DMEs	drug-metabolizing enzymes
DM	data management	DMETS	Division of Medication Errors and Technical Support (FDA)
	dehydrated and malnourished		
	dermatomyositis	DMF	decayed, missing, or filled
	dextromethorphan		dimethylformamide
	diabetes mellitus		distant metastases-free
	diabetic mother		Drug Master File
	diastolic murmur	DMFI	distant metastases free interval
	disease management	DMFS	decayed, missing, or filled surfaces
	distant metastases		
DM-1	diabetes mellitus type 1		distant metastases-free survival
DM-2	diabetes mellitus type 2	DMFT	decayed, missing, and filled teeth
DMA	Director of Medical Affairs	DMH	Department of Mental Health
Dmab	denosumab	DMI	desipramine (Norpramin)
DMAC	disseminated *Mycobacterium avium* complex		diabetic muscle infarction
			diaphragmatic myocardial infarction
DMAD	disease-modifying antirheumatic drug	*D immitis*	*Dirofilaria immitis* (heartworm)
DMAE	dimethylaminoethanol	DM Isch	diaphragmatic myocardial ischemia
DMAIC	disseminated *Mycobacterium avium-intracellulare* complex		
		DMKA	diabetes mellitus ketoacidosis
DMARD	disease modifying antirheumatic drug	DMM	destabilization of the medial meniscus

dMMR	defective (deficient) mismatch repair
DMN	dysplastic melanocytic nevus
DMO	dimethadone
DMOADs	disease-modifying osteoarthritis drugs
DMOOC	diabetes mellitus out of control
DMORTs	Disaster Mortuary Operational Response Teams
DMP	data monitoring plan
	dimethyl phthalate
DMPA	depot-medroxypro-gesterone acetate
DMPC	dimyristoylphosphatidyl choline
DMPG	dimyristoylphosphatidyl glycerol
d-MPH	dexmethylphenidate (Focalin)
DMPK	drug metabolism and pharmacokinetics
DMPM	diffuse malignant peritoneal mesothelioma
DMPS	dimercaptopropane-sulfonic acid
D-MRI	dynamic magnetic resonance imaging
DMS	dimethylsulfide
DMSA	succimer (dimercaptosuccinic acid; Chemet)
DMSO	dimethyl sulfoxide
DMT	dimethyltryptamine
DMTU	dimethylthiourea
DMV	difficult mask ventilation
	disk, macula, and vessels
	Doctor of Veterinary Medicine
DMVP	disc, macula, vessel, periphery
DMX	diathermy, massage, and exercise
DN	denuded
	diabetic nephropathy
	dicrotic notch
	down
	dysplastic nevus (nevi)
D & N	distance and near (vision)
D2N	door-to-needle (time)
DNA	deoxyribonucleic acid
	did not answer
	did not attend
	does not apply
DNA ds	deoxyribonucleic acid double-stranded
DNAR	do not attempt resuscitation
DNase	deoxyribonuclease
DNA ss	deoxyribonucleic acid single-stranded
DNCB	dinitrochlorobenzene
DNC	Dermatology Nurse, Certified
	did not come
	dilatation and curettage (usually written as D&C)
DND	died a natural death
DNE	diabetes nurse educator
DNEPTE	did not exist prior to enlistment
DNET	dysembryoplastic neuroepithelial tumor
DNFB	Discharged, No Final Bill (report)
DNFC	does not follow commands
DNI	do not intubate
DNIC	diffuse noxious inhibitory control
DNIF	duties not including flying
DNKA	did not keep appointment
DNMT	DNA (desoxyribonucleic acid) methyltransferase
DNN	did not nurse
DNP	did not pay
	dinitrophenylhydrazine
	do not publish
	dorsal Nail Plate
DNR	daunorubicin
	did not respond
	do not report
	do not resuscitate
	dorsal nerve root
DNR-CC	do not resuscitate – comfort care
DNS	deviated nasal septum
	Director of Nursing Services
	Doctorate, Nursing Science
	doctor did not see patient
	do not show
	dysplastic nevus syndrome
D_5 1/4 NS	dextrose 5% in 1/4 normal saline (0.225% sodium chloride) injection
D_5 1/2NS	dextrose 5% in 0.45% sodium chloride injection
D_5NS	5% dextrose in normal saline (0.9% sodium chloride) injection
DNT	did not test
	dysembryoplastic neuroepithelial tumor
DNV	Det Norske Veritas (certifying organization)
DNW	did not wait
DO	detrusor overactivity
	diet order
	dissolved oxygen
	distocclusal
	distraction osteogenesis
	Doctor of Osteopathy
	doctor's order
D/O	disorder
✓DO	check doctor's order
DO_2	oxygen delivery
DOA	date of admission
	dead on arrival
	dominant optic atrophy
	driver of automobile
	duration of action
DOA-DRA	dead on arrival despite resuscitative attempts

DOB	dangle out of bed	DOSA	day of surgery admission
	date of birth	DOSAK	Central Tumor Registry operated
	Dobrava hantavirus		by the German-Austrian-Swiss
	dobutamine		Association for Head and Neck
	doctor's order book		Tumors
DOC	date of conception	DOSS	docusate sodium (dioctyl sodium
	diabetes out of control		sulfosuccinate)
	Department of Corrections	DOT	date of transcription
	died of other causes		date of transfer
	diet of choice		died on table
	disorders of consciousness		directly observed therapy
	docetaxel (Taxotere)		Directory of Occupational Titles
	drug of choice		Doppler ophthalmic test
	Drug Optimization Clinic	DOTS	directly observed treatment, short
DOCA	desoxycorticosterone acetate		course
DOCP	desoxycorticosterone pivalate	Doughnut	computed tomography (CT)
DOD	date of death		scanner (slang)
	dead of disease	DOV	date of visit
	Department of Defense		distribution of ventilation
	drug overdose	DOW	discharge order written
DODD	demand oxygen delivery device	DOX	doxepin
DOE	date of examination		doxorubicin (Adriamycin)
	disease-oriented evidence	DOXY	doxycycline
	dyspnea on exertion	doz	dozen
DOES	disorders of excessive somnolence	DP	dental prosthesis
DOH	Department of Health		depersonalization
DOI	date of implant (pacemaker)		diastolic pressure
	date of injury		disability pension
	digital object identifier		discharge planning
DO$_2$I	oxygen delivery index		disease progression
DOJ	Department of Justice		docetaxel and cisplatin
DOL	days of life		dorsalis pedis (pulse)
DOL #2	second day of life	D/P	dialysate-to-plasma ratio
DOLV	double-outlet left ventricle	DPA	Department of Public Assistance
DOM	Doctor of Oriental Medicine		dipropylacetic acid
	domiciliary		D-penicillamine (penicillamine;
	domiciliary care		Cuprimine)
DOMS	delayed-onset muscle soreness		dual photon absorptiometry
DON	Director of Nursing		durable power of attorney
	donepezil HCl (Aricept)	DPAP	diastolic pulmonary artery pressure
DONFL	dissociated optic nerve fiber layer	DPB	days postburn
DOOC	diabetes out of control		diffuse panbronchiolitis
DOOR	deafness, onychodystrophy,	DPBS	Dulbecco phosphate-buffered saline
	osteodystrophy, and mental	DPC	delayed primary closure
	retardation (syndrome)		discharge planning coordinator
DOP	degenerate oligonucleotide-primed		distal palmar crease
	dopamine	DPCP	diphenylcyclopropenone
DOPS	diffuse obstructive pulmonary		(diphencyprone)
	syndrome	DPD	dihydropyrimidine dehydrogenase
	dihydroxyphenylserine	DPDL	diffuse poorly differentiated
	Director of Pharmacy Service(s)		lymphocytic lymphoma
DOR	date of release	DPE	Division of Pharmacovigilance and
	duration of response		Epidemiology (FDA)
DORV	double-outlet right ventricle	DPEJ	direct percutaneous endoscopic
DORx	date of treatment		jejunostomy
DOS	date of surgery	DPF	docetaxel, cisplatin, (Platinol) and
	dead on scene		fluorouracil
	doctor's order sheet	2,3-DPG	2,3-diphosphoglyceric acid

DPGN	diffuse proliferative glomerulonephritis		Driver Performance Test
		DPTM	direct patient tumor model
DPH	Department of Public Health	DPTPM	diphtheria, pertussis, tetanus, poliomyelitis, and measles
	diphenhydramine (Benadryl)		
	Doctor of Public Health	DPU	delayed pressure urticaria
	phenytoin (diphenylhydantoin; Dilantin)	DPUD	duodenal peptic ulcer disease
		DPVSs	dilated perivascular spaces
DPI	days postinfection	DPXA	dual-photon x-ray absorptiometry
	dietary protein intake	DQ	developmental quotients
	Doppler perfusion index	D/Q	deep quiet
	dry powder inhaler	D&Q	deep and quiet
	dry powder for inhalation	DQA	Data Quality Audit
DPIL	dextrose (percentage), protein (grams per kilogram) Intralipid® (grams per kilogram)	DQE	detective quantum efficiency (radiology)
		DQM	data quality manager
DPJ	dislocation of prosthetic joint	DQOL	diabetes quality of life
DPL	diagnostic peritoneal lavage	DQOLS	Dermatology Quality of Life Scales
DPLD	diffuse parenchymal lung disease		
D5PLM	dextrose 5% and Plasmalyte M® injection	DQRS	Drug Quality Reporting System (FDA)
DPM	distintegrations per minute (dpm)	Dr	doctor
	Doctor of Podiatric Medicine	DR	delivery room
	drops per minute		diabetic retinopathy
DPN	deep peroneal nerve		diagnostic radiology
	dermatosis papulosa nigra		dining room
	diabetic peripheral neuropathy		diurnal rhythm
	diabetic polyneuropathy		drug resistant
DPNP	diabetic peripheral neuropathic pain	DRA	Deficit Reduction Act of 2005
			distal rectal adenocarcinoma
DPOA	durable power of attorney		drug-related admissions
DPOAE	distortion-product otoacoustic emission	DRAPE	drug-related adverse patient event
		DRC	dose-response curve
DPOAHC	durable power of attorney for health care	DRE	digital rectal examination
			Drug Recognition Expert (for detection of impaired drivers)
DPP	dentine phosphoproteins		
	dorsalis pedal pulse	DREAM	downstream regulatory element antagonistic modulator (gene)
	duration of positive pressure		
DPP-4	dipeptidyl peptidase IV	DRESS	depth resolved surface coil spectroscopy
DPP-IV	dipeptidyl peptidase IV		
DPPC	colfosceril palmitate (dipalmitoylphosphatidylcholine)		drug rash with eosinophilia and systemic symptoms
DPPE	tesmilifene (diethyl phenylmethyl phenoxy ethanamine)	DREZ	dorsal root entry zone
		DRG	diagnosis-related groups
DPR	Department of Professional Regulation		dorsal root ganglia
		DRGE	drainage
	diagnostic procedure room	DRI	defibrillation response interval
DPS	diaphragm pacing stimulation		Dietary Reference Intakes
	disintegration per second		Disability Rating Index
dps	degrees per second		Discharge Readiness Index
DPSS	Department of Public Social Service		dopamine reuptake inhibitor
		DRIL	distal revascularization internal ligation
DPsy	Doctor of Psychology		
DPT	Demerol, Phenergan, and Thorazine (this is a dangerous abbreviation)	DRL	distal residual limb(s)
		DRM	drug-related morbidity
		DRN	dorsal raphe nucleus
	diphtheria, pertussis, and tetanus (immunization)		drug-related neutropenia
		DrotAA	drotrecogin alfa (activated) (Xigris)
	Doctor of Physical Therapy	DRP	data review plan

	drug-related problem
DRPLA	dentatorubral-pallidolluysian atrophy
DRPn	drug-resistant *Streptococcus pneumoniae*
DRPN	diabetic radiculoplexus neuropathy
DRR	digitally reconstructed radiography
	drug regimen review
DRS	Delirium Rating Scale
	designated record set
	Disability Rating Scale
	disease-related symptoms
	Duane retraction syndrome
DRSG	dressing
DRSI	disease-related symptom improvement
DRSP	drug-resistant *Streptococcus pneumoniae*
DRT	drug-related thrombocytopenia
DrTPar	diphtheria toxoid (reduced antigen quantity for adults), tetanus toxoid, and acellular pertussis (reduced antigen quantity for adults) vaccine, for adult use
DRUB	drug screen-blood
DRUJ	distal or radial ulnar joint
dRVVT	diluted Russell viper-venom time
DS	deep sleep
	Dextrostix
	diaphragmatic surgery
	dietary supplement
	discharge summary
	disoriented
	distant supervision
	double-stapled (suture)
	double strength
	Down syndrome
	drug screen
D/S	5% dextrose and 0.9% sodium chloride (saline) injection
%DS	percent diameter stenosis
D&S	diagnostic and surgical
	dilation and suction
D5S	dextrose 5% in 0.9% sodium chloride (saline) injection
D_5-1/2S	5% dextrose in 0.45% sodium chloride (saline) injection
18Ds	Special Operations Forces medics
DSA	digital subtraction angiography (angiocardiography)
	Donor Sperm Archive
DSAEK	descemet stripping and automated endothelial keratoplasty
DSAP	disseminated superficial actinic porokeratosis
DSB	drug-seeking behavior
DSBs	double-strand (DNA) breaks

DSC	differential scanning calorimeter
	Down syndrome child
	dynamic susceptibility contrast
DSD	degenerative spinal disease
	detrusor sphincter dyssynergia
	digital selenium drum (radiology)
	discharge summary dictated
	dry sterile dressing
DSDB	direct self-destructive behavior
ds DNA	double-stranded desoxyribonucleic acid
DSE	dobutamine stress echocardiography
DSF	doxorubicin, streptozocin, and fluorouracil
DSG	desogestrel
DSG	dressing
DSG	deoxyspergualin
DSHEA	Dietary Supplement Health and Education Act of 1994
DSHR	delayed skin hypersensitivity reaction
DSHS	Department of Social and Health Services
DSI	deep shock insulin
	Depression Status Inventory
DSIAR	double-stapled ileoanal reservoir
DSL	desaturated lecithin
DSM	delayed systolic murmur
	disease state management
	drink skim milk
DSM-IV	Diagnostic and Statistical Manual of Mental Disorders, 4th edition
DSM-IV-TR	Diagnostic and Statistical Manual of Mental Disorders 4th Edition—Text Revision
dSMA	distal spinal muscular atrophy
DSMB	Data and Safety Management Board
	Data and Safety Monitoring Board
DSMC	Data Safety and Monitoring Committee
	double-sinus magnetocardiogram
DSME	Diabetes Self Management Education
DSMO	Designated Standard Maintenance Organization
DSMT	Diabetes Self Management Training
DSO	distal subungual onychomycosis
DSP	diabetic sensorimotor polyneuropathy
	digital signal processor
	disseminated superficial porokeratosis
	distal symmetrical polyneuropathy
DSPC	distearoylphosphatidyl choline

DSPD	dangerous severe personality disorder	D & T	diagnosis and treatment dictated and typed
D-SPINE	dorsal spine	DTaP	Diphtheria toxoid, tetanus toxoid, and acellular pertussis vaccine, adsorbed (Daptacel, Infanrix, and Tripedia for active immunization for infants and children under the age of 7 years)
DSPN	distal sensory polyneuropathy distal symmetric polyneuropathy		
DSPS	delayed sleep phase syndrome		
DSRCT	desmoplastic small round cell tumor		
DSRF	drainage subretinal fluid		
dsRNA	double-stranded deoxyribonucleic acid	DTB	door-to-balloon (time)
DSS	dengue shock syndrome	DTBC	tubocurarine (D-tubocurarine)
	Department of Social Services	DTBE	Division of Tuberculosis Elimination
	Disability Status Scale		
	discharge summary sheet	DTC	day treatment center
	disease-specific survival		differentiated thyroid cancer
	distal splenorenal shunt		direct-to-consumer (advertising)
	docusate sodium (dioctyl sodium sulfosuccinate)		disseminated tumor cells
			diticarb (diethyldiothio-carbamate)
DSSLR	double, seated straight leg raise		tubocurarine (D-tubocurarine)
DSSN	distal symmetric sensory neuropathy	DTCA	direct-to-consumer advertising
		DTD	diastropic dysplasia
DSSP	distal symmetric sensory polyneuropathy	DTD #30	dispense 30 such doses
		DTF	deep transverse friction
DSST	Digit-Symbol Substitution Test		Dental Treatment Facility
DST	daylight saving time	DTH	delayed-type hypersensitivity
	dexamethasone suppression test	DTI	deep tissue injury
	digit substitution test		Department of Trade and Industry (United Kingdom)
	donor-specific (blood) transfusion		
DSTO	dog smarter than owner (Veterinary slang)		diffusion-tensor imaging
			Doppler tissue imaging
DSU	day stay unit	DTIC	dacarbazine (DTIC-Dome)
	day surgery unit	D TIME	dream time
DSUH	direct suggestion under hypnosis	DTIs	direct thrombin inhibitors
D/Sum	discharge summary	DTM	deep tissue massage
DSUR	Development Safety Update Report		dermatophyte test medium
DSV	digital subtraction ventriculography	DTMS	drug therapy management service
DSVP	Dietary Supplement Verification Program (United States Pharmacopeia Purity Compliance)	DTO	danger to others
			deodorized tincture of opium (warning: this is NOT paregoric)
DSW	Doctorate in Social Work	DTOGV	dextral-transposition of great vessels
DSWI	deep sternal wound infection		
	deep surgical wound infection	DTP	differential time to positivity
DSX	dysmetabolic syndrome X		diphtheria, tetanus toxoids, pertussis (antigens unspecified) vaccine
DT	deceleration time		
	delirium tremens		
	destination therapy (refers to heart transplantation)		distal tingling on percussion (+Tinel sign)
		DTPA	pentetic acid (diethylenetriaminepentaacetic acid)
	dietary thermogenesis		
	dietetic technician		
	diphtheria and tetanus toxoids, adsorbed, pediatric strength	DTP$_a$	diphtheria, tetanus toxoids, acellular pertussis vaccine, for pediatric use
	discharge tomorrow		
	docetaxel (Taxotere)	DTPa-HIB	diphtheria toxoid, tetanus toxoid, acellular pertussis, and Haemophilus influenzae type b conjugate vaccine
D/T	date/time		
	due to		
d/t	due to		
d4T	stavudine (Zerit)		

DTPa-HIB-IPV	diphtheria toxoid, tetanus toxoid, acellular pertussis, *Haemophilus influenzae* type b conjugate, and poliovirus inactivated vaccine		duration
		DUS	digital ultrasound
			distal urethral stenosis
			Doppler ultrasound stethoscope
			duplex ultrasonography
DTP$_w$	diphtheria, tetanus toxoids, whole-cell pertussis vaccine	3DUS	three-dimensional ultrasound
		DUSN	diffuse unilateral subacute neuroretinitis
DTR	Dance Therapist, Registered		
	deep tendon reflexes	DV	data verification
	Dietetic Technician Registered		distance vision
dtr	daughter		domestic violence
DTs	delirium tremens		double vision
DTS	danger to self	D&V	diarrhea and vomiting
	digital tomosynthesis		disc and vessels
	donor specific transfusion	DVA	Department of Veterans Affairs
3D TSE	three-dimensional turbo-spin echo (images)		directional vacuum-assisted (biopsy)
DTT	diphtheria tetanus toxoid		distance visual acuity
	dithiothreitol		vindesine (Eldisine; desacetyl vinblastine amide sulfate)
DTUS	diathermy, traction, and ultrasound		
DTV	due to void	DVAB	directional vacuum-assisted biopsy
DTVP	Developmental Test of Visual Perception	DVC	direct visualization of vocal cords
		D V® Cream	dienestrol vaginal cream
DTwP	diphtheria and tetanus toxoids with whole-cell pertussis vaccine	DVD	digital video disc
			dissociated vertical deviation
DTX	detoxification		double-vessel disease
DU	decubitus ulcer	DVG	double vein graft
	depleted uranium	DVH	dose-volume histogram
	developmental unit	DVI	atrioventricular sequential pacing
	diabetic urine		digital vascular imaging
	diagnosis undetermined		direct visual inspection
	dialysis unit	DVIU	direct vision internal urethrotomy
	duodenal ulcer	DVLA	Driver and Vehicle Licensing Agency (United Kingdom)
	duroxide uptake		
DUB	Dubowitz (score)	DVPX	divalproex sodium (Depakote)
	dysfunctional uterine bleeding	DVM	Doctor of Veterinary Medicine
DUBI	dysfunctional urinary bladder instability	DVMP	disc, vessels, and macula periphery
DUCL	dorsal ulnocarpal ligament	DVO	distance vision only (glasses prescription)
DUD	dihydrouracil dehydrogenase		
DUE	drug use evaluation		
D&UE	dilation and uterine evacuation	DVP	digital volume pulse
DUF	Doppler ultrasonic flowmeter		divalproex (Depakote)
DUI	driving under the influence	dVP	da Vinci (robotic) prostatectomy
DUID	driving under the influence of drugs	DVPA	daunorubicin, vincristine, prednisone, and asparaginase
DUII	driving under the influence of intoxicants	DVR	Division of Vocational Rehabilitation
DUIL	driving under the influence of liquor		dose-volume relationship
			double-valve replacement
DUKM	dialysate urea kinetic modeling	DVSA	digital venous subtraction angiography
DUM	drug use monitoring		
DUN	dialysate urea nitrogen	DVT	deep vein thrombosis
DUNHL	diffuse undifferentiated non-Hodgkins lymphoma		digital volume tomography
		DVTS	deep venous thromboscintigram
DUO	Duotube®	DVVC	direct visualization of vocal cords
DUR	drug utilization review	DW	daily weight

	deionized water
	detention warrant
	dextrose in water
	diffusion-weighted (imaging)
	distilled water
	doing well
	double wrap
	dry weight (hemodialysis)
D/W	dextrose in water
	discussed with
D-W	Dandy-Walker (deformity/malformation)
	Danis-Weber (classification for ankle fractures)
D₅W	5% dextrose (in water) injection
D10W	10% dextrose (in water) injection
D20W	20% dextrose (in water) injection
D50W	50% dextrose (in water) injection
D70W	70% dextrose (in water) injection
5 DW	5% dextrose (in water) injection
DWD	died with disease
DWDL	diffuse well-differentiated lymphocytic lymphoma
DWI	diffusion-weighted (magnetic resonance) imaging
	driving while intoxicated
	driving while impaired
DWI/PI	diffusion-weighted imaging/ perfusion imaging
DWMRI	diffusion-weighted magnetic resonance imaging
DWR	deep water running
DWRT	delayed work recall test
DWSCL	daily-wear soft contact lens
DWSMB	Dean-Woodcock Sensory Motor Battery (measures of sensory-motor functioning)
DWV	Dandy-Walker variant (a congenital anomaly)
DWW	dynamic wall walk
Dx	diagnosis
	diagnostic evaluation
	disease
DXA	dual-energy x-ray absorptiometry
DXG	dioxalane guanine
DxLS	diagnosis responsible for length of stay
DXM	dexamethasone
	dextromethorphan
DXR	delayed xenograft rejection
DXT	deep x-ray therapy
DXRT	deep x-ray therapy
DXS	Dextrostix®
DY	dusky (infant color)
	dysprosium
DYF	drag your feet (author's note: see you in court)

DYFS	Division of Youth and Family Services
DYRK1A	dual-specificity tyrosine-(Y)-phosphorylation regulated kinase 1A
DysD	dysthymic disorder
DYTRO	dynamic tone-reducing orthosis
DZ	diazepam (valium)
	disease
	dizygotic
	dozen
DZP	diazepam (Valium)
DZT	dizygotic twins
DZX	dexrazoxane (Zinecard)

D

E

E East (as in the location e.g., 2E, would be second floor, East wing)
 edema
 effective
 eloper
 enema
 engorged
 eosinophil
 Escherichia
 esophoria for distance
 ethambutol [part of tuberculosis regimen, see RHZ(E/S)/HR]
 evaluation
 evening
 expired
 eye
 methylenedioxy-methamphetamine (MDMA; Ecstasy)

E′ elbow
 esophoria for near
e- electron
E_1 estrone
E_2 estradiol
E_3 estriol
4E 4 plus edema
E11 Echovirus 11
 embryonic day 11 (11-day-old embryo)
E20 Enfamil 20®
E → A say E,E,E, comes out as A,A,A upon auscultation of lung showing consolidation
EA early amniocentesis
 elbow aspiration
 electroacoustic analysis
 electroacupuncture
 enteral alimentation
 epidermolytic acanthoma
 epidural anesthesia
 episodic ataxia
 esophageal atresia
E/A ratio of peak mitral early diastolic and atrial contraction velocity
 European American
E&A evaluate and advise
EAA electrothermal atomic absorption
 epidural anesthesia and analgesia
 essential amino acids
 extrinsic allergic alveolitis
EAB elective abortion
 Ethical Advisory Board
EAC erythema annulare centrifugum
 esophageal adenocarcinoma
 external auditory canal
EACA aminocaproic acid (epsilon-aminocaproic acid)
 esophageal adenocarcinoma
EADL extended activities of daily living
EADs early after-depolarizations
EAE experimental allergic encephalomyelitis
 experimental autoimmune encephalomyelitis
EAEC enteroaggregative *Escherichia coli*
eAG estimated average glucose
EAggEC enteroaggregative *Escherichia coli*
EAHF eczema, allergy, and hay fever
EAL electronic artificial larynx
EAM external auditory meatus
EAP Early Access Program (premarketing use of drug)
 Employment (Employee) Assistance Programs
 erythrocyte acid phosphatase
 etoposide, doxorubicin (Adriamycin), and cisplatin (Platinol)
EAR estimated average requirement
 excess absolute risk
EARLIES early decelerations
EART extended abdominal radiation therapy
EAR OX ear oximetry
EAS external anal sphincter
EASC endoscopic ambulatory surgery center
EASE Estimation and Assessment of Substance Exposure (model)
EAST external rotation, abduction stress test
EAT Eating Attitudes Test
 ectopic atrial tachycardia
EATL enteropathy-associated T-cell lymphoma
EAU experimental autoimmune uveitis
EB eosinophilic bronchitis
 epidermolysis bullosa
 Epstein-Barr (virus)
EBA enamel bonding agent
 epidermolysis bullosa acquisita
EBB electron beam boosts
 equal breath bilaterally
EBBS equal bilateral breath sounds
EBC early (stage) breast cancer
 endocrine-responsive breast cancer
 endoscopic brush cytology
 esophageal balloon catheter
EBCPGs evidence-based clinical practice guidelines
EBCT electron-beam computed tomography

EBCTCG	Early Breast Cancer Trialists' Collaborative Group
EBD	endocardial border delineation
	endoscopic balloon dilation
	evidence-based decision (making)
EBE	equal bilateral expansion
EBEA	Epstein-Barr (virus) early antigen
EBF	erythroblastosis fetalis
EBG	evidence-based (practice) guidelines
EBL	endoscopic band ligation
	estimated blood loss
EBL-1	European bat lyssavirus 1
EBLA	expected blood loss anemia
EBLV	European bat lyssavirus
EBM	evidence-based medicine
	expressed breast milk
EBMT	European Bone Marrow Transplant (registry group)
EBNA	Epstein-Barr (virus) nuclear antigen
EBO	evidence-based outcomes
EBOS	early-onset benign occipital seizure
EBOV	Ebola virus
EBO-Z	Ebola Zaire virus
EBP	electric breast pump
	epidural blood patch
	evidence-based practice
EBPM	evidence-based prospective memory
EBR	external beam radiotherapy
	eye-blink rate
EBRs	evidence-based recommendations
EBRT	external beam radiation therapy
EBS	empiric Bayesian screening
	epidermolysis bullosa simplex
EBSB	equal breath sounds bilaterally
EBT	electron beam tomography
	erythromycin breath test
EBUS	endobronchial ultrasonography (ultrasound)
EBUS-TBNA	endobronchial ultrasound-guided transbronchial needle aspiration
EBV	Epstein-Barr virus
EBVCA	Epstein-Barr viral capsid antigen
EBVEA	Epstein-Barr virus, early antigen
EBVNA	Epstein-Barr virus, nuclear antigen
EC	ejection click
	electrical cardioversion
	electrocautery
	emergency contraception
	endocervical
	endometrial cancer
	enteric coated
	epirubicin and cyclophosphamide
	Escherichia coli
	esophageal candidiasis
	ethics committee
	etopside and carboplatin
	European Community
	extracellular
	eye care
	eyes closed
E₂C	estradiol cypionate
E & C	education and counseling
ECA	enteric coated aspirin (tablets)
	Epidemiological Catchment Area
	ethacrynic acid
	external carotid artery
ECAD	extracorporeal albumin dialysis
e-CAM	electronic Compilation of Analytical Methods
ECASA	enteric coated aspirin (tablets)
ECBD	exploration of common bile duct
ECBO	enterocytopathogenic bovine orphan (virus)
ECC	early childhood caries
	edema, clubbing, and cyanosis
	embryonal cell cancer
	emergency cardiac care
	Emergency Communications Center
	endocervical curettage
	estimated creatinine clearance
	external cardiac compression
	extracorporeal circulation
ECCE	extracapsular cataract extraction
ECD	electron capture dissociation
	endocardial cushion defect
	equivalent current dipole
	Erdheim-Chester disease
	expanded criteria donor
E-CD	E-cadherin
ECDB	encourage to cough and deep breathe
ECDC	European Centre for Disease Prevention and Control
ECDPC	European Centre for Disease Prevention and Control (EDCD is used)
ECDs	electronic control devices
ECE	endothelin-converting enzyme
	extracapsular extension
ECEMG	evoked compound electromyography
ECF	epirubicin, cisplatin, and fluorouracil
	extended care facility
	extracardiac Fontan (procedure)
	extracellular fluid
ECF-A	eosinophil chemotactic factors of anaphylaxis
ECFV	extracellular fluid volume
ECG	electrocardiogram
ECGE	extracorporeal gas exchange
ECHINO	echinocyte

ECHO	echocardiogram	ECPD	external counterpressure device
	enterocytopathogenic human orphan (virus)	ECPP	extracorporeal photophoresis
		ECR	emergency chemical restraint
	etoposide, cyclophosphamide, doxorubicin (hydroxydaunomycin), and vincristine (Oncovin)		extensor carpi radialis
		E/C Ratio	estriol/creatinine ratio
		ECRB	extensor carpi radialis brevis
		eCRF	Electronic Case Report Form
ECHO (2D)	echocardiogram (2-dimensional)	ECRL	extensor carpi radialis longus
EChoG	electrocochleography	ECS	elective cosmetic surgery
ECHO/RV	echocardiography/ radionuclide ventriculography		electrocerebral silence
			endometrial-cancer-specific
ECI	extracorporeal irradiation	ECSs	elastic compression stockings
ECIB	extracorporeal irradiation of blood	ECT	electroconvulsive therapy
ECIC	external carotid and internal carotid		emission computed tomography
			enhanced computed tomography
	extracranial to intracranial (anastamosis)	ECTb	Emory Cardiac Toolbox
		eCTD	electronic Common Technical Document
EC/IC	extracranial/intracranial		
ECID	European Centre for Infectious Disease	ECTR	endoscopic carpal tunnel release
		ECU	electrocautery unit
ECK1	*Escherichia coli* K1		emergency care unit
ECL	electrochemiluminescence		emotional care units
	enterochromaffin-like		environmental control unit
	extend of cerebral lesion		extensor carpi ulnaris
	extracapillary lesions		eternal care unit (morgue) (slang)
ECLA	extracorporeal lung assist	ECV	emergency center visits
ECLP	extracorporeal liver perfusion		external cephalic version (obstetrics)
ECM	erythema chronicum migrans		
	esophagocardiomyotomy	ECVD	extracellular volume depletion
	extracellular mass	ECVE	extracellular volume expansion
	extracellular matrix	ECVP	extracellular volume depletion (dehydration)
ECM/BCM	extracellular mass, body cell mass ratio		
		ECW	extracellular water
ECMO	enterocytopathogenic monkey orphan (virus)	ECWHSP	Enhanced Coal Workers' Health Surveillance Program (CDC)
	extracorporeal circulation membrane oxygenation (oxygenator)	ECX	epirubicin, cisplatin, and capecitabine (Xeloda)
		ECZ	eczema
ECN	extended care nursery	ED	eating disorder(s)
ecNOS	endothelial constitutive nitric oxide synthetase		education
			effective dose
ECochG	electrocochleography		elbow disarticulation
ECOG	Eastern Cooperative Oncology Group		emergency department
			emotional disorder
ECoG	electrocochleography		energy density
	electrocorticogram		epidural
E coli	*Escherichia coli*		erectile dysfunction
ECO$_{tox}$	*Escherichia coli* (heat-labile toxin) vaccine		ethynodiol diacetate
			every day (this is a dangerous abbreviation)
ECP	effective conduction period		
	emergency care provider		extensive disease
	emergency contraception pills		extensor digitorum
	eosinophil cationic protein	ED$_{50}$	median effective dose
	external counterpulsation	EDA	elbow disarticulation
	extracorporeal photochemotherapy	EDAC	early definitive abdominal closure
	extracorporeal photopheresis		Early Detection of Alcohol Consumption (test)
ECPL	endocavitary pelvic lymphadenectomy		
		EDAM	edatrexate

EDAP	Emergency Department Approved for Pediatrics	EDP	emergency department physician
			end-diastolic pressure
	etoposide, dexamethasone, cytarabine, (Ara-C and cisplatin (Platinol)	EDQ	extensor digiti quinti (tendon)
		EDQM	European Directorate for the Quality of Medicines
EDAS	encephalodural arterio-synangiosis	EDQV	extensor digiti quinti five
EDAT	Emergency Department Alert Team	EDR	edrophonium (Tensilon)
			escalating dose regimen
EDAX	energy-dispersive analysis of x-rays		extreme drug resistance
		EDRF	endothelium derived relaxing factor (nitric oxide)
EDB	ethylene dibromide		
	extensor digitorum brevis	EDS	Ehlers-Danlos syndrome
EDC	effective dynamic compliance		excessive daytime somnolence
	electrodesiccation and curettage	EDSS	Expanded Disability Status Scale (Score)
	electronic data capture		
	end diastolic counts	EDT	exposure duration threshold
	estimated date of conception	EDTA	edetic acid (ethylenedi-aminetetraacetic acid)
	estimated date of confinement		
	estramustine, docetaxel, and carboplatin	EDTU	emergency diagnostic and treatment unit
	extensor digitorum communis	EDU	education
ED&C	electrodesiccation and curettage		eating disorder unit
EDCF	endothelium-derived constricting factor	EDUC	education
		EDV	end-diastolic velocity
EDCP	eccentric dynamic compression plates		end-diastolic volume
			epidermal dysplastic verruciformis
EDCTP	European and Developing Countries Clinical Trials Partnership	EDW	estimated dry weight
		EDX	edatrexate
			electrodiagnostic
EDD	endothelium-dependent dilation		energy-dispersive X-ray (analysis)
	esophageal detector device		
	expected date of delivery	EDXA	energy dispersive X-ray analysis
EdD	Doctor of Education	EDXRF	energy-dispersive x-ray fluorescence
EDENT	edentulous		
EDF	elongation, derotation, and flexion	EE	emetic episodes
EDH	epidural hematoma		emotional exhaustion
	extradural hematoma		end to end
EDHCA	Emergency Department Health Care Assistant		energy expenditure
			equine encephalitis
EDHF	endothelium-derived hyperpolarizing factor		erosive esophagitis
			esophageal endoscopy
EDI	Eating Disorders Inventory		ethinyl estradiol
	electrodeionization		exchange efficiency (units)
EDITAR	extended-duration topical arthropod repellent		expressed emotion
			external ear
EDL	extensor digitorum longus	E & E	eyes and ears
ED/LD	emotionally disturbed and learning disabled	EEA	electroencephalic audiometry
			elemental enteral alimentation
EDLF	endogenous digitalis-like factors		end-to-end anastomosis
EDLS	endogenous digitalis-like substance		energy expended with activity
EDM	early diastolic murmur	EEC	ectrodactyly-ectodermal dysplasia (cleft syndrome)
	esophageal Doppler monitor		
	extensor digiti minimi		endogenous erythroid colony
EDMD-AD	autosomal dominate Emery-Dreifuss muscular dystrophy	EE/CMA	ethinylestradiol/chlormadinone acetate (Belara; not available in the US)
EDNO	endothelium-related nitric oxide		
ED-OU	emergency department/observation unit	EECP	enhanced external counter-pulsation

E

EE/DRSP	ethinylestradiol/drospirenone (Yasmin)		estimated gestational age
		EGB	endoscopic grasp biopsy
EEE	eastern equine encephalomyelitis	EGb	extract of *Ginkgo biloba*
	edema, erythema, and exudate	EGBUS	external genitalia, Bartholin, urethral, and Skene glands
	external eye examination		
EEG	electroencephalogram	EGC	early gastric carcinoma
EELS	electron energy loss spectrometry	EGCG	epigallocatechin gallate
EEN	estimated energy needs	EGFR	epidermal growth factor receptor
EENT	eyes, ears, nose, and throat	eGFR	estimated glomerular filtration rate
EEP	end expiratory pressure	EGD	esophagogastroduodenoscopy
EER	extended endocardial resection	EGDT	early goal-directed therapy
	extraesophageal reflux		esophagogastric devascularization and transection
EERD	extraesophageal reflux disease		
EES	extraosseous Ewing sarcoma	EGF	epidermal growth factor
EES®	erythromycin ethylsuccinate	EGF-R	epidermal growth factor receptor
EET	early exercise testing	EGG	electrogastrography
EEUS-NA	endoscopic esophageal ultrasound-guided needle aspiration	EGJ	esophagogastric junction
		EGL	eosinophilic granuloma of the lung
EEV	encircling endocardial ventriculotomy	EGS	ethylene glycol succinate
		EGSs	external guide sequences
EF	eccentric fixation	EGTA	esophageal gastric tube airway
	ejection fraction		ethyleneglycoltetracetic acid
	endurance factor	EH	eccentric hypertrophy
	erythroblastosis fetalis		educationally handicapped
	extended-field (radiotherapy)		enlarged heart
EFA	essential fatty acid		essential hypertension
	estimated fetal age		extramedullary hematopoiesis
EFAD	essential fatty acid deficiency	Eh	*Entamoeba histolytica*
E-FAP	Emory Functional Ambulation Profile	EHB	elevate head of bed
			extensor hallucis brevis
EFBW	estimate fetal body weight	EHBA	extrahepatic biliary atresia
EFD	episode free day	EHBF	extrahepatic blood flow
EFDA	Expanded Functions Dental Assistant	EHC	enterohepatic circulation
		EHD	electronic home detention
EFE	endocardial fibroelastosis	EHDA	etidronate sodium
	epidemic fatal encephalopathy	EHDP	etidronate disodium (Didronel)
EFF	effacement	EHE	epithelioid hemangioendothelioma
EFI	extended-field irradiation	EHEC	enterohemorrhagic *Escherichia coli*
EFHBM	eosinophilic fibrohistiocytic lesion of bone marrow	EHF	epidemic hemorrhagic fever
			extremely high frequency
EFM	electronic fetal monitor(ing)	EHH	episodic hypothermia with hyperhidrosis
	external fetal monitoring		
EFMM	external fetal maternal monitor		esophageal hiatal hernia
EFMT	electric field mediated transfer	EHI	exertional heat illness
EFN	effusion	EHL	electrohydraulic lithotripsy
EFPIA	European Federation of Pharmaceutical Industries and Associations		extensor hallucis longus
		EHN	ethotoin
		EHO	extrahepatic obstruction
EFR	effective filtration rate	EHP	eosinophilic hepatic pseudotumor(s)
EFRT	extended field radiotherapy		
EFS	event-free survival	EHPH	extrahepatic portal hypertension
EFV	efavirenz (Sustiva)	EHR	electronic health record(s)
EFW	estimated fetal weight	2EHRZ/	daily ethambutol,
EF/WM	ejection fraction/wall motion	6HE	isoniazid, rifampicin, and
EG	ethylene glycol		pyrazinamide for 2 months,
e.g.	for example		followed by isoniazid and
EGA	esophageal gastric (tube) airway		ethambutol for 6 months

2[EHRZ]₃/ the same as 2EHRZ/6HE
6HE   but given three times weekly in
   the initial intensive phase
2EHRZ/ the same as 2EHRZ/6HE,
4HR   followed by 4 months of daily
   isoniazid and rifampicin
EHS Early Head Start (program)
   electrical hypersensitivity
   employee health service
   Engelbreth-Holm-Swarm (tumor)
   exertional heat stroke
EHT electrohydrothermosation
   essential hypertension
EI early intervention
   entry inhibitor
   environmental illness
   enzyme immunoassay
   extensor indicis
E/I expiratory to inspiratory (ratio)
E & I endocrine and infertility
EIA enzyme immunoassay
   exercise-induced asthma
   external iliac artery
EIAB extracranial-intracranial arterial
   bypass
EIAC enzyme-inducing anticonvulsants
EIACD enzyme-inducing anticonvulsant
   drug
EIAD extended-interval aminoglycoside
   dosing
EIAEDs enzyme-inducing antiepileptic
   drugs
EIAV equine infectious anemia virus
EIB exercise-induced bronchospasm
EIC early ischemic change(s)
   electrical impedance cardiography
   endometrial intraepithelial
   carcinoma
   epidermal inclusion cyst
   extensive intraductal component
EICA extra-intracranial artery (bypass)
EID electroimmunodiffusion
   electronic infusion device
EIDs emerging infectious disease
EIDC extreme intervertebral disk collapse
EIEC enteroinvasive *Escherichia coli*
EIL elective induction of labor
EIN Employer Identification Number
   endometrial intraepithelial
   neoplasia
eIND Electronic Investigational New
   Drug (application)
EIOA excessive intake of alcohol
EIP Early Intervention Program
   elective interruption of pregnancy
   end-inspiratory pressure
   extensor indicis proprius

eIPV enhanced inactivated polio vaccine
EIR entomological inoculation rate
EIS electrical impedance scanning
   endoscopic injection scleropathy
EISR expanded international search
   report
EIT electrical impedance tomography
EITB enzyme-linked immuno-
   electrotransfer blot
EIV external iliac vein
EJ ejection
   elbow jerk
   external jugular
EJB ectopic junctional beat
EJN extended jaundice of newborn
EJP excitatory junction potential
EJV external jugular vein
EK Ektachem 400 (see page 356)
   erythrokinase
EKC epidemic keratoconjunctivitis
EKG electrocardiogram
EKO echoencephalogram
EKY electrokymogram
EL elliptical
   encephalitis lethargica
   exercise limit
   exploratory laparotomy
E-L external lids
ELA Establishment License Application
ELAD extracorporeal liver-assist device
ELAFF extended lateral arm free flap
ELAM endothelial leukocyte adhesion
   molecule
ELAMS Electronic Laboratory Animal
   Monitoring System
ELB early light breakfast
   elbow
ELBW extremely low birth weight (less
   than 1000 g)
ELC earlobe creases
ELCA excimer laser coronary angioplasty
ELCPM endoscopic laser cricopharyngeal
   myotomy
ELD end-of-life decision(s)
ELDs end-of-life decisions
ELDU extralabel drug use
ELEC elective
ELF elective low forceps
   endoscopic laser foraminotomy
   epithelial lining fluid
   etoposide, leucovorin, and
   fluorouracil
   extremely low frequency
ELFA enzyme-linked fluorescent
   immunoassay
ELG endolumenal gastroplication
   endoluminal graft

E

ELH	endolymphatic hydrops		endomysial antibody
ELI	endomyocardial lymphocytic infiltrates	EMA-CO	etoposide, methotrexate, dactinomycin (actinomycin-D), cyclophosphamide, and vincristine (Oncovin)
ELIG	eligible		
ELIOT	electron intraoperative treatment		
ELISA	enzyme-linked immunosorbent assay	eMAR	electronic medication administration record
ELISPOT	enzyme-linked immunospot	EMB	endometrial biopsy
ELITT	endometrial laser intrauterine thermal therapy		endomyocardial biopsy eosin-methylene blue (agar) ethambutol (Myambutol) Explanation of Medicare Benefits
Elix	elixir		
ELLIP	ellipotocytosis		
ELM	epiluminescent microscopy	EMBx	endomyocardial biopsy
	external laryngeal manipulation	EMC	encephalomyocarditis
ELM scale-2	Early Language Milestone Scale - second edition		endometrial currettage essential mixed cryoglobulinemia extraskeletal myxoid chondrosarcoma
ELND	elective lymph node dissection		
ELOP	estimated length of program		
ELOS	estimated length of stay	EMD	electromechanical dissociation
ELP	electrophoresis	EMDA	electromotive drug administration
	eruptive lingual papillitis	EMDR	eye movement desensitization and reprocessing
ELPS	excessive lateral pressure syndrome		
ELR	elevating leg rests (wheelchair description)	EME	early myoclonic encephalopathy extreme medical emergency
ELS	Eaton-Lambert syndrome	EMEA	European Medicines Evaluation Agency
	Editor in the Life Sciences		
	endolymphatic sac	EMERG	emergency
ELSD	evaporative light scattering detection	EMF	elective midforceps electromagnetic field(s) electromagnetic flow electromotive forces endomyocardial fibrosis erythrocyte maturation factor evaporated milk formula
ELSI	ethical, legal, and social implications		
ELSIE	Extractables and Leachables Safety Information Exchange		
ELSS	emergency life support system	EMG	electromyograph
ELST	endolymphatic sac tumor		emergency
ELT	endoscopic laser therapy		essential monoclonal gammopathy
	euglobulin lysis time	EMI	educably mentally impaired
ELTR	European Liver Transplant Registry		elderly and mentally infirm
ELVIS™	Enzyme-Linked Virus Inducible System		electromagnetic interference
EM	early memory	EMIC	emergency maternity and infant care
	ejection murmur		
	electron microscope	E-MICR	electron microscopy
	emergency medicine	EMIT	enzyme-multiplied immunoassay technique (test)
	emmetropia		
	eosinophilia-myalgia (syndrome)	EML	essential medicines lists (World Health Organization)
	episodic migraine		
	erythema migrans	EMLA®	eutectic mixture of local anesthetics (lidocaine and prilocaine in an emulsion base)
	erythema multiforme		
	erythromelalgia		
	esophageal manometry	EMLB	erythromycin lactobionate
	estramustine (Emcyt)	EMMA	eye-movement measuring apparatus
	extensive metabolizers		
	external monitor	EMMV	extended mandatory minute ventilation
E/M	Evaluation and Management (coding system)		
		EMo	ear mold
EMA	early morning awakening	EmOC	emergency obstetric care

EMP	electromolecular propulsion	
	estramustine phosphate (Emcyt)	
EMPD	extramammary Paget disease	
EMPI	enterprise master patient index	
EMR	Eastern Mediterranean Region (WHO)	
	educable mentally retarded	
	electrical muscle stimulation	
	electronic medical record	
	emergency mechanical restraint	
	empty, measure, and record	
	endoscopic mucosal resection	
	eye-movement recording	
EMS	early morning specimen	
	early morning stiffness	
	electrical muscle stimulation	
	emergency medical services	
	eosinophilia myalgia syndrome	
EMSA	electrophoretic mobility shift assay	
EMSU	early morning specimen of urine	
EMT	emergency medical technician	
	epithelial-mesenchymal transformation (transition)	
	estramustine (Emcyt)	
EMTA	Emergency Medical Technician, Advanced	
EMTALA	Emergency Medical Treatment and Active Labor Act	
EMTC	emergency medical trauma center	
EMT-D	emergency medical technician-defibrillation	
EMTP	Emergency Medical Technician, Paramedic	
EMU	early morning urine	
	electromagnetic unit	
	epilepsy monitoring unit	
EMV	equine morbilli virus	
	eye, motor, verbal (grading for Glasgow Coma Scale)	
EMVC	early mitral valve closure	
EMW	electromagnetic waves	
EMZL	extranodal marginal-zone (B-cell) lymphoma	
EN	each nostril	
	enema	
	enteral nutrition	
	erythema nodosum	
E/N	eggnog	
E 50% N	extension 50% of normal	
ENA	extractable nuclear antigen	
ENB	esthesioneuroblastoma	
ENC	encourage	
eNDA	Electronic New Drug Application	
ENDO	endodontia	
	endodontics	
	endoscopy	

	endotracheal
EndoCAB	plasma antiendotoxin core antibody
ENF	Enfamil
ENF c̄ Fe	Enfamil with iron
ENG	electronystagmogram
	engorged
ENL	enlarged
	erythema nodosum leprosum
ENMG	electroneuromyography
ENMT	ears, nose, mouth, and throat
ENOG	electroneurography
eNOS	endothelial nitric oxide synthase
ENP	extractable nucleoprotein
ENRD	endoscopy-negative reflux disease
ENS	enteric nervous system
	exogenous natural surfactant
ENT	ears, nose, throat
ENTIS	European Network of Teratology Information Services
ENTV	enzootic nasal tumor virus
ENUP	European Network of Uropathology
ENV	environment
ENVD	elevated new vessels on the disk
ENVE	elevated new vessels elsewhere
ENVT	environment
ENZ	enzastaurin
EO	early onset
	elbow orthosis
	embolic occlusion
	eosinophilia
	ethylene oxide
	eyes open
e/o	evidence of
E & O	errors and omissions
EOA	erosive osteoarthritis
	esophageal obturator airway
	examine, opinion, and advice
	external oblique aponeurosis
EOAD	early-onset Alzheimer disease
EOAE	evoked otoacoustic emissions
EOB	edge of bed
	end of bed
	explanation of benefits
EOC	Emergency Operations Center
	enema of choice
	epithelial ovarian cancer
EOD	early-onset disease
	end of day
	end organ damage
	every other day (this is a dangerous abbreviation)
	extent of disease
EOE	Equal Opportunity Employer
EOFAD	early-onset form of familial Alzheimer disease

E

123

E of I	evidence of insurability	EPCA	early prostate cancer antigen
EOG	electro-oculogram	Ep-CAM	epithelial cell adhesion molecule
	electro-olfactogram	EPCs	endothelial progenitor cells
	Ethrane, oxygen, and gas (nitrous		Evidence-based Practice Centers
	oxide)	EPCV	engineering, procurement,
EOGBS	early-onset group B streptococcal		construction, and validation
	(sepsis)	EPD	electrode placement device
EOIT	end of initial treatment		equilibrium peritoneal dialysis
EOLC	end-of-life-care	EPDS	Edinburgh Postnatal Depression
EOM	error of measurement		Scale
	external otitis media	EPEC	enteropathogenic *Escherichia coli*
	extraocular movement	EPEG	etoposide (VePesid)
	extraocular muscles	EPEs	extrapyramidal effects
EOMB	explanation of Medicare benefits	EPF	endoscopic plantar fasciotomy
EOMG	early-onset myasthenia gravis		Enfamil Premature Formula®
EOMI	extraocular movements intact		extrapyramidal features
	extraocular muscles intact	EPG	electronic pupillography
EOO	external oculomotor		Episodic Payment Group
	ophthalmoplegia	EPHI	electronic protected health
EOP1	end-of-phase 1		information
EOP2	end-of-phase 2	EPI	echoplanar imaging
EOR	emergency operating room		epinephrine
	end of range		epirubicin (Ellence)
EORA	elderly onset rheumatoid arthritis		epitheloid cells
EORTC	European Organization for		exercise pressure index
	Research and the Treatment of		exocrine pancreatic insufficiency
	Cancer		Expanded Program of
EORTC	European Organisation for		Immunizations, (World Health
QLQ C30	Research and Treatment of		Organization)
	Cancer Quality of Life		Eysenck Personality Inventory
	Questionnaire	EPIC	etoposide, prednisolone,
EOS	end of session		ifosfamide, and cisplatin
	end of study	EPID	epidural
	eosinophil	EPIDs	electronic portal imaging devices
EP	ectopic pregnancy	epiDX	epirubicin (4′-epidoxorubicin;
	electronic prescribing		Ellence)
	electrophysiologic	EPIG	epigastric
	elopement precaution	EPIS	epileptic postictal sleep
	endogenous pyrogen		episiotomy
	Episcopalian	epith.	epithelial
	esophageal pressure	EPL	effective patent life
	etoposide and cisplatin (Platinol)		extensor pollicis longus (tendon)
	evoked potentials	EPM	electronic pacemaker
E&P	estrogen and progesterone	EPMR	electronic patient medical record
EPA	eicosapentaenoic acid	EPN	emphysematous pyelonephritis
	Environmental Protection Agency		ependymoma
EPAB	extracorporeal pneumoperititoneal		estimated protein needs
	access bubble	EPO	epoetin alfa (erythropoietin;
E-Panel	electrolyte panel (See page 356)		Epogen)
EPAP	expiratory positive airway		evening primrose oil
	pressure		exclusive provider organization
EPB	extensor pollicis brevis	EPOCH	etoposide, prednisone, vincristine
EPBD	endoscopic papillary balloon		(Oncovin), cyclophosphamide,
	dilatation		doxorubicin
EPC	emergency protective custody		(hydroxydaunorubicin)
	erosive prephloric changes	EPP	erythropoietic protoporphyria
	external pneumatic compression		extrapleural pneumonectomy

E

EPPID	electronic positive patient and specimen identification	ER+	estrogen receptor-positive
EPPK	epidermolytic palmoplantar keratoderma	ER−	estrogen receptor-negative
		ERA	environmental risk assessment
EPPROM	extremely preterm premature rupture of the membranes (less than or equal to 24 weeks)		estrogen receptor assay
			evoked response audiometry
		%ERAD	eradication rates
EPQ	Exercise Participation Questionnaire	ERAS	Electronic Residency Application Service
EPQ-R	Eysenck Personality Questionnaire—Revised		enhanced recovery after surgery (protocols)
EPR	electronic prescription record	erbB1	estrogen receptor (tyrosine kinase family) type B1
	electron paramagnetic (spin) resonance	ERBD	endoscopic retrograde biliary drainage
	electrophrenic respiration	ERbeta	estrogen receptor beta
	emergency physical restraint	ER by ICA	estrogen receptor immunocytochemistry assay
	epirubicin (Ellence)		
	estimated protein requirement	ERC	endoscopic retrograde cholangiography
	expiratory pressure relief		
EPS	electrolyte-polyethyleneglycol solution	ERCC-1	excision repair cross-complementation group 1
	electrophysiologic study	ERCP	endoscopic retrograde cholangiopancreatography
	expressed prostatic secretions		
	extrapulmonary shunt	ERCT	emergency room computerized tomography
	extrapyramidal syndrome (symptom)		
		ERD	early retirement with disability
EPSA	evoked potential signal averaging		erectile dysfunction
EPSCCA	extrapulmonary small cell carcinoma	ERDP	extended-release dipyridamole
		ERE	external rotation in extension
EPSDT	early periodic screening, diagnosis, and treatment	EREM	extended-release epidural morphine
EPSE	extrapyramidal side effects	ERF	external rotation in flexion
EPSP	excitatory postsynaptic potential	ERFC	erythrocyte rosette forming cells
EPSS	E point septal separation	ERG	electroretinogram
EPT	electroporation therapy	ERI	elective replacement indicator
	endpoint temperature	ERIG	equine-rabies immune globulin
EPT®	early pregnancy test	ERL	effective refractory length
EPTE	existed prior to enlistment	ERLND	elective regional lymph node dissection
EPTS	existed prior to service		
EPV	events/person-year	ERM	epiretinal membrane
eq	equal	ERMBT	erythromycin breath testing
EQC	equivalent quality control	ERMS	embryonal rhabdomyosarcoma
EQ-5D	European Quality of life scale (EuroQol-5) (includes single item measures of: mobility, self-care, usual activities, pain/discomfort, and anxiety/depression)		exacerbating-remitting multiple sclerosis
		ERN	error-related negativity (signal)
		ERNA	equilibrium radionuclide angiocardiography
		ERO	effective regurgitant orifice (cardiology)
equip	equipment		
ER	emergency room	EROS	event-related optical signal
	end range	ERP	effective refractory period
	estrogen receptors		emergency room physician
	extended release		endocardial resection procedure
	external resistance		endoscopic retrograde pancreatography
	external rotation		
E & R	equal and reactive		event-related potentials
	examination and report		estrogen receptor protein

E

exposure and ritual prevention

ERPF   effective renal plasma flow

ER/PR   estrogen receptor/progesterone receptor

ERRT   Exposure, Relaxation, and Rescripting Therapy

ERS   endoscopic retrograde sphincterotomy

evacuation of retained secundines (afterbirth)

extended, rotated, side bent (position of the spine)

ERSR   Electronic Regulatory Submission and Review

ERS-TM   Event Reporting System - Transfusion Medicine

ERT   estrogen replacement therapy

external radiotherapy

ERTD   emergency room triage documentation

ERUS   endorectal ultrasound

ERV   early revascularization

expiratory reserve volume

e-Rx   electronic prescription

Er:YAG   Erbium: yttrium aluminum garnet (laser)

ERYTH   erythromycin

ES   electrical stimulation

Eleutherococcus senticosus (Siberian Ginseng)

embryonic stem (cells)

emergency service

endoscopic sclerotherapy

endoscopic sphincterotomy

end-to-side

epileptic seizure(s)

ever-smokers

Ewing sarcoma

excessive sleepiness

ex-smoker

extra strength

ESA   early systolic acceleration

end-to-side anastomosis

ethmoid sinus adenocarcinoma

ESADDI   estimated safe and adequate daily dietary intake

ESAP   evoked sensory (nerve) action potential

ESAS   Edmonton Symptom Assessment System

ESAs   erythropoietin-stimulating agents

ESAT   extrasystolic atrial tachycardia

ESBL   extended-spectrum beta-lactamases

ESBLKP   extended-spectrum beta-lactamase-producing *Klebsiella pneumoniae*

ESC   embryonic stem cells

end systolic counts

ESCAPE   hospital antibiotic resistant pathogens (*Enterococcus faecium, Staphylococcus aureus, Clostridium difficile, Acinetobacter baumannii, Pseudomonas aeruginosa, and Enterobacteriaceae*)

ESCC   epidural spinal cord compression

esophageal squamous cell carcinoma

ESCOP   European Scientific Cooperative on Phytotherapy

ESCS   electrical spinal cord stimulation

ESD   early supported discharge

Emergency Services Department

endoscopic submucosal dissection

esophagus, stomach, and duodenum

ESE   exon splice enhancer

ES EOC   early-stage epithelial ovarian cancer

ESES   electrical status epilepticus during sleep

eSET   elective single embryo transfer

ESF   external skeletal fixation

ESFT   Ewing sarcoma family of tumors

ESH   endoscopic saphenous (vein) harvest

ESHAP   etopside, methylprednisolone (Solu-Medrol), high-dose cytarabine (ara-C), and cisplatin (Platinol)

ESI   electric source imaging

electrospray ionization

epidural steroid injection

ESI-MS   electrospray ionization-mass spectrometry

ESIN   elastic stable intramedullary nailing

ESKAPE   hospital antibiotic resistant pathogens (*Enterococcus faecium, Staphylococcus aureus, Klebsiella pneumoniae, Acinetobacter baumannii, Pseudomonas aeruginosa, and Enterobacter species*)

ESKD   end-stage kidney disease

ESL   English as a second language

ESLD   end-stage liver disease

end-stage lung disease

ESM   ejection systolic murmur

endolymphatic stromal myosis

ethosuximide (Zarontin)

ESMO   European Society of Medical Oncology

ESN   educationally subnormal

ESN(M)   educationally subnormal-moderate

ESN(S)   educationally subnormal-severe

ESO	esophagus		enterostomal therapy (therapist)
	esotropia		epirubicin and paclitaxel (Taxol)
ESO/D	esotropia at distance		esotropia
ESO/N	esotropia at near		essential thrombocythemia
ESP	endometritis, salpingitis, and peritonitis		essential tremor
	end-systolic pressure		eustachian tube
	especially		evaluation and treatment
	extrasensory perception		Ewing tumor
ESPAC	European Study Group for Pancreatic Cancers		exchange transfusion
			exercise treadmill
ES/PNET	Ewing sarcomas and peripheral neuroectodermal tumor		exposure time
		et	and
ESR	early sheath removal	ET′	esotropia at near
	electron spin resonance	E & T	evaluation and treatment
	erythrocyte sedimentation rate	E/T	evaluation and treatment
ESRD	end-stage renal disease	E(T)	intermittent esotropia at infinity
ESRF	end-stage renal failure	E(T′)	intermittent esotropia at near
ESRS	Extrapyramidal Symptom Rating Scale	ET-1	endothelin-1
		2ET	two embryo transfer
ESS	elastic scattering spectroscopy	ET @ 20′	esotropia at 6 meters (infinity)
	emotional, spiritual, and social	ETA	endotracheal airway
	endometrial stromal sarcoma		estimated time of arrival
	endoscopic sinus surgery		ethionamide (Trecator-SC)
	English springer spaniels	ETAAS	electrothermal atomic absorption spectrometry
	Epworth Sleepiness Scale		
	essential	ETAC	early treatment of the allergic child
	euthyroid sick syndrome	*et al*	and others
EST	early stent thrombosis	ETBD	etiology to be determined
	Eastern Standard Time	EtBr	ethidium bromide
	Emotional Stroop Task	ETC	and so forth
	endodermal sinus tumor		ecarin clotting time
	endoscopic spincterotomy		electrothermal capsulorrhaphy
	electroshock therapy		Emergency and Trauma Center
	electrostimulation therapy		endoscopic tissue culture
	established patient		epirubicin, paclitaxel (Taxol), and cyclophosphamide
	estimated		
	exercise stress test		esophageal-tracheal Combitube
	expressed sequence tag		estimated time of conception
E-stim	electrical stimulation	ETCH-C	Evaluation Tool of Children's Handwriting-Cursive
ESTS	extremity soft tissue sarcoma		
ESTs	expressed sequence tags	ETCO$_2$	end-tidal carbon dioxide
ESU	electrosurgical unit	ETD	electron transfer dissociation
ESWL	extracorporeal shock wave lithotripsy		endoscopic transformational diskectomy
ESWT	extracorporeal shockwave therapy		eustachian tube dysfunction
			eye-tracking dysfunction
ESZ	eszopiclone (Lunesta)	ETDLA	esophageal-tracheal double lumen airway
ET	ejection time		
	electron tomography	ETE	end-to-end
	embryo transfer		extrathyroidal extension
	endocrine therapy	ETEC	enterotoxigenic *Escherichia coli*
	endometrial thickness	ETF	early treatment failure
	endothelin		eustachian tubal function
	endotoxin	ETFN	empiric therapy in a febrile neutropenic (patient)
	endotracheal		
	endotracheal tube	ETG	Episodic Treatment Group
	endurance training	EtG	ethyl glucuronide

E

ETGT	equal to or greater than		extrauterine pregnancy
ETH	elixir terpin hydrate	EuroSIDA	a prospective observational cohort
	ethanol		study to assess the impact of
	Ethrane		antiretroviral drugs on the
ETHc̄C	elixir terpin hydrate with codeine		outcome of the general
ETI	ejective time index		population of 14,200 patients
	endotracheal intubation		HIV-infected patients living in
ETKTM	every test known to man		Europe
ETL	echo train length (radiology)	EUS	endoscopic ultrasonography
ETLE	extratemporal lobe epilepsy		esophageal ultrasound
ETLT	equal to or less than		external urethral sphincter
ETO	estimated time of ovulation	EUS-FNA	endoscopic ultrasonography with
	etoposide (VePesid)		fine-needle aspiration
	eustachian tube obstruction	EUTH	euthanasia
EtO	ethylene oxide	EV	epidermodysplasia verruciformis
EtOH	alcohol (ethyl alcohol)		esophageal varices
	alcoholic		etoposide and vincristine
ETOP	elective termination of pregnancy		eversion
ETP	elective termination of pregnancy	eV	electron volt (unit of radiation
	electronic transmission of		energy)
	prescriptions	EV71	enterovirus-71
ETS	elevated toilet seat	EVA	Entry and Validation Application
	endoscopic transthoracic		ethylene vinyl acetate
	sympathectomy		etoposide, vinblastine, and
	endotracheal suction		doxorubicin (Adriamycin)
	end-to-side	EVAC	evacuation
	environmental tobacco smoke	EVAc	ethylene-vinyl acetate copolymer
	erythromycin topical solution	eval	evaluate (evaluation)
ETS®	urine drug screen for six drugs of	EVAR	endovascular aneurysm repair
	abuse	EVBL	esophageal variceal bleeding
ETT	endotracheal tube	EVC	Ellis-van Creveld (syndrome)
	endurance treadmill test	EVD	external ventricular
	esophageal transit time		(ventriculostomy) drain
	exercise tolerance test		extraventricular drain
	exercise treadmill test (time)	EVE	endoscopic vascular examination
	extrathyroidal thyroxine		evening
ETT-Tl	exercise treadmill test with	EVER	eversion
	thallium	EVG	endovascular grafting
ETU	emergency and trauma unit	EVH	endoscopic (saphenous) vein
	emergency treatment unit		harvesting
ETV	endoscopic third ventriculostomy	EVI	Exposure to Violence Interview
ETX	edatrexate	EVL	endoscopic variceal ligation
ETYA	eicosatetraynoic acid	EVLT	endovenous laser therapy
EU	Ehrlich units	EVS	electronic vessel sealing
	endotoxin units		endoscopic variceal sclerosis
	equivalent units	EVT	endovascular therapy
	esophageal ulcer	EVUS	endovaginal ultrasound
	etiology unknown	EW	expiratory wheeze
	European Union		elsewhere
	excretory urography	EWB	emotional well-being
EUA	examine under anesthesia		estrogen withdrawal bleeding
EUCD	emotionally unstable character	EWBH	extracorporeal whole body
	disorder		hyperthermia
EUD	external urinary device	EWCL	extended-wear contact lens
EUG	extrauterine gestation	EWDs	Ethnic Word Descriptors
EUL	extra uterine life	EWE	Eastern and Western
EUM	external urethral meatus		encephalomyelitis vaccine
EUP	Experimental Use Permit	EWG	Expert Working Group

E

EWHO	elbow-wrist-hand orthosis
EWL	estimated weight loss
EWS	Early Warning Score
	Ewing sarcoma
EWSCLs	extended-wear soft contact lenses
EWT	erupted wisdom teeth
ex	examined
	example
	excision
	exercise
exam	examination
ExB	excisional biopsy
EXC	excision
EXE	exemestane (Aromasin)
EXEC 22	Executive 22 chemistry profile (see page 356)
EXECHO	exercise echocardiography
EXEF	exercise ejection fraction
EXGBUS	external genitalia, Bartholin (glands), urethral (glands), and Skene (glands)
EXH VT	exhaled tidal volume
EXIT	Ex-Utero Intrapartum Treatment
EXIT 25	Executive Interview (cognitive impairment test)
EXL	elixir
EXOPH	exophthalmos
EXP	experienced
	expired
	exploration
	expose
expect	expectorant
exp lap	exploratory laparotomy
EXT	extension
	extensor (tendon)
	external
	extract
	extraction
	extremities
	extremity
Ext mon	external monitor
extrav	extravasation
ext. rot.	external rotation
EXTUB	extubation
EX U	excretory urogram
EZ	Edmonston-Zagreb (vaccine)
EZ-HT	Edmonston-Zagreb high-titer (vaccine)

F

F	facial
	Fahrenheit
	fair
	false
	fasting
	father
	feces
	female
	finger
	firm
	flow
	fluoride
	French
	Friday
	fundi
	fundus
	phenylalanine (also referred to as Phe)
F/	full upper denture
/F	full lower denture
(F)	final
°F	degrees Fahrenheit
F=	firm and equal
F_1	offspring from the first generation
F_2	offspring from the second generation
F_3	Fluothane
14 F	14-hour fast required
F II-F XIII	factor 2 through 13
FA	Fanconi anemia
	fatty acid
	femoral acetabular
	femoral artery
	fetus active
	fibroadenoma
	first aid
	flip angle (radiology)
	fludarabine (Fludara)
	fluorescein angiogram
	fluorescent antibody
	folic acid
	folinic acid (leucovorin calcium) (this is a dangerous abbreviation)
	forearm
	Friedreich ataxia
	functional activities
Fa	father
FAA	febrile antigen agglutination
	folic acid antagonist
FAAAAI	Fellow of the American Academy of Allergy, Asthma & Immunology

FAAD	Fellow American Academy of Dermatology	FACEM	Fellow of the American College of Emergency Medicine
FAAH	fatty acid amide hydrolase	FACEP	Fellow of the American College of Emergency Physicians
FAAM	Functional Ankle Ability Measure		
FAAMT	Fellow of the American Association for Medical Transcription	FACES	pain scale for assessing pain intensity
FAAN	Food Allergy and Anaphylaxis Network	FACG	Fellow of the American College of Gastroenterology
FAAP	family assessment adjustment pass	FACH	forceps to after-coming head
FAAPM	Fellow, American Academy of Pain Management	FACHE	Fellow of the American College of Healthcare Executives
FAA SOL	formalin, acetic, and alcohol solution	FACIT-F	Functional Assessment of Chronic Illness Therapy Fatigue Subscale
FAAN	Fellow of the American Academy of Nursing	FACLM	Fellow of the American College of Legal Medicine
FAAP	Fellow of the American Academy of Pediatrics	FACN	Fellow of the American College of Nutrition
FAB	digoxin immune Fab (Digibind) French-American-British Cooperative group functional arm brace	FACNP	Fellow of the American College of Neuropsychopharmacology
		FACO	Fellow of the American College of Otolaryngology
FABACs	fatty acid bile acid conjugates	FACOG	Fellow of the American College of Obstetricians & Gynecologists
FABER	flexion, abduction, and external rotation	FACOS	Fellow of the American College of Orthopedic Surgeons
FABF	femoral artery blood flow		
FABIANS	Felt awful but I'm alright now syndrome (slang)	FACP	Fellow of the American College of Physicians
FAC	ferrite ammonium citrate fluorouracil, doxorubicin (Adriamycin), and cyclophosphamide	FACPRM	Fellow of the American College of Preventive Medicine
		FACR	Fellow of the American College of Radiology
	fractional area change fractional area concentration functional aerobic capacity	FACS	Fellow of the American College of Surgeons fluorescent-activated cell sorter
FACA	Fellow of the American College of Anaesthetists	FACSM	Fellow of the American College of Sports Medicine
FACAG	Fellow of the American College of Angiology	FACT	focused appendix computed tomography
FACAL	Fellow of the American College of Allergists	FACT-An	Functional Assessment of Cancer Therapy-Anemia
FACAN	Fellow of the American College of Anesthesiologists	FACT-B	....-Breast
		FACT-F	....-Fatigue
FACAS	Fellow of the American College of Abdominal Surgeons	FACT-G	....-General
		FACT-L	.....-Lung
FACC	Fellow of the American College of Cardiology	FACT-O	....-Ovarian
		FACT-P	....-Prostate
FACCP	Fellow of the American College of Chest Physicians	FAD	familial Alzheimer disease Family Assessment Device fetal abdominal diameter fetal activity determination flavin adenine dinucleotide
FACCPC	Fellow of the American College of Clinical Pharmacology & Chemotherapy		
		FADI	Foot and Ankle Disability Index
FACD	Fellow of the American College of Dentists	FADS	fetal akinesia deformation sequences
FACE	Fatality Assessment and Control Evaluation (National Institute for Occupational Safety and Health report)	FAE	fetal alcohol effect
		FAEE	fatty acid ethyl ester
		FAF	frequency-altered feedback

F

FAFSA	Free Application for Federal Student Aid	FAST	facial droop, **a**rm weakness, **s**lurred speech, and **t**ime to call 911 (mnemonic to help recognize and act on seeing stroke symptoms)	
FAGA	full-term appropriate for gestational age			
FAH	fumarylacetoacetase hydrolase		fetal acoustic stimulation testing	
FAI	Functional Assessment Inventory		flow-assisted short-term	
FAK	focal adhesion kinase		fluorescent allergosorbent technique	
FAL	femoral arterial line			
FALL	fallopian		focused assessment with sonography for trauma	
FALS	familial amyotrophic lateral sclerosis			
FAM	family	FAT	Fetal Activity Test	
	fluorouracil, doxorubicin (Adriamycin), and mitomycin		fluorescent antibody test	
			food awareness training	
	full allosteric modulators	FATSAT	fat saturation	
FAMA	fluorescent antibody to membrane antigen	FAV	facio-auricular vertebral	
		FAVD	forceps-assisted vaginal delivery	
FAME	fluorouracil, doxorubicin (Adriamycin), and semustin (methyl CCNU)	FAZ	foveal avascular zone	
		FB	fasting blood (sugar)	
			finger breadth	
FAMMM	familial atypical multiple mole melanoma		flexible bronchoscope	
			foreign body	
FAM-S	fluorouracil, doxorubicin (Adriamycin), mitomycin, and streptozotocin	F/B	followed by	
			forward/backward	
			forward bending	
FAMTX	fluorouracil, doxorubicin (Adriamycin), and methotrexate	FBC	full (complete) blood count	
		FBCOD	foreign body, cornea, right eye	
FANA	fluorescent antinuclear antibody	FBCOS	foreign body, cornea, left eye	
FANG	fluorescent angiography	FBD	familial British dementia	
FANSS&M	fundus anterior, normal size and shape and mobile		fibrocystic breast disease	
			functional bowel disease	
FAO	fatty acid oxidation	FBF	forearm blood flow	
	Food and Agriculture Organization	FBG	fasting blood glucose	
			foreign-body-type granulomata	
FAOS	Foot and Ankle Outcome Score	FBH	hydroxybutyric dehydrogenase	
FAP	Facility Admission Profile	FBHH	familial benign hypocalciuric hypercalcemia	
	familial adenomatous polyposis			
	familial amyloid polyneuropathy	FBI	flossing, brushing, and irrigation	
	femoral artery pressure		full bony impaction	
	fibrillating action potential	FBL	fecal blood loss	
	functional ambulation profile	FBM	felbamate (Felbatol)	
FAQ	frequently asked question(s)		fetal breathing motion	
FAR	frontal arousal rhythm		foreign body, metallic	
F-ara-A	fludarabine phosphate (Fludara)	FBO	for the benefit of	
f-ARPV	fosamprenavir (Lexiva)	FBP	frontal bite plane (dental)	
FARS	Fatality Analysis Reporting System	FBRCM	fingerbreadth below right costal margin	
FAS	fetal alcohol syndrome			
	foreign accent syndrome	FBS	failed back syndrome	
FASAY	functional analysis of separated alleles in yeast		fasting blood sugar	
			fetal bovine serum	
FASC	fluorescent-activated substrate conversion (assay)		foreign body sensation (eye)	
		FBSS	failed back surgery syndrome	
	fasciculations	FBU	fingers below umbilicus	
FASD	fetal alcohol spectrum disorder	FBW	fasting blood work	
FASHP	Fellow of the American Society of Health-System Pharmacists	FC	family conference	
			febrile convulsion	
FASPS	familial advanced sleep-phase syndrome		female child	
			fever, chills	

F

	film coated (tablets)		flow cytometry
	financial class		Foley criteria met
	finger clubbing	FCMC	family centered maternity care
	finger counting	FCMD	Fukiyama congenital muscular
	flexion contractor		dystrophy
	flow compensation (radiology)	FCMN	family centered maternity nursing
	flucytosine (Ancobon)	FCNV	fever, cough, nausea, and vomiting
	foam cuffed (tracheal or	FCOU	finger count, both eyes
	endotracheal tube)	FCP	formocresol pulpotomu
	Foley catheter	FCR	flexor carpi radialis
	follows commands		fractional catabolic rate
	foster care	FCRB	flexor carpi radialis brevis
	French Canadian	FCRT	fetal cardiac reactivity test
	functional capacity		focal cranial radiation therapy
	functional class	FCS	fever, chills, and sweating
F/C	film coated (tablet)	FCSNVD	fever, chills, sweating, nausea,
F + C	flare and cells		vomiting, and diarrhea
F & C	foam and condom	FCSRT	Free and Cued Selective
5FC	flucytosine (this is a dangerous		Reminding Test
	abbreviation as it can be seen as	FCT	fever-clearance time
	5FU)	FCU	flexor carpi ulnaris (tendon)
FCA	Federal False Claims Act	FCV	feline calicivirus
	femoral cortical allograft	FD	Fabry disease
	fetal cardiac activity		familial dysautonomia
FCAS	familial cold autoinflammatory		fetal demise
	syndrome		fetal distress
F. cath.	Foley catheter		focal distance
FCBD	fibrocystic breast disease		food diary
FCC	familial cerebral cavernoma		forceps delivery
	familial colonic cancer		Forestier Disease
	family centered care		free drain
	femoral cerebral catheter		full denture
	follicular center cells		fully dilated
	fracture compound comminuted		functional deficits
FCCA	Final Comprehensive Consensus	F & D	fixed and dilated
	Assessment	FDA	Food and Drug Administration
FCCC	fracture complete, compound, and		fronto-dextra anterior
	comminuted	FDAAA	Food and Drug Administration
FCCL	follicular center cell lymphoma		Amendments Act of 2007
FCCM	Fellow, American College of	FDAMA	Food and Drug Administration
	Critical Care Medicine		Modernization Act (1997)
FCCU	family centered care unit	FDB	first-degree burn
FCD	feces collection device		flexor digitorum brevis
	fibrocystic disease	FDBL	fecal daily blood loss
	focal cortical dysplasia	FDC	familial dilated cardiomyopathy
FCDB	fibrocystic disease of the breast		fixed-dose combination
FCE	fluorouracil, cisplatin, and		(preparations)
	etoposide	FDCA	Food, Drug, and Cosmetic Act
	functional capacity evaluation	FDCS	follicular dendritic cell sarcomas
FCFD	fluorescence capillary-fill device	FDCs	follicular dendritic cells
FCH	familial combined hyperlipidemia	FDD	focus to detector distance
	fibrosing cholestatic hepatitis		(radiology)
FCHL	familial combined hyperlipemia	FDE	fixed-drug eruption
FCI	flow cytometric	FDEIA	food-dependent, exercise-induced
	immunophenotyping		anaphylaxis
FCL	fibular collateral ligament	FDF	flexor digitorum profundus
F-CL	fluorouracil and calcium leucovorin		(tendon)
FCM	facial choreic movements	FDG	feeding

	fluorine-18-labeled deoxyglucose (^{18}fluorodeoxyglucose)
FDGB	fall down, go boom
FDG-PET	positron emission tomography with ^{18}fluorodeoxyglucose
FDGS	feedings
FDI	first dorsal interosseous
	food-drug interaction
	Functional Disability Index
FDIP	fourth dorsal interosseus pedis (muscle)
FDIU	fetal death in utero
FDL	flexor digitorum longus
FDLMP	first day of last menstrual period
FDM	feline diabetes mellitus
	fetus of diabetic mother
	flexor digiti minimi
FDMA	first dorsal metatarsal artery
FD-OCT	Fourier domain optical coherence tomography
FDP	fibrin-degradation products
	fixed dental prosthesis
	fixed-dose procedure
	flexor digitorum profundus
FDPCA	fixed-dose patient-controlled analgesia
FD-PET	fluorodopa-positron emission tomography
FDQB	flexor digiti quinti brevis
FDR	first-dose reaction
FDS	flexor digitorum superficialis
	for duration of stay
FDT	frequency-doubling technology (perimetry for visual field screening)
	fronto-dextra transversa (right frontotransverse)
	Functional Dexterity Test
FE	field echo (radiology)
	flexion and extension
	frequency encode (radiology)
Fe	female
	iron
F & E	full and equal
FEB	febrile
FEC	fluorouracil, epirubicin, and cyclophosphamide
	fluorouracil, etoposide, and cisplatin
	forced expiratory capacity
FEC100	fluorouracil, epirubicin, and cyclophosphamide (the 100 refers to 100 mg/m^2 of epirubicin)
FECG	fetal electrocardiogram
FeCh	ferrochelatase
FECP	free erythrocyte coproporphyrin
FeCrNi	iron-chromium-nickel alloy

FECT	fibroelastic connective tissue
FED	fish eye disease
FEE	Far-Eastern equine encephalitis
FEES	fiberoptic endoscopic evaluation (examination) of swallowing
FEESST	flexible endoscopic evaluation of swallowing with sensory testing
FEF	forced expiratory flow rate
FEF$_{25\%-75\%}$	forced expiratory flow during the middle half of the forced vital capacity
FEF$_{x-y}$	forced expiratory flow between two designated volume points in the forced vital capacity
FEHBP	Federal Employee Health Benefits Plan
FEL	familial erythrophagocytic lymphohistiocytosis
	free electron laser
FeLV	feline leukemia virus
FEM	femoral
FEMA	Federal Emergency Management Agency
FEM-FEM	femoral femoral (bypass)
FEMG	facial electromyography
FEM-POP	femoral popliteal (bypass)
FEM-TIB	femoral tibial (bypass)
femto	prefix for units denoting a factor of 10^{-15} or 0.000,000,000,000,001 (symbol f)
FERGs	focal electroretinograms
FEN	fluid, electrolytes, and nutrition
FENa	fractional extraction of sodium
FENIB	familial encephalopathies with neuroserpin inclusion bodies
FEN-PHEN	fenfluramine and phentermine
FENS	field-electrical neural stimulation
FENs	foreign-educated nurses
FEOM	full extraocular movements
FEP	first-episode psychosis
	free erythrocyte porphyrins
	free erythrocyte protoporphorin
	functional exercise program
FER	flexion, extension, and rotation
FERPA	Family Educational Rights and Privacy Act
FERR	serum ferritin
FES	fat embolism syndrome
	floppy eyelid syndrome
	forced expiratory spirogram
	functional electrical stimulation
FeSO$_4$	ferrous sulfate
FESS	functional endonasal sinus surgery
	functional endoscopic sinus surgery
FET	familial essential tremor
	fixed erythrocyte turnover
	frozen embryo transfer

F

FETI	fluorescence (fluorescent) energy transfer immunoassay		fresh frozen plasma
		FFPE	formalin-fixed, paraffin-embedded
FEU	fibrinogen equivalent units	FFQ	food frequency questionnaire
FEUO	for external use only	FFR	freedom from relapse
FEV	familial exudative vitreoretinopathy		Forward Functional Reach (test)
FEV_1	forced expiratory volume in one second		fractional flow reserve
		FFROM	full, free range of motion
FEVC	forced expiratory vital capacity	FFS	failure-free survival
$FEV_{1\%VC}$	forced expiratory volume in one second as percent of forced vital capacity		fee-for-service
			Fight For Sight
			flexible fiberoptic sigmoidoscopy
FEVR	familial exudative vitreoretinopathy		fall from standing
FF	fat free	FFT	fast-Fourier transforms
	fecal frequency		flicker fusion threshold
	filtration fraction	FFTC	fast-Fourier Transform Convolution
	finger-to-finger	FFTDWB	flat foot touchdown weight bearing
	five-minute format	FFTP	first full-term pregnancy
	flat feet	FFU/1	fundus firm 1 cm below umbilicus
	force fluids	FFU/2	fundus firm 2 cm below umbilicus
	formula fed	FG	fasting glucose
	forward flexion		fibrin glue
	foster father		fusiform gyrus
	Fox-Fordyce (disease)	FGAs	first-generation antihistamines
	fundus firm		first-generation antipsychotics
	further flexion	FGC	familial gigantiform cementoma
F/F	face-to-face		female genital cutting
F&F	filiform and follower		full gold crown
	fixes and follows	FGF	fibroblast growth factor
F→F	finger to finger	FGFR2	fibroblast growth factor receptor 2
FF1/U	fundus firm 1 cm above umbilicus	FGID	functional gastrointestinal disorder(s)
FF2/U	fundus firm 2 cm above umbilicus		
FF@u	fundus firm at umbilicus	FGM	female genital mutilation
FFA	free fatty acid	FGM/C	female genital mutilation/cutting
	fundus fluorescein angiogram	FGP	fundic gland polyps
	fusiform face area	FGR	fetal growth restriction
FFAT	Free Floating Anxiety Test	FGS	fibrogastroscopy
FFB	flexible fiberoptic bronchoscopy		focal glomerulosclerosis
FFCD	French Foundation for Digestive Cancerology	FH	familial hypercholesterolemia
			family history
FFD	fat-free diet		favorable histology
	focal-film distance		fetal head
FFDM	freedom from distant metastases		fetal heart
	full-field digital mammography		Fisher House (housing for hospitalized veterans' families)
FFE	free-flow electrophoresis		
FFF	field-flow fractionation		fundal height
	freedom from (biochemical and/or clinical) failure	FH+	family history positive
		FH−	family history negative
FFI	fast food intake	FHA	filamentous hemagglutinin
	fatal familial insomnia	FHB	flexor hallucis brevis
FFL	flexible fiberoptic laryngoscopy	FHBL	familial hypobetalipoproteinemia
FFM	fat-free mass	FHC	familial hypertrophic cardiomyopathy
	Five-Factor Model (of personality)		
	five-finger movement		family health center
	full-face mask	FHCIC	Fuchs heterochromic iridocyclitis
	freedom from metastases	FHD	family history of diabetes
FFN	fetal fibronectin	FHF	fulminant hepatic failure
FFOV	functional field of view	FHH	familial hypocalciuric hypercalcemia
FFP	free from progression		

	fetal heart heard	FIP	feline infectious peritonitis
FHI	fibrous hamartoma of infancy		flatus in progress
	frontal horn index	FIQ	Fibromyalgia Impact Questionnaire
	Fuchs heterochromic iridocyclitis	FIRDA	frontal intermittent rhythmic delta
FHL	flexor hallucis longus		activity (electroencephalograph)
	functional hallux limitus	FIRI	fasting insulin resistance index
FHM	familial hemiplegic migraine	FISH	fluorescent (fluorescence) *in situ*
FHN	family history negative		hybridization
FHNH	fetal heart not heard	FISH-MD	fluorescence *in situ* hybridization
FHO	family history of obesity		microdissection
FHP	family history positive	FISP	fast imaging with steady state
FHR	fetal heart rate		precision
FHRB	fetal heart rate baseline	FIT	fecal immunochemical test
FHRV	fetal heart rate variability		functional inferior turbinoplasty
FHS	fetal heart sounds	FITC	fluorescein isothiocyanate
	fetal hydantoin syndrome		conjugated
FHT	fetal heart tone	FIV	feline immunodeficiency virus
FHVP	free hepatic vein pressure		in vitro fertilization (French)
FHX	fluorouracil, hydroxyurea, and	FIVC	forced inspiratory vital capacity
	radiotherapy	FIX	factor IX (nine)
FHx	family history	FJB	facet joint block
FI	fecal incontinence	FJN	familial juvenile nephrophthisis
	feeding intolerance	FJP	familial juvenile polyposis
	fiscal intermediary	FJROM	full joint range of motion
FIA	familial intracranial aneurysms	FJS	finger joint size
	Family Independence Agency	FJSI	facet joint steroid injection
	(formerly Department of Social	FJV	first jejunal vein
	Services)	FK506	tacrolimus (Prograf)
FIAC	fiacitabine	FKA	failed to keep appointment
FIAU	fialuridine		formally known as
FIB	fibrillation	FKBP	FK-506 binding protein
	fibula		(tacrolimus; Prograf)
	focused ion-beam	FKD	Kinetic Family Drawing
FICA	Federal Insurance Contributions	FKE	full-knee extension
	Act (Social Security)	FKGL	Flesh-Kincaid Grade Level (score)
FiCO$_2$	fraction of inspired carbon dioxide	FL	fatty liver
FICS	Fellow of the International College		femur length
	of Surgeons		fetal length
FID	father in delivery		fluid
	focus to isocenter distance		fluorescein
	(radiology)		fluorouracil and leucovorin
	free induction decay		flutamide and leuprolide acetate
FIESTA	fast imaging employing steady-		focal laser
	state acquisition (imaging)		focal length
FIF	forced inspiratory flow		follicular lymphoma
FiF	Functional Intact Fibrinogen (test)		full liquids
FIGE	field inversion gel electrophoresis		functional limitations
FIGLU	formiminoglutamic acid	fL	femtoliter (10^{-15} liter)
FIGO	International Federation of	F/L	father-in-law
	Gynecology and Obstetrics	FLA	free-living amebic (ameba)
FIH	first-in-human (trial)		low-friction arthroplasty
FIL	father-in-law	FLACC	Face, Legs, Activity, Cry, and
	Filipino		Consolability (pain assessment
FIM	functional independence measure		scale)
FIN	flexible intramedullary nail	FLAG	**fl**udarabine, a**ra**-C (cytarabine), and
FIND	follow-up intervention for normal		**G**-CSF (filgrastim)
	development	FLAIR	fluid-attenuated inversion recovery
FiO$_2$	fraction of inspired oxygen		(imaging)

FLAP	fluorouracil, leucovorin, doxorubicin (Adriamycin), and cisplatin (Platinol)	FLZ	flurazepam (Dalmane)
		FM	face mask
			family medicine
	5-lipoxygenase activating protein		fat mass
FLASH	fast low-angle shot		fetal movements
FLAVO	flavopiridol		fibromyalgia (syndrome)
FLB	funny looking beat		fine motor
FLBS	funny looking baby syndrome (see note under FLK)		floor manager
			fluorescent microscopy
FLC	follicular large cell lymphoma		follicular mucinosis
	fuzzy logic control		foster mother
FLD	fatty liver disease	F & M	firm and midline (uterus)
	field	F-MACHOP	fluorouracil, methotrexate, cytarabine (ara-C), cyclophosphamide, doxorubicin (hydroxydaunorubicin), vincristine (Oncovin), and prednisone
	fluid		
	flutamide and leuprolide acetate depot		
	full lower denture		
FL Dtr	full lower denture		
FLE	frontal lobe epilepsy	FMC	fetal movement count
FLe	fluorouracil and levamisole		fine motor coordination
flexsig	flexible sigmoidoscopy	FMD	family medical doctor
FLF	funny looking facies (see note under FLK)		fibromuscular dysplasia
			flow-mediated dilatation
FLG	funny looking grin (radiology)		foot-and-mouth disease
FLGA	full-term, large for gestational age	FMDV	foot-and-mouth disease virus
FLI	fluid-line intake	FME	Frühsommer-meningoenzephalitis vaccine
FLIC	Functional Living Index– Cancer		
FLIE	Functional Living Index– Emesis		full-mouth extraction
FLIM	fluorescence lifetime imaging microscopy	FMEA	failure mode and effects analysis
		FMEN-1	familial multiple endocrine neoplasia, type 1
FLIPI	Follicular Lymphoma International Prognostic Index		
		FMF	familial Mediterranean fever
FLK	funny looking kid (should never be used: unusual facial features, is a better expression)		fetal movement felt
			forced midexpiratory flow
		FMG	fine mesh gauze
FLM	fetal lung maturity		foreign medical graduate
fl. oz.	fluid ounce (approximately 30 mL)	FMH	family medical history
FLP	fasting lipid profile		fibromuscular hyperplasia
	Functional Limitations Profile	FM 100-hue	Farnsworth-Munsell 100-hue test
FL REST	fluid restriction	FmHx	family history
FLS	fibroblast-like synoviocytes	FML	familial multiple lipomatosis
	flashing lights and/or scotoma	FML®	fluorometholone
	flu-like symptoms	FMLA	Family and Medical Leave Act of 1993
FLT	fluorothymidine		
FLU	fluconazole (Diflucan)	FMN	first malignant neoplasm
	fludarabine (Fludara)		flavin mononucleotide
	flunisolide (Aero Bid)	FMO	fluence map optimization
	fluoxetine (Prozac)	FMOA	full-mouth odontectomy and alveoloplasty
	fluticasone propionate (Flonase)		
	influenza	FMOL	femtomole (10^{-15} mole)
FLU A	influenza A virus	FMP	fasting metabolic panel
FLUO	Fluothane		first menstrual period
fluoro	fluoroscopy		functional maintenance program
FLUT	flutamide (Eulexin)	FMPA	full-mouth periapicals
FLV	Friend leukemia virus	FMR	fetal movement record
FLW	fasting laboratory work		focused medical review
FLX	flexion		functional magnetic resonance (imaging)
	fluoxetine (Prozac)		

	functional mitral regurgitation	FNS	food and nutrition services
FMR1	fragile X mental retardation 1		functional neuromuscular stimulation
FMRD	full-mouth restorative dentistry		
fMRI	functional magnetic resonance imaging	F/NS	fever and night sweats
		FNT	finger-to-nose (test)
FMRP	fragile X mental retardation protein(s)	FNTC	fine-needle transhepatic cholangiography
FMS	fast macula scans	FO	foot orthosis
	fibromyalgia syndrome		foramen ovale
	fluorouracil, mitomycin, and streptozocin		foreign object
			fronto-occipital
	full-mouth series	FOB	father of baby
F & MS	frontal and maxillary sinuses		fecal occult blood
FMT	fluorescein meniscus time (dry-eye test)		feet out of bed
			fiberoptic bronchoscope
	functional muscle test		foot of bed
FMTC	familial medullary thyroid carcinoma	FOBT	fecal occult blood test
		FOC	father of child
FMTM	fast macular thickness maps		fluid of choice
FMU	first morning urine		fronto-occipital circumference
FMV	flow-mediated vasodilation	FOCF	first observation carried forward
	fluorouracil, semustine (methyl-CCNU), and vincristine	FOD	fixing right eye
			free of disease
FMX	full-mouth x-ray	FOE	functionally-oriented exercises
FMZ	flumazenil (Romazicon)	FOEB	feet over edge of bed
FN	facial nerve	FOF	fell on floor
	false negative	FOG	Fluothane, oxygen and gas (nitrous oxide)
	febrile neutropenia		
	femoral neck		full-on gain
	finger-to-nose (test)	FOH	family ocular history
	flight nurse	FOI	fiberoptic intubation
F/N	fluids and nutrition		flight of ideas
F to N	finger-to-nose	FOIA	Freedom of Information Act
FNA	femoral neck anteversion	FOID	fear of impending doom
	fine-needle aspiration	FOK	feeling-of-knowing (episodic memory procedure)
FNa	filtered sodium		
FNAB	fine-needle aspiration biopsy	FOL	fiberoptic laryngoscopy
FNAC	fine-needle aspiratory cytology	FOLFIRI	leucovorin, (**fol**inic acid) **fluoro**uracil, and **iri**notecan
FNB	femoral nerve block		
FNC	Family Nurse Clinician	FOLFOX	leucovorin calcium (folinic acid), fluorouracil, and oxaliplatin
	femoral nerve catheter		
FNCJ	fine-needle catheter jejunostomy	FOM	floor of mouth
FND	fludarabine, mitoxantrone (Novantrone), and dexamethasone	FOMi	fluorouracil, Oncovin, (vincristine), and mitomycin
		FONSI	finding of no significant impact
	focal neurological deficit	FOO	family of origin
FNF	femoral-neck fracture	FOOB	fell out of bed
	finger-nose-finger (test)	FOOSH	fell on outstretched hand
FNH	focal nodular hyperplasia	FOP	fasting office profile
FNHL	follicular non-Hodgkin lymphoma		fibrodysplasia ossificans progressiva
FNHTR	febrile nonhemolytic transfusion reaction	FOPS	fiberoptic proctosigmoidoscopy
		FORMIL	foreign military
FNMTC	familial nonmedullary thyroid carcinoma	FOS	fiberoptic sigmoidoscopy
			fixing left eye
FNP	Family Nurse Practitioner		force of stream (urology)
FN-PSG	full-night polysomnograms		fosphenytoin (Cerebyx)
FNR	false-negative rate		fructooligosaccharides

F

	full of stool (slang)	FPNP	Family Planning Nurse Practitioner
	future order screen	FPO	fetal pulse oximetry
FOSC	freestanding outpatient surgery center	FPOR	follicle puncture for oocyte retrieval
FOSS	Functional Outcome Swallowing Scale	FPPI	first postpacing interval
FOT	forced oscillation technique	FPR	fluoroscopy programmed radiography
	form of thought	FPS	frames per second (radiology)
	frontal outflow tract	FPU	family participation unit
FOV	field of view	FPV	fosamprenavir (Lexiva)
FOVI	field of vision intact	FPZ	fluphenazine (Prolixin; Permitil)
FOW	fenestration of oval window	FPZ-D	fluphenazine decanoate (Prolixin Decanoate)
FOZ	functional optical zone	FQ	fluoroquinolones
FP	fall precautions		frequency
	false positive	FQHC	Federally Qualified Health Center(s)
	familial porencephaly		
	family planning	FQRPA	fluoroquinolone-resistant *Pseudomonas aeruginosa*
	family practice		
	family practitioner	FR	failure rate
	family presence		fair
	fibrous proliferation		father
	flat plate		Father (priest)
	fluorescence polarization		Federal Register
	fluticasone propionate		first responder
	food poisoning		flow rate
	frozen plasma		fluid restriction
F/P	fluid/plasma (ratio)		fluid retention
F-P	femoral popliteal		fractional
fpA	fibrinopeptide A		fractional reabsorption
FPAL	full term, premature, abortion, living		freestyle, no head or lower-extremity fixation (aquatic therapy)
FPB	femoral-popliteal bypass		
	flexor pollicis brevis		frequent relapses
FPC	familial pancreatic cancer		Friends
	familial polyposis coli		frothy
	family practice center		full range
FPD	feto-pelvic disproportion	Fr	French (catheter gauge)
	fixed partial denture	F/R	fire/rescue
FPDL	flashlamp-pumped pulsed dye laser	F & R	force and rhythm (pulse)
FPE	first-pass effect	FRA	fall risk assessment
FPG	fasting plasma glucose		femoral ring allograft
FPHx	family psychiatric history		fluorescent rabies antibody
FPIA	fluorescence-polarization immunoassay	FRAC	fracture
FPIES	food protein-induced enterocolitis syndrome	FRACTS	fractional urines
		FRAG	fragment
FPL	federal poverty level	FRAG-X	Fragile X Syndrome
	final printed labeling (FDA document)	FRAP	family risk assessment program
			ferric-reducing antioxidant power (assay)
	flexor pollicis longus (tendon)		
	final printed labeling		fluorescence recovery after photobleaching
	forward pressure level		
FPLD	familial partial lipodystrophy	FRAX	fracture risk assessment tool from the World Health Organization
FPLV	feline panleucopenia virus		
FPM	full passive movements	FRC	frozen red cells
FPN	ferroportin		functional residual capacity
FPNA	first-pass nuclear angiocardiography	FRCPC	Fellow of the Royal College of Physicians of Canada

FRCPE	Fellow of the Royal College of Physicians of Edinburgh	FSC	Fatigue Symptom Checklist
			flexible sigmoidoscopy
FRCSC	Fellow of the Royal College of Surgeons of Canada		Forensic Science Center
			fracture, simple, and comminuted
FRCSE	Fellow of the Royal College of Surgeons of Edinburgh		fracture, simple, and complete
		FSCC	fracture, simple, complete, and comminuted
FRCSI	Fellow of the Royal College of Surgeons of Ireland	FSD	female sexual dysfunction
FRE	flow-related enhancement		focal-skin distance
FREQ	frequency		fracture, simple, and depressed
FRET	fluoresence resonance energy transfer	FSE	fast spin-echo
			fetal scalp electrode
FRF	filtration replacement fluid	FSF	fibrin stabilizing factor
FRG	Functional Related Groups	FSG	fasting serum glucose
FRH	febrile-range hyperthermia		focal and segmental glomerulosclerosis
FRJM	full range of joint movement		
FRN	fetal rhabdomyomatous nephroblastoma	FSGA	full-term, small for gestational age
		FSGN	focal segmental glomerulonephritis
FRNT	focus-reduction neutralization test	FSGS	focal segmental glomerulosclerosis
FROA	full range of affect	FSH	facioscapulohumeral
FROM	full range of motion		follicle-stimulating hormone
FROMAJE	functioning, reasoning, orientation, memory, arithmetic, judgment, and emotion (mental status evaluation)	FSHD	facioscapulohumeral (muscular) dystrophy
		FSHMD	facioscapulohumeral muscular dystrophy
FRP	follicle regulatory protein	FSIQ	Full-Scale Intelligence Quotient (part of Wechsler test)
	functional refractory period		
FRS	first-rank symptoms	FSL	fasting serum level
	flexed, rotated, side-bent (position of the spine)	FSM	functional status measures
		F-SM/C	fungus, smear and culture
	Framingham risk scores	FSME	Frühsommer-meningoencephalitis
	Functional Rating Scale	FSO	for screws only (prosthetic cups)
FRSN	fluoroquinolone-resistant *Streptococcus pneumoniae*		frontal sinus obliteration
		FSOP	French Society of Pediatric Oncology
FRSS	forward resuscitative surgery system	FSP	Family Service Plan
			fibrin split products
Fru	fructose	FSR	fractionated stereotactic radiosurgery
FS	fetoscope		
	fibromyalgia syndrome		fusiform skin revision
	field size	FSRP	Framingham Stroke Risk Profile
	fingerstick	FSRS	fractionated stereotactic radiosurgery
	flexible sigmoidoscopy		
	food stamps	FSRT	fractionated stereotactic radiotherapy
	foreskin		
	fractional shortenings	FSS	Fatigue Severity Scale
	frozen section		federal supply schedule (cost source)
	full strength		
	functional status		fetal scalp sampling
F & S	full and soft		fetal scalp stimulation
FSA	Family Services Association		Flinders Symptom Score
FSAD	female sexual arousal disorder(s)		Forensic Science Service (United Kingdom)
FSALO	Fletcher suite after loading ovoids		
FSALT	Fletcher suite after loading tandem		Freeman-Sheldon syndrome
FSB	fetal scalp blood		French steel sound (dilated to #24FSS)
	full spine board		
FSBG	fingerstick blood glucose		frequency-selective saturation
FSBM	full-strength breast milk		full-scale score
FSBS	fingerstick blood sugar		

F

	functional somatic symptoms	FTIUP	full-term intrauterine pregnancy
FST	forward surgical team(s)	FTKA	failed to keep appointment
FSW	feet of sea water (pressure)	FTLB	full-term living birth
	field service worker	FTLD	frontotemporal lobar degeneration
FSWs	female sex workers		frontotemporal lobar dementia
	focal slow waves	FTLFC	full-term living female child
	(electroencephalograph)	FTLMC	full-term living male child
FT	family therapy	FTM	female-to-male (transmission)
	fast-twitch		fluid thioglycollate medium
	feeding tube	FTMH	full-thickness macular hole(s)
	filling time	FTMS	Fourier-transform mass
	finger tip		spectrometer
	flexor tendon	FTN	finger-to-nose
	fluidotherapy		full-term nursery
	follow through	FTNB	full-term newborn
	foot (ft)	FTND	Fagerstrom Test for Nicotine
	Fourier transform (radiology)		Dependence
	free testosterone		full-term normal delivery
	full-term	FTNSD	full-term, normal, spontaneous
F$_3$T	trifluridine (Viroptic)		delivery
FT$_3$	free triiodothyronine	FTO	full-time occlusion (eye patch)
FT$_4$	free thyroxine	FTOZ	frontotemporal orbitozygomatic
FT$_4$I	free thyroxine index	FTOZ1	one-piece frontotemporal
FTA	femorotibial angle		orbitozygomatic
	fluorescent titer antibody	FTP	failure to progress
	fluorescent treponemal antibody		full-term pregnancy
FTA-ABS	fluorescent treponemal antibody	FTR	father
	absorption		failed to report
FTAGA	full-term average gestational age		failed to respond
FTB	fingertip blood		for the record
FTBD	full-term born dead	FTRAM	free transverse rectus abdominis
FTBI	fractionated total body irradiation		myocutaneous (flap)
FTC	emtricitabine (Emtriva)	FTSD	full-term spontaneous delivery
	fallopian tube carcinoma	FTSG	full-thickness skin graft
	Federal Trade Commission	FTT	failure to thrive
	follicular thyroid carcinoma		fetal tissue transplant
	frames to come		Finger-Tapping Test
	full to confrontation	Ftube	feeding tube
FTD	failure to descend	FTUPLD	full-term uncomplicated pregnancy,
	frontotemporal degeneration		labor, and delivery
	frontotemporal dementia	FTV	Fortovase (saquinavir, soft gel cap)
	full-term delivery		functional trial visit
FTE	failure to engraft	FTW	failure to wean
FTEs	full-time equivalents	FU	Farmacopeia Ufficiale (Italian
FTF	failure to fly (for attempted		Pharmacopoeia)
	suicide) (slang)		fraction unbound
	finger-to-finger		fluorouracil
	free thyroxine fraction	F & U	flanks and upper quadrants
FTFTN	finger-to-finger-to-nose	F/U	follow-up
FTG	full-thickness graft		fundus at umbilicus
FTI	farnesyltransferase inhibitor	F↑U	fingers above umbilicus
	force-time integral	F↓U	fingers below umbilicus
	free thyroxine index	5-FU	fluorouracil
FTICR-MS	Fourier-transform ion cyclotron	FUA	flat and upright (x-ray of the)
	resonance-mass spectrometry		abdomen
F TIP	finger tip	FUB	functional uterine bleeding
FTIR	Fourier-transform infrared	FUCO	fractional uptake of carbon
	spectroscopy		monoxide

F

FUD	fear, uncertainty, and doubt		flutter waves
	frequency, urgency, and dysuria	FWB	fetal well-being
	full upper denture		free water bolus
FUDR(r)	floxuridine		fresh whole blood
FU Dtr	full upper denture		full-weight bearing
FUFA	fluorouracil and leucovorin (folinic acid)		functional well-being
		FWCA	functional work capacity assessment
FU/FL	full upper denture, full lower denture	FWD	fairly well developed
FUFOL	fluorouracil and leucovorin calcium (folinic acid)	FWHM	full-width at half maximum (radiology)
Fugl	Fugl-Meyer Assessment of Motor Recovery After Stroke	FWS	fetal warfarin syndrome
		FWW	front-wheel walker
FUL	federal upper limit (price list)	Fx	fraction
FULG	fulguration		fractional urine
5FU/LV	fluorouracil and leucovorin		fracture
FUN	follow-up note	FXa	activated factor X
FUNASA	Fundão Naçional de Sade (Brazil's national health agency)	FXaI	activated factor X inhibitor
		Fx-BB	fracture both bones
FUNG-C	fungus culture	Fx-dis	fracture-dislocation
FUNG-S	fungus smear	F XI	Factor XI (eleven)
FUO	fever of undetermined origin	FXL	functional
FUOV	follow-up office visit	FXN	function
FU/LP	full upper denture, partial lower denture	FXR	fracture
		FXS	fragile X syndrome
FUP	follow-up	FXTAS	fragile X associated tremor/ataxia syndrome
FUS	focused ultrasound		
	Fuchs uveitis syndrome	FY	fiscal year
	fusion	FYC	facultative yeast carrier
FUT	fibrinogen update test	FYI	for your information
FUV	follow-up visit	FZ	flutamide and goserelin acetate (Zoladex)
FV	femoral vein		
F & V	fruits and vegetables	FZRC	frozen red (blood) cells
FVBG	free vascularized bone graft		
FVC	false vocal cord(s)		
	forced vital capacity		
FVCA	four-vessel cerebral angiography		
FVD	fever, vomiting, and diarrhea		
FVFR	filled voiding flow rate		
FVH	focal vascular headache		
F VII	factor VII (antihemophilic factor 7)		
F VIII	factor VIII (factor eight; antihemophilic factor)		
FVL	factor V-Leiden (mutation)		
	femoral vein ligation		
	flow volume loop		
	functional visual loss		
FVM	fetal ventriculomegaly		
FVP	foot venous pressure		
FVR	feline viral rhinotracheitis		
	forearm vascular resistance		
FVS	field verification simulation		
FVT	fast ventricular tachycardia		
FVWs	flow-velocity waveforms (umbilical artery Doppler)		
FW	fetal weight		
F/W	followed with		
F waves	fibrillatory waves		

F

G

G	gallop
	gastrostomy
	gauge
	gauss (a unit of magnetic flux density in radiology)
	gavage feeding
	gingiva
	good
	grade
	gram (g) (28.35 g = 1 ounce)
	grass (allergies)
	gravida
	guaiac
	guanosine
	riboflavin (vitamin G)
G +	gram-positive
	guaiac positive
G −	gram-negative
	guaiac negative
↑g	increasing
↓g	decreasing
G1-4	grade 1-4
G-11	hexachlorophene
GA	Gamblers Anonymous
	gastric analysis
	general anesthesia
	general appearance
	geographic atrophy
	gestational age
	ginger ale
	glycyrrhetinic acid
	glucose/acetone
	granuloma annulare
Ga	gallium
67Ga	gallium citrate Ga 67
GAA	alpha-glucosidase (gene)
	glacial acetic acid
GAAS	generally accepted as safe
GABA	gamma-aminobutyric acid
GABHS	group A beta hemolytic streptococci
GABS	group A beta (hemolytic) streptococci
GAD	generalized anxiety disorder
	glutamic acid decarboxylase
GAE	granulomatous amebic encephalitis
GAEB	good air entry bilaterally
GAF	geographic adjustment factors
	Global Assessment of Functioning (scale)
GAG	glycosaminoglycan
GAGS	global acne grading system

GAGPS	glycosaminoglycan polysulfate
GAGS	global acne grading system
GAHM	genioglossus advancement and hyoid myotomy
GAL	galanthamine hydrobromide (Razadyne)
	gallon (1 gallon US = 3.8 L; 1 gallon UK = 4.5 L)
	Guardian *ad Litem* (court appointed guardian)
GalC	galactocerebrosidase
G'ale	ginger ale
GALI-PUT	galactose-1-phosphate uridye transferase enzyme
GALT	galactose-1-phosphate uridyltransferase (gene)
	gut-associated lymphoid tissue
GAM	Gamma Knife
	gene-activated matrices
Gamma-GT	gamma-glutamyl transpeptidase
GAMT	guanidinoacetate methyltransferase
GAN	giant axonal neuropathy
GAO	General Accounting Office
GAP	GTPase activating protein
GAP-43	growth-associated protein-43
GAR	gonnococcal antibody reaction
GARFT	glycinamide ribonucleotide formyl transferase
GARP	Genetic Algorithm Rule-Set Prediction
GAS	general adaption syndrome
	ginseng-abuse syndrome
	Glasgow Assessment Schedule
	Global Assessment Scale
	group A streptococcal (*Streptococcus pyogenes*) disease vaccine
	group *A* streptococci
Gas Anal F&T	gastric analysis, free and total
Ga scan	gallium scan
Gastroc	gastrocnemius
GAT	geriatric assessment team
	Goldmann applanation tonometry
	group adjustment therapy
GATB	General Aptitude Test Battery
GAU	geriatric assessment unit
GAVE	gastric antral vascular ectasia
GAVI	Global Alliance for Vaccines and Immunization
Gaw	airway conductance
GB	gallbladder
	gingival bleeding
	Ginkgo biloba
	Guillain-Barré (syndrome)
G & B	good and bad
GBA	gingivobuccoaxial
	ganglionic-blocking agent

	glucocerebrosidase		grid conversion factor (radiology)
GBBS	group B beta hemolytic streptococcus	GC/FID	gas chromatography/flame ionization detection
GBD	global burden of disease	GCI	General Cognitive Index
GBE	*Ginkgo biloba* extract	GCIIS	glucose control insulin infusion system
GBEF	gallbladder ejection fraction		
GBG	gonadal-steroid binding globulin	GCKD	glomerulocystic kidney disease
GBH	gamma benzene hexachloride (lindane)	GCL	generalized congenital lipodystrophy
GBIA	Guthrie bacterial inhibition assay	GCM	giant cell myocarditis
GBL	gamma butyrolactone		good central maintained
GBM	glioblastoma multiforme	GCMD	generalized cardiovascular metabolic disease
	glomerular basement membrane		
GBMI	guilty but mentally ill	GCMN	giant congenital melanocytic nevus
GBP	gabapentin (Neurontin)		
	gastric bypass	GC-MS	gas chromatography-mass spectroscopy
	gated blood pool (imaging)		
GBPS	gated blood pool scan	GC-O	gas chromatography-olfactometry
GBR	gamma band response (audiology)	GCP	gentamicin, clindamycin, and polymyxin topical preparation
	good blood return		
	guided bone regeneration		good clinical practice
GBS	gallbladder series	GCPFL	grid-controlled variable-rate pulsed fluoroscopy
	gastric bypass surgery		
	group B streptococcal (*Streptococcus agalactiae*) disease vaccine	GCPS	Greig cephalopolysyndactyly syndrome
		GCR	gastrocolonic response
	group B streptococci		glucocerebrosidase
	Guillain-Barré syndrome	GCS	Glasgow Coma Scale
GBs	Glasgow-Blatchford bleeding score		glucocorticosteroid(s)
			graduated compression stockings
GBV-C	GB virus type C (also known as hepatitis G virus)	GCSE	generalized convulsive status epilepticus
GBW	generalized body weakness	GCSP	glycine cleavage system protein
GBX	gall bladder extraction (cholecystectomy)	G-CSF	filgrastim (Neupogen; granulocyte colony-stimulating factor)
GC	gas chromatography	GCST	Gibson-Cooke sweat test
	gastric cancer	GCT	general care and treatment
	geriatric chair (Gerichair)		germ-cell tumor
	gingival curettage		giant-cell tumor
	gliomatosis cerebri		glucose challenge test
	glucocorticoid		granulosa cell tumor
	gonococci (gonorrhea)	GCU	gonococcal urethritis
	good condition	GCV	ganciclovir (Cytovene)
	graham crackers		great cardiac vein
G−C	gram-negative cocci	GCVF	great cardiac vein flow
G+C	gram-positive cocci	GD	gastric distension
GCA	ghost cell ameloblastoma		Gaucher disease
	giant cell arteritis		gemcitabine (Gemzar) and docetaxel (Taxotere)
GCB	germinal center B-cell-like (lymphoma)		
			generalized delays
	gradient compression bandaging		gestational diabetes
GCBP	gated cardiac blood pool		good
GCC	glassy cell carcinoma		gravely disabled
	guanylyl cyclase C		Graves disease
GCE	general conditioning exercise	Gd	gadolinium
GCDFP	gross cystic disease fluid protein	G & D	growth and development
GCF	giant cell fibroblastoma	GDA	gastroduodenal artery
	gingival crevicular fluid	GDB	Guide Dogs for the Blind

G

Gd-BOPTA	gadolinium benzyloxypropionic tetra acetate	GEH	generalized eruptive histiocytosis
GDC	Guglielmi detachable coil	GEICAM	Grupo Español de Investigacion en Cancer de Mama (the Spanish Group for the Investigation of Breast Cancer)
GDD	glaucoma drainage devices		
Gd-DTPA	gadopentetate (Magnevist)		
Gd-DTPA-BMA	gadodiamide (Omniscan)	GEJ	gastroesophageal junction
		GEL	giant esophageal leiomyoma
GdE	gadolinium enhancing	GEM	gemcitabine (Gemzar)
GD FA	grandfather		gemfibrozil (Lopid)
GDGT	granddaughter		general equivalence mapping
GDH	glutamic dehydrogenase		generalized erythema multiforme
Gd-HPD03A	gadoteridol	GEMOX	gemcitabine and oxaliplatin
		GEMU	geriatric evaluation and management unit
GDJ	gastroduodenal junction		
g/dl	grams per deciliter	GEN	general
GDM	gestational diabetes mellitus		general anesthesia
GDM A-1	gestational diabetes mellitus, insulin controlled, Type I		genital
		GenD	genetic doping
GDM A-2	gestational diabetes mellitus, diet controlled, Type II	GEN/ENDO	general anesthesia with endotracheal intubation
GD MO	grandmother	GENT	gentamicin
Gd-MRI	gadolinium-enhanced magnetic resonance imaging	GENTA/P	gentamicin-peak
		GENTA/T	gentamicin-trough
GDNF	glial (cell line) derived neurotrophic factor	GEP	gastroenteropancreatic
			gene expression profiles
Gd$_2$O$_2$S	gadolinium oxysulphide	GEQ	generic equiavalent
GDP	gamma-detecting probe	GER	gastroesophageal reflux
	gel diffusion precipitin	GERD	gastroesophageal reflux disease
GDPs	general dental practitioners	GES	gastric emptying scintigraphy
GDR	glucose disposal rate	GEST	gestational
GDS	Geriatric Depression Scale	GET	gastric emptying time
	Global Deterioration Scale		graded exercise test
GDS-15	15-item Geriatric Depression Scale	GET 1/2	gastric emptying half-time
GDx®	a scanning laser polarimeter	GETA	general endotracheal anesthesia
GE	gainfully employed	GETS	Glasgow and Edinburgh Throat Scale
	gastric emptying		
	gastroenteritis	GETV	gadolinium-enhancing tumor volume
	gastroenterology		
	gemcitabine (Gemzar) and erlotinib (Tarceva)	GEU	geriatric evaluation unit
		GF	gastric fistula
	General Electric		girlfriend
	gastroesophageal		gluten free
	geometric efficiency (radiology)		grandfather
	gradient echo (radiology)	GFAAS	graphite furnace atomic absorption spectrometry
	group exercise		
GEA	gastroepiploic artery	GFAP	glial fibrillary acidic protein
GEC	galactose elimination capacity	GF-BAO	gastric fluid, basal acid output
GED	General Educational Development (Test)	GFCL	Goldmann fundus contact lens
		GFD	gluten-free diet
	General Equivalency Diploma	GFFF	gravitational field-flow fractionation
GEE	gait energy expenditure		
	generalized estimating equations (statistics)	GFJ	grapefruit juice
		GFM	good fetal movement
	Global Evaluation of Efficacy	GFP	green fluorscent protein
	glycine ethyl ester	GFR	glomerular filtration rate
	graft-enteric erosion		grunting, flaring, and retractions
GEF	graft-enteric fistula	GFS	gel-forming solution

	glaucoma filtering surgery	GIFT	gamete intrafallopian (tube) transfer
GG	gamma globulin		
	Gates-Glidden (dental drills)	GIH	gastrointestinal hemorrhage
	guaifenesin (glyceryl guaiacolate)	GIK	glucose-insulin-potassium
G=G	grips equal and good	GIL	gastrointestinal (tract) lymphoma
GGDS	global genome damage score	GILZ	glucocorticoid-induced leucine zipper
GGE	Gastrografin enema		
	generalized glandular enlargement	GING	gingiva
GGF	great grandfather		gingivectomy
GGM	great grandmother	G1K	greater than one thousand
GGO	ground-glass opacity	GIO	glucocorticoid-induced osteoporosis
GGS	glands, goiter, and stiffness		
	group G streptococci	GIOP	glucocorticoid-induced osteoporosis
GGT	gamma-glutamyl-transferase		
GGTP	gamma-glutamyl-transpeptidase	GIP	gastric inhibitory peptide
GH	general health		giant cell interstitial pneumonia
	genetic hemochromatosis		glucose-dependent insulinotropic polypeptide
	gingival hyperplasia		
	glenohumeral	GIPU	gastrointestinal procedure unit
	good health	GIR	glucose infusion rate
	group home	GIRDCA	Gruppo Italiano Ricerca Dermatiti da Contatto e Ambientali (patch test series)
	growth hormone		
GH₃	Gerovital		
GHAA	Group Health Association of America	GIS	gas in stomach
			gastrointestinal series
GHB	gamma hydroxybutyrate (sodium oxybate; Xyrem)	GISA	glycopeptide intermediate-resistant *Staphylococcus aureus*
GHb	glycosylated hemoglobin	GIST	gastrointestinal stromal tumor
GHD	growth hormone deficiency	GIT	gastrointestinal tract
GHDA	growth hormone deficiency (syndrome) in adults	GITS	gastrointestinal therapeutic system
			gut-derived infectious toxic shock
GHG	greenhouse gases	GITSG	Gastrointestinal Tumor Study Group
GHI	growth hormone insufficiency		
GHJ	glenohumeral joint	GITT	glucose insulin tolerance test
G-H jt	glenohumeral joint	GIWU	gastrointestinal work-up
GHLC	glenohumeral ligament complex	giv	given
GHM	gynecological health maintenance	GJ	gastrojejunal
GHP(S)	gated heart pool (scan)		gastrojejunostomy
GHQ	General Health Questionnaire		grapefruit juice
GHQ-30	General Health Questionnaire	GJH	generalized joint hypermobility
GHRF	growth hormone releasing factor	GJIC	gap junction intercellular communication
GHT	glaucoma hemifield test		
GI	gastrointestinal	GJT	gastrojejunostomy tube
	gingival index (dental)	G1K	greater than one thousand
	glycemic index	GK	Gamma Knife
	granuloma inguinale	GKRS	gamma-knife radiosurgery
GIA	gastrointestinal anastomosis	GKS	gamma-knife surgery
GIB	gastric ileal bypass	GKT	gamma-knife thalamotomy
	gastrointestinal bleeding	GL	gastric lavage
GIC	general immunocompetence		glaucoma
	Global Impression of Change		greatest length
GICOR	The Spanish Group of Clinical Research in Radiation Oncology	GLA	gamolenic acid
			gingivolinguoaxial
			glucose-lowering agents
GID	gastrointestinal distress	GLAD	glenoid labrum articular disruption
	gender identity disorder		
GIDA	Gastrointestinal Diagnostic Area	GLB	Graham-Leach-Bliley Act of 1999
GIFD #3	colonoscope		

G

GLC	gas-liquid chromatography	GMLOS	geometric mean length of stay
	glaucoma	GMOs	genetically modified organisms
GLD	Glanders (*Actinobacillus mallei*) vaccine	GMP	general medical panel (see page 356)
	globoid cell leukodystrophy (Krabbe disease)		Good Manufacturing Practices guanosine monophosphate
GLF	ground-level fall	GMR	gallop, murmur or rub
GLIO	glioblastoma	GMS	galvanic muscle stimulation
GLL	green-light laser		general medical services
GLM	general linear model		general medicine and surgery
GLN	glomerulonephritis		Gomori methenamine silver (stain)
GLOC	gravity-induced loss of consciousness	GM&S	general medicine and surgery
GLP	Gambro Liendia Plate	GMSPS	Glasgow Meningococcal Septicemia Prognostic Score
	Good Laboratory Practice (Principles of)	GMTs	geometric mean antibody titers
	group-living program	GN	gastrocnemius
GLP-1	glucagon-like peptide-1		glomerulonephritis
GLR	gravity lumbar reduction		graduate nurse
GLU	glucose		gram-negative
GLU 5	five-hour glucose tolerance test	GNA	*Galanthus nivalis* agglutinin
GLUC	glucose	GNB	ganglioneuroblastoma
GLYCOS Hb	glycosylated hemoglobin		gram-negative bacilli
			gram-negative bacteremia
GM	gastric mucosa	GNBM	gram-negative bacillary meningitis
	general medicine	GNC	gram-negative cocci
	genetically modified	GND	gram-negative diplococci
	geometric mean	GNDS	Guy Neurological Disability Scale
	gram (g)	GNG	gluconeogenesis
	grand mal		go/no-go (frontal executive function test)
	grandmother		
	gray matter	GNID	gram-negative intracellular diplococci
G-M	Geiger-Müller (counter)		
GM +	gram-positive	GNP	Gerontological Nurse Practitioner
GM −	gram-negative	GNR	gram-negative rods
gm%	grams per 100 milliliters	GnRH	gonadotropin-releasing hormone
GMA	grand mal attack	GNS	gram-negative sepsis
GmbH	*Gesellschaft mit beschränkter Haftung* (a corporation with restricted liability or a private limited liability company)		oblimersen sodium (Genasense)
		GnSAF	gonadotropin surge attenuating factor
		GNT	Graduate Nurse Technician
GMC	general medical clinic	GNYHA	Greater New York Hospital Association
	general medical condition		
	geometric mean concentration	GO	gemtuzumab ozogamicin (Mylotarg)
	gross-motor coordination		
GMCD	grand mal convulsive disorder		Graves ophthalmopathy
GM-CSF	sargramostim (granulocyte-macrophage colony-stimulating factor; Leukine)		Greek Orthodox
		GOAT	Galveston Orientation and Amnesia Test
GME	gaseous microemboli	GOBI	*growth* monitoring, *oral* rehydration, *breast* feeding, and *immunization*
	graduate medical education		
GMF	general medical floor		
GMFCS	Gross Motor Function Classification System	GOCS	Global Obsessive-Compulsive Scale
GMFM	gross motor function measure	GOD	glucose oxidase
GMH	germinal matrix hemorrhage	GOG	Gynecologic Oncology Group
GML	gingival margin levels (dental)	GOJ	gastro-oesophageal junction (UK and other countries)
GMLT	Groton Maze Learning Test		

G

GOK	God only knows (slang)	GPC/TP	glycerylphosphorylcholine to total phosphate
GOLD	Global Initiative for Chronic Obstructive Lung Disease (guidelines)	G6PD	glucose-6-phosphate dehydrogenase
GOM	granular osmiophilic material	GPEDs	generalized periodic eleptiform discharges
GOMER	get out of my emergency room		
GON	gonococcal ophthalmia neonatorum	GPGL	gamma probe guided lymphoscintigraphy
	greater occipital nerve	GPI	general paralysis of the insane
	greater occipital neuritis		glucose-6-phosphate isomerase
GONA	glaucomatous optic nerve atrophy		glycoprotein IIb/IIIa receptor inhibitor(s)
GONIO	gonioscopy		
GOO	gastric outlet obstruction	GPi	globus pallidus interna
GOR	gastro-oesophageal reflux (United Kingdom)	G-PLT	giant platelets
		GPMAL	gravida, para, multiple births, abortions, and live births
	general operating room		
GORD	gastro-oesophageal reflux disease (United Kingdom)	GPN	General Pediatric Nurse
			glossopharyngeal neuralgia
GORK	God only really knows (slang)		graduate practical nurse
GOS	gadolinium oxyorthosilicate	GPO	group purchasing organization
	galactose oxidase and Schiff reagent (test)	GPP	Good Programming Practice
		GPRD	General Practice Research Database (United Kingdom)
	Glasgow Outcome Scale		
GOSE	Glasgow Outcome Scale-Extended	GPS	Gamma Poisson Shrinker
			Goodpasture syndrome
GOT	glucose oxidase test	GPS™	Gravitational Platelet Separation (System)
	glutamic-oxaloacetic transaminase (aspartate aminotransferase)		
		GPT	glutamic pyruvic transaminase
	goals of treatment		Grooved Pegboard Test (of hand function)
GOX	glucose oxidation		
GP	gabapentin (Neurontin)	GPU	geriatric psychiatric unit
	gastroparesis	GPVP	good pharmacovigilance process
	general practitioner		
	globus pallidus	GPX	glutathione peroxidase
	glucose polymers	GPx-1	glutathione peroxidase-1
	glycoprotein	GR	gastric resection
	gram-positive		growth rate
	grandparent	gr	grain (approximately 65 mg) (this is a dangerous abbreviation)
	gutta percha		
G/P	gravida/para	G−R	gram-negative rods
G$_4$P$_{3104}$	four pregnancies (gravid), 3 went to term, one premature, no abortion (or miscarriage), and 4 living children (p = para)	G+R	gram-positive rods
		GRA	granisetron (Kytril)
			glucocorticoid remediable aldosteronism
GPA	gelatin particle agglutination	gravida 6, para 4-0-2-3	6 pregnancies resulting in 4-full term deliveries with 0 premature births and 2 abortions or miscarriages and 3 living children
	global program on AIDS		
G#P#A#	gravida (number of pregnancies)		
	para (number of live births)		
	abortion (number of abortions)		
G6Pase	glucose-6-phosphatase		
GPB	gram-positive bacilli	GRAS	generally recognized as safe
GPC	gel-permeation chromatography	GRASE	Generally Recognized as Safe and Effective
	giant papillary conjunctivitis		
	glycerophosphorylcholine	GRASS	gradient recalled acquisition in a steady state
	G-protein coupled		
	gram-positive cocci	Grav.	gravid (pregnant)
GPCL	gas-permeable contact lens	GRC	gastric remnant cancers
GPCR	G protein-coupled receptors	GRD	gastroesophageal reflux disease

G

GRD DTR	granddaughter	GSK	GlaxoSmithKline
GRD SON	grandson	GSM	Global System of Mobile
GRE	glycopeptide-resistant enterococci		Communication
	graded resistive exercise		grey-scale median
	gradient-recalled echo	GSMD	gestational sack and maternal date
	gradient refocused echo	GSP	generalized social phobia
GR-FR	grandfather		general survey panel
GRKP	gentamicin-resistant *Klebsiella*		Good Statistical Practice
	pneumoniae	GSPN	greater superficial petrosal
GR-MO	grandmother		neurectomy
GRN	granules	GSR	galvanic skin resistance (response)
	green		gastrosalivary reflex
GRO	growth-related oncogene	GSS	genotypic-sensitivity scores
GRP	Good Regulatory Practice		Gerstmann-Sträussler-Scheinker
	group		(syndrome)
Gr$_1$P$_0$AB$_1$	one pregnancy, no births, and one	GST	glutathione S-transferase
	abortion		gold sodium thiomalate
GRP HM	group home		(Myochrysine)
GRR	gross reproduction rate	GSTM	gold sodium thiomalate
GRT	gastric residence time		(Myochrysine)
	gene replacement therapy	GSUI	genuine stress urinary
	glandular replacement therapy		incontinence
	Graduate Respiratory Therapist	GSV	greater saphenous vein
	grasp and release test	GSW	gunshot wound
	group-randomized trial	GSWA	gunshot wound to abdomen
GRTT	Graduate Respiratory Therapist	GT	gait
	Technician		gait training
GRV	gastric residual volume		gastrostomy
GS	gallstone		gastrotomy tube
	generalized seizure		gene therapy
	general surgery		Glanzmann thrombasthenia
	Gleason score		glucose tolerance
	gliosarcoma		great toe
	glucosamine sulfate		greater trochanter
	gluteal sets		green tea
	Gram stain		group therapy
	grip strength	GTA	glutaraldehyde
G/S	5% dextrose (glucose) and 0.9%	GTB	gastrointestinal tract bleeding
	sodium chloride (saline)	GTC	generalized tonic-clonic (seizure)
	injection	GTCS	generalized tonic-clonic seizure
G & S	gait and stance	GTCs	green tea catechins
GSAP	greatest single allergen present	GTD	gestational trophoblastic disease
G-SAS	Gambling Symptom Assessment	GTE	general therapeutic exercise
	Scale		Green tea extract
GS-Cbl	glutathionylcobalamin	GTF	gastrostomy tube feedings
GSCs	glioblastoma stem cells		glucose tolerence factor
GSCU	geriatric skilled care unit	GTH	gonadotropic hormone
GSD	gallstone disease	GTN	gestational trophoblastic neoplasms
	German shepherd dogs		glomerulo-tubulo-nephritis
	globule-size distribution		glyceryl trinitrate (name for
	glucogen storage disease		nitroglycerin in the United
GSD-1	glycogen storage disease, type 1		Kingdom)
GSE	genital self-examination	GTO	Golgi tendon organ(s)
	gluten sensitive enteropathy	GTP	glutamyl transpeptidase
	grip strong and equal		green tea polyphenols
GSH	glutathione		guanosine triphosphate
GSI	genuine stress incontinence	GTPAL	gestation, term, preterm, abortion
GSIS	glucose-stimulated insulin secretion		and living

G

GTR	granulocyte turnover rate	GXT	graded exercise test
	gross total resection	Gy	gray (radiation unit)
	guided tissue regeneration	GYN	gynecology
GTS	Gilles de la Tourette syndrome	GYO	gynecology-oncology
gtt.	drops	GZTS	Guilford-Zimmerman Temperament Survey
GTT	gestational transient thyrotoxicosis		

GTR　granulocyte turnover rate
　　　gross total resection
　　　guided tissue regeneration
GTS　Gilles de la Tourette syndrome
gtt.　drops
GTT　gestational transient thyrotoxicosis
　　　gestational trophoblastic tumor
　　　glucose tolerance test
GTT agar　gelatin-tellurite-taurocholate agar
GTT3H　glucose tolerence test, 3 hours (oral)
gtts.　drops
G-tube　gastrostomy tube
GTV　gross tumor volume
GU　gastric upset
　　genitourinary
　　gonococcal urethritis
GUAG　Get-up-and-Go (test)
GUAR　guarantor
GUD　genital ulcer disease
GUI　genitourinary infection
GUM　Genitourinary Medicine (clinics)
GUS　genitourinary sphincter
　　　genitourinary system
GUSTO　Global Utilization of Streptokinase and TPA for Occluded Arteries
GV　gentian violet
　　growth velocity
GVF　Goldmann visual fields
　　　good visual fields
GVG　vigabatrin (gamma-vinyl GABA)
GVH　generalized visceral hypersensitivity
GVHD　graft-versus-host disease
GVL　graft-versus leukemia
GVM　Graft-versus malignancy
GVN　gentamicin, vancomycin, and nystatin
GVS　gastric vertical stapling
GVSDS　growth velocity standard deviation score
GVT　graft-versus-tumor
GW　Gulf War
G/W　dextrose (glucose) in water
G&W　glycerin and water (enema)
GWA　genome-wide association
　　　gunshot wound of the abdomen
GWAS　genome-wide association studies
GWBI　General Well-Being Index
GWD　Guinea-worm disease
GWMFT　Graded Wolf Motor Function Test
GWS　Gulf-war syndrome
GWT　gunshot wound of the throat
GWTG　Get With The Guidelines (American Heart Association program)
GWX　guide-wire exchange
GXP　graded exercise program

GXT　graded exercise test
Gy　gray (radiation unit)
GYN　gynecology
GYO　gynecology-oncology
GZTS　Guilford-Zimmerman Temperament Survey

G

H

H Haemophilis
Haldol (haloperidol); as in vitamin
H (slang)
head
heart
height
Helicobacter
heroin
high
Hispanic
hour
husband
hydrogen
hyperopia
hypermetropia
hyperphoria
hypodermic
isoniazid [part of tuberculosis
regimen, see RHZ(E/S)/HR]
objective angle
trastuzumab (Herceptin)
H′ hip
Ⓗ hypodermic injection
H² hiatal hernia
H₂ hydrogen
3H high, hot, and a helluva lot
H24 24 hour
356h Application to Market a New
Drug, Biologic or an Antibiotic
Drug for Human Use (FDA form
number)
HA headache
hearing aid
heart attack
hemadsorption
hemagglutination
hemolytic anemia
Hispanic American
hospital-acquired
hospital admission
hyaluronan
hyaluronic acid
hyperalimentation
hypermetropic astigmatism
hypothalmic amenorrhea
hydroxyapatite
H/A head-to-abdomen (ratio)
holding area
HA-1A® nebacumab
HAA haloacetic acid
hepatitis-associated antigen
HAAB hepatitis A antibody

HAAF hypoglycemia-associated
autonomic failure
HAART highly active antiretroviral
treatment
HAAs haloacetic acids
HABF hepatic artery blood flow
HAC hand-assisted colectomy
hospital acquired condition
hydroxyapatite cement
HAc acetic acid
HACA human antichimeric antibodies
HACCP Hazard Analysis Critical Control
Point(s)
HACE hepatic artery chemoembolization
high-altitude cerebral edema
HACEK Haemophilus
group parainfluenzae, H. aprophilus,
and H. paraphrophilus,
Actinobacillus
actinomycetemcomitans,
Cardiobacterium hominis,
Eikenella corrodens, and
Kingella kingae
HACS hyperactive child syndrome
HAD HIV (human immunodeficiency
virus)-associated dementia
human adjuvant disease
hypertonic acetate dextran
HADH the reduced form of nicotinamide-
adenine dinucleotide (hydride
donors in biochemical redox
reactions)
HADS Hospital Anxiety and Depression
Scale
HAE hearing aid evaluation
hepatic artery embolization
herb-related adverse event
hereditary angioedema
HAEC Hirschprung associated
enterocolitis
HAF hyperalimentation fluid
HAFM hospital-acquired Plasmodium
falciparum malaria
HAGG hyperimmune antivariola gamma
globulin
HAGHL humeral avulsion of the
glenohumeral ligament
HAGL humeral avulsion of the
glenohumeral ligament
HAH high-altitude headache
HAI hemagglutination inhibition
assay
hepatic arterial infusion
HAIC hepatic arterial infusional
chemotherapy
HAIR-AN hyperandrogenism insulin
resistance-acanthosis nigricans

HAK	hyperalimentation kit	
	hyperkeratotic actinic keratosis	
HAL	hemorrhoidal artery ligation	
	hip axis length	
	hyperalimentation	
HALC	hand-assisted laparoscopic colectomy	
HALDN	hand-assisted laparoscopic donor nephrectomy	
HALE	health-adjusted life expectancy	
HALN	hand-assisted laparoscopic (radical) nephrectomy	
HALO	halothane (Fluothane)	
	hours after light onset	
HALRI	hospital-acquired lower respiratory infections	
HALRN	hand-assisted laparoscopic radical nephrectomy	
HALS	hand-assisted laparoscopic surgery	
HALSR	hand-assisted laparoscopic sigmoid resection	
HAM	Haldol, Ativan, and morphine	
	high-alert medication(s) (medications where recurring reported errors have had serious consequences and warrant special attention)	
	high-dose cytarabine (ara-C) and mitoxantrone	
	HTLV-1-associated myelopathy	
	human albumin microspheres	
HAMA	human antimurine antibody	
HAM-A	Hamilton Anxiety (scale)	
HAM D	Hamilton Depression (scale)	
HAMLET	human alpha-lactalbumin made lethal to tumor cells	
HA-MRSA	healthcare-associated methicillin-resistant *Staphylococcus aureus*	
HAMS	hamstrings	
HAN	heroin-associated nephropathy	
HAND	HIV (human immunodeficiency virus)-associated neurocognitive-disorder(s)	
HANE	hereditary angioneurotic edema	
HANI	head and neck injury	
HAO	hearing aid orientation	
HAP	hearing aid problem	
	heredopathia atactica polyneuritiformis	
	hospital-acquired pneumonia	
	hydroxyapatite	
HAp	hydroxyapatite	
HAPC	hospital-acquired penetration contact	
HAPD	home-automated peritoneal dialysis	
HAPE	high-altitude pulmonary edema	

HapMap	A catalog of common genetic variants that occur in human beings. It describes what these variants are, where they occur in our DNA, and how they are distributed among people within populations and among populations in different parts of the world. (The International Haplotype Map Project) (www.hapmap.org)	
HAPS	hepatic arterial perfusion scintigraphy	
HAPTO	haptoglobin	
HAQ	Headache Assessment Questionnaire	
	Health Assessment Questionnaire	
HAR	high-altitude retinopathy	
	hyperacute rejection	
HARD	heartworm-associated respiratory disease	
HARDI	high-angular resolution diffusion-weighted imaging	
HARH	high-altitude retinal hemorrhage	
HARP	hypoprebetalipoproteinemia, acanthocytosis, retinitis pigmentosa, and pallidale degeneration (syndrome)	
HARS	Hamilton Anxiety Rating Scale	
	HIV-associated adipose redistribution syndrome	
HAS	Hamilton Anxiety (Rating) Scale	
	headache associated with sexual activity	
	hemangiosarcoma	
	Holmes-Adie syndrome	
	home assessment service	
	hyperalimentation solution	
hASC	human adipose-derived stem cells	
HASCI	head and spinal cord injury	
HASCVD	hypertensive arteriosclerotic cardiovascular disease	
HASHD	hypertensive arteriosclerotic heart disease	
HASTE	half-Fourier acquisition single-shot turbo spin-echo	
HAT	head, arms, and trunk	
	hepatic artery thrombosis	
	heterophile antibody titer	
	histone acetyltransferase	
	hormone ablative therapy	
	hospital arrival time	
	human African trypanosomiasis (sleeping sickness)	
HATU	2-(1H-7-Azabenzotriazol-1-yl)—1,1,3,3 tetramethyl uranium hexafluorophosphate (a peptide-coupling reagent)	

H

HAV	hallux abducto valgus	HBID	hereditary benign intraepithelial
	hepatitis A vaccine		dyskeratosis
	hepatitis A virus	HBIG	hepatitis B immune globulin
HAV-HBV	hepatitis A virus, and hepatitis B	Hb	mutant hemoglobin with a
	virus vaccine	Kansas	low affinity for oxygen
HAZWO	Hazardous Waste	HBLs	hemangioblastomas
PER	Operations and Emergency	HBLV	B-lymphotropic virus human
	Response	HBM	Health Belief Model
HB	heart-beating (donor)		human biomonitoring
	heart block		human bone marrow
	heel-to-buttock		human breast milk
	hemoglobin (Hb)	HBNK	heparin-binding neurotrophic factor
	hepatitis B	hBNP	human B-type natriuretic peptide
	high calorie		(nesiritide [Natrecor])
	hold breakfast	HBO	hit by owner (Veterinary slang)
	housebound		hyperbaric oxygen (HBO_2
	hydrocodone bitartrate		preferred)
1°HB	first degree heart block	HBO_2	hyperbaric oxygen
HB1°	first degree heart block	HbO_2	hemoglobin, oxygenated
HB2°	second degree heart block		hyperbaric oxygen (HBO_2
HB3°	third degree heart block		preferred)
HBAB	hepatitis B antibody	HBOC	hemoglobin-based oxygen carrier
Hb A_{1c}	glycosylated hemoglobin		hereditary breast and ovarian
HBAC	hyperdynamic beta-adrenergic		cancer
	circulatory	HBOT	hyperbaric oxygen
HbAS	sickle cell trait		treatment/therapy (HBO_2T
HBB	hospital blood bank		preferred)
HBBW	hold breakfast for blood work	HBO_2T	hyperbaric oxygen treatment
HBC	health and beauty care	HBoV	human bocavirus
	hereditary breast cancer	HBP	hand breast pump
	hit by car		high blood pressure
HBcAb	hepatitis B core antibody	HBPM	home blood pressure monitoring
	(antigen)	HBR	half-body radiation
HBc AB	hepatitis B core antibody	HBr	hydrobromide
HBc Ag	hepatitis B core antigen	HBRs	human biting rates
HbCO	carboxyhemoglobin	HBRT	horseback riding therapy
HB core	hepatitis B core antigen	HBS	Health Behavior Scale
HBC	hit by car		human body shape
HbCV	*Haemophilus* b conjugate vaccine		hungry bone syndrome
HBD	has been drinking	HbS	sickle cell hemoglobin
	hydroxybutyrate dehydrogenase	HBsAg	hepatitis B surface antigen
HBDH	hydroxybutyrate dehydrogenase	HbSC	sickle cell hemoglobin C
HBE	hepatitis B epsilon	HBSS	Hank balanced salt solution
	human bronchial epithelial (cells)	HbSS	sickle cell anemia
	hypopharyngoscopy, bronchoscopy,	HBT	hydrogen breath test
	and esophagoscopy		hypertrophy of the base of the
HBeAb	hepatitis Be antibody (antigen)		tongue
HBED	hydroxybenzylethylene-diamine	HbT	total hemoglobin concentration
	diacetic acid	HBV	hepatitis B vaccine
H Bee	honey bee (allergies)		hepatitis B virus
HbF	fetal hemoglobin		honey-bee venom
HBF	hepatic blood flow	HBVig	hepatitis B virus immune globulin
HBGA	had it before, got it again	HBVP	high biological value protein
HBGM	home blood glucose monitoring	HBW	high birth weight
HBH	Health Belief Model	H/BW	heart-to-body weight (ratio)
HBHC	hospital based home care	HBEX	home-based exercise
HBI	Harvey-Bradshaw Index	HC	hair count
	hemibody irradiation		hairy cell

H

	handicapped		hydrochloride (when part of a drug
	head circumference		name, as in thiamine HCl
	health coaching		[thiamine hydrochloride])
	healthy controls	HCLF	high carbohydrate, low fiber (diet)
	heart catheterization	HCLs	hard contact lenses
	heel cords	HCLV	hairy cell leukemia variant
	hemicrania continua	HCM	health care maintenance
	Hickman catheter		heterogeneous cation-exchange
	home care		membrane
	hospital course		hypercalcemia of malignancy
	hot compress		hypertrophic cardiomyopathy
	housecall	HCMV	human cytomegalovirus
	Huntington chorea	HCO$_3$	bicarbonate
	hydrocephalus	HCP	handicapped
	hydrocortisone		healthcare provider
4-HC	4-hydroperoxycyclo-phosphamide		healthcare proxy
H & C	hot and cold		hearing conservation programs
HCA	continuous heated aerosol		hereditary coporphyria
	health care aide		hexachlorophene
	heterocyclic antidepressant		home chemotherapy program
	High-Content Analysis		hospital chemistry profile
	hypercapnic acidosis		hydrocephalus
	hypercalcemia	HCPCS	HCFA (Health Care Financing
	hypothermic circulatory arrest		Administration) Common
HCAO	hepatitis C-associated		Procedural Coding System
	osteosclerosis	HCPG	Hutchinson-Gilford Progeria
HCAP	healthcare-associated pneumonia		syndrome
H-CAP	altretamine (hexamethyl-	HCPOA	healthcare power of attorney
	melamine), cyclophosphamide,	HCQ	hydroxychloroquine (Plaquenil)
	doxorubicin (Adriamycin), and	HCR	health care review
	cisplatin (Platinol)	hCRF	human corticotropin-releasing
HCB	hexachlorobenzene		factor (Xerecept)
HC-BPPV	horizontal canal benign paroxysmal	HCS	healthcare surrogate
	positional vertigo		heel-cord stretches
HCBR	human carbonyl reductase		human chorionic
HCBS	home and community-based		somatomammotropin
	services		hypercoagulable states
HCC	Hearing Coordination Center	17-HCS	17-hydroxycorticosteroids
	hepatocellular carcinoma	HCSE	horse chestnut seed extract
	Hürthle cell carcinoma	HCSS	hypersensitive carotid sinus
HCCL	heavily calcified coronary lesions		syndrome
HCD	herniate cervical disk	HCT	head computerized (axial)
	hydrocolloid dressing		tomography
HCFA	Health Care Financing		hematopoietic cell transplantation
	Administration		hematocrit
HCFC	hydrochlorofluorocarbon		histamine challenge test
HCFU	1-hexylcarbamoyl-5-fluorouracil		human chorionic thyrotropin
	(Camofur)		hydrochlorothiazide (this is a
hCG	human chorionic gonadotropin		dangerous abbreviation)
HCH	hexachlorocyclohexane		hydrocortisone
	hygroscopic condenser humidifier	HCTU	home cervical traction unit
HCI	home care instructions	HCTZ	hydrochlorothiazide (this is a
HCL	hairy cell leukemia		dangerous abbreviation)
	hemorrhagic corpus luteum	HCV	hepatitis C vaccine
	hydrogel contact lens		hepatitis C virus
HCl	hydrochloric acid (when it appears	HCVD	hypertensive cardiovascular disease
	separately [not as part of a drug	HCWs	healthcare workers
	name])	HCY	homocysteine

H

HCYS	homocysteine
HD	haloperidol decanoate
	Hansen disease
	hearing distance
	heart disease
	Heller-Dor (procedure)
	heloma durum
	hemodialysis
	herniated disk
	high definition
	high dose
	hip disarticulation
	Hirschsprung disease
	Hodgkin disease
	hospital day
	hospital discharge
	house dust
	Huntington disease
HDA	heteroduplex analysis
	high-dose arm
HDAC	histone deacetylase
HD-AC	high-dose cytarabine
HDAC2	histone deacetylase 2
HD-ara-C	high-dose cytarabine (ara-C)
HDBQ	Hilton Drinking Behavior Questionnaire
HD-Bu	high-dose busulfan
HDC	habilitative day care
	high-dose chemotherapy
	histamine dihydrochloride
HDC-ASCS	high-dose chemotherapy with autologous stem cell support
HDCC	high-dose combination chemotherapy
HD-CPA	high-dose cyclophosphamide
HDCPT	high-dose cyclophosphamide therapy
HDC-SCR	high-dose chemotherapy with stem-cell rescue
HDCT	high-dose chemotherapy
HDCV	rabies virus vaccine, human diploid (human diploid cell vaccine)
HDD-CKD	hemodialysis dependent-chronic kidney disease
HDE	Humanitarian Device Exemption (FDA)
H/D-Ex	hydrogen/deuterium amide exchange
HDF	hemodiafiltration
HDG	hydrogel (dressing)
HDGC	hereditary diffuse gastric cancer
HDH	high-density humidity
HDI	high-definition image
HDIs	histone deacetylase inhibitors
HDK	high-dose ketoconazole
HDL	high-density lipoprotein
HDL-C	high-density lipoprotein cholesterol

HDLW	hearing distance for watch to be heard in left ear
HDM	home-delivered meals
	house dust mite
HDMEC	human dermal microvascular endothelial cells
HDMP	high-dose methylprednisolone
HD-MTX	high-dose methotrexate
HD-MTX-CF	high-dose methotrexate and leucovorin (citrovorum factor)
HD-MTX/LV	high-dose methotrexate and leucovorin
HDN	hemolytic disease of the newborn
	heparin dosing nomogram
	high-density nebulizer
HDNS	Hodgkin disease, nodular sclerosis
HD-OCT	high-definition optical coherence tomography
HDP	high-density polyethylene
	hydroxymethyline diphosphonate
HDPA	high-dose pulse administration
HDPAA	heparin-dependent platelet-associated antibody
HDPC	hand piece
HDPE	high-density polyethylene
HDR	head-down rest
	heparin dose response
	high-dose rituximab
	husband to delivery room
HDRA	histoculture drug response assay
HDRB	high-dose rate brachytherapy
HDRS	Hamilton Depression Rating Scale
HDRW	hearing distance for watch to be heard in right ear
HDS	Hamilton Depression (Rating) Scale
	herniated disk syndrome
HDSCR	health deviation self-care requisite
HDT	habilitative day treatment
	hearing distraction test
HDU	hemodialysis unit
	high-dependency unit (an intensive care unit)
HDV	hepatitis D virus
HDW	hearing distance (with) watch
HDYF	how do you feel
HE	hard events
	hard exudate
	health educator
	hepatic encephalopathy
H&E	hematoxylin and eosin
	hemorrhage and exudate
	heredity and environment
HEA	health
HEAR	hospital emergency ambulance radio

HEAT	human erythrocyte agglutination test	HES	hetastarch (hydroxyethyl starch; Hespan)
HEB	hydrophilic emollient base		hypereosinophilic syndrome
HEC	Health Education Center	HEs	hypertensive emergencies
HeCOG	Hellenic Cooperative Oncology Group	hES	human embryonic stem
		hESCs	human embryonic stem cells
HEDIS	Health Employer Data and Information Set	20-HETE	20-hydroxyeico-satetraenoic acid
		HETF	home enteral tube feeding
HEENT	head, eyes, ears, nose, and throat	HEV	hepatitis E vaccine
HeFH	heterozygous familial hypercholesterolemia		hepatitis E virus
			high-endothelial venule
HEI	Health Eating Index (US Department of Agriculture)	Hex	altretamine (hexamethylmelamine; Hexalen)
HEICS	Hospital Emergency Incident Command System	Hexa-CAF	altretamine (hexamethylmelamine), cyclophosphamide, methotrexate (amethopterin), and fluorouracil
HEK	human embryonic kidney		
HEL	*Helicobacter pylori* vaccine		
	human embryonic lung	HF	Hageman factor
HeLa	Helen Lake (tumor cells)		hard feces
HELLP Syn- drome	hemolysis, elevated liver enzymes, and low platelet count		hay fever
			head of fetus
			heart failure
HEM	hematology		high frequency
	hypertensive emergency		Hispanic female
HEMA	hydroxyethylmethacrylate		hot flashes
HEMI	hemiparesis		house formula
	hemiplegia	HFA	health facility administrator
hemoc	hematology/oncology		high-functioning autism
Hem/Onc	Hematology/Oncology		hydrofluoroalkane-134a
HEMOSID	hemosiderin	H-FABP	heart-type fatty acid-binding protein
HEMPAS	hereditary erythrocytic multinuclearity with positive acidified serum test		
		HFAP	Healthcare Facilities Accreditation Program
HEMS	helicopter emergency medical services	HFAS	hereditary flat adenoma syndrome
		HFB	high-frequency band
HEN	hemorrhages, exudates, and nicking	HFC	hydrofluorocarbon
		HFCB	horizontal flow clean bench
	home enteral nutrition	HFCC	high-frequency chest compression
He-Ne	helium-neon	HFCN	high-flow nasal cannula
HEP	hemoglobin electrophoresis	HFD	high-fiber diet
	hemorrhage, exudates, and papilledemaa		high-forceps delivery
			high-frequency discharges
	heparin	HFE	hemochromatosis gene
	hepatic	hFH	heterozygous familial hypercholesterolemia
	hepatoerythropoietic porphyria		
	hepatoma	HFHD	high-flux hemodialysis
	histamine equivalent prick	HFHL	high-frequence hearing loss
	home exercise program	HFI	hereditary fructose intolerance
HEPA	hamster egg penetration assay	HFIP	hexafluoro-isopropranolol
	high-efficiency particulate air (filter)	HFJV	high-frequency jet ventilation
		H flu	*Haemophilus influenzae*
HepB	hepatitis B	HFM	hand-foot-and-mouth (disease) (often caused by coxsackievirus A16)
hep cap	heparin cap		
HER2	human epidermal growth factor 2		hemifacial microsomia
hERG	human ether-a-go-go-related gene	HFMD	hand-foot-and-mouth disease (often caused by coxsackievirus A16)
HERP	human exposure (dose)/ rodent potency (dose)		

H

HFMSE	Hammersmith Functional Motor Scale-Expanded		hip guidance orthosis
		HGP	Human Genome Project
HFO	high-frequency oscillation	HGPIN	high-grade prostatic intraepithelial neoplasia
	hold for observation		
HFOV	high-frequency oscillatory ventilation	HGPRT	hypoxanthine-guanine phosphoribosyl-transferase
HFP	hepatic function panel (see page 356)	HGS	hand-grip strength
			human genome sequence
	Hoffa fat pad	HGSIL	high-grade squamous intraepithelial lesion
HFPPV	high-frequency positive pressure ventilation		
		HGV	hepatitis G vaccine
HFR	hemorrhagic fever with renal syndrome vaccine		hepatitis G virus
		HH	hard of hearing
HFRS	hemorrhagic fever with renal syndrome		head hood
			heart healthy
HFRT	hyperfractionated radiotherapy		hereditary hemochromatosis
HFS	hand-foot skin (reaction)		hiatal hernia
	hand-foot syndrome		home health
	hemifacial spasm		homonymous hemiopia
	hot flash score		household
HFs	hair follicles		hyperhidrosis
HFSH	human follicle-stimulating hormone		hyperhomocystinemia
			hypogonadotropic hypogonadism
HFSRT	hypofractionated stereotactic radiotherapy		hypoeninemic hypoaldosteronism
		H/H	hemoglobin/hematocrit
HFST	hearing-for-speech test	H&H	hemoglobin and hematocrit
HFUPR	hourly fetal urine production rate	HHA	health hazard appraisal
HFUS	high-frequency ultrasound		hereditary hemolytic anemia
HFV	high-frequency ventilation		home health agency
	high-fruit/vegetable (diet)		home health aid
HFX RT	hyperfractionated radiation therapy	HH Assist	hand-held assist
HG	handgrasp	HHC	hereditary hemochromatosis
	handgrip		home health care
	Harris-Galante (cups used in hip replacements; types I or II)	HHCA	home health care agency
			hypothermic hypokalemic cardioplegic arrest
	hemoglobin		
	hyperemesis gravidarum	HHcy	hyperhomocystinemia
Hg	mercury	HHD	Doctor of Holistic Health
HGA	high-grade astrocytomas		hand-held dynamometer
Hgb	hemoglobin		home hemodialysis
Hgb ELECT	hemoglobin electrophoresis		household distance (physical therapy goal of mobility)
Hgb F	fetal hemoglobin		hypertensive heart disease
Hgb S	sickle cell hemoglobin	HHFM	high-humidity face mask
HGD	high grade dysplasia	HHH	hypermethionemia, hyperammonemia, and homocitrolinemia (syndrome)
HGE	human granulocytic ehrlichiosis		
HGES	handgrasp equal and strong		
HGF	hepatocyte growth factor	HHHFNC	heated, humidified, high-flow, nasal cannula
	hereditary gingival fibromatosis		
HGG	high-grade glioma	HHHQ	Health Habits and History Questionnaire (Block-National Cancer Institute)
	human gamma globulin		
HGH	human growth hormone		
HGI	high-glycemic index	HHIE-S	hearing handicap inventory for the elderly-short form
	Human Genome Initiative		
HGM	home glucose monitoring	HHM	high-humidity mask
HGN	hypogastric nerve		humoral hypercalcemia of malignancy
HGNT	high-grade neuroendocrine tumors		
HGO	hepatic glucose output	HHN	hand-held nebulizer

H

HHNC	hyperosmolar hyperglycemic nonketotic coma	HIB_{ps}	*haemophilus influenzae* type b polysaccharide vaccine
HHNK	hyperglycemic hyperosmolar nonketotic (coma)	HIC	Hearing Impaired Clinic Human Investigation Committee
HHNS	hyperosmolar-hyperglycemic nonketotic syndrome		Humphriss immediate contrast (astigmatism test)
HHPPS	home health prospective payment system	hi-cal HICF	high caloric high-information-content
HHRG	Home Health Resource Group (reimbursement categories for home health)	HICPAC	fingerprinting Hospital Infection Control Practices Advisory Committee (Centers for Disease Control and
HHS	hand-held shower Health and Human Service (US Department of)		Prevention guidelines)
	Hypothenar Hammer syndrome	HID	headache, insomnia, and depression herniated intervertebral disk
HHT	hereditary hemorrhagic telangiectasis	HIDA	hepato-iminodiacetic acid (lidofenin)
HHTC	high-humidity trach collar	HiDAC	high-dose cytarabine (ara-C)
HHTM	high-humidity trach mask	HIDS	hyperimmunoglobulinemia D
HHTS	high-humidity tracheostomy shield		syndrome
HHV-8	human herpesvirus 8	HIE	hyperimmunoglobulinemia E
HHVG	human herpes virus G		hypoxic-ischemic encephalopathy
HI	*Haemophilus influenzae*	HIES	hyper-immunoglobulin E syndrome
	head injury	HIF	*Haemophilus influenzae*
	health insurance		higher integrative functions
	hearing impaired		hypoxia-inducible factor
	hemagglutination inhibition	HIFU	high-intensity focused
	homicidal ideation		ultrasonography
	hospital insurance	HIHA	high impulsiveness, high anxiety
	human insulin	HIHARS	hyperventilation-induced high-
	hypomelanosis of Ito		amplitude rhythmic slowing
	hypopnea index	HII	hepatic-iron index
	hypoxic-ischemic	HIIC	heated intraoperative
Hi5	HIV positive ("V" being Roman numeral for 5) (slang)		intraperitoneal chemotherapy
HIA	hemagglutination inhibition	HIL	hypoxic-ischemic lesion
	antibody	HILA	high impulsiveness, low anxiety
HIAA	hydroxyindoleacetic acid	HILIC	hydrophilic interaction
5-HIAA	5-hydroxyindoleacetic acid		chromatography
HIAP	human intracisternal A-type particle	HILP	hyperthermic isolated limb perfusion
HIB	*Haemophilus influenzae* type b (vaccine)	HIM	health information management helium ion microscope hexyl-insulin monoconjugate
HIB_{cn}	*haemophilus influenzae* type b conjugate vaccine	HIN	*haemophilus influenzae* nontypable strain(s) vaccine
HIBGIA	had it before, got it again (slang)	HINI	hypoxic-ischemic neuronal injury
HIB_{HbOC}	*haemophilus influenzae* type b vaccine, HbOC conjugate vaccine	HINN	Hospital-issued Notice of Noncoverage
HIB_{PRP-D}	*haemophilus influenzae* type b vaccine, PRP-D conjugate vaccine	HINT HIO	Harris Infant Neuromotor Test health insuring organization hepatic iron overload
$HIB_{PRP-OMP}$	*haemophilus influenzae* type b vaccine, PRP-OMP conjugate vaccine	HIP HIPA	health insurance plan heparin-induced platelet aggregation
HIB_{PRP-T}	*haemophilus influenzae* type b vaccine, PRP-T conjugate vaccine	HIPAA	Health Insurance Portability and Accountability Act of 1996
		HIPC	hormone-independent prostate cancer

H

HIPEC	hyperthermic intraperitoneal chemotherapy	HKS	heel-knee-shin (test)
HIPJ	hallux interphalangeal joint	HKT	heterotopic kidney transplant
HIPPS	Health Insurance Prospective Payment System	HL	hairline
			half-life
hi-pro	high-protein		hallux limitus
HIR	head injury routine		haloperidol
HIS	Hanover Intensive Score		harelip
	Health Intention Scale		hearing level
	high-intermittent suction		hearing loss
	histidine		heavy lifting
	Home Incapacity Scale		hemilaryngectomy
	hospital (healthcare) information system		heparin lock
			hepatic lipase
HISA	Home Improvement and Structural Alterations (grant)		Hickman line
			Hodgkin lymphoma
HISMS	How I See Myself Scale		hyperlipidemia
Hisp	Hispanic	H&L	heart and lung
HIST	histamine	HL7	Health Level Seven International (standards for health information) (www.hl7.org)
HISTO	histoplasmin skin test		
	histoplasmosis		
HIT	heparin-induced thrombocytopenia	HLA	human leukocyte antigen
	histamine-inhalation test		human lymphocyte antigen
	home infusion therapy	HLADR	human leukocyte antigen, type DR
HITS	high-intensity transient signals	HLA nega-	heart, lungs, and
HITTS	heparin-induced thrombotic thrombocytopenia syndrome	tive	abdomen negative
		HLB	head, limbs, and body
HIU	head injury unit	HLCs	human landing catches
HIV	human immunodeficiency virus	HLD	haloperidol decanoate (Haldol)
	human immunodeficiency virus vaccine		herniated lumbar disk
			high-level disinfection
HIV-1	human immunodeficiency virus type 1		high-lipid disorder
			hyperlipidemia
HIV-2	human immunodeficiency virus type 2	HLDP	hypoglossia-limb deficiency phenotype
HIVAN	human immunodeficiency virus-associated nephropathy	HLES	hypertensive lower esophageal sphincter
HIVAT	home intravenous antibiotic therapy	HLGD	higher-level gait disorder
		HLGR	high-level gentamicin resistance
HIVD	herniated intervertebral disk	HLGT	high-level group term
HIV-D	human immunodeficiency virus-related dementia	HLH	helix-loop-helix
			hemophagocytic lymphohistiocytosis
hi-vit	high-vitamin		human luteinizing hormone
HIVMP	high-dose intravenous methylprednisolone	HLHS	hypoplastic left-heart syndrome
		HLI	head lice infestation
HIVN	human immunodeficiency virus nephropathy	HLK	heart, liver, and kidneys
		HLM	heart-lung machine
HJB	Howell-Jolly bodies		hemosiderin-laden macrophages
HJR	hepatojugular reflux	HLOS	hypertensive lower oesophageal sphincter (United Kingdom and other countries)
HK	hand-to-knee		
	heel-to-knee		
	hexokinase	HLP	hyperlipoproteinemia
hK6	human kallikrein 6	HLRCC	hereditary leiomyomatosis renal cell cancer
HKAFO	hip-knee-ankle-foot orthosis		
HKAO	hip-knee-ankle orthosis	hLS	human lung surfactant
HKD	hyperkinetic disorder	HLT	heart-lung transplantation (transplant)
HKMN	Hickman (catheter)		
HKO	hip-knee orthosis		high-level term

H

HLV	herpes-like virus		Hoechst Marion Roussel
	hypoplastic left ventricle	^{1}H-MRS	proton magnetic resonance
HM	hand motion		spectroscopy
	head movement	HMS	Hunter-MacDonald syndrome
	health maintenance		hyper-reactive malarial
	heart murmur		splenomegaly
	heavily muscled		hypodermic morphine sulfate (this
	heloma molle		is a dangerous abbreviation)
	Hispanic male	HMS®	medrysone
	Holter monitor	hMSCs	human mesenchymal stem cells
	home	HMSN I	hereditary motor and sensory
	human milk		neuropathy type I
	human semisynthetic insulin	HMSR	high medical-social risk
	humidity mask	HMSS	hyperactive malarial splenomegaly
HMA	hemorrhages and microaneurysms		syndrome
	heteroduplex mobility assay	HMV	home mechanical ventilation
HMB	beta-hydroxy-beta methylbutyrate	HMWCK	high-molecular weight cytokeratin
	(a leucine metabolite)	HMWK	high-molecular weight kininogen
	homatropine methylbromide	HMX	heat massage exercise
	hypersensitivity to mosquito bites	HN	head and neck
HMBA	hexamethylene bisacetamide		head nurse
HMD	hyaline membrane disease		high nitrogen
HMDP	hydroxymethyline diphosphonate		home nursing
HME	heat and moisture exchanger	H&N	head and neck
	heat, massage, and exercise	HN2	mechlorethamine HCl (Mustargen)
	hereditary multiple exostoses	H1N1	Spanish influenza virus
	home medical equipment	H2N2	Asian influenza virus
	human monocytic ehrlichiosis	H3N2	Hong Kong influenza virus
HMEF	heat moisture exchanging filter	H5N1	avian influenza A virus
HMETSC	heavy metal screen	HNC	head and neck cancer
HMF	human milk fortifier		Holistic Nurse, Certified
HMG	human menopausal gonadotropin		human neutrophil collagenase
HMGB1	high-mobility group box 1		hyperosmolar nonketotic coma
	(chromosomal protein)	HNCa	head and neck cancer
HMG CoA	hydroxymethyl glutaryl coenzyme A	HNCCG	Head and Neck Cancer
HMI	healed myocardial infarction		Cooperative Group
	history of medical illness	HNE	human neutrophil elastase
HMIS	hospital medical information	HNI	hospitalization not indicated
	system	HNKDC	hyperosomolar nonketotic diabetic
HMK	homemaking		coma
HM & LP	hand motion and light perception	HNKDS	hyperosmolar nonketotic diabetic
HMM	altretamine (hexamethyl-melamine;		state
	Hexalen)	HNL	histiocytic necrotizing
HMO	Health Maintenance Organization		lymphadenitis (Kikuchi-Fujimoto
	human milk oligosaccharides		disease)
	hypothetical mean organism	HNLN	hospitalization no longer necessary
HMP	health maintenance plan	HNMM	mucosal melanomas of the head
	hereditary metabolic profile		and neck
	hexose monophosphate	^{1}H-NMR	proton nuclear magnetic resonance
	hot moist packs		(spectroscopy)
HMPAO	hexylmethylpropylene amineoxine	HNN	hybrid neural network
HMPC	Committee on Herbal Medicinal	HNP	herniated nucleus pulposus
	Products (EMEA)	HNPCC	heredity nonpolyposis colorectal
HMPS	hereditary mixed polyposis		cancer
	syndrome	HNPP	hereditary neuropathy with liability
HMPs	herbal medicinal products		to pressure palsies
HMPV	human metapneumovirus	HNRNA	heterogeneous nuclear ribonucleic
HMR	histocytic medullary reticulosis		acid

H

HNS	0.45% sodium chloride injection (half-normal saline)	HORS	Hemiballism/Hemichorea Outcome Rating Score
	head and neck surgery	HOS	Health Outcomes Survey
	head, neck, and shaft		Holt-Oram syndrome
HNSCC	squamous cell carcinoma of the head and neck		hybrid orthosis system
			hypo-osmotic swelling
HNSN	home, no services needed	HOSP	hospital
HNT	hantaan (hantavirus) vaccine		hospitalization
HNV	has not voided	HOT	home oxygen therapy
HNWG	has not worn glasses	HOTV	letter symbols used in pediatric visual acuity testing
HO	hand orthosis		
	heme oxygenase	HOVT	letter symbols used in pediatric visual acuity testing
	Hemotology-Oncology		
	heterotropic ossification	Ho:YAG	holmium: yttrium-aluminum-garnet
	hip orthosis	HP	hard palate
	house officer		Harvard pump
H/O	history of		*Helicobacter pylori*
+HO	hemoccult positive		hemipelvectomy
H₂O	water		hemiplegia
H₂O₂	hydrogen peroxide		herbal products
HOA	hip osteoarthritis		high-protein (supplement)
	hypertropic osteoarthropathy		home program
HOB	head of bed		hot packs
HOB UPSOB	head of bed up for shortness of breath		house physician
			hydrogen peroxide
HOC	Health Officer Certificate		hydrophilic petrolatum
HOCM	high-osmolality contrast media		hypersensitivity pneumonitis
	hypertrophic obstructive cardiomyopathy		hypertrophic pachymeningitis
		Hp	*Helicobacter pylori*
HOD	heroin overdose	H&P	history and physical
HOG	halothane, oxygen, and gas (nitrous oxide)	HPA	hybridization protection assay
			hypothalamic-pituitary-adrenal (axis)
	Hoosier Oncology Group		
HOH	hand-over-hand (rehabilitation term)	HPAE-PAD	high-pH anion exchange chromatography coupled with pulsed amperometric detection
	hard of hearing		
	head of household	HPAI	highly pathogenic avian influenza A virus
HOI	history of immunization		
	hospital onset of infection	HPAT	home parenteral antibiotic therapy
HOM	high-osmolar contrast media	HPB	Health Protection Branch (the Canadian equivalent of the U.S. Food and Drug Administration)
HOMA	homeostatic assessment model algorithm (index)		
	homeostatic model assessment	HPC	hemangiopericytoma
HOME	Home Observation for Measurement of the Environment		hematopoietic progenitor cell
			hereditary prostate cancer
			history of present condition (complaint)
HOMU	history of medication use		
HONC	Hooked on Nicotine Checklist	HPCE	high-performance capillary electrophoresis
	hyperosmolar, nonketotic coma		
Honda	hypertensive obese non-compliant diabetic adult (slang)	HPD	hearing protection device
			high-protein diet
HONK	hyperosmolar nonketotic		home peritoneal dialysis
HOP	hourly output		hours post dose
HOPI	history of present illness	HpD	hematoporphyrin derivative
Hopkins-25	Hopkins Symptom Checklist-25	HP&D	hemoprofile and differential
HOR	higher-order repeat	HPDP	health promotion and disease prevention
HORF	high-output renal failure		

H

HPE	hemorrhage, papilledema, exudate	hPTH	human parathyroid hormone I$_{34}$ (teriparatide)
	history and physical examination	HPTM	home prothrombin time monitoring
	holoprosencephaly	HPTX	hemopneumothorax
HPET	*Helicobacter pylori* eradication therapy	HPV	human papilloma virus
			human papilloma virus vaccine
HPF	high-power field		human parvovirus
HPFB	Health Products and Food Branch (Canada)	*H pylori*	*Helicobacter pylori*
		HPZ	high-pressure zone
HPFH	hereditary persistence of fetal hemoglobin	HQC	hydroquinone cream
		HQL	health-related quality of life
HPG	human pituitary gonadotropin	HR	hallux rigidus
2hPG	2-hour post-challenge glucose		Harrington rod
HPH	Hashimoto-Pritzker histiocytosis		hazard ratio
HPI	history of present illness		health related
HPIP	history, physical, impression, and plan		heart rate
			hemorrhagic retinopathy
HPK	hyperkeratosis		histamine release
HPL	human placenta lactogen		hospital record
	hyperlipidemia		hour
	hyperplexia	Hr 0	zero hour (when treatment starts)
HPLC	high-performance (pressure) liquid chromatography	Hr -2	minus two hours (two hours prior to treatment)
HPM	hemiplegic migraine	H & R	hysterectomy and radiation
HPMC	high-performance membrane chromatography	HRA	high-right atrium
			histamine-releasing activity
	hydroxypropyl methylcellulose	H2RA	histamine$_2$-receptor antagonist
HPMG	hard palate mucosal graft	HRC	Human Rights Committee
HPN	home parenteral nutrition	HRCT	high-resolution computed tomography
HPNI	hemodialysis prognostic nutrition index		
		HRD	hazard ratios of death
HPNS	high-pressure nervous syndrome		human retroviral disease
HPO	hydrophilic ointment		hypertension renal disease
	hypertrophic pulmonary osteoarthropathy		hypoparathyroidism, retardation, and dysmorphism (syndrome)
HPOA	hypertrophic pulmonary osteoarthropathy	HRE	high-resolution electrocardiography
		HRECG	high-resolution electrocardiography
HPP	hypophosphatasia	HRF	Harris return flow
2HPP	2-hour postprandial (blood sugar)		health-related facility
2HPPBS	2-hour postprandial blood sugar		histamine-releasing factor
HPPM	hyperplastic persistent pupillary membrane		hypertensive renal failure
			hypoxic respiratory failure
HPRC	hereditary papillary renal carcinoma	HRI	HMG-CoA (3-hydroxy-3-methylglutaryl-coenzyme A) reductase inhibitors
hPRL	prolactin, human		
HPS	hantavirus pulmonary syndrome	HRIF	histamine inhibitory releasing factor
	hepatopulmonary syndrome		
	Helicobacter pylori serology	HRIG	human rabies immune globulin
	hypertrophic pyloric stenosis	HRL	head rotated left
HpSA	*Helicobacter pylori* stool antigen	HRLA	human reovirus-like agent
HPT	heparin protamine titration	HRLM	high-resolution light microscopy
	histamine provocation test	hRLX-2	synthetic human relaxin
	home pregnancy test	HRMPC	hormone-refractory metastatic prostate cancer
	hyperparathyroidism		
9HPT	9-hole Peg Test	HRMS	high-resolution mass spectrometry
HPTD	highly permeable transparent dressing	HRMT	human resting muscle (myofascial) tone

HRNB	Halstead-Reitan Neuropsychological Battery		hysterectomy and sterilization
HROs	high-reliability organizations	HSA	Health Services Administration (Administrator)
HRP	high-risk pregnancy		Health Systems Agency
	horseradish peroxidase		human serum albumin
HRP-2	histidine-rich protein-2		hypersomnia-sleep apnea
HRPC	hormone-refractory prostate cancer	HSAN	hereditary sensory and autonomic neuropathy (types I-IV)
HRQL	health-related quality of life		
HRQOL	health-related quality of life	HSB	husband
HRR	head rotated right	HSBS	evening blood sugar
	heart rate recovery	HSBG	heel-stick blood gas
HRRC	Human Research Review Committee	HSC	hematopoietic stem cell
		HSCL	Hopkins Symptom-Check List
HRS	Haw River syndrome	HSCR	Hirschsprung disease
	hepatorenal syndrome	hs-CRP	high-sensitivity C-reactive protein
	Hodgkin-Reed-Sternberg (cells)	HSCSS	hypersensitive carotid sinus syndrome
	hours		
HRSD	Hamilton Rating Scale for Depression	HSCT	hematopoietic stem cell transplant
		HSD	Honestly Significant Difference (test) (Turkey)
HRSEM	high-resolution scanning electron microscopy		
			hypoactive sexual desire (disorder)
HRST	heat, reddening, swelling, or tenderness	HSDD	hypoactive sexual desire disorder
		HSE	herpes simplex encephalitis
	heavy-resistance strength training		human skin equivalent
HRSV	human respiratory syncytial virus		hypertonic saline-epinephrine
HRT	heart rate	HSEES	Hazardous Substances Emergency Events Surveillance
	heart rate turbulence		
	Heidelberg retina tomograph	HSES	hemorrhagic shock and encephalopathy
	heparin-response test		
	high-risk transfer	HSG	herpes simplex genitalis
	hormone replacement therapy		hysterosalpingogram
	hyperfractioned radiotherapy	HSGYV	heat, steam, gum, yawn, and Valsalva maneuver (for otitis media)
HRU	health resource utilization		
HRV	heart rate variability		
	heterogeneous resistance to vancomycin	H-SIL	high-grade squamous intraepithelial lesions
HS	bedtime	HSJ	hepatic schistosomiasis japonica
	half-strength	HSK	herpes simplex keratitis
	hamstrings		hyperkeratotic seborrheic keratosis
	hamstring sets	HSL	herpes simplex labialis
	handsewn (suture)		hormone-sensitive lipase
	Harmonic scalpel	HSM	hepatosplenomegaly
	Hartman solution (lactated Ringers)		holosystolic murmur
	heart size	HSN	Hansen-Street nail
	heart sounds		heart sounds normal
	heavy smoker		hereditary sensory neuropathy
	heel spur	HSOs	health services organizations
	heel stick	HSP	heat shock protein
	hereditary spherocytosis		Henoch-Schönlein purpura
	herpes simplex		hereditary spastic paraparesis
	hidradenitis suppurativa		hereditary spastic paraplegia
	high school		hypersensitivity pneumonitis
	hippocampal sclerosis		hysterosalpingography
	house staff	HSPC	hydrogenated soy phosphatidyl choline
	Hurler syndrome		
H → S	heel-to-shin	HSPE	high-strength pancreatic enzymes
H&S	hearing and speech	HSQ	Health Status Questionnaire
	hemorrhage and shock	HSR	heated serum reagin

	hypersensitivity reaction
	hypofractionated stereotactic radiotherapy
HSRC	Human Subjects Review Committee
HSS	half-strength saline (0.45% Sodium Chloride)
	Hospital Surgical Service
	hypertonic saline solution (3%, 5% or 7.5% sodium chloride injection) (This is a dangerous abbreviation)
HSSE	high soap-suds enema
HST	horseshoe tear (retina)
HS-tk	herpes simplex thymidine kinase
hsUHR-OCT	high-speed ultra-high-resolution optical coherence tomography
HSV	herpes simplex virus
	highly selective vagotomy
HSV-1	herpes simplex virus type 1
	herpes simplex virus type 1 vaccine
HSV$_2$	herpes simplex virus type 2 vaccine
HSV$_{12}$	herpes simplex virus types 1, 2 vaccine
HSV-2	herpes simplex virus type 2
HSVE	herpes simplex virus encephalitis
HT	hammertoe
	head trauma
	healing time
	Health Technician
	hearing test
	heart
	heart transplant
	height
	heparin trap (hep-trap; heparin lock; a venous access device)
	high temperature
	hormonotherapy
	Hubbard tank
	hypermetropia
	hyperopia
	hypertension
	hyperthermia
	hyperthyroid
H/T	heel and toe (walking)
H&T	hospitalization and treatment
H(T)	intermittent hypertropia
HT-1	hereditary tyrosinemia type 1
5-HT$_1$	serotonin (5-hydroxytryptamine)
HTA	Health Technology Assessment (Program)
	hydrothermal ablation
	hypertension (French)
ht. aer.	heated aerosol
HTAT	human tetanus antitoxin
HTB	hot tub bath

HTBF	high-throughput blood fractionation
HTBZ	dihydrotetrabenazine
HTC	heated-tracheostomy collar
	high-throughput (protein) crystallization
	hypertensive crisis
HTDS	high-throughput drug screening
HTE	highly-treatment experienced (patients)
hTERT	human telomerase reverse transcriptase
HTF	house tube feeding
HTGL	hepatic triglyceride lipase
HTK	heel-to-knee (test)
	histidine-tryptophan-ketoglutarate (Bretschneider solution)
HTL	hearing threshold level
	honey-thick liquid (diet consistency)
	human T-cell leukemia
	human thymic leukemia
HTLV III	human T-cell lymphotrophic virus type III
HTM	*Haemophilus* test medium
	high threshold mechanoceptors
	human tropomyosin
HTML	hypertext markup language
HTN	hypertension
HTNV	Hantaan virus
HTO	high tibial osteotomy
HTP	House-Tree-Person-test
5-HTP	serotonin (5-hydroxytryptophan)
HTR	hard tissue replacement
hTRT	human telomerase reverse transcriptase
HTS	head traumatic syndrome
	heel-to-shin (test)
	Hematest(r) stools
	high-throughput screening
HTSCA	human tumor stem cell assay
HtSDS	height standard deviation score
H-TSH	human thyroid-stimulating hormone
HTT	hand thrust test
	hyalinizing trabecular tumor
HTV	herpes-type virus
HTVD	hypertensive vascular disease
HTX	hemothorax
HTx	hand transplantation
	heart transplant
HU	head unit
	Hounsfield units
	hydroxyurea
	hypertensive urgencies
Hu	Hounsfield units
HUAEC	human umbilical endothelial cells
HUCB	human umbilical cord blood

H

HUD	humanitarian use device (FDA designation)	HVOD	hepatic veno-occlusive disease
HUH	Humana Hospital	HVOO	hepatic venous outflow obstruction
HUI	Health Utilities Index	HVPC	high-voltage pulsed current
HUI2	Health Utilities Index Mark 2	HVPG	hepatic venous pressure gradient
HUI3	Health Utilities Index Mark 3	HYPT	hyperventilation provocation test
HUIFM	human leukocyte interferon meloy	HVR	hypoxic ventilatory response
HUK	human urinary kallikrein	HVS	hyperventilation syndrome
HUM	heat, ultrasound, and massage	HVS-TK	herpes simplex virus thymidine kinase
HUM 70/30	human insulin, regular 30 units/mL with human insulin isophane suspension 70 units/mL (Humulin® 70/30 insulin)	HW	hemiwalker heparin well homework housewife
HUMARA	human androgen receptor assay	HWB	hot water bottle
HUM L	human insulin zinc suspension (Humulin® L Insulin)	HWE	hot water epilepsy
		HWFE	housewife
HUM N	human insulin isophane suspension (Humulin® N Insulin)	HWG	has worn glasses
		HWH	halfway house
HUM R	human insulin, regular (Humulin® R Insulin)	HWP	hot wet pack
		HWPG	has worn prescription glasses
HUR	hydroxyurea	Hx	history
HUS	head ultrasound hemolytic uremic syndrome Hospital Unit Secretary husband		hospitalization
		HXM	altretamine (hexamethylmelamine; Hexalen)
		Hx & Px	history and physical (examination)
husb	husband	Hy	hypermetropia
HUT	head-upright tilt (test) hyperplasia of usual type	HyCoSy	hysterosalpingo-contrast sonography
HUTT	head-up tilt-table testing	HYDRO	hydronephrosis
HUV	human umbilical vein		hydrotherapy
HUVEC	human umbilical vein endothelial cells	HYG	hygiene
		HYPER	above higher than
HV	hallux valgus Hantavirus has voided healthy volunteers Hemovac® hepatic vein herpesvirus home visit hypervariable	Hyper Al	hyperalimentation
		Hyper K	hyperkalemia
		HYPER T & A	hypertrophic tonsils and adenoids
		HYPO	below hypodermic injection lower than
		HYPOFx	hypo-fraction
H&V	hemigastrecotomy and vagotomy	hypo K	hypokalemia
HVII	hypervariable segment II	hypoMAG	hypomagnesemia
HVA	homovanillic acid	hypoNa	hyponatremia
HVD	hypertensive vascular disease	hypopit	hypopituitarism
HVDO	hypovitaminosis D osteopathy	HYs	healthy years of life
HVE	high-voltage electrophoresis	Hyst	hysterectomy
HVES	high-voltage electrical stimulation	HYVET	Hypertension in the Very Elderly Trial
HVF	Humphrey visual field		
HVFD	homonymous visual field defects	Hz	Hertz
HVGS	high-voltage galvanic stimulation	HZ	herpes zoster
HVI	high-voltage ICD (implantable cardioverter-defibrillator) hollow viscus injury	HZD	herpes zoster dermatitis
		HZO	herpes zoster ophthalmicus
		HZV	herpes zoster virus
HVL	half-value layer hippocampal volume loss		
HVLT	Hopkins Verbal Learning Test-Revised		

I

I	impression
	incisal
	incontinent
	independent
	initial
	inspiration
	intact (bag of waters)
	intermediate
	iris
	one
Ⓘ	independent
I_2	iodine
I^{131}	radioactive iodine
I-3+7	idarubicin and cytarabine
IA	ideational apraxia
	idiopathic anaphylaxis
	incidental appendectomy
	incurred accidentally
	indigenous Australian(s)
	intra-amniotic
	intra-arterial
	invasive aspergillosis
I & A	irrigation and aspiration
IAA	ileoanal anastomosis
	insulin autoantibodies
	interrupted aortic arch
	intra-abdominal abscess
	intra-abdominal adiposity
	intra-arterial angiography
IAAA	inflammatory abdominal aortic aneurysms
IAAT	intra-abdominal adipose tissue
IAB	incomplete abortion
	induced abortion
	intermittent androgen blockade
IABC	intra-aortic balloon counterpulsation
IABCP	intra-aortic balloon counterpulsation
IABP	intra-aortic balloon pump
	intra-arterial blood pressure
IAC	internal auditory canal
	intra-arterial chemotherapy
	isolated adrenal cell
IACC	intra-arterial cytoreductive chemotherapy
IAC-CPR	interposed abdominal compressions—cardiopulmonary resuscitation
IACG	intermittent angle-closure glaucoma
IACNS	isolated angiitis of central nervous system

IACP	intra-aortic counterpulsation
IAD	implantable atrial defibrillator
	intermittent androgen deprivation
	intractable atopic dermatitis
	intraoperative autologous (blood) donation
IADHS	inappropriate antidiuretic hormone syndrome
IADL	Instrumental Activities of Daily Living
IA DSA	intra-arterial digital subtraction arteriography
IADT	intermittent androgen deprivation therapy
IAEA	International Atomic Energy Agency
IAET	International Association for Enterostomal Therapy (Standards of Care Dermal Wounds: Pressure Ulcers)—see WOCN
IAF	intra-abdominal fat
IAG	indolyl-3-acryloylglycine
IAGT	indirect antiglobulin test
IAHA	immune adherence hemagglutination
IAHC	intra-arterial hepatic chemotherapy
IAHD	idiopathic acquired hemolytic disease
IAI	intra-abdominal infection
	intra-abdominal injury
	intra-amniotic infection
IALD	instrumental activities of daily living
IAM	internal auditory meatus
IAN	indinavir (Crixivan) associated nephrolithiasis
	inferior alveolar nerve
	intern's admission note
IAO	immediately after onset
	inferior anterior oblique
IAP	independent adjudicating panel
	intermittent acute porphyria
	intra-abdominal pressure
	intracarotid amobarbital procedure
IAPP	islet amyloid polypeptide
IAQ	indoor air quality
IARC	International Agency for Research on Cancer
IART	intra-atrial reentrant tachycardia
IAS	idiopathic ankylosing spondylitis
	intermittent androgen suppression
	internal anal sphincter
	Interpersonal Adjective Scales
IASD	interatrial septal defect
IAT	immunoaugmentive therapy
	Implicit Association Test
	indirect antiglobulin test

	intracarotid amobarbital test	IBTR	intrabreast-tumor recurrence
	intraoperative autologous transfusion		ipsilateral breast tumor recurrence
IATT	intra-arterial thrombolytic therapy	IBU	ibuprofen
IAV	infraclavicular axillary vein	IBW	ideal body weight
	intermittent assist ventilation	IC	between meals
IAVC	intrinsic atrioventricular conduction		iliac crest
IB	ileal bypass		immune complex
	insulin-receptor binding test		immunocompromised
	isolation bed		incipient cataract (grade 1+ to 4+)
	investigator's brochure		incomplete
IB1A	interferon beta-1a (Avonex)		indirect calorimetry
IBAM	idiopathic bile acid malabsorption		indirect Coombs (test)
IBBB	intra-blood-brain barrier		individual counseling
IBBBB	incomplete bilateral bundle branch block		informed consent
			inspiratory capacity
IBC	Institutional Biosafety Committee		intensive care
	invasive bladder cancer		intercostal
	iron binding capacity		intercourse
IBCLC	International Board-Certified Lactation Consultant		intermediate care
			intermittent catheterization
IBD	identity-by-descent		intermittent claudication
	infectious bursal disease		interstitial changes
	inflammatory bowel disease		interstitial cystitis
	isosulfan blue dye		irinotecan and carboplatin
IBDQ	Inflammatory Bowel Disease Questionnaire		intracerebral
			intracranial
IBE	individual bioequivalence		intraincisional
IBG	iliac bone graft		ion chromatography
IBI	intermittent bladder irrigation		irritable colon
ibid	at the same place	I/C	imipenem-cilastatin (Primaxin)
IBILI	indirect bilirubin	I3C	indole-3-carbinol
IB-IVUS	integrated backscatter intravascular ultrasound	IC_{50}	half maximal inhibitory concentration
IBM	ideal body mass	ICA	ileocolic anastomosis
	inclusion body myositis		intermediate care area
IBMI	initial body mass index		internal carotid artery
IBMIR	instant blood-mediated inflammatory reaction		intracranial abscess
			intracranial aneurysm
IBMTR	International Bone Marrow Transplant Registry		islet-cell antibody
		ICa	calcium, ionized
IBNR	incurred but not reported	ICAAC	Interscience Conference on Antimicrobial Agents and Chemotherapy
IBOW	intact bag of waters		
IBP	ibuprofen		
	intrableb pigmentation	ICAD	intracranial atherosclerotic disease
IBPB	interscalene brachial plexus block	ICAM	intracellular adhesion molecule
IBPS	Insall-Burstein posterior stabilizer	ICAM-1	intercellular adhesion molecule-1
IBR	immediate breast reconstruction	ICAMA	Interstate Compact on Adoption and Medical Assistance
	infectious bovine rhinotracheitis	ICAO	internal carotid artery occlusion
IBRS	Inpatient Behavior Rating Scale	ICAS	intermediate coronary artery syndrome
IBS	irritable bowel syndrome		
IBS-C	irritable bowel syndrome, constipation-predominant	ICAT	infant cardiac arrest tray
			isotope-coded affinity tag
IBS-D	Irritable Bowel Syndrome–Diarrhea Type	ICB	intracranial bleeding
		ICBG	iliac crest bone graft
IBT	ink blot test (Rorschach test)	ICBT	intercostobronchial trunk
	interblinking time	ICC	idiopathic chronic cough
	immune-based therapy		immunocytochemistry

	Indian childhood cirrhosis
	Infection Control Committee
	interstitial cells of Cajal
	intracluster correlation coefficient
	intraclass correlation coefficient
	invasive cervical carcinoma
	islet cell carcinoma
ICCD	intensified charge-coupled device
ICCE	intracapsular cataract extraction
ICC-MY	myenteric interstitial cells of Cajal
ICCU	intensive coronary care unit
	intermediate coronary care unit
ICD	implantable cardioverter defibrillator
	indigocarmine dye
	informed consent document
	instantaneous cardiac death
	intercusp distance (dental)
	isocitrate dehydrogenase
	irritant contact dermatitis
ICDA	International Classification of Disease, Adapted
ICDB	incomplete database
ICDC	implantable cardioverter defibrillator catheter
ICD 9 CM	International Statistical Classification of Diseases, 9th Revision, Clinical Modification
ICD-10	International Classification of Diseases and Related Health Problems, 10th revision
ICD-10-PCS	International Statistical Classification of Diseases, 10th Revision, Procedure Coding Classification System
ICDO	International Classification of Diseases for Oncology
ICDSC	Intensive Care Delirium Screening Checklist
ICE	ice, compression, and elevation
	ifosfamide, carboplatin, and etoposide
	Immigration and Customs Enforcement
	individual career exploration
	interleukin-1 alpha converting enzyme
	interleukin-1 beta converting enzyme
	intracardiac echocardiography
+ ice	add ice
ICECI	International Classification of External Causes of Injuries
icEEG	intracranial electroencephalography
ICER	incremental cost-effectiveness ratio
ICES	ice, compression, elevation, and support
	intracranial electrical stimulation

ICF	intermediate care facility
	intracellular fluid
ICFDH	International Classification of Functioning, Disability, and Health
ICG	impedance cardiography
	indocyanine green
ICGA	indocyanine green angiography
ICH	immunocompromised host
	International Conference on Harmonization (of Technical Requirements for Registration of Pharmaceuticals for Human Use)
	intracerebral hemorrhage
	intracranial hemorrhage
ICHD-II	International Classification of Headache Disorders, 2nd Edition
ICHI	International Classification of Health Interventions
ICHT	immuno-chemotherapy
ICI	intracavernosal injection
	intracranial injury
ICIQ-SF	International Consultation on Incontinence Questionnaire
ICISG	International Cancer Information Service Group
ICIT	intensified conventional insulin therapy
ICL	intracorneal lens
	isocitrate lyase
ICLE	intracapsular lens extraction
ICM	intercostal margin
	intercostal muscle
	ischemic cardiomyopathy
ICMP	ischemic cardiomyopathy
ICN	infection control nurse
	intensive care nursery
ICN2	neonatal intensive care unit level II
ICP	inductively coupled plasma
	infantile cerebral palsy
	intercostal position (for chest lead)
	intracranial pressure
	intrahepatic cholestasis of pregnancy
ICPC	International Classification of Primary Care
	Interstate Compact on the Placement of Children
ICPC-2	International Classification of Primary Care, 2nd revision
ICP-MS	inductively-coupled plasma—mass spectrometer
ICP-OES	inductively-coupled plasma—optical emission spectrometry
ICPP	intubated continuous positive pressure
ICR	intercaudate nucleus ratio
	intercostal retractions

I

	intrastromal corneal ring		irrigation and debridement
ICRC	International Committee of the Red Cross	IDA	idarubicin (Idamycin) iron deficiency anemia
ICRF-159	razoxane	IDAM	infant of drug abusing mother
ICRP	International Commission on Radiological Protection	IDAST	identification and antimicrobial susceptibility testing
ICRS	intrastromal corneal ring segments	IDB	incomplete database
ICS	ileocecal sphincter	IDC	idiopathic dilated cardiomyopathy
	inhaled corticosteroid(s)		invasive ductal cancer
	intercostal space	IDCF	immunodiffusion complement
ICSC	idiopathic central serous choroidopathy		fixation
		IDCM	idiopathic dilated cardiomyopathy
ICSD	International Classification of Sleep Disorders	IDC-P	intraductal carcinoma of the prostate
ICSH	interstitial cell-stimulating hormone	IDD	insulin-dependent diabetes
ICSI	intracytoplasmic sperm injection		intervertebral disk disease
ICSR	Individual Case Safety Reports		iodine-deficiency disorders
	intercostal space retractions	I/DD	intellectual and developmental
ICT	icterus		disabilities
	indirect Coombs test	IDDD	Interview for Deterioration in
	inflammation of connective tissue		Daily Life in Dementia
	immunochromatographic test	IDDM	insulin-dependent diabetes mellitus
	induction chemotherapy	IDDS	implantable drug delivery system
	intensive conventional therapy		intrathecal drug delivery systems
	intermittent cervical traction	IDE	insulin degrading enzyme
	intracranial tumor		Investigational Device Exemption
	intracutaneous test	IDEA	Individuals with Disabilities
	iron chelation therapy		Education Act
	islet cell transplant	IDET	intradiskal electrothermal therapy
ICTP	C-terminal telopeptide of type I collagen	IDF	International Diabetes Federation
		IDFC	immature dead female child
ICTX	intermittent cervical traction	ID-GDM	insulin-dependent gestational
ICTx	intensive chemotherapy		diabetes mellitus
ICU	intensive care unit	IDH	intramural duodenal hematoma
	intermediate care unit		isocitric dehydrogenase
ICV	intracerebroventricular	IDI	Interpersonal Dependency
ICVH	ischemic cerebrovascular headache		Inventory
ICW	in connection with		intrathecal drug infusion
	intact canal wall	IDIS	Iowa Drug Information System
	intercellular water	IDK	internal derangement of knee
ID	identification	IDL	intermediate-density lipoprotein
	identify		ischemic digital loss
	idiotype	IDLH	immediately dangerous to life or
	ifosfamide, mesna uroprotection, and doxorubicin		health
		IDM	infant of a diabetic mother
	immunodiffusion		intermediate diastolic murmur
	induction delivery	IDMC	immature dead male child
	infectious disease (physician or department)		Independent Data Monitoring Committee
	initial diagnosis	IDMP	International Drug Monitoring
	initial dose		Program
	intellectual disability	IDMS	isotope dilution mass spectrometry
	internal derangement	IDNA	iron-deficient, not anemic
	intradermal	ID-NAT	individual donation nucleic acid
	iron deficiency		(amplification) testing
id	the same	IDO	idiopathic detrusor overactivity
I & D	incision and debridement	IDP	initiate discharge planning
	incision and drainage		inosine diphosphate

IDPN	intradialytic parenteral nutrition	IELT	Intravaginal Ejaculatory Latency Time
IDR	idarubicin (Zavedos)	IEM	immune electron microscopy
	idiosyncratic drug reaction		inborn errors of metabolism
	intradermal reaction		inherited erythromelalgia
IDS	infectious disease service	iEMG	integrated electromyography
	integrated delivery system	IEMR	integrated electronic medical records
	intradermal smears		
IDSA	Infectious Disease Society of America (guidelines)	IEN	intraepithelial neoplasia
IDT	intensive diabetes treatment	IENFD	intraepidermal nerve fiber density
	interdisciplinary team	IEP	idiopathic eosinophilic pneumonia
	intradermal test		immunoelectrophoresis
IDTF	independent diagnostic testing facility		Individualized Education Plan
		IEPA	immunoelectrophoresis analysis
ID-TLR	ischemia-driven target lesion revascularization	I:E ratio	inspiratory to expiratory time ratio
		IES	Impact of Event Scale
IDTP	immunodiffusion tube precipitin	IET	infantile estropia
IDU	idoxuridine	IEX	ion exchange
	infectious disease unit	IF	idiopathic flushing
	injecting drug user		ifosfamide (Ifex)
IDV	indinavir (Crixivan)		immunofluorescence
	intermittent demand ventilation		impaired fecundity
IDVC	indwelling venous catheter		index finger
IE	ifosfamide, and etoposide with mesna		injury factor
			interferon
	immunoelectrophoresis		interfrontal
	induced emesis		intermaxillary fixation
	infectious enteritis		internal fixation
	infective endocarditis		intrinsic factor
	inner ear		involved field (radiotherapy)
	internal/external (rotation)	IFA	immunofluorescent assay
	international unit (European abbreviation)		imported fire ants
			indirect fluorescent antibody
I/E	inspiratory/expiratory ratio		iron and folic acid
I & E	ingress and egress (tubes)	IFAT	immunofluorescence antibody test (technique)
	internal and external		
i.e.	that is	IFC	interferential current
IEC	independent ethics committee		intravital flow cytometry
	inpatient exercise center	IFCC	International Federation of Clinical Chemistry (units)
	intradiskal electrothermal coagulation		
		IFE	immunofixation electrophoresis
IED	immune-enhancing diet		in-flight emergency
	improvised explosive device	IFG	impaired fasting glucose
	interictal epileptic discharge		inferior frontal gyrus
	intermittent explosive disorder	IFI	invasive fungal infection
IEE	idiopathic eosinophilic esophagitis	IFIS	intraoperative floppy-iris syndrome
		IFL	indolent follicular lymphoma
IEED	involuntary emotional expression disorder		irinotecan, fluorouracil, and leucovorin
IEEG	intracranial electroencephalogram	IFM	Intergroupe Francophone du Myélome (myeloma French-speaking group)
IEF	isoelectric focusing		
IEH	involuntary emergency hospitalization		internal fetal monitoring
		IFN	interferon
IEI	idiopathic environmental intolerance	IFN α-1	interferon alfa-1
		IFNB	interferon beta-1 b (Betaseron)
IEL	internal elastic lamina	IFO	ifosfamide (Ifex)
	intestinal-intraepithelial lymphocyte		in front of

iFOBT	immunochemical fecal occult blood tests		infectious hepatitis
			inguinal hernia
IFOP	infrared fiber-optic probe		inhaled (this is a dangerous abbreviation)
IFOS	ifosfamide (Ifex)		
IFP	inflammatory fibroid polyps		in-house
IFPMA	International Federation of Pharmaceutical Manufacturers Associations	IHA	immune hemolytic anemia
			indirect hemagglutination
			infusion hepatic arteriography
IFRT	involved-field radiotherapy		intrahepatic arterial
IFSAC	Inventory of Functional Status After Childbirth	IHC	idiopathic hypercalciuria
			immobilization hypercalcemia
IFSE	internal fetal scalp electrode		immunohistochemistry
IFSP	individualized family service plan		inner hair cell (in cochlea)
IFVA	intraoperative fluorescence vascular angiography	IHCP	idiopathic hypertrophic cranial pachymeningitis
IG	image-guided	IHD	intermittent hemodialysis
	immunoglobulin		intraheptic duct (ule)
Ig	immunoglobulin		ischemic heart disease
IgA	immunoglobulin A	IHDN	integrated health delivery network
IgAN	immunoglobulin A nephropathy	IHES	idiopathic hypereosinophilic syndrome
IGC	Impairment Group Code(s)		
	intermediate glucose control	IHGK	immortalized human gingival keratinocytes
IGCCC	International Germ Cell Consensus Classification	IHH	idiopathic hypogonadotrophic hypogonadism
IGCS	inpatient geriatric consultation services		
		IHHE	infantile hepatic hemangioendothelioma
IgD	immunoglobulin D		
IGDE	idiopathic gait disorders of the elderly	IHHS	idiopathic hyperkinetic heart syndrome
IGDM	infant of gestational diabetic mother	IHI	Institute for Healthcare Improvement
IGE	idiopathic generalized epilepsy	IHO	idiopathic hypertrophic osteoarthropathy
	impaired gas exchange		
IgE	immunoglobulin E	IHP	idiopathic hypertrophic pachymeningitis
IGF-1	insulin-like growth factor 1		
IGFA	indocyanine-green fundus angiography		idiopathic hypoparathyroidism
			inferior hypogastric plexus
IGFBP-3	insulin-like growth factor-binding protein 3		isolated hepatic perfusion
		IHPH	intrahepatic portal hypertension
IG-FESS	image-guided funduscopic nasal surgery	IHPS	infantile hypertrophic pyloric stenosis
IGF1R	insulin-like growth factor 1 receptor	IHR	inguinal hernia repair
			intrinsic heart rate
IgG	immunoglobulin G	IHS	Indian Health Service
IGHL	inferior glenohumeral ligament		integrated healthcare system
IGI	image guided implantology		International Headache Society (criteria)
IGIM	immune globulin intramuscular		
IGIV	immune globulin intravenous		Idiopathic Headache Score
IgM	immunoglobulin M	IHs	iris hamartomas
IGP	interstitial glycoprotein	IHSA	iodinated human serum albumin
IGR	intrauterine growth retardation	IHSS	idiopathic hypertrophic subaortic stenosis
IGRT	image-guided radiation therapy		
IGT	impaired glucose tolerance		in-home supportive services
IGTN	impaired glucose tolerance and neuropathy	IHT	insulin hypoglycemia test
		IHTSDC	International Health Terminology Standard Organization
	ingrown toenail		
IH	indirect hemagglutination	IHU	inpatient hospice unit

IHW	inner-heel wedge	ILB	incidental Lewy body
II	image intensifier (radiology)	ILBBB	incomplete left bundle branch block
	internal iliac (artery)		
IIA	internal iliac artery	ILBW	infant, low birth weight (less than 2,500 g)
IICP	increased intracranial pressure		
IICU	infant intensive care unit	ILC	interstitial laser coagulation
IID	infectious intestinal disease		invasive lobular cancer
IIDD	idiopathic inflammatory demyelinating diseases	ILCOR	International Liaison Committee on Resuscitation
IIEF	International Index of Erectile Function	ILD	immature lung disease
			implantable loop device
IIF	indirect immunofluorescence		indentation load deflection
IIH	idiopathic infantile hypercalcemia		interlaminar distance in flexion
	idiopathic intracranial hypertension		intermediate density lipoproteins
			interstitial lung disease
	iodine-induced hyperthyroidism		ischemic leg disease
IIHT	iodide-induced hyperthyroidism	ILE	infantile lobar emphysema
IIM	idiopathic inflammatory myopathies		involutional lateral entropion
		ILF	indicated low forceps
	intracortical interaction mapping	ILFC	immature living female child
IINB	iliohypogastric ilioinguinal nerve block	ILHP	ipsilateral hemidiaphragmatic paresis
IIP	idiopathic interstitial pneumonitis	ILI	influenza-like illness
IIPF	idiopathic interstitial pulmonary fibrosis		isolated limb infusion
		ILK	intralesional Kenalog
IIQ	Incontinence Impact Questionnaire	ILM	internal limiting membrane
IIS	immunization information system	ILMC	immature living male child
IITs	investigator-initiated trials	ILMI	inferolateral myocardial infarct
IJ	ileojejunal	ILP	independent living program
	internal jugular		interstitial laser photocoagulation
I&J	insight and judgment		isolated limb perfusion
IJC	internal jugular catheter	ILQTS	idiopathic long QT (interval) syndrome
IJD	inflammatory joint disease		
IJO	idiopathic juvenile osteoporosis	ILR	implantable loop recorder
IJP	internal jugular pressure	ILS	increased life span
IJR	idiojunctional rhythm		intralabyrinthine schwannomas
IJT	idiojunctional tachycardia	ILT	interstitial laser therapy
IJV	internal jugular vein	ILVEN	inflammatory linear verrucal epidermal nevus
IK	immobilized knee		
	interstitial keratitis	IM	ice massage
IKDC	International Knee Documentation Committee (evaluation; score; form)		imatinib mesylate (Gleevec) (This is a very dangerous abbreviation)
			infant mortality
IL	immature lungs		infectious mononucleosis
	interleukin (1, 2, etc.)		intermetatarsal
	intralesional		internal margin (for radiotherapy)
	Intralipid®		internal medicine
IL-2	aldesleukin (Proleukin; interleukin-2)		intramedullary
			intramuscular
IL-11	oprelvekin (Neumega; interleukin-11)	IMA	inferior mesenteric artery
			internal mammary artery
ILA	iliolumbar artery	IMAC	ifosfamide, mesna uroprotection, doxorubicin (Adriamycin), and cisplatin
	inferior lateral angle		
	insulin-like activity		
ILAEC	Intersocietal Commission for Accreditation of Echocardiography Laboratories		immobilized metal affinity chromatography

I

IMAE	internal maxillary artery embolization	IMRA	immunoradiometric assay
IMAG	internal mammary artery graft	IMRaD	introduction, methods, results, and discussion (format)
IMARD	immunomodulating antirheumatic drugs	iMRI	intraoperative magnetic resonance imaging
IMAT	intensity-modulated arc therapy	IMRS	intensity-modulated radiosurgery
IMB	intermenstrual bleeding	IMRT	intensity-modulated radiation therapy
IMBP	immobilized mismatch binding protein	IMS	immunosuppressants
IMC	intermediate care		incurred in military service
	intermittent catheterization		involuntary movements
	intramedullary catheter		ion mobility spectrometry
IMCI	Integrated Management of Childhood Illness	IMSS	Mexican Institute for Social Security (*Instituto Mexicano del Seguro Social*)
IMCU	intermediate care unit		
IMDs	inherited metabolic disorders	IMT	inspiratory muscle training
IME	important medical event		intimal medial thickness
	independent medical examination (evaluation)	IMU	intermediate medicine unit
	isometric exercise	IMV	inferior mesenteric vein
IMF	idiopathic myelofibrosis		intermittent mandatory ventilation
	ifosfamide, mesna uroprotection, methotrexate, and fluorouracil		intermittent mechanical ventilation
	immobilization mandibular fracture	IMVP-16	ifosfamide, mesna uroprotection, methotrexate, and etoposide
	inframammary fold	IN	insulin (it is dangerous to use abbreviations for insulin therapy)
	intermaxillary fixation		
IMG	internal medicine group		intranasal (this is a dangerous abbreviation as it can be read as IV [intravenous] or IM [intramuscular]; use nasally or intranasal)
IMGU	insulin-mediated glucose uptake		
IMH	idiopathic myocardial hypertrophy		
	intramural hematoma		
IMH	indirect microhemagglutination (test)	In	indium
		in.	inch
IMI	imipramine	INAD	in no apparent distress
	impending myocardial infarction		Investigational New Animal Drug
	inferior myocardial infarction	INB	intercostal nerve blockade
	intramuscular injection	INC	incisal
^{131}I-MIBG	iodine^{131}-metaiodobenzyl-guanidine (iobenguane ^{131}I)		incision
			incomplete
IMIG	intramuscular immunoglobulin		incontinent
IMLC	incomplete mitral leaflet closure		increase
IMM	immunizations		inside-the-needle catheter
	Important Message from Medicare	INCC	Institut National du Cancer du Canada
IMN	idiopathic membranous nephropathy		
	immune modulating nutrition (immunonutrition)	INCMNSZ	Instituto Nacional de Ciencias Médicas y Nutrición (Mexico)
	internal mammary (lymph) node	Inc Spir	incentive spirometer
	intramedullary nail	INCSs	intranasal corticosteroids
IMP	impacted	IND	incision and drainage
	important		indinavir (Crixivan)
	impression		induced
	improved		Investigational New Drug (application)
	inosine monophoshate		
IMPX	impaction	INDA	Investigational New Drug Application
IMQ	Infant/Child Monitoring Questionnaires	INDIGO	interstitial laser ablation of the prostate
IMR	infant mortality rate	INDM	infant of nondiabetic mother

INDO	indomethacin	INST	instrumental delivery
^{111}In-DTPA	indium pentetate	INT	intermittent needle therapy internal
INE	infantile necrotizing encephalomyelopathy	Int mon	internal monitor
		interp	interpretation
INEX	inexperienced	interv	intervention
INF	infant	Int Med	internal medicine
	infarction	intol	intolerance
	infected	int-rot	internal rotation
	infection	int trx	intermittent traction
	inferior	intub	intubation
	influenza virus vaccine, not otherwise specified	INV	Invirase (saquinavir, hard gel cap)
		inver	inversion
	information	INVOS	in vivo optical spectroscopy
	infused	IO	inferior oblique
	infusion		initial opening
	intravenous nutritional fluid		inoperable
INF$_a$	influenza virus, attenuated live vaccine		intestinal obstruction
			intraocular pressure
INFas	influenza virus attenuated live vaccine, intranasal		intra-Ommaya
			intraoperative
INFC	infected		intraosseous
	infection	I&O	intake and output
INFi	influenza virus inactivated vaccine	IOA	intact on admission
info	information	IOC	intern on call
INFs	influenza virus vaccine, split viron		intraoperative cholangiogram
INFs-AB3	influenza virus inactivated vaccine, split virion, types A and B, trivalent	IOCG	intraoperative cholangiogram
		IOD	implant-supported overdenture
			interorbital distance
INF$_w$	influenza virus vaccine, whole viron	IODM	infant of diabetic mother
		IOF	intraocular fluid
ING	inguinal	IOFB	intraocular foreign body
✓ing	checking	IOFNA	intraoperative fine needle aspiration
INH	inhalation		
	isoniazid (isonicotinic acid hydrazide)	IOH	idiopathic orthostatic hypotension
		IO-HDRBT	intraoperative high-dose-rate brachytherapy
INI	intranuclear inclusion		
inj	injection	IOI	idiopathic orbital inflammation
	injury		intraosseous infusion
INK	injury not known	IOL	induction of labor
iNKT	invariant natural killer T (cell)		intraocular lens
INN	International Nonproprietary Name		intraocular lymphoma
INO	inhaled nitrous oxide	IOLI	intraocular lens implantation
	internuclear ophthalmoplegia	IOLM	intraoperative lymphatic mapping
INOP	internodal ophthalmoplegia	IOM	Institute of Medicine
iNOS	inducible nitric oxide synthase		internuclear ophthalmoplegia
inpt	inpatient		intraoperative monitor(ing)
INQ	inferior nasal quadrant	ION	ischemic optic neuropathy
INR	international normalized ratio (for anticoagulant monitoring)	IONIS	indirect optic nerve injury syndrome
INS	idiopathic nephrotic syndrome	IONTO	iontophoresis
	inspection	IOOA	inferior oblique overaction
	insurance	IOP	iontophoresis
	intranasal corticosteroids (steroids)		intensive outpatient program
in situ	in the natural or normal place		intraocular pressure
INSS	International Neuroblastoma Staging System		intraosseous puncture
		IOR	ideas of reference

I

	immature oocyte retrieval	
	inferior oblique recession	
IO-RB	intraocular retinoblastoma	
IORT	intraoperative radiation therapy	
IOS	intraoperative sonography	
IOSH	Institute for Occupational Safety and Health	
IOT	intraocular tension	
IOTEE	intraoperative transesophageal echocardiography	
IOTT	intensification-of-treatment trigger (criteria)	
IOUS	intraocular ultrasound	
IOV	initial office visit	
IP	ice pack	
	incubation period	
	individualized plan	
	Infrapatellar	
	inpatient	
	in plaster	
	interpersonal (therapy)	
	interphalangeal	
	interstitial pneumonia	
	intestinal permeability	
	intraperitoneal	
	invasive procedures	
	inverted (inverting) papilloma	
I/P	iris/pupil	
IP3	inositol triphosphate	
IPA	independent practice association	
	interpleural analgesia	
	invasive pulmonary aspergillosis	
	isopropyl alcohol	
IPAA	ileo-pouch anal anastamosis	
IPAH	idiopathic pulmonary arterial hypertension	
IPAP	inspiratory positive airway pressure	
IPB	infrapopliteal bypass	
IPC	indirect pulp cavity	
	intermittent pneumatic compression (boots)	
	intraperitoneal chemotherapy	
IPCD	idiopathic paroxysmal cerebral dysrhythmia	
	infantile polycystic disease	
IPCK	infantile polycystic kidney (disease)	
IPCR	inpatient cardiac rehabilitation	
IPCT	intraperitoneal chemotherapy	
IPD	idiopathic Parkinson disease	
	immediate pigment darkening	
	inflammatory pelvic disease	
	intermittent peritoneal dialysis	
	interpupillary distance	
	interspinous process decompression	
	invasive pneumococcal disease	

IPEX	immune dysregulation, polyendocrinopathy, enteropathy, X-linked (syndrome)
IPF	idiopathic pulmonary fibrosis
	inpatient psychiatric facility
	interstitial pulmonary fibrosis
IPFD	intrapartum fetal distress
IPG	immobilized pH gradient
	impedance plethysmography
	implantable pulse generator
	individually polymerized grass
IPH	idiopathic pulmonary hemosiderosis
	interphalangeal
	intraparenchymal hemorrhage
	intraperitoneal hemorrhage
IPHC	intraperitoneal hyperthermic chemotherapy
IPHEP	independent progressive home exercise program
IPHP	intraperitoneal hyperthermic chemotherapy
IPI	International Prognostic Index
IPJ	interphalangeal joint
IPK	intractable plantar keratosis
IPL	intense pulsed light
IPM	intranodal-palisaded myofibroblastoma
	intrauterine pressure monitor
	interventional pain management
IPMI	inferoposterior myocardial infarct
IPMN	intraductal papillary mucinous neoplasm
IPN	infantile periarteritis nodosa
	intern's progress note
	interstitial pneumonia
IPO	inferior posterior oblique
IPOF	immediate postoperative fitting
IPOM	intraperitoneal onlay mesh
IPOP	immediate postoperative prosthesis
IPP	inflatable penile prosthesis
	intrapleual pressure
	intravesical protrusion of the prostate
	isolated pelvic perfusion
IPPA	inspection, palpation, percussion, and auscultation
IPPB	intermittent positive-pressure breathing
IP-PDT	intraperitoneal photodynamic therapy
IPPE	initial preventive physical examination
IPPF	immediate postoperative prosthetic fitting
IPPI	interruption of pregnancy for psychiatric indication

IPPR	inpatient pulmonary rehabilitation	IRAD	International Registry of Acute Aortic Dissection
IPPV	intermittent positive pressure ventilation	IRA-EEA	ileorectal anastomoses with end-to-end anastomosis
IPRG	Interdisciplinary Pharmacogenomics Review Group (FDA)	IRAP	interleukin-1 receptor antagonist protein
IPS	idiopathic pneumonia syndrome	IRB	Institutional Review Board
	infundibular pulmonic stenosis	IRBBB	incomplete right bundle branch block
	initial prognostic score		
	intermittent photic stimulation	IRBC	immature red blood cell
	intraparietal sulcus		irradiated red blood cells
iPs	induced pluripotent stem (cells)	iRBCs	*Plasmodium falciparum*-infected red blood cells
iPSCs	induced pluripotent stem cells		
	islet-producing stem cells	IRBP	implantable rotary blood pump
IPSF	immediate postsurgical fitting		interphotoreceptor retinoid-binding protein
IPSID	immunoproliferative small intestinal disease		
		IRC	indirect radionuclide cystography
IPSP	inhibitory postsynaptic potential		infrared coagulation
IPSS	inferior petrosal sinus sampling		Institutional Review Committee (Board)
	International Prostate Symptom Score		
		IRCU	intensive respiratory care unit
IPST	intraprocedural stent thrombosis	IRD	immune renal disease(s)
I PSY	intermediate psychiatry	IRDA	intermittent rhythmic delta activity
IPT	intended primary treatment	IRDM	insulin-requiring diabetes mellitus
	intermittent pelvic traction		insulin-resistant diabetes mellitus
iPTH	parathyroid hormone by radioimmunoassay	IR-DRGs	International Refined Diagnosis Related Groups
IPTX	intermittent pelvic traction	IRDS	idiopathic respiratory distress syndrome
IPV	inactivated poliovirus vaccine		
	intimate partner violence		infant respiratory distress syndrome
	intrapulmonary percussive ventilation	IRE	internal rotation in extension
IPVC	interpolated premature ventricular contraction	IRED	infrared-emission detection
		IRF	impaired renal function
IPW	interphalangeal width		inpatient rehabilitation facilities
IQ	intelligence quotient		internal rotation in flexion
IQR	interquartile range	IRH	intraretinal hemorrhage
	intraquartile range (statistical term)	IRI	immunoreactive insulin
IQWiG	Leiter des Institus für Qualität and Wirtschaftlichkeit im Gesundheitswesen (Institute for Quality and Economy in Healthcare)		irinotecan (Camptosar)
			ischemic reperfusion injury
		IRIS	immune reconstitution inflammatory syndrome
		IRIV	immunopotentiating reconstituted influenza virosomes
IR	immediate-release (tablets)	IRM	magnetic resonance imaging (French)
	immunoreactive		
	inferior rectus	IRMA	immediate response mobile analysis (blood analysis system)
	infrared		
	insulin resistance		immunoradiometric assay
	internal reduction		intraretinal microvascular abnormalities
	internal resistance		
	internal rotation	IRMS	isotope-ratio mass spectrometry
	inversion recovery (radiology)	IRN	iterated rippled noise
	intraoral radiography (dental)	IRNS	intercostal repetitive nerve stimulation
	interventional radiology		
I&R	insertion and removal	IROS	ipsilateral routing of signals
IRA	infarct-related artery	IROX	irinotecan and oxaliplatin
IRAAF	intraoperative radiofrequency ablation for chronic atrial fibrillation	IRP	intellectual property rights

IRR	infrared radiation		isolette servo-control
	intrarenal reflux	ISCM	intramedullary spinal cord
	irregular rate and rhythm		metastases
IRRC	Institutional Research Review	I/SCN	urinary iodine/thiocyanate ratio
	Committee	ISCOM	immunostimulating complex
irreg	irregular	ISCP	infection surveillance and control
IRR HYDRO	irreversible hydrocolloid		program
		ISCs	irreversible sickle cells
IRRs	incidence rate ratios	ISCU	infant special care unit
IRS	Information and Referral Society	ISD	inhibited sexual desire
	insulin receptor substrate		initial sleep disturbance
	insulin-resistance syndrome		intrinsic (urethral) sphincter
IRSB	intravenous regional sympathetic		deficiency
	block		isosorbide dinitrate (Isordol)
IRSG	Intergroup Rhabdomyosarcoma	ISDN	isosorbide dinitrate (Isordol)
	Study Group	ISE	Integrated Safety Summary
IRT	immunoreactive trypsin		internal scalp electrode
	incident response team		ion-sensitive electrode
	Intermittent Recovery Test	ISEL	*in situ* end labeling
IRU	intensive rehabilitation unit	ISF	interstitial fluid
IRV	inspiratory reserve volume	ISFET	ion-selective field effect transistor
	inverse ratio ventilation	ISG	immune serum globulin (immune
IS	incentive spirometer		globulin)
	induced sputum	ISH	isolated systolic hypertension
	Infant Star (ventilator)	ISHH	*in situ* hybridization
	infarct size		histochemistry
	Information Services (Department)	ISHLT	International Society for Heart and
	in situ		Lung Transplantation
	intercostal space	ISHT	isolated systolic hypertension
	inventory of systems	ISI	Insomnia Severity Index
	ipecac syrup		Insulin Sensitivity Index
I-S	Ionescu-Shiley (prosthetic heart		International Sensitivity Index
	valve)	ISK	inflamed seborrheic keratosis
I & S	intact and symmetrical		isokinetic
I/S	instruct/supervise	ISMA	infantile spinal muscular atrophy
I2S	iduronate-2-sulfatase	ISMN	isosorbide mononitrate
ISA	ileosigmoid anastomosis	ISMO®	isosorbide mononitrate
	Incest Survivors Anonymous	ISMP	Institute for Safe Medication
	intrinsic sympathomimetic activity		Practices
ISAAC	International Study of Asthma and	ISNA	iron-sufficient, not anemic
	Allergies in Childhood	ISO	International Organization for
	(questionnaire; protocol)		Standardization
ISADH	inappropriate secretion of		isocenter
	antidiuretic hormone		isodose
ISAM	infant of substance abusing		isolette
	mother		isoproterenol
ISB	inappropriate sexual behaviors	ISOE	isoetharine
	incentive spirometry breathing	ISOF	isoflurane (Florane)
ISBN	International Standard Book	ISOK	isokinetic
	Number	ISOM	isometric
ISBP	interscalen brachial plexus	ISOs	isoenzymes
ISC	carcinoma *in situ* (also CIS)	ISP	Individual Service Plan
	indwelling subclavian catheter		inferior spermatic plexus
	infant servo-control		interspace
	infant skin control	ISPP	individualized sleep promotion
	intermittent self-catheterization		plan
	intermittent straight	*ISQ*	as before; continue on (*in status*
	catheterization		*quo*)

ISR	injection site reaction	ITA	individual treatment assessment
	in situ reconstruction		inferior temporal artery
	in-stent restenosis		itasetron
	integrated secretory response	ITAG	internal thoracic artery graft
ISRCTN	International Standard Randomized	ITAL	intrathoracic artificial lung
	Controlled Trial Number	ITB	iliotibial band
ISS	idiopathic short stature		intrathecal baclofen
	Individual Self-Rating Scale	ITBC	intraluminal typical bronchial
	Injury Severity Score		carcinoid
	Integrated Summary of Safety	ITBS	iliotibial band syndrome
	irritable stomach syndrome		Iowa Tests of Basic Skills
	ischial spine sign	ITC	Incontinence Treatment Center
IS10S	10% invert sugar in 0.9% sodium		in-the-canal (hearing aid)
	chloride (saline) injection		isothermal titration calorimetry
ISSHL	idiopathic sudden sensorineural	ITCP	idiopathic thrombocytopenic
	hearing loss		purpura
ISSP	Infant Support Services Program	ITCs	isolated tumor cells
ISSSTE	The Institute of Social Security and	ITCU	intensive thoracic cardiovascular
	Services for Civil Servants		unit
	(*Instituto de Seguridad y*	ITD	impedance threshold device
	Servicios Sociales de los	ITDD	intrathecal drug delivery
	Trabajadores del Estado)	ITE	insufficient therapeutic effect
	(Mexico)		in-the-ear (hearing aid)
IST	immunosuppressive therapy	ITF	inpatient treatment facility
	inappropriate sinus tachycardia	ITFF	intertrochanteric femoral fracture
	injection sclerotherapy	ITGV	intrathoracic gas volume
	insulin sensitivity test	ITM	Institute of Tropical Medicine,
	insulin shock therapy		(Antwerp, Belgium)
ISU	intermediate surgical unit	ITMTX	intrathecal methotrexate
ISW	interstitial water	ITN	irinotecan (Camptosar)
IS10W	10% invert sugar injection	ITNs	insecticide-treated nets
	(in water)	ITOC	intratracheal oxygen catheter
ISWI	incisional surgical wound	ITOP	intentional termination of
	infection		pregnancy
IT	iliotibial	ITOU	intensive therapy observation unit
	incentive therapy	ITP	idiopathic thrombocytopenic
	individual therapy		purpura
	inferior-temporal		immune thrombocytopenia
	inferior turbinate		immune thrombocytopenic
	information technology		purpura
	Information Technology		interim treatment plan
	(Department)	ITPA	Illinois Test of Psycholinguistic
	Inhalation Therapist		Ability
	inhalation therapy	ITQ	inferior temporal quadrant
	inspiratory time	ITR	isotretinoin (Accutane)
	intensive therapy	ITRA	itraconazole (Sporanox)
	intermittent traction	ITS	intelligent testing strategies
	interpreted		internal transcribed spacer
	intertrochanteric		iontophoretic transdermal system
	intertuberous		isometric trunk stabilization
	intrathecal (dangerous		intratympanic steroids
	abbreviation)	ITSCU	infant-toddler special care unit
	intratracheal (dangerous, could be	ITT	identical twins (raised) together
	interupted as intrathecal)		incremental treadmill test
	intratumoral		insulin tolerance test
	intratympanic (this is a dangerous		intention-to-treat (analysis)
	abbreviation that could be	ITTF	intra-operative transit time
	interpreted as intrathecal)		flowmetry

I

ITU	infant-toddler unit	IVA	Intervir-A
	intensive therapy unit	IVAD	implantable venous access device
	intensive treatment unit		implantable vascular access device
ITVAD	indwelling transcutaneous vascular access device	IVBAT	intravascular bronchoalveolar tumor
ITX	immunotoxin(s)	IVC	inferior vena cava
ITx	intestinal transplantation		inspiratory vital capacity
ITZ	itraconazole (Sporanox)		intravenous chemotherapy
IU	internal urethrotomy		intravenous cholangiogram
	international unit (this is a dangerous abbreviation as it is read as intravenous; use "units")		intraventricular catheter
			intraventricular conduction
		IVCCM	in-vivo corneal confocal microscopy
IUBT	intrauterine blood transfusion		
IUC	intrauterine catheter	IVCD	intraventricular conduction defect (delay)
IUCD	intrauterine contraceptive device		
IUD	intrauterine death	IVCF	inferior vena cava filter
	intrauterine device	IVCI	intravenous continuous infusion
IUDE	intrauterine drug exposure	IVCP	inferior vena cava pressure
	intravenous drug exposure	IVCS	intravenous conscious sedation
IUDR	idoxuridine (Herplex)	IVCV	inferior venacavography
IUFB	intrauterine foreign body	IVD	instrumental vaginal delivery
IUFD	intrauterine fetal death (demise)		intervertebral disk
	intrauterine fetal distress		intravenous drip
IUFT	intrauterine fetal transfusion		in vitro diagnostic
IUGR	intrauterine growth retardation (restriction)		ischemic vascular dementia
		IVDA	intravenous drug abuse
IUI	intrauterine insemination	IVDK	Information Network of Departments of Dermatology (Göttingen University) (http://www.ivdk.org)
IUI/COH	intrauterine insemination with controlled ovarian hyperstimulation		
IULN	institutional upper limit of normal	IVDMIAs	in vitro diagnostic multivariate index assays
IUMR	intrauterine myelomeningocele repair		
		IVDSA	intravenous digital subtraction angiography
IUP	intrauterine pregnancy		
IUPAC	International Union of Pure and Applied Chemistry	IVDU	intravenous drug user
		IVELT	intravaginal ejaculation latency time
IUPAT	intrauterine pregnancy at term		
IUPB	infected units per billion	IVET	in vivo expression technology
IUPC	intrauterine pressure catheter	IVF	intervertebral foramina
IUPD	intrauterine pregnancy delivered		intravenous fluid(s)
IUP,TBCS	intrauterine pregnancy, term birth, cesarean section		intraventricular fibrinolysis
			in vitro fertilization
IUP,TBLC	intrauterine pregnancy, term birth, living child	IVFA	intravenous fluorescein angiography
IUR	intrauterine retardation	IVFBT	*in vitro* fertilization boosted tree (model)
IUS	intrauterine system		
IUT	intersection-union test	IVFE	intravenous fat emulsion
	intrauterine transfusion	IVF-ET	in vitro fertilization-embryo transfer
IUTD	immunizations up to date		
IV	four	IVFT	intravenous fetal transfusion
	interview	IVGG	intravenous gamma globulin
	intravenous (i.v.)	IVGTT	intravenous glucose tolerance test
	intravertebral	IVH	intravenous hyperalimentation
	invasive		intraventricular hemorrhage
	inversion	IVID	intravenous iron dextran (INFeD; DexFerrum)
	symbol for class 4 controlled substances		
		IVIG	intravenous immunoglobulin

IVJC	intervertebral joint complex	IWI	inferior wall infarction
IVK	intravitreal injection of triamcinolone acetonide (Kenalog) (also IVTA)	IWL	insensible water loss involuntary weight loss
		IWMI	inferior wall myocardial infarct
IVL	intravascular lymphomatosis intravenous lock	IWML	idiopathic white matter lesion
		IWT	ice-water test impacted wisdom teeth
IVLBW	infant of very low birth weight (less than 1,500 g)	Ixa	ixabepilone
IVMP	intravenously administered methylprednisolone	IXT	intermittent exotropia
IVNC	isolated ventricular noncompaction		
IVO	intraoral vertical osteotomy		
IVOX	intravascular oxygenator (oxygenation)		
IVP	intravenous push (this is a dangerous meaning as it is read as intravenous pyelogram) intravenous pyelogram		
IVPB	intravenous piggyback		
IVPF	isovolume pressure flow		
IVPU	intravenous push		
IVR	idioventricular rhythm interactive voice-response (system) intravaginal ring intravenous retrograde intravenous rider (this is a dangerous abbreviation as it has been read as IVP-intravenous push) isovolumic relaxation (time)		
IVRA	intravenous regional anesthesia		
IVRAP	intravenous retrograde access port		
IVRG	intravenous retrograde		
IV-RNV	intravenous radionuclide venography		
IVRO	intraoral vertical ramus osteotomy		
IVRS	interactive voice response system		
IVRT	isovolumic relation time		
IVS	intraventricular septum irritable voiding syndrome		
IVSD	intraventricular septal defect		
IVSE	interventricular septal excursion		
IVSO	intraoral vertical segmental osteotomy		
IVSS	intravenous Soluset®		
IVST	interventricular septum thickness		
IVT	intravenous transfusion intraventricular		
IVTA	intravitreal injection of triamcinolone acetonide		
IVTTT	intravenous tolbutamide tolerance test		
IVU	intravenous urography (urogram)		
IVUC	intravenous ultrasound catheter		
IVUS	intravascular ultrasound		
IW	inspiratory wheeze		
IWD	individual with a disability		

J

J	Jaeger measure of near vision with 20/20 about equal to J1
	jejunostomy
	Jewish
	joint
	joule
	juice
J 1-16	Jaeger near acuity notation (1 to 16 scale)
JA	joint aspiration
Jack	jackknife position
JAFAR	Juvenile Arthritis Functional Assessment Report
JAMA	*Journal of the American Medical Association*
JAMG	juvenile autoimmune myasthenia gravis
JAN	Japanese Accepted Name
JAR	junior assistant resident
JARAN	junior assistant resident admission note
JBE	Japanese B encephalitis
JBS	Johanson Blizzard syndrome
JC	Joint Commission (www.jointcommission.com)
	junior clinicians (medical students)
JCA	juvenile chronic arthritis
JCAHO	Joint Commission on Accreditation of Healthcare Organizations (this has been changed to TJC, The Joint Commission)
JCC	Jackson cross cylinder (astigmatism test)
JCO	Journal of Clinical Oncology
	Juvenile Court Order
JCOG	Japanese Clinical Oncology Group
JCQ	Job Content Questionnaire
JD	Doctor of Jurisprudence (a law degree)
	jaundice
JDG	jugulodigastric
JDLR	Just doesn't look right (something is wrong, but no diagnosis has been made yet) (slang)
JDM	juvenile diabetes mellitus
JDMS	juvenile dermatomyositis
JE	Japanese encephalitis
JEB	junctional epidermolysis bullosa
	junctional escape beat
JEJ	jejunum
JEN	Japanese encephalitis vaccine
JER	junctional escape rhythm
JET	jejunal extension tube
	junctional ectopic tachycardia

JEV	Japanese encephalitis virus
JF	joint fluid
JFS	Jewish Family Service
JGCT	juvenile granulosa cell tumor
JGI	jejunogastric intussusception
JHR	Jarisch-Herxheimer reaction
JHS	joint hypermobility syndrome
JI	jejunoileal
JIA	juvenile idiopathic arthritis
JIB	jejunoileal bypass
JIS	juvenile idiopathic scoliosis
JJ	jaw jerk
J & J	Johnson & Johnson Health Care Systems, Inc.
JLD	just like dad; an explanation for a child's unusual facial features (slang)
JLIS	Jessner lymphocytic infiltration of the skin
JLO	Judgment of Line Orientation (test)
JLP	juvenile laryngeal papillomatosis
JM-9	iproplatin
JME	juvenile myoclonic epilepsy
JMI	Jones Medical Inc.
JMML	juvenile myelomonocytic leukemia
JMS	junior medical student
JNA	juvenile nasopharyngeal angiofibroma
JNB	jaundice of newborn
JNCL	juvenile-onset neuronal ceroid lipofuscinosis
JND	just noticeable difference
JNR	Just not right (something is wrong, but no diagnosis has been made yet) (slang)
JNT	joint
JNVD	jugular neck vein distention
JODM	juvenile-onset diabetes mellitus
JOF	juvenile ossifying fibroma
JOLs	judgments of learning
JOMAC	judgment, orientation, memory, abstraction, and calculation
JOMACI	judgment, orientation, memory, abstraction, and calculation intact
JOR	jaw-opening reflex
JORRP	juvenile-onset recurrent respiratory papillomatosis
JP	Jackson-Pratt (drain)
	Jobst pump
	joint protection
JPA	joint position awareness
	juvenile pilocytic astrocytoma
JPB	junctional premature beats
JP BS	Jackson-Pratt to bulb suction
JPC	junctional premature contraction

JPOF	juvenile psammomatoid ossifying fibroma
JPS	joint position sense
	juvenile polyposis syndrome
JPT	Japanese from Tokyo (populations included in HapMap - see HapMap)
JR	junctional rhythm
JRA	juvenile rheumatoid arthritis
JRAN	junior resident admission note
Jr BF	junior baby food
JRC	joint replacement center
JSF	Japanese spotted fever
JSPE	Jefferson Scale of Physician Empathy
JSRV	jaagziekte sheep retrovirus
JSW	joint space width
JT	jejunostomy tube
	joint
	junctional tachycardia
JTF	jejunostomy tube feeding
JTH	Jebsen Test of Hand (Function)
JTJ	jaw-to-jaw (position)
JTP	joint projection
JTPS	juvenile tropical pancreatitis syndrome
J-Tube	jejunostomy tube
JUV	juvenile
JV	jugular vein
JVC	jugular venous catheter
JVD	jugular venous distention
JVI	jugular-valve incompetencce
JVP	jugular venous pressure
	jugular venous pulsation
	jugular venous pulse
JVPT	jugular venous pulse tracing
JW	Jehovah's Witness
Jx	joint
JXG	juvenile xanthogranuloma

K	cornea
	kelvin
	ketamine (Ketalar, Vitamin K, Special K, and Super K)
	kilodalton
	Kosher
	potassium
	thousand
	vitamin K
K'	knee
K^+	potassium
K_1	phytonadione (Methyton)
K_2	menatetrenone
K_3	menadione
K_4	menadiol sodium diphosphate
17K	17-ketosteroids
510(k)	Medical Device Premarket Notification
KA	kainic acid
	kala-azar
	keratoacanthoma
	ketoacidosis
Ka	first order absorption constant in $hr.^{-1}$
KAB	knowledge, attitude, and behavior
K-ABC	Kaufman Assessment Battery for Children
KABINS	knowledge, attitude, behavior, and improvement in nutritional status
KACT	kaolin-activated clotting time
Kaizen	Good Change (Japanese)
KAFO	knee-ankle-foot orthosis
KAO	knee-ankle orthosis
KAS	Katz Adjustment Scale
KASH	knowledge, abilities, skills, and habits
kat	katal
K-A units	King-Armstrong units
KB	ketone bodies
	knee-bearing
Kb	kilobase (genetics; 1,000 base pairs)
KBD	Kashin-Beck disease
KBG	a rare genetic disease (syndrome) whose name was derived from the initials of the affected patients in the original report. Characterized by a distinct facial phenotype, macrodontia, short stature, developmental delay, and/or mental retardation.
KC	kangaroo care
	keratoconjunctivitis

	keratoconus	KGD	ketogenic diet
	kinship care	KGF	keratinocyte growth factor
	knees-to-chest	KGC	Keflin, gentamicin, and
	Korean conflict		carbenicillin
kcal	kilocalorie	17-KGS	17-ketogenic steroids
KCCQ	Kansas City Cardiomyopathy	KGy	kiloGray
	Questionnaire	K24H	potassium, urine 24-hour
KCCT	kaolin cephalin clotting time	KHF	Korean hemorrhagic fever
KChIPs	potassium channel-interacting	KHQ	King's Health Questionnaire
	proteins	kHz	kilohertz
kCi	kilocurie	KI	karyopyknotic index
KCl	potassium chloride		knee immobilizer
	keratoconus		potassium iodide
KCO	potassium channel opener	KID	keratitis, ichthyosis, and deafness
KCS	keratoconjunctivitis sicca		(syndrome)
KCZ	ketoconazole (Nizoral)		kidney
KD	Kawasaki disease	kilo	kilogram
	Keto Diastix®		thousand
	ketogenic diet	KIN	kinetic
	kidney donors	KISS	saturated solution of potassium
	knee disarticulation		iodide
	knowledge deficit	KIT	Kahn Intelligence Test
kd	kilodalton		a cytokine receptor expressed on
KDA	known drug allergies		the surface of hematopoietic
kDa	kilodalton		stem cells as well as other cell
KDC®	brand name of infant warmer		types (also known as C-kit
KDQ	Kidney Disease Questionnaire		receptor and CD117)
KDQOL	Kidney Disease Quality of Life	KIU	kallikrein inhibitor units
KDU	Kidney Dialysis Unit	KJ	kilojoule
KE	first order elimination rate constant		knee jerk
	in hr.$^{-1}$	KJR	knee-jerk reflex
KED	Kendrick extrication device	KK	knee kick
KEEP	Kidney Early Evaluation Program		knock-knee
	(National Kidney Foundation)	KKS	kallikrein-kinin system
k_{el}	elimination rate constant	K & L	Kellgren and Lawrence (scale for
KELS	Kohlman Evaluation of Living		osteoarthritis assessment)
	Skills	KLB	klebsiella vaccine
KET	ketamine (Ketalar)	KL-BET	Kleihauer-Betke
	ketoconazole (Nizoral)	Kleb	*Klebsiella*
	ketones	KLF	Krüppel-like factor
KETO	ketoconazole (Nizoral)	KLH	keyhole limpet hemocyanin
17 Keto	17 ketosteroids	K-Lor®	potassium chloride tablets
keV	kilo-electron volts	KLS	kidneys, liver, and spleen
KEVD	Krupin eye valve with disc		Kleine-Levin syndrome
KF	kidney function	KM	kanamycin
KFA	kinetic fibrinogen assay	KMC	kangaroo-mother care
KFAB	kidney-fixing antibodies	KMnO$_4$	potassium permanganate
KFAO	knee-foot-ankle orthosis	KMO	Kaiser-Meyer-Olkin (measure of
KFD	Kikuchi-Fujimoto disease		statistical sampling adequacy)
	Kyasanur Forrest disease	KMV	killed measles vaccine
KFE	knee flexion and extension	KN	knee
KFR	Kayser-Fleischer ring	KNO	keep needle open
KFS	Klippel-Feil syndrome	KNSA	Kron Nutritive Sucking Apparatus
KFSD	keratosis follicularis spinulosa	KO	keep open
	decalvans		knee orthosis
kg	kilogram (1 kg = 2.2 pounds)		knocked out
K-G	Kimray-Greenfield (filter)	KOH	potassium hydroxide

K

KOL	key opinion leader	KUS	kidney(s), ureter(s), and spleen
KOOS	Knee Injury and Osteoarthritis Outcome Score	KV	kilovolt
		KVAs	vitamin k antagonists
KOR	keep open rate	KVFD	Kelvin-Voigt Fractional Derivative
KOSCHI	King Outcome Scale for Closed Head Injury	KVO	keep vein open
		KVP	kilovolt peak
KP	hot pack	KW	Keith-Wagener (ophthalmoscopic finding, graded I-IV)
	keratoprecipitate		
	kinetic perimetry		Kimmelstiel-Wilson
kPa	kilopascal	KWB	Keith, Wagener, Barker
KPC	Klebsiella pneumoniae carbapenemase	KWIC	keywork in context
		K-wire	Kirschner wire
KPCA	Kernel Principal Component Analysis	KXRF	K-shell X-ray Fluorescence
		KYPHO	kyphoplasty

KPD   kidney paired donation
KPE   Kelman phacoemulsification
KPM   kilopounds per minute
KPS   Karnofsky performance status
           (scores) (scale)
KQI   key quality indicators
Kr   krypton
KRAS   V-Ki-ras2 Kirsten rat sarcoma viral
           oncogene homolog (a protein
           which in humans is encoded by
           the *KRAS* gene)
K-rod   Küntscher rod
KS   Kawasaki syndrome
           Kaposi sarcoma
           kidney stone
           Klinefelter syndrome
17-KS   17-ketogenic steroids
           17-ketosteroids
KSA   knowledge, skills, and abilities
K-SADS   Kiddie Schedule for Affective
           Disorders and Schizophrenia
KSE   knee sling exercises
KSHV   Kaposi sarcoma-associated
           herpesvirus
KS/OI   Kaposi sarcoma and opportunistic
           infections
KSP   Karolinska Scales of Personality
KSR   potassium chloride sustained
           release (tablets)
KSS   Kearns-Sayre syndrome
KSW   knife stab wound
KT   kidney transplant
           kinesiotherapy
           known to
KTC   knee-to-chest
KTP   potassium-titanyl-phosphate (laser)
KTS   Klippel-Trenaunay syndrome
KTU   kidney transplant unit
           known to us
KTx   kidney transplantation
KTZ   ketoconazole (Nizoral)
KUB   kidney(s), ureter(s), and bladder
           kidney ultrasound biopsy

K

L

L fifty
  Laribacter
  left (this is a dangerous
   abbreviation; spell out "left" to
   avoid surgical errors)
  lente insulin (this is a dangerous
   abbreviation, since there is also
   a Lantus insulin available)
  levorotatory
  lingual
  Listeria
  liter (1 L = 1,000 mL = 1 quart
   plus about 2 ounces)
  liver
  low
  lumbar
  lung
l levorotatory
L′ lumbar
Ⓛ left (this is a dangerous
   abbreviation; spell out "left" to
   avoid surgical errors)
L1 first language
L₁...L₅ lumbar nerve 1 through 5
  lumbar vertebra 1 through 5
L1-2 lumbar spine, between first and
   second vertebrae (the disk space)
L2 second language
LA language age
  laryngeal amyloid
  latex agglutination
  Latin American
  left arm
  left atrial
  left atrium
  leukoaraiosis (a radiologic finding)
  light adaptation
  linguoaxial
  linoleic acid
  lives alone
  local anesthesia
  long acting
  lupus anticoagulant
L + A light and accommodation
  living and active
LAA large artery atherosclerosis
  left atrium and its appendage
LAAM levomethadyl acetate (L-alpha
   acetylmeth-adol, Orlaam)
LAAs leukemia-associated antigens
LAAT left atrial appendage thrombus
LAB laboratory
  left abdomen (LAb)

LABA laser-assisted balloon angioplasty
  long-acting beta-2 agonist
LABBB left anterior bundle branch block
LABC locally advanced breast cancer
LABD linear immunoglobulin A bullous
   dermatosis
LABR laparoscopic-assisted bowel
   resection
LAC laceration
  lactobacillus acidophilus vaccine
  laparoscopic-assisted colectomy
  left antecubital
  left atrial catheter
  locally advanced cancer
  long arm cast
  lupus anticoagulant
LAc Licensed Acupuncturist
LACC locally advanced cervical
   carcinoma
LACE listening and communication
   enhancement
LACI lacunar circulation infarct
  lipoprotein-associated coagulation
   inhibitor
LACS laser-assisted capsular shrinkage
LACT- lactate arterial
ART
LAD laser anesthesia device
  left anterior descending
  left atrial diameter
  left atrial dimension
  left axis deviation
  leukocyte adhesion deficiency
  ligament augmentation device
LADA left anterior descending (coronary)
   artery
LADCA left anterior descending coronary
   artery
LADD left anterior descending diagonal
LADG laparoscopy-assisted distal
   gastrectomy
LAD-MIN left axis deviation minimal
LADPG laparoscopically assisted distal
   partial gastrectomy
LAE left atrial enlargement
  long above elbow
LAEC locally advanced esophageal cancer
LAEI large artery elasticity index
LAEs liver-associated enzymes
LAF laminar air flow
  Latin-American female
  low animal fat
  lymphocyte-activating factor
LAFB left anterior fascicular block
LAFF lateral arm free flap
LAFM locally acquired *Plasmodium*
   falciparum malaria
LAFR laminar airflow room

LAG	lymphangiogram	chole	cholecystectomy
LAGB	laparoscopic-adjustable gastric banding	LAPMS	long arm posterior molded splint
		LAPW	left atrial posterior wall
LAH	left anterior hemiblock	LAQ	long arc quad
	left atrial hypertrophy	LAR	laryngeal adductor reflex
LAHB	left anterior hemiblock		left arm, reclining
LAHNC	locally advanced (squamous cell) head and neck cancer		long-acting release
			low anterior resection
LAI	left atrial isomerism	LARC	Locally-advanced rectal cancer
LAIC	left anterior interior chain (of muscles)	LARM	left arm
		LARS	laparoscopic antireflux surgery
LAIT	latex agglutination inhibition test	LARSI	lumbar anterior-root stimulator implants
LAIV	live, attenuated influenza vaccine		
LAK	lymphokine-activated killer	LAS	lactic acidosis syndrome
LAL	left axillary line		laxative abuse syndrome
	limulus amebocyte lysate		left arm, sitting
LALLS	low-angle laser light scattering		leucine acetylsalicylate
LALT	larynx-associated lymphoid tissue		long arm splint
	low-air loss therapy (mattress)		low-amplitude signal
LAM	lactational anovulatory method (birth control)		lymphadenopathy syndrome
			lymphangioscintigraphy
	laminectomy		lysine acetylsalicylate
	laminogram	LASA	Linear Analogue Self-Assessment (scales)
	laparoscopic-assisted myomectomy		
	laser-assisted myringotomy		lipid-associated sialic acid
	Latin-American male	LASCC	locally advanced squamous cell carcinoma
	lymphangioleiomyomatosis		
lam✓	laminectomy check	LASCCHN	locally advanced squamous cell carcinoma of the head and neck
LAMA	laser-assisted microanastomosis		
LAMB	mucocutaneous lentigines, atrial myxoma, and blue nevus (syndrome)		
		LASEC	left atrial spontaneous echo contrast
L-AMB	liposomal amphotericin B	LASER	light amplification by stimulated emission of radiation
LAMI	laminectomy		
LAMMA	laser microprobe mass analysis	LASGB	laparoscopic-adjustable silicone gastric banding
LAN	lymphadenopathy		
LANA	latency-associated nuclear antigen	LASIK	laser *in situ* keratomileusis
LANC	long arm navicular cast	LASO	left anterior superior oblique
LA-NSCLC	locally-advanced nonsmall-cell lung cancer	L-ASP	asparaginase (Elspar)
		LAST	left anterior small thoracotomy
LAO	left anterior oblique	LASW	Licensed Advanced Social Worker
	long-acting opioid(s)	LAT	lateral
LAP	laparoscopy		latex agglutination test
	laparotomy		left anterior thigh
	left abdominal pain		lidocaine, epinephrine, (Adrenalin) and tetracaine
	left atrial pressure		
	leucine amino peptidase	LATCH	literature attached to chart
	leukocyte alkaline phosphatase	lat.men.	lateral meniscectomy
	lower abdominal pain	LATS	long-acting thyroid stimulator
LAPA	locally-advanced pancreatic adenocarcinoma	LATVH	laparoscopic-assisted total vaginal hysterectomy
lap-appy	laparoscopic appendectomy	LAUP	laser-assisted uvula-palatoplasty
		LAV	left atrial volume
Lap-Band®	laparoscopic-adjustable gastric banding		live attenuated flavivirus
			lymphadenopathy associated virus
LAPC	locally advanced pancreatic cancer	LAVA	laser-assisted vasal anastomosis
	locally-advanced prostate cancer	LAVH	laparoscopically assisted vaginal hysterectomy
lap	laparoscopic		

L

LAVHLSO	laparoscopically assisted vaginal hysterectomy, left salpingo-oophorectomy		LBO	large bowel obstruction
LAVHRSO	laparoscopically assisted vaginal hysterectomy, right salpingo-oophorectomy		LBOTC	laryngeal and base-of-tongue carcinomas
			LBP	low back pain
				low blood pressure
LAVM	laparoscopic-assisted vaginal myomectomy		LBQC	large base quad cane
			LBRF	louse-borne relapsing fever
LAW	left atrial wall		LBS	low back syndrome
LAWER	life-terminating acts without the explicit request			pounds
			LBT	low back tenderness
LAX	laxative			low back trouble
LAZ	length-for-age Z-score		LBV	left brachial vein
LB	large bowel			Lewy body variant
	lateral bend			low biological value
	left breast		LBVO	left brachial vein occlusion
	left buttock		LBW	lean body weight
	live births			low birth weight (less than 2,500 g)
	low back		LBWI	low birth weight infant
	lower body		LC	Lactation Consultant
	lung biopsy			Laënnec cirrhosis
	lymphoid body			laparoscopic cholecystectomy
lb	pound (1 lb = 0.454 Kg)			lapatinib (Tykerb) and capecitabine (Xeloda)
L&B	left and below			lethal concentration
LB3	colonoscope			left circumflex
4LB	four-layer bandages			leisure counseling
LBA	laser balloon angioplasty			level of consciousness
	lower-body adiposity			levocarnitine (Carnitor)
	lymphocyte blastogenesis assay			living children
LBB	left breast biopsy			low calorie
	long-back board			lung cancer
LBBB	left bundle branch block		L & C	lids and conjunctivae
LBBx	left breast biopsy		3LC	triple-lumen catheter
LBC	liquid-based cytology		LC50	median lethal concentration
LBCD	left border of cardiac dullness		LCA	latent class analysis (a statistical tool)
L/B/Cr	electrolytes, blood urea nitrogen, and serum creatinine (see page 356)			Leber congenital amaurosis
				left circumflex artery
LBD	large bile duct			left coronary artery
	left border dullness			leukocyte common antigen
	left brain-damaged			life cycle assessment
	Lewy body dementia			light contact assist
	ligand-binding domain		LCAD	long-chain acyl-coenzyme A dehydrogenase
	low back disability			
	low bone density		LCAH	life-care at home
LBE	long below elbow		LCAL	large-cell anaplastic lymphoma
LBG	Landry-Guillain-Barré (syndrome)		LCaP	localized prostate cancer
			LCAR	L-carnitine
LBH	length, breadth, and height		LCAT	lecithin cholesterol acyltransferase
LBI	Lewy body-like inclusions		LCB	left costal border
	low back injury		LCC	left cranial-caudal (mammogram view)
LBM	last bowel movement			
	lean body mass		LCCA	left circumflex coronary artery
	loose bowel movement			left common carotid artery
LBMD	low bone mineral density			leukocytoclastic angiitis
LBMI	last body mass index		LCCE	Lamaze-Certified Childbirth Educator
LBNA	lysis bladder neck adhesions			
LBNP	lower-body negative pressure		LCCS	low cervical cesarean section

LCD	coal tar solution (*liquor carbonis detergens*)	
	lattice corneal dystrophy	
	liquid crystal display (radiology)	
	local coverage determination	
	localized collagen dystrophy	
	low-calcium diet	
	low contrast detail (radiology)	
LCDC	Laboratory Centre for Disease Control (Canada)	
LCDCP	low-contact dynamic compression plate	
LCDD	light chain deposition disease	
LCDE	laparoscopic common duct exploration	
LCDs	local coverage determinations	
LCE	laparoscopic cholecystectomy	
	left carotid endarterectomy	
	leukocyte esterase	
LC-EI-MS	liquid chromatography-electron impact-mass spectrometry	
LCF	late clinical failure	
	left circumflex	
LCFA	long-chain fatty acid	
LCFM	left circumflex marginal	
LCGU	local cerebral glucose utilization	
LCH	Langerhans cell histiocytosis	
	local city hospital	
LCINS	lung cancer in never-smokers	
LCIS	lobular cancer *in situ*	
LCL	lateral collateral ligament	
	localized cutaneous leishmaniasis	
	lymphoblastoid cell line	
LCLC	large-cell lung carcinoma	
LCLF	low-cholesterol, low-fat (diet)	
LCM	laser-capture microdissection	
	left costal margin	
	lower costal margin	
	lymphocytic choriomeningitis	
LCMI	left ventricular mass index	
LC-MS-MS	liquid chromatography coupled to tandem mass spectrometry	
LCN	lidocaine	
LCNB	large-core needle biopsy	
LCNEC	large-cell neuroendocrine carcinoma	
LCO	low cardiac output	
LCOS	low cardiac output syndrome	
LCP	leg calve perthes	
	Leishmaniasis Control Program	
	long, closed, posterior (cervix)	
LCPD	Legg-Calvé-Perthes disease	
LCPUFAs	long-chain polyunsaturated fatty acids	
LCR	cerebrospinal fluid (French)	
	late cortical response	
	late cutaneous reaction	

	ligase chain reaction
	locus control region
	low contrast resolution
LCRS	Living Conditions Rating Scale
LCRs	low-copy repeats
LCS	Leydig cell stimulation
	lids, conjunctiva, and sclera
	low constant suction
	low continuous suction
	Lung Cancer Subscale
LCSG	left cardiac sympathetic ganglionectomy
	lost child support group
LCSS	Lung Cancer Symptom Score
LCSW	Licensed Clinical Social Worker
	low continuous wall suction
LCT	long-chain triglyceride
	low cervical transverse
	lymphocytotoxicity
LCTA	lungs clear to auscultation
LCTAB	lungs clear to auscultation bilaterally
LCTCS	low cervical transverse cesarean section
LCTD	low-calcium test diet
LCV	leucovorin
	leukocytoclastic vasculitis
	low cervical vertical
LCX	left circumflex coronary artery
LD	laboratory departmemnt
	lactic dehydrogenase (formerly LDH)
	laser Doppler
	last dose
	latissimus dorsi
	learning disability
	learning disorder
	left deltoid
	Legionnaires disease
	lethal dose
	levodopa
	Licensed Dietician
	liver disease
	living donor
	loading dose
	long dwell
	low density
	low dosage
	lumbar drain (drainage)
	Lyme disease
L&D	labor and deliver
L/D	labor and delivery
	light to dark (ratio)
LD-1	lactic dehydrogenase 1
LD-5	lactic dehydrogenase 5
LD_{50}	median lethal dose
LDA	laser-Doppler anemometry
	linear discriminant analysis

	low density areas	LDV	laser-Doppler velocimetry
	low-dose arm		laser Doppler vibrometry
LDB	Legionnaires disease bacterium	LE	labor epidural
LDCOC	low-dose combination oral contraceptive		lateral epicondylitis (tennis elbow)
			left ear
LD-CT	low-dose (spiral) computed tomography		left eye
			lens extraction
LDD	laser disk decompression		leptin
	Lee and Desu D (test)		leukocyte esterase
	Lhermitte-Duclos disease		limbic encephalitis
	light-dark discrimination		live embryo
	lumbar disk disease		local excision
LDDS	local dentist		lower extremities
LDEA	left deviation of electrical axis		lupus erythematosus
LDEI	large-dose extended-interval (dosing)	LEA	lower-extremity amputation
			lumbar epidural anesthesia
LDF	laser-Doppler flowmetry	LEAD	lower-extremity arterial disease
LDH	lactic dehydrogenase	LEAP	Lower-Extremity Amputation Prevention (program)
	lumbar disk herniation		
LDIH	left direct inguinal hernia	LEAS	Lower-Extremity Activity Scale
LDIR	low-dose of ionizing radiation	LEB	lumbar epidural block
LDI-TOF-MS	laser desorption/ionization time-of-flight-mass spectrometer	LEC	lens epithelial cell
			low-emetogenic chemotherapy
LDK	low-dose ketoconazole	LECA	left external carotid artery
LDL	limitation of daily life	LECBD	laparoscopic exploration of the common bile duct
	low-density lipoprotein		
LDL-C	low-density lipoprotein cholesterol	LE-CEMRA	lower extremity contrast-enhanced magnetic resonance angiography
LDLT	living donor liver transplantation		
LDM	lorazepam, dexamethasone, and metoclopramide		
		LED	liposomal encapsulated doxorubicin (Doxil)
	low-dose metronomic (chemotherapy)		
			lowest effective dose
LDMRT	low-dose mediastinal radiation therapy		lupus erythematosus disseminatus
		LEE	lower extremity edema
LDN	laparoscopic donor nephrectomy	LEEP	loop electrosurgical excision procedure
	Licensed Dietitian Nutritionist		
	living-donor nephrectomy	LEF	lower extremity fracture
	low-dose naltrexone (ReVia)	LEH	liposome-encapsulated hemoglobin
LDNF	lung-derived neurotrophic factor	LEHPZ	lower esophageal high pressure zone
LDO	Licensed Dispensing Optician		
l-dopa	levodopa	LEJ	ligation of the esophagogastric junction
LDP	laparoscopic distal pancreatectomy		
LD-PCR	limiting dilution polymerase chain reaction	LEL	low-energy laser
		LELs	lymphoepithelial lesions
LDPM	laser Doppler perfusion monitoring	LEM	lateral eye movements
LDQA	laboratory-developed quadruplex assay		light electron microscope
		LEMS	Lambert-Eaton myasthenic syndrome
LDR	labor, delivery, and recovery		
	length-to-diameter ratio	LEN	lenalidomide (Revlimid)
	long-duration response	LENT-SOMA	Late Effect of Normal Tissue—Subjective Objective Management Analytic (toxicity table)
LDR/P	labor, delivery, recovery, and postpartum		
LDS	Language Development Survey		
	locked-door seclusion	LEP	leptospirosis
LDT	left dorsotransverse		limited English proficiency
LD-T	lactic dehydrogenase total		liposome-encapsulated paclitaxel
LDUB	long double upright brace		lower esophageal pressure
LDUH	low-dose unfractionated heparin	LEP 2	leptospirosis 2

L

LE prep	lupus erythematosus preparation	LFGNR	lactose fermenting gram-negative rod
L-ERX	leukoerythroblastic reaction		
LES	local excitatory state	LFI	local-field irradiation
	lower esophageal sphincter	LFL	left frontolateral
	lumbar epidural steroids	LFM	lateral force microscopy
	lupus erythematosus systemic	LFP	left frontoposterior
LESEP	lower extremity somatosensory evoked potential		Low-Fowler position
		LFPN	large-fiber peripheral neuropathy
LESG	Late Effects Study Group	LFS	leukemia-free survival
LESI	lumbar epidural steroid injection		Li-Fraumeni syndrome
LESP	lower esophageal sphincter pressure		liver function series
		LFT	latex flocculation test
LESS	laparoscopic single-site surgery		left fronto-transverse
LET	lateral elbow tendinopathy		liver function tests
	left esotropia		low-flap transverse
	leukocyte esterase test	LFU	limit flocculation unit
	lidocaine, epinephrine and tetracaine gel		lost to follow-up
		LG	large
	linear energy transfer		laryngectomy
	lupus erythematosus tumidus		left gluteal
LEU	leucine		linguogingival
LEV	levamisole (Ergamisol)		lymphography
	levator muscle	L-G	Lich-Gregoire (ureteroneocystostomy)
LEVA	levamisole (Ergamisol)		
LeY	Lewis Y (antigen)	LGA	large for gestational age
LF	laparoscopic fundoplications		left gastric artery
	Lassa fever		localized granuloma annulare
	left foot	LGBP/LC	laparoscopic gastric bypass with simultaneous cholecystectomy
	left frontal		
	little finger	LGBT	lesbian, gay, bisexual, and transsexual
	living female		
	long finger	LGFD	looks good from doorway (patient who complains but looks fine) (slang)
	low fat		
	low forceps		
	low frequency	LGG	low-grade gliomas
	lymphatic filariasis	L-GG	*Lactobacillus rhamnosus* strain GG
L/F	Latin female	LGI	lower gastrointestinal (series)
LFA	left femoral artery		low-glycemic index
	left forearm	LGIOS	low-grade intraosseous-type osteosarcoma
	left fronto-anterior		
	leukocyte function-associated antigen	LGL	large granular lymphocyte
			low-grade lymphoma(s)
	low-friction arthroplasty		Lown-Ganong-Levine (syndrome)
	lumbar facet arthropathy	LGLS	Lown-Ganong-Levine syndrome
	lymphocyte function-associated antigen	LGM	left gluteus medius (maximus)
		LGMD21	limb-girdle muscular dystrophy type 21
LFA-1	leukocyte function-associated antigen-1		
		LGN	lateral geniculate leaflet
LFB	low-frequency band		lobular glomerulonephritis
LFC	lateral femoral condyle	LGNET	low grade neuroendocrine carcinoma
	living female child		
	low-fat and cholesterol	LG-NHL	low-grade non-Hodgkin lymphoma
LFCS	low-flap cesarean section	LGS	Lennox-Gastaut syndrome
LFD	lactose-free diet		low-Gomco suction
	low-fat diet	LGSIL	low-grade squamous intraepithelial lesion
	low-fiber diet		
	low-forceps delivery	LGV	lymphogranuloma venerum
	lunate fossa depression	LH	learning handicap

L

	left hand
	left hemisphere
	left hyperphoria
	luteinizing hormone
	lymphoid hyperplasia
LHA	left hepatic artery
LHB	long head of the biceps
LHC	left heart catheterization
LHCJ	left heart catheterization, Judkins approach
LHD	left-hand dominant
	left hepatic duct
LHF	left heart failure
LHG	left hand grip
LHH	left homonymous hemianopsia
LHI	Labor Health Institute
LHL	left hemisphere lesions
	left hepatic lobe
LHON	Leber hereditary optic neuropathy
LHP	left hemiparesis
LHR	legal health record
	leukocyte histamine release
	long-handled reacher
LHRH	luteinizing hormone-releasing hormone
LHRH-A	luteinizing hormone-releasing hormone analogue
LHRT	leukocyte histamine release test
LHS	left hand side
	long-handled sponge
LHSH	long-handled shoe horn
	long-handled shower head
LHT	left hypertropia
LI	lactose intolerance
	lamellar ichthyosis
	large intestine
	laser iridotomy
	learning impaired
	linear interpolator (radiology)
	linguoincisal
	liver involvement
Li	lithium
LIA	laser interference acuity
	left iliac artery
LIB	left in bottle
	local in breast
LIC	left iliac crest
	left internal carotid
	leisure interest class
LICA	left internal carotid artery
LICD	lower intestinal Crohn disease
LICM	left intercostal margin
LiCO3	llithium carbonate (the proper designation is Li_2CO_3)
Li_2CO_3	lithium carbonate
LICS	left intercostal space
LID	levodopa-induced dyskinesia
Lido	lidocaine

LIF	laser-induced fluorescence
	left iliac fossa
	left index finger
	leukemia-inhibiting factor
	liver (migration) inhibitory factor
LIFE	laser-induced fluorescence emission
	lung imaging fluorescence endoscopy
LIFT	ligation of intersphincteric fistula tract
LIG	ligament
	lymphocyte immune globulin
LIGHTS	phototherapy lights
LIH	laparoscopic inguinal herniorrhaphy
	last image hold (radiology)
	left inguinal hernia
LIHA	low impulsiveness, high anxiety
LIID	latanoprost-induced iris darkening
LIJ	left internal jugular
LILA	low impulsiveness, low anxiety
LILT	low-intensity laser therapy
LIM	limited toxicology screening
LIMA	left internal mammary artery (graft)
LIMS	laboratory information management system(s)
LIN	liquid nitrogen
	lobular intraepithelial neoplasia
LINAC	linear accelerator
LINCL	late-infantile neuronal ceroid lipofuscinosis
LINDI	lithium-induced nephrogenic diabetes insipidus
LING	lingual
LIO	laser-indirect ophthalmoscope
	left inferior oblique (muscle)
LIOU	laparoscopic intraoperative ultrasound
LIP	licensed independent practitioner
	lithium-induced polydipsia
	lymphocytic interstitial pneumonia
LIPV	left inferior pulmonary vein
LIQ	liquid
	liquor
	lower inner quadrant
LIR	left iliac region
	left inferior rectus
LIR-1	leucocyte immunoglobulin-like receptor-1
LIS	late-onset idiopathic scoliosis
	lateral internal sphincterotomy
	left intercostal space
	locked-in syndrome
	low intermittent suction
	lung injury score
LISO	left inferior superior oblique

L

LISS	low ionic strength saline		Lewis lung carcinoma
LISW	Licensed Independent Social Worker		limited liability corporation
			long leg cast
LIT	literature	LLBCD	left lower border of cardiac dullness
	liver injury test		
	low-intensity (resistance) training	LLCH	localized Langerhans' cell histiocytosis
LITA	left internal thoracic artery		
LITH	lithotomy	LLD	late-life depressions
LITHO	lithotripsy		left lateral decubitus
LITT	laser-induced thermotherapy		left length discrepancy
LIV	left innominate vein		leg length differential
L-IVP	limited intravenous pyelogram	LLE	left lower extremity
LIVB	live birth		little league elbow
LIVC	left inferior vena cava	LLETZ	large-loop excision of the transformation zone
LIVPRO	liver profile (see page 356)		
LIWS	low intermittent wall suction	LLFG	long leg fiberglas (cast)
LJ	left jugular	LLG	left lateral gaze
	lockable joints	LL-GXT	low-level graded exercise test
LJL	lateral joint line	LLI	leg-length inequality
LJM	limited joint mobility	LLINs	long-lasting insecticidal (bed) nets
LK	lamellar keratoplasty	LLITN	long-lasting insecticide-treated nets
	left kidney	LLL	left lower lid
LKA	Lazare-Klerman-Armour (Personality Inventory)		left lower lobe (lung)
		LLLE	lower lid, left eye
LKM-3	liver-kidney microsomal antibodies type 3	LLLNR	left lower lobe, no rales
		LLLT	low-level laser therapy
LKS	Landau-Kleffner syndrome	LLN	lower limit of normal
	liver, kidneys, spleen	LLO	Legionella-like organism
LKSB	liver, kidneys, spleen, and bladder	LLOD	lower lid, right eye
LKSNP	liver, kidneys, and spleen not palpable		lower limit of detection
		LLOQ	lower limit of quantitation
LL	large lymphocyte	LLOS	lower lid, left eye
	left lateral	LLP	Limited Liability Partnership
	left leg		long leg plaster
	left lower	LLPDD	late luteal phase dysphoric disorder
	left lung	LLPS	low-load prolonged stress
	lepromatous leprosy	LLQ	left lower quadrant (abdomen)
	lid lag		lower limit of quantitation
	long leg (brace or cast)	LLR	left lateral rectus
	lower lid	LLRE	lower lid, right eye
	lower limb	LLS	lazy leukocyte syndrome
	lower lip	LLSB	left lower sternal border
	lower lobe	LLSD	laser light scattering detector
	lumbar laminectomy	LLT	left lateral thigh
	lumbar length		lowest level term
	lymphocytic leukemia	LLWC	long leg walking cast
	lymphoblastic lymphoma	LLX	left lower extremity
L&L	lids and lashes	LM	landmarks
LL2	limb lead two		left main
LLA	lids, lashes, and adnexa		lentigo maligna
	limulus lysate assay		light microscopy
LLAs	lipid-lowering agents		linguomesial
LLAT	left lateral		living male
LLB	last living breath		lower midline
	left lateral bending		lung metastases
	left lateral border		lymphatic malformation
	long leg brace	L/M	Latin male
LLC	laparoscopic laser cholecystectomy		liters per minute

LMA	laryngeal mask airway	LMWD	low molecular weight dextran
	left mentoanterior	LMWH	low molecular weight heparins
	liver membrane autoantibody	LMX-4®	4% lidocaine topical cream
LMAM	left message on answering machine	LN	latent nystagmus
			left nostril (nare)
LMB	Laurence-Moon-Biedl syndrome		lymph nodes
	left main bronchus	LN₂	liquid nitrogen
LMC	living male child	LNA	alpha-linolenic acid
LMCA	left main coronary artery	LNB	lymph node biopsy
	left middle cerebral artery	LNC	Legal Nurse Consultant
LMCAT	left middle cerebral artery thrombosis	LNCaP	lymph node carcinoma of the prostate
LMCL	left midclavicular line	LNCC	Legal Nurse Consultant, Certified
LMD	Langer mesomelic dysplasia	LNCs	lymph node cells
	local medical doctor	LND	lateral neck dissection
	low molecular weight dextran		light-near dissociation
	lumbar microdiskectomy		living non-directed (donors)
LME	left mediolateral episiotomy		lonidamine
LMEE	left middle ear exploration		lymph node dissection
LMF	left middle finger	LNE	lymph node enlargement
	melphalan (L-PAM), methotrexate, and fluorouracil		lymph node excision
		LNEC	laryngeal neuroendocrine carcinoma
LMFT	Licensed Marriage and Family Therapist	LNF	laparoscopic Nissen fundoplication
LMHC	Licensed Mental Health Counselor	LNG	levonorgestrel
LMI	large multivalent immunogen	LNI	lymph node involvement
L/min	liters per minute	LNM	Lansinoh for Nursing Mothers (ointment used for sore nipples)
LML	left medial lateral		
	left middle lobe		lymph node metastases
LMLE	left mediolateral episiotomy	LNMC	lymph node mononuclear cells
LMLO	left medial-lateral oblique (mammogram view)	LNMP	last normal menstrual period
		LNNB	Luria-Nebraska Neuropsychological Battery
LMM	lentigo maligna melanoma		
LMN	letter of medical necessity	LNS	lymph node sampling
	lower motor neuron	LNT	late neurological toxicity
LMNL	lower motor neuron lesion	LNU	laparoscopic nephroureterectomy
LMOM	left message on (answering) machine		learned nonuse (splint)
		LO	lateral oblique (x-ray view)
LMOR	left message on recorder		linguo-occlusal
LMP	last menstrual period		lumbar orthosis
	left mentoposterior	5-LO	5-lipoxygenase
	low malignant potential	LOA	late-onset agammaglobulinemia
LMP1	latent membrane protein 1		leave of absence
LMPC	laser microdissection and pressure catapulting		left occiput anterior
			Letter of Agreement
LMR	left medial rectus		long-acting opioid
LMRM	left modified radical mastectomy		looseness of associations
LMRP	Local Medical Review Policy		lumbar osteoarthritis
LMS	lateral medullary syndrome		lysis of adhesions
	leiomyosarcomas	LOAD	late-onset Alzheimer disease
LMST	leptomeningeal metastasis in solid tumors	LOAEL	lowest observed adverse effect level
LMT	lateral meniscal tear	LOB	loss of balance
	left main trunk	LOBNH	lights on but nobody home (slang for intellectually challenged)
	left mentotransverse		
	Licensed Massage Therapist	LOC	laxative of choice
	light moving touch		level of care
LMW	low molecular weight		level of comfort

	level of concern
	level of consciousness
	local
	localization
	loss of consciousness
LOCF	last observation carried forward (used for inputting data missing due to dropouts in longitudinal clinical trials)
LOCM	low-osmolality contrast media
LOCS	Lens Opacities Classification System (score)
LOD	late-onset disease
	limit of detection
	line of duty
	log of odds
LOE	lack of efficacy
	left otitis externa
	level of evidence
LOEL	lowest-observed-effect level
LOF	lack of function
	leaking of fluids
	leave on floor
	loss of fit
LOFD	low-outlet forceps delivery
LOG	Logmar chart
log	logarithm any base
log$_{10}$	logarithm base 10
log$_2$	logarithm base 2
log$_e$	logarithm base 3 (natural)
logMAR	logarithm of the minimum angle of resolution
LOH	loss of heterozygosity
LOHF	late-onset hepatic failure
LOHP	oxaliplatin (Eloxatin)
LOIH	left oblique inguinal hernia
LOI	level of injury
	Leyton Obsessional Inventory
	loss of imprinting
LOINC	Logical Observation Identifier Names and Codes
LOL	laughing out loud (slang)
	left occipitolateral
	little old lady
LOLINAD	little old lady in no apparent distress
LOM	left otitis media
	limitation of motion
	little old man
	loss of motion
	low-osmolar (contrast) media
LOMSA	left otitis media, suppurative, acute
LOMSC	left otitis media, suppurative, chronic
LoNa	low sodium
LOO	length of operation
LOOCV	leave-one-out cross-validation
LOP	laparoscopic orchiopexy

	leave on pass
	left occiput posterior
	level of pain
LOPS	loss of protective sensation
LOQ	limit(s) of quantitation
	lower outer quadrant
LOR	loss of resistance
LORETA	low-resolution electromagnetic tomography
LORS-I	Level of Rehabilitation Scale-I
LOS	length of stay
	limits of stability (test)
	loss of sight
	lower oesophageal sphincter (United Kingdom and other countries)
	low-output syndrome
lo-SES	lower socioeconomic status
LOT	left occiput transverse
	Licensed Occupational Therapist
LOU	level of understanding
LOV	loss of vision
LOVA	loss of visual acuity
Low T	low testosterone
LOX	lipid oxidation
	lysyl oxidase
LOZ	lozenge
LP	lamina propria
	laparoscopic pyeloplasty
	lash ptosis
	Licensed Psychologist
	light perception
	linguopulpal
	lipid panel (see page 356)
	lipoprotein
	low protein
	lumbar puncture
L5%P	lidocaine 5% patch (Lidoderm)
L/P	lactate-pyruvate ratio
	lidocaine and prilocaine
LP5	Life-Pak 5
LPA	left pulmonary artery
Lp(a)	lipoprotein (a)
LPA%	left pulmonary artery oxygen saturation
L-PAM	melphalan (Alkeran)
LPC	laser photocoagulation
	Licensed Professional Counselor
	leukocyte-depleted packed cells
LPCC	Licensed Professional Certified Counselor
LPC-L	lymphoplasmacytoid lymphoma
LPcP	light perception with projection
LPD	leiomyomatosis peritonealis disseminata
	low-potassium dextran
	low-protein diet
	luteal phase defect

L

	luteal phase deficiency	LPV	left portal vein
	lymphoproliferative disease		left pulmonary vein
LPDA	left posterior descending artery		lopinavir (Kaletra)
LPEP	left pre-ejection period	LPV/RTV	lopinavir and ritonavir
LPF	late parasitological failure	LPZ	lateral peripheral zone (prostate
	liver plasma flow		needle biopsy location)
	low-power field	LQT1	a specific type of long QT
	lymphocytosis-promoting factor		(interval) syndrome. There are
LPFB	left posterior fascicular block		10 types
LPFL	lateral patellofemoral ligament	LQTS	long QT (interval) syndrome
LPH	left posterior hemiblock	LR	labor room
	lumbar puncture headache		lactated Ringer (injection)
LPHB	left posterior hemiblock		laser resection
LPI	laser peripheral iridectomy		lateral rectus
	last patient in		late relapse
	leukotriene pathway inhibitor		left-right
	lysinuric protein intolerance		light reflex
LPICA	left posterior internal carotid artery		likelihood ratios
LPIH	left-posterior-inferior hemiblock		local recurrence
LPIT	lumbar puncture and intrathecal	L&R	left and right
	(chemotherapy or other agents)	L → R	left to right
LPL	laparoscopic pelvic	LR1A	labor room 1A
	lymphadenectomy	LRA	left radial artery
	left posterolateral		left renal artery
	lipoprotein lipase	LRAD	least restrictive assistive device
	lymphoplasmacytic lymphoma	LRC	locoregional control
LPLC	low-pressure liquid		lower rib cage
	chromatography	LRCP	Licentiate of the Royal College of
LPLND	laparoscopic pelvic lymph node		Physicians
	dissection	LRCS	Licentiate of the Royal College of
LPM	latent primary malignancy		Surgeons
	liters per minute	LRD	limb reduction defects
LPME	liquid-phase microextraction		living-related donor
LPN	laparoscopic partial nephrectomy		living renal donor
	Licensed Practical Nurse	LRDT	living-related donor transplant
LPO	left posterior oblique	LRE	localization-related epilepsy
	light perception only	LREH	low-renin essential hypertension
LPPC	leukocyte-poor packed cells	LRF	left rectus femoris
LPPH	late postpartum hemorrhage		left ring finger
Lp-PLA2	lipoprotein-associated		local-regional failure
	phospholipase A2	L&R gtt	Levophed and Regitine drip
LPR	laryngopharyngeal reflux		(infusion)
	leprosy (Hansen disease) vaccine	LRHT	living-related hepatic
LPS	last Pap smear		transplantation
	latency to persistent sleep	LRI	lower respiratory infection
	lipopolysaccharide	LRK TX	living related kidney transplant
LPSDT	laryngopharyngeal sensory	LRLT	living-related liver transplantation
	discrimination testing	LRM	left radical mastectomy
LP SHUNT	lumboperitoneal shunt		local regional metastases
		LRMP	last regular menstrual period
LPSO	left posterior superior oblique	LRN	laparoscopic radical nephrectomy
LPsP	light perception without projection	LRND	left radical neck dissection
LPT	leptospirosis (Leptospira-	LRO	long-range objective
	Leptospires sp.) vaccine	LROM	limited range of motion
	Licensed Physical Therapist	Lrot	left rotation
	low-pain threshold	LRP	laparoscopic radical prostatectomy
LPTN	Licensed Psychiatric Technical		lipoprotein receptor-related protein
	Nurse		lung-resistance protein

LRPRBC	leucocytes-reduced packed red blood cells	late systolic click
		least significant change
LRQ	lower right quadrant	left subclavian (artery) (vein)
LROU	lateral rectus, both eyes	leukemia stem cells
LRR	light reflection rheography	lichen simplex chronicus
	local recurrence rates	liquid scintillation counting
	locoregional recurrences	LSCA left scapuloanterior
LRRT	locoregional radiotherapy	LSCC laryngeal squamous cell carcinoma
LRS	lactated Ringer solution	LSCCB limited-state small-cell cancer of the bladder
	lumbosacral radicular syndrome	
LRT	likelihood ratio test	LSCM laser-scanning confocal microscopy
	living renal transplant	LSCP left scapuloposterior
	local radiation therapy	LSCS lower segment cesarean section
	lower respiratory tract	LSD least significant difference
LRTD	living relative transplant donor	low-salt diet
	lower respiratory tract disease	lumbosacral derangement
LRTI	ligament reconstruction with tendon interposition	lysergide
		lysosomal storage disorder
	lower respiratory tract infection	LSD1 lysine-specific demethylase 1
LRV	left renal vein	LSE local side effects
	log reduction value	LSed level of sedation
LRW	LAL (*Limulus* amebocyte lysate) reagent water	LSF line spread function (radiology)
		low-saturated fat
LRYGB	laparoscopic Roux-en-Y gastric bypass	LSFA low-saturated fatty acid (diet)
		LSG laparoscopic sleeve gastrectomy
LRZ	lorazepam (Ativan)	LSH laparoscopic supracervical hysterectomy
LS	left side	
	legally separated	leishmaniasis vaccine
	Leigh syndrome	LSHR laparoscopic suprapubic hernia repair
	liver scan	
	liver-spleen	LSI levonorgestrel subdermal implant
	loose stool	L-SIL low-grade squamous intraepithelial lesions
	low salt	
	lumbosacral	LSK liver, spleen, and kidneys
	lung sounds	LSKM liver-spleen-kidney-megalgia
	Lynch syndrome	LSL left sacrolateral
L/S	lecithin-sphingomyelin ratio	left short leg (brace)
L&S	ligation and stripping	LSLF low sodium, low fat (diet)
	liver and spleen	LSM laser scanning microscope
L5-S1	lumbar fifth vertebra to sacral first vertebra (where the lumbar and sacral spines join)	late systolic murmur
		least squares mean
		limited sampling model
LSA	left sacrum anterior	liver, spleen masses
	left subclavian artery	LSMFT liposclerosing myxofibrous tumor
	lipid-bound sialic acid	LSMT life-sustaining medical treatment
	lymphosarcoma	LSO left salpingo-oophorectomy
LSAs	low-sedating antihistamines	left superior oblique
LSB	left scapular border	lumbosacral orthosis
	left sternal border	LSP left sacrum posterior
	local standby	liver-specific (membrane) lipoprotein
	lumbar spinal block	
	lumbar sympathetic block	L–Spar Elspar (asparaginase)
LSBP	lateralized single-bundle patellar (tendon graft)	L-spine lumbar spine
		LSPO left superior posterior oblique
LS BPS	laparoscopic bilateral partial salpingectomy	LSQ Life Situation Questionnaire
		LSR laser skin resurfacing
LSC	laser-scanning cytometry	left superior rectus
	last sexual contact	L/S ratio lecithin/sphingomyelin ratio

L

LSS	limb-sparing surgery	LTCH	long-term care hospital (average
	liver-spleen scan		length of stay greater than
	lumbar spinal stenosis		25 days)
LSSS	large, simple safety study	LTC-IC	long-term culture-initiating cells
	Liverpool Seizure Severity Scale	LTCL	lateral talocalcaneal ligament
LST	left sacrum transverse	LTCR	long-term complete remission(s)
LSTAT	life support for trauma and	LTCS	low-transverse cesarean section
	transport	LTD	largest tumor dimension
LSTC	laparoscopic tubal coagulation		leg transfer device
LSTL	laparoscopic tubal ligation		line, tube, and drain (incident)
LSTM	lean soft tissue mass		lipid tear deficiency
L's & T's	lines and tubes		long-term depression
LSU	life support unit		long-term disability
LSV	left subclavian vein	LTD$_4$	leukotriene D$_4$
	lesser saphenous vein	LTE	less than effective
LSVC	left superior vena cava	LTE$_4$	leukotriene E$_4$
LSW	left-side weakness	LTED	long-term estrogen deprivation
	Licensed Social Worker	LTF	lost to follow-up
LT	laboratory technician	LTFU	long-term follow-up
	left	LTG	lamotrigine (Lamictal)
	left thigh		long-term goal
	left triceps		low-tension glaucoma
	leukotrienes	LTGA	left transposition of great artery
	Levin tube	LTH	left total hip (arthroplasty)
	light		luteotropic hormone
	light touch	LTK	laser thermal keratoplasty
	liver transplantation		left total knee (arthroplasty)
	low transverse	LTL	laparoscopic tubal ligation
	lumbar traction		left temporal lobectomy
	lung transplantation		leukocyte telomere length
	lunotriquetral	LTLD	lyso-thermosensitive liposomal
	lymphotoxin		doxorubicin
L/T	long term	LTM	long-term memory
L&T	lettuce and tomato		long-term monitoring
LT3	liothyronine sodium (Cytomel)	LTNPs	long-term nonprogressors (HIV
LT4	levothyroxine		infections)
LTA	laryngotracheal applicator	LTOT	long-term oxygen therapy
	laryngeal tracheal anesthesia	LTP	laser trabeculoplasty
	lateral thoracic arteries		lateral tibial plateau
	local tracheal anesthesia		lateral trochanteric pain
LTAC	long-term acute care		long-term plan
LTACHs	long-term acute care hospitals		long-term potentiation
LTAS	left transatrial septal	LTPA	leisure-time physical activity
LTB	laparoscopic tubal banding	LTR	laryngotracheal reconstruction
	laryngotracheobronchitis		long terminal repeats
LTB$_4$	leukotriene B$_4$		lower trunk rotation
LTBI	latent tuberculosis infection	LTRA	leukotriene receptor antagonist
LTC	Lapra-Ty (suture) clip	LTS	laparoscopic tubal sterilization
	left to count		laryngotracheal stenosis
	long-term care		long-term survivors
	long thick closed	LTT	lactose tolerance test
LTC$_4$	leukotriene C$_4$		lymphocyte transformation test
LTC-101	long-term care form-101	LTUI	low transverse uterine incision
LTCBDE	laparoscopic transcystic common	LTV	long-term variability
	bile duct exploration		long-term ventilation
LTCCS	low-transverse cervical cesarean		Luche tumor virus
	section	LTV+	long-term variability– average to
LTCF	long-term care facility		moderate

L

LTV 0	long-term variability–absent	L-VAM	leuprolide acetate, vinblastine, doxorubicin (Adriamycin), and mitomycin
LTVC	long-term venous catheter		
LTWN	long-term low-level white noise		
LTx	liver transplant	LVAS	left ventricular assist system
	lung transplantation	LVAT	left ventricular activation time
LTZ	letrozole (Femara)	LVBP	left ventricle bypass pump
LU	left upper	LVD	left ventricular dimension
	left ureteral		left ventricular dysfunction
	living unit	LVDD	left ventircular diastolic dysfunction
	Lutheran		
L & U	lower and upper	LVDd	left ventricular end-diastolic diameter
LUA	left upper arm		
LUD	laparoscopic ulnar drainage	LVDP	left ventricular diastolic pressure
	left uterine displacement	LVDs	left ventricular systolic diameter
LUE	left upper extremity	LVDT	linear variable differential transformer
Lues I	primary syphilis		
Lues II	secondary syphilis	LVDV	left ventricular diastolic volume
Lues III	tertiary syphilis	LVE	left ventricular enlargement
LUFF	lateral upper arm free flap (reconstruction of pharyngeal defect)	LVEDD	left ventricular end-diastolic diameter
		LVEDP	left ventricular end diastolic pressure
LUL	left upper lid		
	left upper lobe (lung)	LVEDV	left ventricular end-diastolic volume
LUM	laparoscopic-ultraminilaparotomic myomectomy		
		LVEF	left ventricular ejection fraction
Lum Lam	lumbar laminectomy	LVEP	left ventricular end pressure
LUNA	laparoscopic uterosacral nerve ablation	LVESD	left ventricular end-systolic dimension
LUOB	left upper outer buttock	LVESV	left-ventricular end-systolic volumes
LUOQ	left upper outer quadrant		
LUQ	left upper quadrant	LVESVI	left ventricular end-systolic volume index
LURD	living-unrelated donor		
LUS	laparoscopic ultrasonography	LVET	left ventricular ejection time
	lower uterine segment	LVF	left ventricular failure
LUSB	left upper scapular border		left visual field
	left upper sternal border	LVFP	left ventricular filling pressure
LUST	lower uterine segment transverse	LVFU	leucovorin and fluorouracil
LUT	look-up table (radiology)	LVFWR	left ventricular free wall rupture
	lower urinary tract	LVG	left ventrogluteal
LUTD	lower urinary tract dysfunction	LVH	left ventricular hypertrophy
LUTS	lower urinary tract symptoms	LVHR	laparoscopic ventral hernia repair
LUTT	lower urinary tract tumor		
LuTX	lung transplantation	LVID	left ventricular internal diameter
LUW	lungworm vaccine	LVIDd	left ventricle internal diameter at end-diastole
LUX	left upper extremity		
LV	leave	LVIDs	left ventricle internal dimension systole
	left ventricle		
	left ventricular	LVL	large volume leukapheresis
	leucovorin		left vastus lateralis
	live virus	LVM	left ventricular mass
LVA	left ventricular aneurysm	LVMI	left ventricular mass index
LVAS	large vestibular aqueduct syndrome	LVMM	left ventricular muscle mass
		LVN	Licensed Visiting Nurse
LVC	laser vision correction		Licensed Vocational Nurse
	low-viscosity cement	LVO	left ventricular opacification
	low-vision clinic		left ventricular output
LVAD	left ventricular assist device		left ventricular overactivity
LV Angio	left ventricular angiogram	LVOT	left ventricular outflow tract

L

LVOTO	left ventricular outflow tract obstruction	LX	larynx local irradiation lower extremity
LVP	large volume parenteral left ventricular pressure	LXC	laxative of choice
		LXT	left exotropia
LVPW	left ventricular posterior wall	LYCD	live-yeast cell derivative
LVR	leucovorin	LyE	lymphedema
LVRS	lung-volume reduction surgery	LYEL	lost-years of expected life
LVRT	liver-volume replaced by tumor	LYG	lymphomatoid granulomatosis
LVS	laryngeal videostroboscopy left ventricular strain	LYM	Lyme disease vaccine lymphocytes
LVS EMI	left ventricular subendocardial myocardial ischemia	lymphs	lymphocytes
		LYS	large yellow soft (stools) life-year saved (cost of) lysine
LVSD	left ventricular systolic dysfunction	lytes	electrolytes (Na, K, Cl, etc.) electrolyte panel (see page 356)
LVSF	left ventricular systolic function		
LVSI	lymph-vascular space invasion (involvement)	LZ	landing zone
LVSP	left ventricular systolic pressure	LZM	lysozyme
LVSW	left ventricular stroke work	LZP	lorazepam (Ativan)
LVSWI	left ventricular stroke work index		
LVT	levetiracetam (Keppra)		
LVV	left ventricular volume live varicella vaccine		
LVW	left ventricular wall		
LVWI	left ventricular work index		
LVWMA	left ventricular wall motion abnormality		
LVWMI	left ventricular wall motion index		
LVWT	left ventricular wall thickness		
LW	lacerating wound living will		
L & W	Lee and White (coagulation) living and well		
LWAQ	Living with Asthma Questionnaire		
LWCT	Lee-White clotting time		
LWBS	left without being seen. This implies the patient was registered but not triaged or assessed. Check to see if this confirms to your facility's definition. (see LWBT and AMA)		
LWBT	left without being treated. Patients who have been seen and triaged, but are waiting to be evaluated further; they leave without being further treated – there absence is without notification. Check to see if this conforms to your facility's definition (see LWBS and AMA)		
LWC	leave without consent		
LWCT	left without completing treatment		
LWD	Leri-Weill dyschondrosteosis		
LWDC	Leri-Weill dyschondrosteosis		
LWOP	leave without pay		
LWOT	left without treatment		
LWP	large whirlpool		

L

M

M	male
	manual
	marital
	married
	masked (audiology)
	mass
	medial
	memory
	mesial
	meta
	meter (m)
	mild
	million
	minimum
	moderate
	molar
	Monday
	monocytes
	mother
	mouth
	M sign—patient just utters "Mmmm" (slang)
	murmur
	muscle
	Mycobacterium
	Mycoplasma
	myopia
	myopic
	thousand
Ⓜ	murmur
M₁	first mitral sound
M1	left mastoid
	tropicamide 1% ophthalmic solution (Mydriacyl)
M1 to M7	categories of acute nonlymphoblastic leukemia
M₂	second mitral sound
m²	square meters (body surface)
M2	right mastoid
M-2	vincristine, carmustine, cyclophosphamide, melphalan, and prednisone
M3	third molar
M₃	third mitral sound
M-3	medical student 3rd year
3M	mitomycin, mitoxantrone, and methotrexate
M-3+7	mitoxantrone and cytarabine
M-4	medical student 4th year
M200	voloximab
MA	machine
	Marketing Authorization (EU)
	Master of Arts

	mean arterial (blood pressure)
	medical assistance
	medical authorization
	megestrol acetate
	menstrual age
	mental age
	meter angle
	Mexican American
	microalbuminuria
	metabolic acidosis
	microaneurysms
	Miller-Abbott (tube)
	milliamps
	monoclonal antibodies
	motorcycle accident
mA	milliamperage (radiology)
M/A	mood and/or affect
MA-1	Bennett volume ventilator
MAA	macroaggregates of albumin
	Marketing Authorization Application (European Union)
MAARI	medically attended acute respiratory illness
MAAS	Motor Activity Assessment Scale
MAB	Massachusetts Biologic Laboratories
	maximum androgen blockade
Mab	monoclonal antibody
MABC	Movement Assessment Battery for Children
MABM	mandibular alveolar bone mass
MABP	mean arterial blood pressure
MAC	Macintosh laryngoscope blade
	macrocytic erythrocytes
	macrophage
	macula
	maximal allowable concentration
	medial arterial calcification
	Medicare Appeals Council
	membrane attack complex
	Mental Adjustment to Cancer (scale)
	methotrexate, dactinomycin (Actinomycin D), and cyclophosphamide
	microcystic adnexal carcinoma
	mid-arm circumference
	minimum alveolar concentration
	monitored anesthesia care
	multi-access catheter
	Mycobacterium avium complex
MACC	methotrexate, doxorubicin, (Adriamycin) cyclophosphamide, and lomustine (Cee Nu)
MACCC	Master Arts, Certified Clinical Competence
MACCE	major adverse cardiac and cerebrovascular event

M

MACE	major adverse cardiac (cardiovascular) event(s)		minor acute illness multiphoton autofluorescence imaging
	Malon antegrade continence (colonic) enema		*Mycobacterium avium-intracellulare*
MACI	Master of Arts in Clinical Investigation	MAIC	*Mycobacterium avium-intracellulare* complex
MACIS	Metastases, Age, Completeness of Resection, Invasion, and Size (cancer staging system)	MAID	mesna, doxorubicin (Adriamycin), ifosfamide, and dacarbazine monofocal acute inflammatory demyelinating (lesions)
MACOP-B	methotrexate, doxorubicin, (Adriamycin) cyclophosphamide, vincristine (Oncovin), prednisone, and bleomycin with leucovorin rescue	MAIR	metabolic acidosis-induced retinopathy
		MAL	malaria vaccine
MACRO	macrocytes		malignant
MACS	magnetic activated cell sorting		methyl aminolevulinate
MACs	malignancy-associated changes		midaxillary line
MACTAR	McMaster-Toronto Arthritis Patient Reference (Disability Questionnaire)		Motor Activity Log
		MALDI	matrix-assisted laser desorption ionization
MAD	major affective disorder	MALDI-	matrix-assisted laser
	mandibular advancement device	TOFMS	desorption ionization-
	mind altering drugs		time-of-flight mass spectrometry
	moderate atopic dermatitis	MALG	Minnesota antilymphoblast
Mad2	mitotic arrest defective protein 2		globulin
MADD	Mothers Against Drunk Driving	malig	malignant
	multiple acyl-CoA dehydrogenase deficiency	MAL-PDT	methyl aminolevulinic acid photodynamic therapy
MADL	mobility activities of daily living	M alpha (1)	alpha (1)-microglobulin
MADRS	Montgomery-Åsburg Depression Rating Scale	MALS	multiangle light scattering
		MALT	mucosa-associated lymphoid tissue
MAE	medical air evacuation		
	moves all extremities	MALToma	lymphoma of mucosa-associated lymphoid tissue
MAES	moves all extremities slowly		
MAEEW	moves all extremities equally well	MAM-36	Manual Ability Measure-36
MAEW	moves all extremities well	MAM	mammogram
MAF	malignant ascites fluid		Mexican-American male
	metabolic activity factor		monitored administration of medication
	Mexican-American female		
MAFAs	movement-associated fetal (heart rate) accelerations	MAMC	Madigan Army Medical Center mid-arm muscle circumference
MAFO	molded ankle/foot orthosis	Mammo	mammography
MAFP	maternal alpha-fetoprotein	MAMP	methamphetamine
MAG	magnesium (Mg)		milliampere
	medication administration guideline (record)	m-AMSA	amsacrine
		MAMTT	minimal active muscle tendon tension
mag cit	magnesium citrate		
MAGIC	mouth and genital ulcers with inflamed cartilage (syndrome)	MAN	malignancy associated neutropenia
MAGP	meatal advancement glandulophaleoplasty		malignant acanthosis nigricans massive aspiration of newborn
mag sulf	magnesium sulfate	MAND	McCarron Assessment of Neuromuscular Development
MAHA	macroangiopathic hemolytic anemia	Mand	mandibular
MAHS	malignancy-associated hemophagocytic syndrome	MANE	Morrow Assessment of Nausea and Emesis
MAI	maximal aggregation index	MANIP	manipulation
	Medication Appropriateness Index	MANOVA	multivariate analysis of variance

MAO   maximum acid output
     methylaminolevulinate
MAO-A   monoamine oxidase type A
MAO-B   monoamine oxidase type B
MAOI   monoamine oxidase inhibitor
MAOP   Mid-Atlantic Oncology Program
MAP   magnesium, ammonium, and
     phosphate (Struvite stones)
     malignant atrophic papulosis
     mean airway pressure
     mean arterial pressure
     Medical Assistance Program
     megaloblastic anemia of
     pregnancy
     Miller Assessment for Preschoolers
     (test for developmental delays)
     mitogen-activated protein
     mitomycin, doxorubicin
     (Adriamycin), and cisplatin
     (Platinol)
     morning after pill (oral
     contraceptives)
     muscle-action potential
     Mycobacterium avium subspecies
     paratuberculosis
     MYH (MutY homolog) - associated
     polyposis
MAPC   multipotent adult progenitor cell
MA-PD   Medicare Part C prescription drug
     plan
MAPI   Millon Adolescent Personality
     Inventory
MAPS   Make a Picture Story
MAR   marital
     medication administration record
     melanoma-associated retinopathy
     mineral apposition rates
     missing at random (incomplete
     data)
MARE   manual active-resistive exercise
MARSA   methicillin-aminoglycoside-
     resistant *Staphylococcus aureus*
MARV   Marburg virus
MAS   macrophage activation syndrome
     McClune-Albright syndrome
     meconium aspiration syndrome
     Memory Assessment Scale
     minimum-access surgery
     mobile arm support
     Modified Ashworth Scale
     0 = No increase in muscle tone
     1 = Slight increase in muscle
     tone, manifested by a catch and
     release or by minimal resistance
     at the end range of motion when
     the part is flexion or
     extension/abduction or
     adduction, etc.

     1+ = Slight increase in muscle
     tone, manifested by a catch,
     followed by minimal resistance
     throughout the remainder (less
     than half) of the range of motion
     2 = More marked increase in
     muscle tone through most of the
     range of motion, but the affected
     part is easily moved
     3 = Considerable increase in
     muscle tone, passive movement
     is difficult
     4 = Affected part is rigid in
     flexion or extension (abduction
     or adduction, etc.)
mAs   milliampere seconds
MASA   mutant allele-specific amplification
MASDA^{SM}   Multiple-Allele-Specific Diagnostic
     Assay
MASER   microwave amplification
     (application) by stimulated
     emission of radiation
MASH   mobile Army surgical hospital
MASHPOT   mashed potatoes
MAST   mastectomy
     medical antishock trousers
     Michigan Alcoholism Screening
     Test
     military antishock trousers
MAT   manual arts therapy
     maternal
     maternity
     mature
     medication administration team
     metabolic activation therapy
     microscopic agglutination test
     Miller-Abbott tube
     Miller Analogies Test
     multifocal atrial tachycardia
MATGF   maternal grandfather
MATGM   maternal grandmother
MATHS   muscle pain, allergy, tachycardia
     and tiredness, and headache
     syndrome
MATTB   Manufacturers Assistance and
     Technical Training Branch
     (FDA)
MAU   microalbuminuria
MAUDE   Manufacturer and User Facility
     Device Experience (FDA)
MAVR   mitral and aortic valve replacement
MAWL   maximum acceptable weight of lift
max   maxillary
     maximal
MAX A   maximum assistance (assist)
MAXCONT   maximum contrast method
MAxL   midaxillary line
MAYO   mayonnaise

M

MB	buccal margin	MBOS	multivalent binding oligomers
	mandible	MBOT	mucinous borderline ovarian
	Mallory body		tumors
	Medical Board	MBP	malignant brachial plexopathy
	medulloblastoma		mannan-binding protein
	mesiobuccal		mannose-binding protein
	methylene blue		mechanical bowel preparation
	myocardial bands		medullary bone pain
M/B	mother/baby		mesiobuccopulpal
MBA	Master of Business Administration		myelin basic protein
	Mini Battery of Achievement	MBPM	Medicare Benefit Policy Manual
M-BACOD	methotrexate (high-dose),	MBq	megabecquerels
	bleomycin, doxorubicin	MBR	major breakpoint region
	(Adriamycin),		Medical Birth Registry
	cyclophosphamide, vincristine	MBS	modified barium swallow
	(Oncovin), and dexamethasone	MBT	maternal blood type
	with leucovorin rescue		2-mercaptobenzothiazole
2-MBAD	2-methylbutyryl-CoA		multiple blunt trauma
	dehydrogenase	MBTS	modified Blalock-Taussig shunt
MBC	male breast cancer	MC	male child
	maximum bladder capacity		Medicare
	maximum breathing capacity		medium-chain (triglycerides)
	metastatic breast cancer		metacarpal
	methotrexate, bleomycin, and		metatarso - cuneiform
	cisplatin		microcalcifications (breast)
	minimal bactericidal concentration		mini-laparotomy cholecystectomy
MB-CK	a creatinine kinase isoenzyme		miscarriage
MBD	Marchiafava-Bignami disease		mitoxantrone and cytarabine
	metabolic bone disease		mitral commissurotomy
	metastatic bone disease		mixed cellularity
	methyl-binding domain		mixed cryoglobulinemia
	methylene blue dye		molluscum contagiosum
	minimal brain damage		monocomponent highly purified
	minimal brain dysfunction		pork insulin
MBE	may be elevated		*Moraxella catarrhalis*
	medium below elbow		mouth care
MBF	meat-base formula		multicenter (study)
	myocardial blood flow		myocarditis
MBFC	medial brachial fascial	m + c	morphine and cocaine
	compartment	MC3	third metacarpal
MBEST	modulus blipped echo-planar	MCA	Medicines Control Agency (United
	single-pulse technique		Kingdom)
MBG	myocardial blush grade		megestrol, cyclophosphamide, and
MBHI	Millon Behavioral Health		doxorubicin (Adriamycin)
	Inventory		metacarpal amputation
MBI	Maslach Burnout Inventory		micrometastases clonogenic assay
	methylene blue installation		middle cerebral aneurysm
	Modified Barthel Index		middle cerebral artery
	molecular breast imaging		monoclonal antibodies
MBL	mannose-binding lectin		motorcycle accident
	menstrual blood loss		multichannel analyzer
	metallo-beta-lactamases		multiple congenital anomalies
MBL-D	mannan-binding lectin deficiency	2-MCA	2-methyl citric acid
MBM	mind-body medicine	MCAD	medium-chain acyl-CoA
	mother's breast milk		dehydrogenase
MBNW	multiple-breath nitrogen washout	MCAF	monocyte chemoattractant and
MBO	malignant bowel obstruction		activity factor
	mesiobuccal occulsion	MCAID	Medicaid

MCAO	middle cerebral artery occlusion	MCHC	mean corpuscular hemoglobin concentration
MCAP	middle cerebral artery pressure		
MCAR	missing completely at random (incomplete data)	MCHL	medial head of the coracohumeral ligament
MCARE	Medicare	MCI	mild cognitive impairment
McAS	McCune-Albright syndrome	mCi	millicurie
MCAT	Medical College Admission Test	μCi	microcurie
MCB	Medicines Control Board (United Kingdom's equivalent to the United States Food and Drug Administration)	MCID	minimum clinically important difference(s)
		mckat	microkatal (1 millionth [10^{-6}] of a katal)
	midcycle bleeding	MCL	mantle cell lymphoma
	middle chamber bubbling		maximum comfort level
MCBDD	National Center on Birth Defects and Developmental Disabilities		medial collateral ligament
			midclavicular line
McB pt	McBurney point		midcostal line
MCBS	Medicare Current Beneficiary Survey		modified chest lead
			most comfortable level
MCC	meningococcal serogroup C conjugate	mcL	microliter (1/1,000 of an mL)
		MCLL	most comfortable listening level
	Merkel cell carcinoma	MCLNS	mucocutaneous lymph node syndrome
	microcrystalline cellulose		
	midstream clean-catch	MCMI	Millon Clinical Multiaxial Inventory
	motorcycle crash		
MCCU	mobile coronary care unit	mcmol	micromoles (one millionth [10^{-6}] of a mole)
MCD	macular corneal dystrtoophy		
	malformation of cortical development	MCN	minimal change nephropathy
		MCNS	minimal change nephrotic syndrome
	mean cell diameter		
	Medicaid	MCO	managed care organization
	microvascular coronary dysfunction		mupirocin calcium ointment (Bactroban Nasal)
	minimal-change disease	Mco2	carbon dioxide excretion
	multicentric Castleman disease	MCOT	mobile cardiac outpatient telemetry
	multicystic dysplasia	MCP	mean carotid pressure
	multiple consecutive discharges (pacemaker related)		metacarpophalangeal joint
			metoclopramide (Reglan)
MCDK	multicystic dysplasia of the kidney		monocyte chemotactic protein
		MCR	Medicare
MCDT	mast cell degranulation test		metabolic clearance rate
MCE	major coronary event		minor cluster region
	myocardial contrast echocardiography		myocardial revascularization
		MC=R	moderately constricted and equally reactive
MCF	multicentric foci		
MCFA	medium-chain fatty acid	MCRC	metastatic colorectal cancer
mcg	microgram (1,000 mcg = 1 milligram) (do not hand write μg, as it is mistakenly read as milligram [mg])	MCS	manufacturer cannot supply
			maternal cigarette smoking
			mental component summary
			microculture and sensitivity
MCG	magnetocardiogram		minimally conscious state
	magnetocardiography		moderate constant suction
MCGN	minimal-change glomerular nephritis		motor cortex stimulation
			multiple chemical sensitivity
MCH	mean corpuscular hemoglobin		myocardial contractile state
	microfibrillar collagen hemostat	MCs	mast cells
	muscle contraction headache	MCSA	minimal cross-sectional area
M-CHAT	Modified Checklist for Autism in Toddlers	M-CSF	macrophage colony-stimulating factor

MC-SR	moderately constricted and slightly reactive	MDASI	MD Anderson Symptom Inventory
MCT	manual cervical traction	MDASI-BT	MD Anderson Symptom Inventory-Brain Tumor Module
	mean circulation time	MDC	Major Diagnostic Category
	medial canthal tendon		medial dorsal cutaneous (nerve)
	medium chain triglyceride	MDCM	mildly dilated congestive cardiomyopathy
	medullary carcinoma of the thyroid		
	microwave coagulation therapy	MDCT	multidetector computed tomography
	multislice computed tomography		
MCTC	metrizamide computed tomography cisternogram	MDCTA	multidetector computed tomographic angiography
MCTD	mixed connective tissue disease	MDD	major depressive disorder
MCTZ	methyclothiazide (Enduron)		manic-depressive disorder
MCU	micturating cystourethrogram		Medical Device Directive (EU)
MCUG	micturating cystourethrogram	MDE	major depressive episode
MCV	mean corpuscular volume	MDF	myocardial depressant factor
	measles-containing vaccine	MDG4	Millennium Development Goal 4
	microvolt	MDGF	macrophage-derived growth factor
MCV4	meningococcal conjugate vaccine		
MCVRI	minimal coronary vascular resistance index	MDGs	Millennium Development Goals
		MDI	manic-depressive illness
MCYLS	marginal cost per year of life saved		mental developmental index
MD	macula degeneration		metered-dose inhaler
	maintenance dialysis		methylenedioxyindenes
	maintenance dose		multi-directional instability
	major depression		multiple daily injection
	mammary dysplasia		multiple dosage insulin
	manic depression	MDIA	Mental Development Index, Adjusted
	mean deviation		
	medical doctor	MDII	multiple daily insulin injection
	mediodorsal	MDIS	metered-dose inhaler-spacer (device)
	Menière disease		
	mental deficiency	MDiv	Master of Divinity
	mesiodistal	MDL	microdirect laryngoscopy
	microdialysis	MDLFC	mid-dorsolateral prefrontal cortex
	movement disorder	MDM	medical decision making
	multiple dose		mid-diastolic murmur
	muscular dystrophy		minor determinant mix (of penicillin)
	myocardial damage		
MD1	myotonic dystrophy type 1	MDM2	an oncogenic homologue protein
MD-50®	diatrizoate sodium injection 50%	MDMA	methylenedioxy-methamphetamine (ecstasy)
MDA	malondialdehyde		
	manual dilation of the anus	MDMX	an oncogenic homologue protein
	mass drug administrations (diethylcarbamazine plus albendazole to stop transmission of filariasis)	MDNT	midnight
		MDO	mentally disordered offender
		MDOT	modified directly observed therapy
		MDP	methylene diphosphonate
	Medical Devises Agency (United Kingdom)	MDPH	Michigan Department of Public Health
	methylenedioxyamphetamine	MDPI	maximum daily permissible intake
	micrometastases detection assay	MDR	Medical Device Reporting (regulation)
	motor discriminative acuity		minimum daily requirement
	Multichannel Discrete Analyzer		multidimensionality reduction
	Muscular Dystrophy Association		multidrug resistance
MDAC	multiple-dose activated charcoal	MD=R	moderately dilated and equally reactive
MDACC	MD Anderson Cancer Center		
MDA LDL	malondialdehydeconjugated low-density lipoprotein	MDR-1	multidrug resistance gene

M

MDRD	Modification of Diet in Renal Disease		middle ear canal(s)
MDRE	multiple-drug-resistant enterococci		mitoxantrone, etoposide, and cytarabine
MDREF	multidrug resistant enteric fever		moderately emetogenic chemotherapy
MDRO	multidrug resistant organism		
MDRS I/P	Mattis Dementia Rating Scale-Initiation/Perseveration subscale	MeCCNU	semustine
		MECG	maternal electrocardiogram
MDRSP	multidrug resistant *Streptococcus pneumoniae*	MECH	mechanical
		mech soft	mechanical soft
MDRT	multiple-drug rescue therapy	MeCP	semustine (methyl CCNU) cyclophosphamide, and prednisone
MDRTB	multidrug resistant tuberculosis		
MDS	maternal deprivation syndrome		
	Miller-Dieker syndrome	MECs	measured environmental concentrations
	Minimum Data Set		
	myelodysplastic syndromes	MED	male erectile dysfunction
MDSC	myeloid-derived suppressor cells		maximal (maximum) economic dose
MD-SR	moderately dilated and slightly reactive		
			medial
MDTS®	Metered Dose Transdermal Spray system		median erythrocyte diameter
			medical
MDSU	medical day stay unit		medication
MDT	maggot debridement therapy		medicine
	Mechanical Diagnostic Therapist		medium
	motion detection threshold		medulloblastoma
	multidisciplinary team		minimal erythema dose
	multidrug therapy		minimum effective dose
MDTM	multidisciplinary team meeting		multiple epiphyseal dysplasia
MDTP	multidisciplinary treatment plan	MEd	Master of Education
MDU	maintenance dialysis unit	MEDAC	multiple endocrine deficiency Addison disease (autoimmune) candidiasis
	microvascular Doppler ultrasonography		
MDUO	myocardial disease of unknown origin	MEDCO	Medcosonolator
		MedDRA	Medical Dictionary for Regulatory Activities
MDV	Marek disease virus		
	multiple dose vial	MEDEX	medication administration record
MDY	month, date, and year	MEDIC	multiecho data image combination
ME	macular edema		
	manic episode	MED-LARS	Medical Literature Analysis and Retrieval System
	medical events		
	medical evidence	MEDLINE	National Library of Medicine medical database
	medical examiner		
	mestranol	MED NEC	medically necessary
	Methodist	MedPAC	Medicare Payment Advisory Commission
	middle ear		
	myalgic encephalomyelitis	MedPAR	Medicare Provider Analysis Review File
M/E	metabolic/endocrine		
	monitor and evaluate	MEDS	medications
	myeloid-erythroid (ratio)	MEE	maintenance energy expenditure
M&E	Mecholyl and Eserine		measured energy expenditure
	mucositis and enteritis		middle ear effusion
MEA	microwave endometrial ablation	MEE/OC	middle ear exploration with ossicular chain reconstruction
	measles virus vaccine		
MEA-I	multiple endocrine adenomatosis type I	MEF	maximum expired flow rate
			middle ear fluid
MEB	Medical Evaluation Board	MEFR	mid expiratory flow rate
	methylene blue	MEFV	maximum expiratory flow-volume
MEC	meconium	MEG	magnetoencephalogram
	medical eligibility criteria		magnetoencephalography

M

Meg-CSF	megakaryocytic colony-stimulating factor	MEP	maximal expiratory pressure
			meperidine (Demerol)
MEGX	monoethylglycinexylidide		motor-evoked potential
MeHg	methylmercury		multimodality-evoked potential
MEI	magnetic endoscope imaging	MEPA	Medication Error Prevention
	medical economic index		Analysis (FDA)
MEIA	microparticle enzyme	MEPS	Mayo Elbow Performance Score
	immunoassay		Medical Expenditure Panel Survey
MEKC	micellar electrokinetic	mEq	milliequivalent
	chromatography	mEq/24 H	millequivalents per 24 hours
MEL	maximum exposure limit	mEq/L	milliequivalents per liter
	melatonin	MER	medical evidence of record
	melphalan (Alkeran)		methanol-extracted residue (of
MELAS	mitochondrial encephalomyopathy with lactic acidosis, and stroke-like episodes (syndrome)		phenol-treated BCG)
			milk ejection reflex
		M/E ratio	myeloid/erythroid ratio
MEL B	melarsoprol (Arsobal)	MERRF	myoclonic epilepsy and ragged red
MELD	Model for End-Stage Liver Disease (score)		fibers
		MERS-TM	Medical Event Reporting System -
MEM	memory		Transfusion Medicine
	monocular estimate method (near retinoscopy)	MES	maximal electroshock
			mesial
MEMB	modified eosin-methylene blue (agar)		myoelectric signals
		MESA	microsurgical epididymal sperm
MEMG	masseter (muscle) electromyographic (events)		aspiration
		MESCC	metastatic epidural spinal cord
MEN	medically-enhanced normality		compression
	meningeal	MeSH	Medical Subject Headings of the
	meninges		National Library of Medicine
	meningitis	MESS	Mangled Extremity Severe Score
	meningococcal (*Neisseria meningitidis*) (serogroups unspecified) vaccine	MEST	mesodermal specific transcript (gene)
		MET	medical emergency team
MEN (II)	multiple endocrine neoplasia (type II)		medical emergency treatment
			metabolic
MEN$_{cn-AC}$	meningococcal (*Neisseria meningitidis*) serogroups A, C conjugate vaccine		metamyelocytes
			metastasis
			metronidazole
MEN$_{cn-B}$	meningococcal (*Neisseria meningitidis*) serogroup B conjugate vaccine	meT	methyltestosterone
		META	metamyelocytes
		METH	methamphetamine
MEN$_{ps}$	meningococcal (*Neisseria meningitidis*) polysaccharide vaccine, not otherwise specified		methicillin
		MetHb	methemoglobin
			methemoglobinemia
MEN$_{ps-ACYW}$	meningococcal (*Neisseria meningitidis*) serogroups A, C, Y, W-135 polysaccharide vaccine	methyl CCNU	semustine
		methyl G	mitroguazone dihydrochloride (Zyrkamine)
MEN$_{ps-B}$	meningococcal (*Neisseria meningitidis*) serogroup B polysaccharide vaccine	methyl GAG	mitroguazone dihydrochloride (Zyrkamine)
		METS	metabolic equivalents (multiples of resting oxygen uptake)
MENS	microcurrent electrical neuromuscular stimulation		metastases
	mini-electrical nerve stimulator	MetS	metabolic syndrome
MEO	malignant external otitis	METT	maximum exercise tolerance test
	Medical Examiner's Office	MEV	million electron volts
MeOH	methyl alcohol	MEWDS	multifocal evanescent white dot
MEOS	microsomal ethanol oxidizing system		syndrome

M

MEX	Mexican	MFT	muscle function test
MF	Malassezia folliculitis	MFU	medical follow-up
	Malassezia furfur	MFVNS	middle fossa vestibular nerve section
	masculinity/femininity		
	meat-free	MFVPT	Motor Free Visual Perception Test
	median frequency (anesthesia-depth monitor)	MFVR	minimal forearm vascular resistance
	mesial facial		
	methotrexate and fluorouracil	MG	malignant glioma
	midcavity forceps		mammography
	middle finger		Marcus Gunn
	midforceps		Michaelis-Gutmann (bodies)
	mother and father		milligram (mg)
	mycosis fungoides		myasthenia gravis
	myelofibrosis	mg	milligram (1,000 mg = 1 gram)
	myocardial fibrosis	Mg	magnesium
M/F	male-female ratio	mG	milligauss
M & F	male and female	μg	microgram (1/1000 of a milligram) (This is a dangerous abbreviation when handwritten, as it is read as mg. Use mcg)
	mother and father		
MFA	malaise, fatigue, and anorexia		
MFAT	multifocal atrial tachycardia		
MFB	metallic foreign body		
	multiple-frequency bioimpedance	M&G	myringotomy and grommets
MFC	medial femoral condyle	mg%	milligrams per 100 milliliters
	multifocal choroiditis	MGA	Myasthenia Gravis Association
MfC	*Medicines for Children*	MGBG	mitoguazone (Zyrkamine)
MFCU	Medicaid Fraud Control Unit	MGCT	malignant glandular cell tumor
MFD	Memory for Designs	MGD	mammography-detected (breast cancer)
	midforceps delivery		
	milk-free diet		meibomian gland dysfunction
	multiple fractions per day	MGd	motexafin gadolinium (Xcytrin)
MFEM	maximal forced expiratory maneuver	MGDF	megakaryocyte growth and development factor
mfERG	multifocal electroretinography	mg/dl	milligrams per 100 milliliters
MFFT	Matching Familiar Figures Test	MGF	macrophage growth factor
MFH	malignant fibrous histiocytoma		mast cell growth factor
MFI	mean fluorescent intensity		maternal grandfather
	Multidimensional Fatigue Inventory	MGG	May-Grünwald-Giemsa (stain)
		MGGM	maternal great grandmother
		MGHL	middle glenohumeral ligament
MFIQ	Mandibular Function Impairment Questionnaire	mgl	milligrams of iodine
M-FISH	multicolor fluorescence in situ hybridization	MGIT	mycobacteria growth indicator (incubator) tube
		mg/kg	milligram per kilogram
MFM	maternal fetal medicine	mg/kg/d	milligram per kilogram per day
	multifidus muscle	mg/kg/hr	milligram per kilogram per hour
MF/MC	multifocal and multicentric	MGM	maternal grandmother
MFNS	mometasone furoate nasal spray (Nasonex)		milligram (mg is correct)
		MGMA	Medical Group Management Association
MFPS	myofascial pain syndrome		
MFR	mid-forceps rotation	Mgmt	Management
	myofascial release	MGN	membranous glomerulonephritis
MFS	Marfan syndrome	MGO	methylglyoxal
	maternal-fetal surgery	MgO	magnesium oxide
	Medicare Fee Schedule	MG/OL	molecular genetics/oncology laboratory
	metastases free survival		
	Miller-Fisher syndrome	MGP	Marcus Gunn pupil
	mitral first sound		maternal grandparents
	monofixation syndrome		medical group practice

M

MGPS	Multi-item Gamma Poisson Shrinker	MH/MR	mental health and mental retardation
MGR	murmurs, gallops, or rubs	MHN	major hepatic necrosis
MGS	magnetic guidance system		massive hepatic necrosis
	malignant glandular schwannoma		mental health nurse
MgSO₄	magnesium sulfate (Epsom salt) (this is dangerous terminology as it can be interpreted as morphine sulfate)	MHO	medical house officer
		MHP	moist heat packs
		MHRA	Medicines and Healthcare Products Regulatory Agency (United Kingdom)
MGT	management		
mgtt	minidrop (60 minidrops = 1 mL)	MHRI	Mental Health Research Institute
MGUS	monoclonal gammopathy of undetermined significance	MHS	major histocompatibility system
			malignant hyperthermia susceptible
MGW	multiple gunshot wound		mental health services
MGW enema	magnesium sulfate, glycerin, and water enema		monomethyl hydrogen sulfate
			multihospital system
M-GXT	multistage graded exercise test	MHsFHF	malarial hepatitis-simulating fulminant-hepatic failure
mGy	milligray (radiation unit)		
MH	macular hemorrhage	MHSI	medical hyperspectral imaging
	macular hole	MHT	malignant hypertension
	malignant hyperthermia		mental health team
	marital history		Mental Health Technician
	medical history	MHTAP	microhemagglutination assay for antibody to *Treponema pallidum*
	menstrual history		
	mental health		
	moist heat	MHV	mechanical heart valves
MHA	Mental Health Assistant		middle hepatic vein
	methotrexate, hydrocortisone, and cytarabine (ara-C)	MHW	medial heel wedge
			mental health worker
	microangiopathic hemolytic anemia	MHX	methohexital sodium
	microhemagglutination	MHx	medical history
	migraine headache	MHxR	medical history review
MHA-TP	microhemagglutination-*Treponema pallidum*	MHz	megahertz
		MI	membrane intact
MHB	maximum hospital benefits		mental illness
MHb	methemoglobin		mental institution
MHBSS	modified Hank balanced salt solution		mesial incisal
			mitral insufficiency
MHC	major histocompatibility complex		myocardial infarction
	mental health center (clinic)	MIA	medically indigent adult
	mental health counselor		minimally-invasive anesthesia
M/hct	microhematocrit		missing in action
MHD	10-hydroxycarbazepine (oxcarbazepine metabolite)	MIBE	measles inclusion body encephalitis
		MIBI	technetium Tc99m sestamibi (a myocardial perfusion agent; Cardiolite)
	maintenance hemodialysis		
	maximum heart distance (radiation therapy)		
		MIBG	iobenguane sulfate I 123 (meta-iodobenzyl guanidine I 123)
MHE	minimal hepatic encephalopathy		
mHg	millimeters of mercury	MIBK	methylisobutylketone
MHH	mental health hold	MIC	maternal and infant care
MHI	Mental Health Index (information)		methacholine inhalation challenge
MHL	maximum heart length (radiation therapy)		medical intensive care
			microscope
	mesenchymal hamartoma of the liver		microcytic erythrocytes
			minimum inhibitory concentration
MHIP	mental health inpatient	MICA	mentally ill, chemical abuser
MHLW	Ministry of Health, Labor, and Welfare (Japan)	MICAR	Mortality Medical Indexing, Classification, and Retrieval

M

MICE	mesna, ifosfamide, carboplatin, and etoposide		mineral
			minimum
MICN	Mobile Intensive Care Nurse		minor
MICR	methacholine inhalation challenge response		minute (min)
		MIN A	minimal assistance (assist)
MICRO	microcytes	MIME	mitoguazone, ifosfamide,
MICROG	microgram		methotrexate, and etoposide with
micromet	micrometastasis		mesna
microV	microvolt	MINE	Medical Information Network of
MICS	microincision cataract surgery		Europe
	minimally invasive cardiac surgery		mesna, ifosfamide, mitoxantrone
MICU	medical intensive care unit		(Novantrone), and etoposide
	mobile intensive care unit		medical improvement not
MID	mesioincisodistal		expected
	microvillus inclusion disease	MINI	Mini International
	minimal ineffective dose		Neuropsychiatric Interview
	multi-infarct dementia	MinIP	minimum intensity projection
MIDAS	migraine disability assessment scale		(radiology)
		MIO	minimum identifiable odor
MIDCAB	minimally invasive direct coronary artery bypass		monocular indirect ophthalmoscopy
MIDD	maternally inherited diabetes and deafness	MIP	macrophage inflammatory protein
			maximum inspiratory pressure
MID EPIS	midline episiotomy		maximum-intensity projection
MIDI	myocardial infarction during intercourse		(radiology)
			mean intrathoracic pressure
Mid I	middle insomnia		mean intravascular pressure
MIE	maximim inspiratory effort		medical improvement possible
	meconium ileus equivalent (cystic fibrosis)		metacarpointerphalangeal
			Michigan Biologic Products
	medical improvement expected		Institute
MIEI	medication-induced esophageal injury	MIPP	maximum-intensity pixel projection (images for MRI)
MIF	Merthiolate, iodine, and formalin	MIPPA	Medicare Improvements for
	mifepristone (RU 486; Mifeprex)		Patients and Providers Act of
	migration inhibitory factor		2008
MIFR	midinspiratory flow rate	MIRD	medical internal radiation dose
MIF 50% VC	midinspiratory flow at 50% of vital capacity	miRNA	micro ribonucleic acid
		MIRP	myocardial infarction rehabilitation
MIG	measles immune globulin		program
	monokine induced by gamma	MIRS	Medical Improvement Review
MIGET	multiple inert gas elimination technique		Standard
		MIRU-VNTR	mycobacterial interspersed
MIH	medication-induced headache		repetitive units containing
	migraine with interparoxysmal headache		variable number of tandem repeats
	myointimal hyperplasia	MIS	management information systems
MII	multichannel intraluminal impedance		melanoma *in situ*
			minimally invasive surgery
MIL	military		mitral insufficiency
	mesial incisal lingual (surface)		moderate intermittent suction
	mother-in-law	MISA	mentally ill and substance abusing
MILD	minimally invasive lumbar decompression	MISC	miscarriage
			miscellaneous
MIMCU	medical intermediate care unit	M Isch	myocardial ischemia
MIN	mammary intraepithelial neoplasia	MISH	multiple *in situ* hybridization
	melanocytic intraepidermal neoplasia	MISO	misonidazole
		MISS	minimally invasive spine surgery

M

	Modified Injury Severity Score (Scale)	MLC	metastatic liver cancer
	Mothers in Sympathy and Support		minimal lethal concentration
MIT	meconium in trachea		mixed lymphocyte culture
	miracidia immobilization test		multilevel care
	mono-iodotyrosine		multileaf collimator
	multiple injection therapy (of		multilumen catheter
	insulin)		myelomonocytic leukemia, chronic
MITO-C	mitomycin (Mutamycin)	MLD	manual lymph drainage
MITOX	mitoxantrone (Novantrone)		masking level difference
MITT	modified intent-to-treat		melioidosis (*Pseudomonas*
MIU	million international units		*pseudomallei*) vaccine
	minor injury unit		metachromatic leukodystrophy
mIU	milli-international unit (one-		microlumbar diskectomy
	thousandth of an International		microsurgical lumbar diskectomy
	unit)		minimal lethal dose
MIVA	mivacurium (Mivacron)		minimal luminal diameter
MIVE	maximum isometric voluntary	MLDA	Mutational Load Distribution
	extension		Analysis
MIVF	maintenance intravenous fluids	MLDT	Manual Lymph Drainage Therapist
	maximum isometric voluntary	MLE	major line extension
	flexion		maximum likelihood estimation
MIW	mental inquest warrant		midline (medial) episiotomy
mix mon	mixed monitor	MLEE	multilocus enzyme electrophoresis
MJ	marijuana	MLF	median longitudinal fasciculus
	megajoule	MLHFQ	Minnesota Living With Heart
MJD	Machado-Joseph Disease		Failure Questionnaire
MJL	medial joint line	MLL	mixed-lineage leukemia
MJS	medial joint space	MLL5	mixed-lineage leukemia 5 (gene)
MJT	Mead Johnson tube	MLN	manifest latent nystagmus
MK	microbial keratitis		mediastinal lymph node
μkat	microkatal (micro-moles/sec)		melanoma vaccine
MKAB	may keep at bedside		mesenteric lymph node
MKB	married, keeping baby	MLNS	minimal lesions nephrotic
MK-CSF	megakaryocyte colony-stimulating		syndrome
	factor		mucocutaneous lymph node
MKI	mitotic-karyorrhectic index		syndrome (Kawasaki syndrome)
MKM	Mehrkoordinaten Manipulator	MLO	medial-lateral oblique
	microgram per kilogram per		(mammogram view)
	minute		mesiolinguo-occlusal (dental)
ml	myoinositol	MLP	mento-laeva posterior
ML	malignant lymphoma		mesiolinguopulpal
	mediolateral		midlevel provider
	middle lobe	MLPA	multiple ligation probe
	midline		amplification
	mucosal leishmaniasis	MLPJ	mechanical loosening of prosthetic
mL	milliliter (1,000 mL = 1 liter)		joint
M/L	monocyte to lymphocyte (ratio)	MLPN	Medical Licensed Practical Nurse
	mother-in-law	MLPP	maximum loose-packed position
MLA	medical laboratory assay	MLPs	mid-level providers
	mento-laeva anterior	MLR	middle latency response
MLAC	minimum local analgesic		mixed lymphocyte reaction
	concentration		multiple logistic regression
MLAP	mean left atrial pressure	MLRA	multiple linear-regression analysis
MLB	microlaryngoscopy and	MLS	macrolides, lincosamides, and
	bronchoscopy		streptogramins
	microlaryngobronchoscopy		Maroteaux-Lamy syndrome
MLBW	moderately low birth weight		match-line shift
			maximum likelihood score

M

	mediastinal B-cell lymphoma with sclerosis		mechanomyography
		mm Hg	millimeters of mercury
MLST	multi-locus sequence typing	MMI	maximal medical improvement
MLT	melatonin	MMK	Marshall-Marchetti-Krantz (cystourethropexy)
	mento-laeva transversa		
MLU	mean length of utterance	MML	minimal masking level (audiology)
MLV	monitored live voice	MMM	metastatic malignant melanoma
MLWHF	Minnesota Living with Heart Failure (questionnaire)		mitoxantrone, methotrexate, and mitomycin
MM	major medical (insurance)		mucous membrane moist
	malignant melanoma		myelofibrosis with myeloid metaplasia
	malignant mesothelioma		
	Marshall-Marchetti	mMMSE	modified version of the mini mental status examination
	medial malleolus		
	medication management	MMMT	malignant mixed mesodermal tumor
	member months		
	meningococcic meningitis		metastatic mixed müllerian tumor
	mercaptopurine and methotrexate	MMN	mismatch negativity
	methadone maintenance		multifocal motor neuropathy
	micrometastases		multiple micronutrients
	millimeter (mm)	MMO	maximum mouth opening
	mismatch (ing)	MMOA	maxillary mandibular odontectomy alveolectomy
	mist mask		
	morbidity and mortality	mmol	millimole
	motor meal	μmol	micromole
	mucous membrane	MMORPGs	massively multiplayer online role-playing games
	multiple myeloma		
	muscle movement	MMP	matrix metalloproteinase
	muscularis mucosae		mitochondrial myopathy
	myelomeningocele		mucous membrane pemphigoid
mM.	millimole (mmol)		multiple medical problems
mm	millimeter		multiplexed molecular profiling (system)
M&M	milk and molasses		
	morbidity and mortality	MMP-8	metalloproteinase-8
MMA	maxillomandibular advancement	MMPI	matrix metalloproteinase inhibitor
	methylmalonic acid		Minnesota Multiphasic Personality Inventory
	methylmethacrylate		
	middle meningeal artery	MMPI-A	Minnesota Multiphasic Personality Inventory - Adolescent version
MMC	migrating motor complex		
	mitomycin (mitomycin C)	MMPI-D	Minnesota Multiphasic Personality Inventory-Depression Scale
	myelomeningocele		
	myoelectrical migrating complex	6-MMPR	6-methylmercaptopurine riboside
MMCP	mumps, measles, chickenpox	MMPs	membership medical practices
MMCT	mitomycin C trabeculectomy	MMR	measles, mumps, and rubella
MMD	malignant metastatic disease		menometrorrhagia
	moyamoya disease		midline malignant reticulosis
	mucus membranes dry		mild mental retardation
	myotonic muscular dystrophy		mismatch repair
MME	membrane metalloendopeptidase	MMRISK	a mnemonic for judging who is at high risk for melanomas: greater than 3 atypical **m**oles, **m**oles that are many in number, **r**ed hair and/or freckles, **i**nability to tan, **s**evere sunburn before age 14, **k**indred (family history of melanoma)
MMECT	multiple monitor electroconvulsive therapy		
MMEFR	maximal mid-expiratory flow rate		
MMF	maxillomandibular fixation		
	mean maximum flow		
	mismatch field		
	mycophenolate mofetil (CellCept)		
MMFR	maximal mid-expiratory flow rate	MMRM	Mixed-effects Models Repeated Measures (analysis)
MMG	mammography		

M

MMRS	Metropolitan Medical Response System	MNNB	Monas-Nitz Neuropsychological Battery
MMR-VAR	measles virus, mumps virus, rubella virus, and varicella virus vaccine	MnP2	mandibular second premolar
		MNPRT	mixed neutron and photon radiotherapy
MMS	Medication Management Standards	MNR	marrow neutrophil reserve
	Mini-Mental State (examination)	MNS	mean nocturnal saturation
	Mohs micrographic surgery		mediastinal nodal sterilization
MMSAs	metropolitan and micropolitan statistical areas		Melnick Needles syndrome
		MNSc	Master of Nursing Science
		MnSOD	manganese superoxide dismutase
MMSE	Mini-Mental State Examination	Mn SSEPS	median-nerve somatosensory-evoked potentials
MMT	malignant mesenchymal tumors		
	manual muscle test	MNT	medical nutrition therapy
	meal-tolerance test	MNTB	medial nucleus of the trapezoid body
	medial meniscal tear		
	methadone maintenance treatment	MNX	meniscectomy
	Mini Mental Test	MNZ	metronidazole (Flagyl)
	mixed müllerian tumors	MO	medial oblique (x-ray view)
MMTP	Methadone Maintenance Treatment Program		medication overdose
			menhaden oil
MMTS	micrometastases		mesio-occlusal
MMTV	malignant mesothelioma of the tunica vaginalis		mineral oil
			monocyte
	monomorphic ventricular tachycardia		month (mo)
			months old
	mouse mammary tumor virus		morbidly obese
MMV	mandatory minute volume		mother
MMWR	*Morbidity and Mortality Weekly Report*		myositis ossificans
		Mo	molybdenum
MMx	multimatrix; a tablet formulation designed to begin dissolution in the terminal ileum	M/O	morning of
		MOA	mechanism of action
			metronidazole, omeprazole, and amoxicillin
MN	Master's Degree in Nursing		
	midnight	MoAb	monoclonal antibody
	mononuclear	MOAHI	mixed obstructive apnea and hypopnea index
Mn	manganese		
M&N	morning and night	MOAS	Modified Overt Aggression Scale
	Mydriacyl and Neo-Synephrine	MOB	medical office building
MNAR	missing not at random (incomplete data)		mobility
			mobilization
MNC	monomicrobial necrotizing cellulitis		mother of baby
		MOB-PT	mitomycin, vincristine (Oncovin), bleomycin, and cisplatin (Platinol)
	mononuclear leukocytes		
MNCH	maternal, newborn, and child health		
		MOC	maintenance of certification
MNCV	motor nerve conduction velocity		medial olivocochlear
MND	minor neurological dysfunction		Medical Officer on Call
	modified neck dissection		metronidazole, omeprazole, and clarithromycin
	motor neuron disease		
MNF	myelinated nerve fibers		mother of child
MNG	multinodular goiter	MoCA	Montreal Cognitive Assessment (to measure cognitive impairment)
MNGIE	mitochondrial neurogasterointestinal encephalomyopathy (syndrome)		
		MOCI	Maudsley Obsessive-Compulsive Inventory
MNM	mononeuritis multiplex	MOD	magneto-optical disc (radiology)
MNMCB	motor neuropathy with multifocal conduction block		maturity onset diabetes
			medical officer of the day

	mesio-occlusodistal	mono,	monochorionic,
	moderate	mono	monoamniotic
	mode of death	MONOS	monocytes
	moment of death	MOP	medical outpatient
	multiorgan dysfunction	8 MOP	methoxsalen (Oxsorlen)
MOD A	moderate assistance (assist)	MOPD II	Majewski osteodysplastic
MODEMS	Musculoskeletal Outcomes Data		primordial dwarfism type II
	Evaluation and Management	MOPP	mechlorethamine, vincristine
	Scale		(Oncovin), procarbazine, and
MOD I	modified independent (for		prednisone
	example, a patient who is	MOPV	monovalent oral poliovirus
	independent, but requires a		vaccine
	walker)	mOPV1	monovalent oral type 1 poliovirus
MOD	modified independent		vaccine
INDEP		MOR	morphine (This is a dangerous
MODM	mature-onset diabetes mellitus		abbreviation)
MODS	microscopic-observation drug-		mortality odds ratio
	susceptibility (assay)	mOR	matched odds ratio
	multiple-organ dysfunction	MOS	Medical Outcome Study
	syndrome (score)		mirror optical system
MODY	maturity-onset diabetes of youth		months
MOE	movement of extremities	mOS	median overall survival
MOEMs	micro-opto-electro-mechanical	MOSES	Multidimensional Observational
	systems		Scale for Elderly Subjects
MOF	mesial occlusal facial	MOSF	multiple-organ system failure
	methotrexate, vincristine	MOSFET	metal oxide semiconductor field-
	(Oncovin), and fluorouracil		effect transistor (dosimeter)
	methoxyflurane (Penthrane)	MOS sf-20	Medical Outcomes Study, short
	multiple-organ failure		form 20 items
MOFS	multiple-organ failure syndrome	MOS sf-36	Medical Outcomes Study, short
MOG	myelin oligodendrocyte		form, 36 items
	glycoprotein	mOsm	milliosmole
MOH	medication overuse headache	mOsmol	milliosmole
	Ministry of Health	MOT	motility examination
MoH	Ministry of Health (Canada)	MOTA	Method Other Than Acceleration
Mohs	Mohs technique; serial excision	MOTS	mucosal oral therapeutic system
	and microscopic examination of	MOTT	mycobacteria other than tubercle
	skin cancers	MOU	medical oncology unit
MOI	mechanism of injury		memorandum of understanding
	multiplicity of infection	MOUS	multiple occurrences of
MoICU	mobile intensive care unit		unexplained symptoms
MOID	Mammalian Orthologous Intron	MOV	minimum obstructive volume
	Database		multiple oral vitamin
MOJAC	mood orientation, judgement,	MOW	Meals on Wheels
	affect, and content	MP	malignant pyoderma
MOL	method of limits		melphalan and prednisone
MOM	metal-on-metal (arthroplasty)		menstrual period
	milk of magnesia		mercaptopurine (Purinethol)
	mother		metacarpal phalangeal joint
	mucoid otitis media		methylprednisolone
MoM	multiples of the median		mitoxantrone and prednisone
MOMP	major outer membrane protein		moist pack
MON	maximum observation nursery		monitor pattern
	monitor		monophasic
MONO	infectious mononucleosis		motor potential
	monocyte		mouthpiece
	monospot		muscularis propria
mono, di	monochorionic, diamniotic		myocardial perfusion

M

M:P	milk to plasma ratio (related to breast feeding concentrations of drug)	m-PFL	methotrexate, cisplatin (Platinol), fluorouracil, and leucovorin
M & P	Millipore and phase	MPFS	Medicare Physician Fee Schedule
4 MP	methylpyrazole (fomepizole; Antizol)	MPG	mean pressure gradient
		MPGN	membranoproliferative glomerulonephritis
6-MP	mercaptopurine (Purenthol)		
MPA	main pulmonary artery	MPH	massive pulmonary hemorrhage
	Medical Products Agency (Sweden; Switzerland)		Master of Public Health
			methylphenidate (Ritalin)
	medroxyprogesterone acetate		miles per hour
MPa	megapascal	MPHD	multiple pituitary hormone deficiencies
MPAC	Memorial Pain Assessment Card	MPI	manufacturer's package insert
MPA/E₂C	medroxyprogesterone acetate; estradiol cypionate (Lunelle)		master patient index
			Maudsley Personality Inventory
MPAP	mean pulmonary artery pressure		milk-product intolerance
MPAQ	McGill Pain Assessment Questionnaire		myocardial perfusion imaging
		MPIF-1	myeloid progenitor inhibitory factor-1
MPAS	Masters of Physician Assistant Studies		
		MPJ	metacarpophalangeal joint
MPB	male-pattern baldness	MPK	milligram per kilogram
	mephobarbital	MPL	maximum permissable level
MPBFV	mean pulmonary-blood-flow velocity		mesiopulpolingual
		MPL®	monophosphoryl lipid A
MPBNS	modified Peyronie bladder neck suspension	MPLC	medium pressure liquid chromatography
MPC	meperidine, promethazine, and chlorpromazine	MPM	malignant peritoneal mesothelioma
			malignant pleural mesothelioma
	mucopurulent cervicitis		Mortality Prediction Model
MPCC	Medical Policy Coordinating Committee	MPN	monthly progress note
			most probable number
MPCN	microscopically positive and culturally negative		multiple primary neoplasms
		MP-NAT	minipool nucleic acid (amplification) testing
M-PCR	multiplex polymerase chain reaction	MPNST	malignant peripheral nerve sheath tumor
MPCU	medical progressive care unit		
MPD	maximum permissable dose	MPO	male-pattern obesity
	methylphenidate (Ritalin)		myeloperoxidase
	moisture permeable dressing	MPOA	medial preoptic area
	multiple personality disorder	MPOD	macular pigment optical density
	myeloproliferative disorder	MPP	massive periretinal proliferation
	myofascial pain dysfunction (syndrome)		maximum pressure picture
		MPP	multiple presentation phenotype
mPD	minimal peripheral dose	MPQ	McGill Pain Questionnaire
MPDPS	multiparous desires permanent sterilization	MPPT	methylprednisolone pulse therapy
		MPR	massive periretinal retraction
MPE	malignant pleural effusion		medication possession ratio
	massive pulmonary embolism		multiplanar reconstruction
	mean prediction error	MPS	Maternal Perinatal Scale
	multiphoton excitation		mean particle size
	myxopapillary ependymoma		mononuclear phagocyte system
MPEC	multipolar electrocoagulation		mucopolysaccharidosis
MPEG	methoxypolyethylene glycol		multiphasic screening
MPF	methotrexate, cisplatin (Platinol), and fluorouracil	MPS-1	mucopolysaccharidosis I
		MPS-II	mucopolysaccharidosis II (Hunter syndrome)
	methylparaben free		
MPFC	medial prefrontal cortex	MPSS	massively parallel signature sequencing
MPFL	medial patellofemoral ligament		

M

	methylprednisolone sodium succinate	MRCT	multiregional clinical trials
MPSV4	meningococcal polysaccharide vaccine	MRD	margin reflex distance
			matched related donor(s)
MPT	melphalan, prednisone, and thalidomide		Medical Records Department
			Minimal Record of Disability
	multiple parameter telemetry		minimal residual disease
MPTRD	motor, pain, touch, and reflex deficit	MRDD	maximum recommended daily dose
			Mental Retardation and Development Disabilities
MPTT	malignant proliferating trichilemmal tumor		mentally retarded and developmentally disabled
MPU	maternal pediatric unit	MRDM	malnutrition-related diabetes mellitus
	medical progressive unit		
MPV	mean platelet volume	MRDSA	magnetic resonance digital subtraction angiography
MPXV	monkeypox virus		
MPZ	midperipheral zone (prostate needle biopsy location)	MRE	magnetic resonance elastography
			manual resistance exercise
MQ	mefloquine (Lariam)		most recent episode
	memory quotient	MRFC	mouse rosette-forming cells
MQOL	McGill Quality of Life Questionnaire	MR FIT	Multiple Risk Factor Intervention Trial
MR	Maddox rod	MRG	mortality reference group
	magnetic resonance		murmurs, rubs, and gallops
	manifest refraction	MRH	Maddox rod hyperphoria
	may repeat		multicentric reticulohistiocytoses
	mean ranking	MRHD	maximum recommended human dose
	measles-rubella		
	medial rectus	MRHT	modified rhyme hearing test
	medical record	MRI	magnetic resonance imaging
	mental retardation	M & RI	measure and record input
	milliroentgen	& O	and output
	mitral regurgitation	MRK	Merck & Co., Inc.
	moderate resistance	MRKH	Mayer-Rokitansky-Kuster-Hauser (syndrome)
M&R	measure and record		
MR × 1	may repeat times one (once)	MRL	minimal response level
MRA	magnetic resonance angiography		moderate rubra lochia
	main renal artery	MRLVD	maximum residue limits of veterinary drugs
	medical record administrator		
	medical research associate	MRLT	mesalamine-related lung toxicity
	midright atrium	MRM	magnetic resonance microimaging
	multivariate regression analysis		modified radical mastectomy
mrad	millirad	MRN	magnetic resonance neurography
MRAN	medical resident admitting note		malignant renal neoplasm
MRAP	mean right atrial pressure		medical record number
MRAS	main renal artery stenosis		medical resident's note
MRC	Master of Rehabilitation Counseling	mRNA	messenger ribonucleic acid
MRCA	magnetic resonance coronary angiography	MRO	multidrug resistant organism(s)
		MROU	medial rectus, both eyes
MRCC	metastatic renal cell carcinoma	MRP	multidrug resistance-associated protein
MRCP	magnetic resonance cholangiopancreatography		
		MP-RAGE	magnetization prepared rapid acquisition gradient-echo
	Member of the Royal College of Physicians		
		MRPN	medical resident progress note
	mental retardation, cerebral palsy	MRPs	medication-related problems
MRCPs	movement-related cortical potentials	MRR	medical record review
			Medication Reconciliation Record
MRCS	Member of the Royal College of Surgeons	MRS	macular raster scan
			magnetic resonance spectroscopy

M

	Melkersson Rosenthal Syndrome		metropolitan statistical area
	mental retardation syndrome		microsomal autoantibodies
	methicillin-resistant *Staphylococcus aureus*		multiple system atrophy
MRSA	methicillin-resistant *Staphylococcus aureus*	MSAD	multiple scan average dose (radiology)
MRSE	methicillin-resistant *Staphylococcus epidermidis*	MSAF	meconium-stained amniotic fluid
		MSAFP	maternal serum alpha-fetoprotein
MRSI	magnetic resonance spectroscopic imaging	MSAP	mean systemic arterial pressure
		MSAS	Mandel Social Adjustment Scale
MRSS	methicillin-resistant *Staphylococcus* species	MSAS-SF	Memorial Symptom Assessment Scale–short form
	modified Rodnan skin-thickness score	MSB	mainstem bronchus
		MSBOS	maximum surgical blood order schedule
MRT	magnetic resonance tomography	MSBP	Munchausen syndrome by proxy
	malignant rhabdoid tumor	MSC	major symptom complex
	mean response time		Medical Service Corps
	modified rhyme test		mesenchymal stromal cells
MRTA	magnetic resonance tomographic angiography		midsystolic click
			MS Contin®
MRTI	magnetic resonance thermal imaging	MSCA	McCarthy Scales of Children's Abilities
MRU	medical resource utilization	MSCC	malignant spinal cord compression
MRV	magnetic resonance venography		metastatic spinal cord compression
MRV(r)	mixed respiratory vaccine		midstream clean-catch (urine culture)
MRX	*Moraxella catarrhalis* vaccine		
MRx	manifest refraction	MSCCC	Master Sciences, Certified Clinical Competence
MR × 1	may repeat once		
MS	mass spectroscopy	MSCR-AMMS	microbial surface component reacting with adhesive matrix molecules
	Master of Science		
	median sternotomy		
	medical student		
	medical/surgical	MSCs	mesenchymal stem cells
	mental status	MSCT	multislice computed tomography
	milk shake	MSCU	medical special care unit
	milliseconds (ms)	MSCWP	musculoskeletal chest wall pain
	minimal support	MSD	male sexual dysfunction
	mitral sounds		microsurgical diskectomy
	mitral stenosis		midsleep disturbance
	moderately susceptible		musculoskeletal disorder
	morning stiffness	MSDBP	mean sitting diastolic blood pressure
	morphine sulfate (This is a dangerous abbreviation)	MS-DRG(s)	Medicare Severity Diagnosis-related Group(s)
	motile sperm		
	motility study	MSDS	material safety data sheet
	motion sickness	MSE	mean squared error
	multiple sclerosis		Mental Status Examination
	muscle spasm		multiscale entropy
	muscle strength	msec	milliseconds
	musculoskeletal	MSEL	myasthenic syndrome of Eaton-Lambert
ms	milliseconds		
M & S	microculture and sensitivity	MSER	mean systolic ejection rate
3MS	Modified Mini-Mental Status (examination)		Mental Status Examination Record
		MSF	meconium-stained fluid
MS III	third-year medical student		Médicins Sans Frontières (Doctors Without Borders)
MSA	Medical Savings Accounts		
	membrane-stabilizing activity		Mediterranean spotted fever
	methane sulfonic acid		megakaryocyte stimulating factor

M

MSG	massage	MSSO	Maintenance and Support Services Organization
	methysergide (Sansert)		
	monosodium glutamate	MSSP	Maternal Support Services Program
MSGT	malignant salivary gland tumor		
MSH	melanocyte-stimulating hormone	MSSU	midstream specimen of urine
MSHA	mannose-sensitive hemagglutinin	MST	maladies sexuellement transmissibles (French for sexually transmitted diseases)
MSI	magnetic source imaging		
	mass sociogenic illness		
	microsatellite instability		mean survival time
	multiple subcortical infarction		median survival time
	musculoskeletal impairment		mental stress test
MSIA	mass spectrometric immunoassay		modified Schirmer test
MSIR®	morphine sulfate immediate release tablets		multiple subpial transection
		MSTA®	mumps skin test antigen
MSIS	Multiple Severity of Illness System	MSTI	multiple soft tissue injuries
		MSTS	American Musculoskeletal Tumor Society (functional rating system)
MSK	medullary sponge kidney		
	musculoskeletal		
MSKCC	Memorial Sloan-Kettering Cancer Center	MSU	maple-syrup urine
			midstream urine
MSL	maximum step length (test)		monosodium urate
	midsternal line	MSUD	maple-syrup urine disease
	multiple symmetrical lipomatosis	MSUS	musculoskeletal ultrasound
MSLT	multiple sleep latency test	MSUs	midstream specimens of urine
MSM	magnetic starch microspheres	mSv	millisievert (radiation unit)
	men who have sex with men	MSW	Master of Social Work
	methsuximide (Celontin)		multiple stab wounds
	methylsulfonylmethane	MT	empty
	midsystolic murmur		macular target
MSN	Master of Science in Nursing		maggot therapy
MSNA	muscle sympathetic nerve activity		maintenance therapy
MSO	managed services organization		malaria therapy
	mentally stable and oriented		malignant teratoma
	mental status, oriented		manual therapy
	most significant other		Medical Technologist
MSO$_4$	morphine sulfate (this is a dangerous abbreviation)		metatarsal
			middle turbinate
MSOD	multisystem organ dysfunction		monitor technician
MSOF	multisystem organ failure		mucosal thickening
MSP	Medoff sliding plate		muscles and tendons
MS-PCR	methylation-specific polymerase chain reaction		muscle tone
			music therapy (Therapist)
MSPN	medical student progress notes		myringotomy tube(s)
MSPU	medical short procedure unit	M/T	masses of tenderness
MSQ	Mental Status Questionnaire		myringotomy with tubes
	meters squared	M & T	*Monilia* and *Trichomonas*
MSR	muscle stretch reflexes		muscles and tendons
MSRPP	Multidimensional Scale for Rating Psychiatric Patients		myringotomy and tympanostomy tube insertion
		MTA	Medical Technical Assistant
MSS	Marital Satisfaction Scale		metatarsal adduction
	maternal serum screening		mineral trioxide aggregate
	mean sac size		multi-targeted antifolate (pemetrexed disodium [Alimta])
	microsatellite stable		
	minor surgery suite	4-MTA	4-methylthioamphetamine
MSSA	methicillin-susceptible *Staphylococcus aureus*	MTA1	metastasis-associated protein 1
MSS-CR	mean sac size and crown-rump length	MTAD	tympanic membrane of the right ear

MT/AK	music therapy/ audiokinetics	MTNX	methylnaltrexone
MTAS	tympanic membrane of the left ear	mTOR	mammalian target of rapamycin
MTAU	tympanic membranes of both ears	MTP	master treatment plan
MTB	*Mycobacterium tuberculosis*		medial tibial plateau
MTBC	Music Therapist-Board Certified		medical termination of pregnancy
	Mycobacterium tuberculosis		metatarsophalangeal
	complex		microsomal triglyceride transfer
MTBE	methyl tert-butyl ether		protein
MTBI	mild traumatic brain injury	MTPJ	metatarsophalangeal joint
MTC	magnetization transfer contrast	MTR	microtubal reanastomosis
	(radiology)		mother
	medullary thyroid carcinoma	MTR-Ō	no masses, tenderness, or rebound
	metoclopramide	MTRS	Licensed Master Therapeutic
	mitomycin (Mutamycin)		Recreation Specialist
	Multi-tiered Co-Pay (Programs)	MTS	May-Thurner syndrome
MTCSA	mid-thigh muscle cross-sectional		mesial temporal sclerosis
	area		Muir-Torre syndrome
MTCT	mother-to-child transmission	mTSS	menstrual toxic shock syndrome
MTD	maximum tolerated dose	MTST	maximal treadmill stress test
	metastatic trophoblastic disease	MTT	mamillothalamic tract
	methadone		mean transit time
	Monroe tidal drainage		methylthiotetrazole
	Mycobacterium tuberculosis direct	MTU	malignant teratoma undifferentiated
	(test)		methylthiouracil
MTDDA	Minnesota Test for Differential	MTWA	microvolt T-wave alternans
	Diagnosis of Aphasia	MTX	methotrexate
MTDI	maximum tolerable daily intake	MTZ	mirtazapine (Remeron)
MTDT	*Mycobacterium* tuberculosis direct		mitoxantrone (Novantrone)
	test	MU	million units
MTE	multiple trace elements		monitor unit
MTE-4®	trace metal elements injection		Murphy unit
	(there was also a #5, #6, and #7)	mU	milliunits
	(no longer marketed)	MUA	manipulation under anesthesia
mTECs	medullary thymic epithelial cells	MUAC	middle upper arm circumference
MTET	modified treadmill exercise testing	MUAP	motor unit action potential
MTF	male-to-female (transmission)	MUD	matched-unrelated donor
	medical treatment facility	MUDDLES	miosis, urination, diarrhea,
	modulation transfer function		diaphoresis, lacrimation,
	(radiology)		excitation of central nervous
MTG	middle temporal gyrus (gyri)		system, and salivation (effects of
	midthigh girth		cholinesterase inhibitors)
MTHFR	methylene tetrahydrofolate	MUDPILES	*m*ethanol, metformin; *u*remia;
	reductase		*d*iabetic ketoacidosis;
MTI	magnetization transfer imaging		*p*henformin, paraldehyde; *i*ron,
	malignant teratoma intermediate		*is*oniazid, ibuprofen; *l*actic
MTJ	midtarsal joint		acidosis; *e*thanol, ethylene
MTL	medial temporal lobe		glycol; and *s*alicylates, sepsis
	mediastinal tuberculous		(causes of metabolic acidosis)
	lymphadenitis	MUE	medication use evaluation
	Metropolitan Life (Insurance	MUFA	monounsaturated fatty acid
	Company) Table (for desirable	MUG	microgram (mcg is preferred)
	weight)	MUGA	multigated (radionuclide)
MTLE	medial (mesial) temporal-lobe		angiogram
	epilepsy		multiple gated acquisition (scan)
MTLV	midtidal lung volume	MUGX	multiple gated acquisition exercise
MTM	medication therapy management	MUHH	Marie Unna hereditary
	modified Thayer-Martin medium		hypotrichosis
	mouth-to-mouth (resuscitation)	MUI	mixed urinary incontinence

M

MULE	microcomputer upper limb exerciser	MVI 12®	brand name for parenteral multivitamins
MULTIP	multipara	MVIC	maximum voluntary isometric contractions
MuLV	murine leukemia virus		
MUM	mumps virus vaccine	MVID	microvillus inclusion disease
MUNE	motor unit estimates	MVO	mixed venous oxygen saturation
MUNSH	Memorial University of Newfoundland Scale of Happiness	MVO₂	myocardial oxygen consumption
		MVP	mean venous pressure
			mitomycin, vinblastine, and cisplatin (Platinol)
MUO	metastasis of unknown origin		
MUPAT	multiple-site perineal applicator technique		mitral valve prolapse
		MVPA	moderate-to-vigorous physical activity
MUPIT	Martinez Universal Perineal Interstitial Template		
		MVPP	mechlorethamine, vinblastine, procarbazine, and prednisone
MUPS	melanoma of unknown primary site		
MUS	mid-urethral slang	MVPS	mitral valve prolapse syndrome
MUSE®	Medicated Urethral System for Erection (alprostadil urethral suppository)	MVR	massive vitreous retraction
			micro-vitreoretinal (blade)
			mitral valve regurgitation
mus-lig	musculoligamentous		mitral valve replacement
MUU	mouse uterine units	MVRI	mixed vaccine respiratory infections
MV	manual ventilation		
	mechanical ventilation	MVS	mitral valve stenosis
	megavolts		motor, vascular, and sensory
	mesenteric vasculitis		Multichannel Verification System
	millivolts	MVT	movement
	minute volume		multiform ventricular tachycardia
	mitoxantrone and etoposide (VePesid)		multivisceral transplant
			multivitamin
	mitral valve	MVU	Montevideo units
	mixed venous	MVV	maximum ventilatory volume
	multivesicular		maximum voluntary ventilation
MVA	malignant ventricular arrhythmias		mixed vespid venom
	manual vacuum aspiration	6-MW	6-minute walk (test)
	mitral valve area	12-MW	12-minute walk (test)
	modified vaccinia ankara	MWA	migraine with aura
	motor vehicle accident	MWB	minimal weight bearing
M-VAC	methotrexate, vinblastine doxorubicin (Adriamycin), and cisplatin	MWC	major wound complications
		MWCO	molecular weight cutoff
		MWD	maximum walking distance
MVB	methotrexate and vinblastine		microwave diathermy
	mixed venous blood	6-MWD	6-minute walking distance
MVC	maximal voluntary contraction	M-W-F	Monday-Wednesday-Friday
	motor vehicle collision (crash)	MWI	Medical Walk-In (Clinic)
MVc	mitral valve closure	MWL	massive weight loss
MV-CBCT	meta-voltage cone-beam computed tomography	MWOA	migraine without aura
		MWS	Mickety-Wilson syndrome
MVD	microvascular decompression	MWT	maintenance of wakefulness test
	microvessel density		Mallory-Weiss tear
	mitral valve disease		malpositioned wisdom teeth
	multivessel disease		maximal walking time
MVE	mitral valve (leaflet) excursion	6-MWT	6-minute walk test
	Murray Valley encephalitis	MWTP	municipal wastewater treatment plants
MV Grad	mitral valve gradient		
MVI	malignant vascular injury	Mx	mammography
	multiple vitamin injection		manifest refraction
MVI®	brand name for parenteral multivitamins		mastectomy
			maxilla

	movement
	myringotomy
MxA	myxovirus resistance protein A
My	myopia
MYD	mydriatic
myelo	myelocytes
	myelogram
MyG	myasthenia gravis
MYOP	myopia
MYR	myringotomy
MYS	medium yellow soft (stools)
MZ	monozygotic
Mz	magnetization vector (radiology)
M/Z	mass/charge
MZL	marginal zone lymphocyte
MZT	monozygotic twins

N

N	nausea
	negative
	Negro
	Neisseria
	nerve
	neutrophil
	never
	newton
	night
	nipple
	nitrogen
	no
	nodes
	nonalcoholic
	none
	normal
	North (as in the location 2N, would be second floor, North wing)
	not
	notified
	noun
	NPH insulin (it is dangerous to use abbreviations for insulin therapy)
	size of sample
N1	study night 1
N I . . . . N XII	first through twelfth cranial nerves
O.1 N	tenth-normal
N_2	nitrogen
N 2.5	phenylephrine HCl 2.5% ophthalmic solution (Neo-Synephrine)
n-3	omega-3
5'-N	5'-nucleotidase
N-9	nonoxynol 9
NA	Narcotics Anonymous
	Native American
	Negro adult
	new admission
	nicotinic acid
	nonadherence
	nonalcoholic
	norethindrone acetate
	normal axis
	not admitted
	not applicable
	not available
	nurse aide
	nurse's aid
	Nurse Anesthetist
	nursing assistant
Na	sodium
Na^+	sodium

M

N & A	normal and active	NAEPP	National Asthma Education and Prevention Program (guidelines)
NAA	*N*-acetylaspartate		
	National Average Allowance (federal physician office visit cost guide)	NAET	Nambudripad allergy elimination technique
		NAF	nafcillin
	neutron activation analysis		Native-American female
	no apparent abnormalities		Negro adult female
	nucleic acid amplification		normal adult female
NAAA	neo-adjuvant androgen ablation		Notice of Adverse Findings (FDA post-audit letter)
NAAC	no apparent anesthesia complications		
		NaF	sodium fluoride
NAA/Cr	N-acetylaspartate/creatine ratio	NaFeEDTA	sodium iron (III) ethylenediaminetetraacetic acid (sodium iron edetic acid)
NAAD	neoadjuvant androgen deprivation (therapy)		
NAAT	nucleic acid amplification techniques (testing)	NAFLD	nonalcoholic fatty liver disease
		NAG	N-acetyl-beta-d-glucosaminidase
NAATPT	not available at the present time		narrow angle glaucoma
NAB	Neuropsychological Assessment Battery	NaHCO₃	sodium bicarbonate
		NAHI	nonaccidental head injury
	not at bedside	NAI	no action indicated
Nab-P	nanoparticles albumin-bound paclitaxel		no acute inflammation
			nonaccidental injury
NABS	normoactive bowel sounds		Nuremberg Aging Inventory
NAbs	neutralizing antibodies	NaI	sodium iodide
NABT	normal-appearing brain tissue	NAION	nonarteritic anterior ischemic optic neuropathy
NABTC	North American Brain Tumor Consortium		
		NAIT	neonatal alloimmune thrombocytopenia
NABX	needle aspiration biopsy		
NAC	acetylcysteine (N-acetylcysteine; Mucomyst)	NAL	nasal angiocentric lymphoma
		NAM	nail-apparatus melanoma
	neoadjuvant chemotherapy		Native-American male
	nipple-areola complex		no abnormal masses
	no acute changes		normal adult male
	no anesthesia complications	NAMCS	National Ambulatory Medical Care Survey
NACD	no anatomical cause of death		
NaCIO	sodium hypochlorite	nAMD	neovascular age-related macular degeneration
NaCl	sodium chloride (salt)		
NaCMC	sodium carboxymethyl cellulose	NANB	non-A, non-B (hepatitis) (hepatitis C)
NACS	Neurologic and Adaptive Capacity Score		
		NANBH	non-A, non-B hepatitis (hepatitis C)
NACT	neoadjuvant chemotherapy		
NAD	nicotinamide adenine dinucleotide	NANC	nonadrenergic, noncholinergic
		NANDA	North American Nursing Diagnosis Association (taxonomy)
	no active disease		
	no acute distress	NaNP	sodium nitroprusside (Nipride)
	no apparent distress	NANSAIDs	nonaspirin, nonsteroidal anti-inflammatory drugs
	no appreciable disease		
	normal axis deviation	NANT	New Approaches to Neuroblastoma Therapy (consortium)
	nothing abnormal detected		
NADA	New Animal Drug Application	NaOCl	sodium hypochlorite
NADase	nicotinamide adenine dinucleotide glycohydrolase	NaOH	sodium hydroxide
		NAP	narrative, assessment, and plan
NADCs	non-AIDS-defining cancers		no apparent pathology
NADE	New Animal Drug Evaluation		nosocomial acquired pneumonia
NADPH	nicotinamide adenine dinucleotide phosphate	NAPA	N-acetyl procainamide
		NAPD	no active pulmonary disease
NADSIC	no apparent disease seen in chest	Na Pent	Pentothal Sodium
NaE	exchangeable sodium	NAR	nasal airflow resistance

	no action required	NBI	no bone injury
	no adverse reaction	NBICU	newborn intensive care unit
	nonambulatory restraint	nBiPAP	nasal bilevel (biphasic) positive
	not at risk		airway pressure
	nursing assessment record	NBIs	nosocomial bloodstream infections
NARC	narcotic(s)	NBL/OM	neuroblastoma and opsoclonus-
NaRI	noradrenaline reuptake inhibitor		myoclonus
NARP	neuropathy, (neurogenic muscle	NBM	no bowel movement
	weakness) ataxia and retinitis		normal bone marrow
	pigmentosa (syndrome)		normal bowel movement
NART	National Adult Reading Test		nothing by mouth
	(United Kingdom)	NBME	National Board of Medical
NAS	nasal		Examiners
	neonatal abstinence syndrome	NBN	newborn nursery
	new active substance	NBP	needle biopsy of prostate
	no abnormality seen		no bone pathology
	no added salt	NBQC	narrow base quad cane
NASBA	nucleic-acid sequencing based	NBR	no blood return
	amplification	NBRM	negative binomial regression model
NaSCN	sodium thiocyanate	NBS	newborn screen (serum thyroxine
NASH	nonalcoholic steatohepatitis		and phenylketonuria)
NAS-NRC	National Academy of Sciences –		Nijmegen breakage syndrome
	National Research Council		no bacteria seen
NaSSA	noradrenergic and specific		normal bowel sounds
	serotonergic antidepresssant	NBT	nitroblue tetrazolium reduction
NASTT	nonspecific abnormality of ST		(tests)
	segment and T wave		normal breast tissue
NAT	N-acetyltransferase	NBTE	nonbacterial thrombotic
	no action taken		endocarditis
	no acute trauma	NBTNF	newborn, term, normal female
	nonaccidental trauma	NBTNM	newborn, term, normal, male
	nonspecific abnormality of T wave	NBW	normal birth weight (2,500–3,999 g)
	nucleic acid test (testing)	N/C	no change
Na^{99m}	sodium pertechnetate	NC	nasal cannula
TcO_4^-	Tc 99m		Negro child
NAUC	normalized area under the curve		neurologic check
NAUTI	nosocomially-associated urinary		no change
	tract infections		no charge
NAW	nasal antral window		no complaints
NAWM	normal-appearing white matter		noncontributory
NB	nail bed		normocephalic
	needle biopsy		nose clamp
	neuroblastomas		nose clips
	newborn		not classified
	nitrogen balance		not completed
	note well		not cultured
NB-BAL	nonbronchoscopic-bronchoalveolar	9 NC	rubitecan (9-nitrocamptothecin;
	lavage		Orathecin)
NBC	newborn center	NCA	neurocirculatory asthenia
	nonbed care		no congenital abnormalities
	nuclear, biological, and chemical	NCAM	neuronal cell adhesion molecule
NBCCS	nevoid basal-cell carcinoma	N/CAN	nasal cannula
	syndrome	NCAP	nasal continuous airway pressure
NBD	neurologic bladder dysfunction		noncalcified coronary artery plaque
	no brain damage	NCAS	zinostatin (neocarzinostatin)
NBF	not breast fed	NC/AT	normocephalic atraumatic
NBH	new bag (bottle) hung	NCB	natural childbirth
NBHH	newborn helpful hints		no code blue

NCBI	National Center for Biotechnology Information (NIH)	NCID	National Center for Infectious Diseases (CDC)
NCC	neurocysticercosis no concentrated carbohydrates nursing care card	NCIE	nonbullous congenital ichthyosiform erythroderma
NCCAM	National Center for Complementary and Alternative Medicine (NIH)	NCIPC	National Center for Injury Prevention and Control (CDC)
		NCIS	National Coroners Information System (Australia)
NCCDPHP	National Center for Chronic Disease and Prevention and Health Promotion (CDC)		nursing care information sheet
		NCIT	Nursing Care Intervention Tool
		NCJ	needle catheter jejunostomy
NCCI	National Correct Coding Initiative	NCL	neuronal ceroid lipofuscinosis
NCCLS	National Committee for Clinical Laboratory Standards		no cautionary labels nuclear cardiology laboratory
NCCN	National Comprehensive Cancer Network	NCKX	sodium-calcium-potassium exchanger
NCCP	noncardiac chest pain	NCLD	neonatal chronic lung disease
NCCT	noncontrast computed tomography	NCM	nailfold capillary microscope
NCCTG	North Central Cancer Treatment Group		nonclinical manager
		NCNC	normochromic, normocytic
NCCU	neurosurgical continuous care unit	NCNR	National Center for Nursing Research (NIH)
NCD	National Coverage Determination (Manual)		
		NCNS	no complications, no sequelae
	neck-capsule distance no congenital deformities	NCO	no complaints offered noncommissioned officer
	normal childhood diseases	NCOG	North California Oncology Group
	not considered disabling not considered disqualifying Nursing-Care Dependency (scale)	NCP	no caffeine or pepper noncancer patients nursing care plan
NCDB	National Cancer Data Base	nCPAP	nasal continuous positive airway pressure
NCDR	new case-detection rate		
NCDs	national coverage determinations	NCPB	neurolytic celiac plexus block
NCE	new chemical entity	NCPE	noncardiogenic pulmonary edema
NCEH	National Center for Environmental Health (CDC)	NcpPCu	nonceruloplasmin plasma copper
		NCPR	no cardiopulmonary resuscitation
NCEP	National Cholesterol Education Program	NCQA	National Commission for Quality Assurance
NCF	neurocognitive function neutrophilic chemotactic factor no cold fluids	NCR	no carbon (paper) required (treated paper which produces a copy of what was written on the paper above)
NC=F	noncompleter=failure		
NCHGR	National Center for Human Genome Research (NIH)	nCR	nodular complete response
		NCRA	National Cancer Registrars Association
NCHS	National Center for Health Statistics	NCRAD	National Cell Repository for Alzheimer Disease
NCICB	National Cancer Institute Center for Bioinformatics		
		NCRC	nonchild-resistant container
NCI	National Cancer Institute	NCRI	National Cancer Research Institute (United Kingdom)
NCICB	National Cancer Institute Center for Bioinformatics		
		NCRR	National Center for Research Resources (NIH)
NCIC	National Cancer Institute of Canada		
		NCRT	neoadjuvant chemoradiation therapy
NCI-CTC	National Cancer Institute Common Toxicity Criteria		
		NCS	nerve conduction studies
NCI-CTCAE	National Cancer Institute Common Toxicity Criteria Adverse Event		no concentrated sweets noncontact supervision
NCIC-CTG	National Cancer Institute of Canada Clinical Trials Group		not clinically significant Nutcracker syndrome

	zinostatin (neocarzinostatin)		nephrogenic diabetes insipidus
NCSE	nonconvulsive status epilepticus	NDIR	nondispersive infrared
NCSN	National Certified School Nurse	NDIRS	nondispersive infrared spectrometer
NCT	neoadjuvant chemotherapy	NDM	neonatal diabetes mellitus
	neutron capture therapy	NDMS	National Disaster Medical System
	noncontact tonometry	Nd/NT	nondistended, nontender
	noncontrast computed tomography	NDO	neurogenic detrusor overactivity
	number connection test	NDP	nedaplatin
	Nursing Care Technician		net dietary protein
NCTR	National Center for Toxicological		Nurse Discharge Planner
	Research	NDPH	new daily persistent headache
NCV	nerve conduction velocity	NDR	neurotic depressive reaction
	nuclear venogram		normal detrusor reflex
NCVHS	National Committee on Vital and	NDRI	norepinephrine and dopamine
	Health Statistics		reuptake inhibitor
NCX	sodium-calcium exchanger	NDS	Neurologic Disability Score
ND	Doctor of Naturopathy		neuropathy disability score
	(Naturopathic Physician)		New Drug Submission
	nasal deformity	NDSC	nasal dermoid sinus cyst
	nasal discharge	NDSO	nasolacrimal drainage system
	nasoduodenal		obstruction
	natural death	NDST	neurodevelopmental screening test
	neck dissection	NDT	nasal duodenostomy tube
	neonatal death		Neurocognitive Driving Test
	neurological development		neurodevelopmental techniques
	neurotic depression		neurodevelopmental treatment
	Newcastle disease		noise detection threshold
	no data	NDV	Newcastle disease virus
	no disease	NDVI	normalized difference vegetation
	nondisabling		index
	nondistended	Nd:YAG	neodymium:yttrium-aluminum-
	none detectable		garnet (laser)
	normal delivery	Nd:YLF	neodymium: yttrium-lithium-
	normal development		fluoride (laser)
	nose drops	NE	nasoenteric
	not detected		nausea and emesis
	not diagnosed		nephropathica epidemica
	not done		neurological examination
	nothing done		never exposed
	Nursing Doctorate		no effect
N&D	nodular and diffuse		no enlargement
Nd	neodymium		norethindrone
NDA	New Drug Application		norepinephrine
	no data available		not elevated
	no demonstrable antibodies		not estimable
	no detectable activity		not examined
NDC	National Drug Code	NEAA	nonessential amino acids
	Nicotine Dependence Center	NEAC	norethindrone acetate
	nondigestible carbohydrates	NEAD	nonepileptic attack disorder
NDD	no dialysis days	NEAT	nonexercise activity thermogenesis
NDD-CKD	nondialysis dependent-chronic		not evaluated at triage
	kidney disease	NEB	hand-held nebulizer
NDE	near-death experience	NEC	necrotizing entercolitis
NDEA	no deviation of electrical axis		noise equivalent counts
NDF	neutral density filter (test)		nonesterified cholesterol
	no disease found		not elsewhere classified
NDGA	nordihydroguaiaretic acid	NECT	nonenhanced computed
NDI	National Death Index		tomography (scan)

N

NED	neuroendocrine differentiation	NETA	norethindrone acetate (Aygestin)
	no evidence of disease	NETSS	National Electronic
NEDSS	National Electronic Disease		Telecommunications System for
	Surveillance System		Surveillance
NEE	neonatal epileptic encephalopathy	NETT	nasal endotracheal tube
NEEG	normal electroencephalogram	NETZ	needle (diathermy) excision of the
NEEP	negative end-expiratory pressure		transformation zone
Ne/ERN	error negativity/error-related	NEURO	neurologic
	negativity		neurological
NEF	negative expiratory force		neurologist
NEFA	nonesterified fatty acid(s)	NEVA	nocturnal electrobioimpedance
NEFG	normal external female genitalia		volumetric assessment (penile
NEFT	nasoenteric feeding tube		measurement)
NEG	negative	NEX	nose-to-ear-to-xiphoid
	neglect		number of excitations (radiology)
NEI	National Eye Institute (NIH)	NEXUS	National Emergency X-
NEISS-AIP	National Electronic Injury		Radiography Utilization Study
	Surveillance System—All Injury		(criteria)
	Program (Database, CDC)	NF	National Formulary
NEJM	*New England Journal of Medicine*		necrotizing fasciitis
NEM	neurotrophic enhancing molecule		Negro female
	no evidence of malignancy		neurofibromatosis
	nucleoside excision mutation		night frequency (of voiding)
NEMD	nonexudative macular degeneration		nodular fasciitis
	nonspecific esophageal motility		none found
	disorder		nonfasting
NENT	nasal endotracheal tube		not found
NEO	necrotizing external otitis		nursed fair
NEOH	neonatal high risk		nursing facility
NEOM	neonatal medium risk	Nf	*Naegleria fowleri*
	normal extraocular muscles	NF1	neurofibromatosis type 1
NEP	needle-exchange program	NF2	neurofibromatous type 2
	neutral endopeptidase	NF90	nuclear factor 90
	no evidence of pathology	NFA	Nerve Fiber Analyzer®
NEPD	no evidence of pulmonary disease	NFALO	Nerve Fiber Analyzer laser
NEPHRO	nephrogram		oththalmoscope
NEPPK	nonepidermolytic palmoplantar	NFAP	nursing facility-acquired
	keratoderma		pneumonia
NEQ	noise equivalent quanta (radiology)	NFAR	no further action required
NEQAS	National External Quality	NFC	nailfold capillaroscopy
	Assurance Scheme (United	NFCS	Neonatal Facial Coding System
	Kingdom)	NFD	nephrogenic fibrosing dermopathy
NER	no evidence of recurrence		no family doctor
NERD	no evidence of recurrent disease	NFFD	not fit for duty
	nonerosive reflux disease	NFI	nerve-function impairment
NES	nonepileptic seizure		no-fault insurance
	nonstandard electrolyte solution		no further information
	not elsewhere specified		normal female infant
NESP	novel erythropoiesis stimulating	NFL	nerve fiber layer
	protein (darbepoetin [Aranesp])		Novantrone (mitoxantrone),
NESTT	nonhazardous explosives for		fluorouracil, and leucovorin
	security training and testing	NFLE	nocturnal frontal lobe epilepsy
NET	choroidal or subretinal	NFLX	norfloxacin (Noroxin)
	neovascularization	NFP	natural family planning
	Internet		no family physician
	naso-endotracheal tube		not-for-profit
	neuroectodermal tumor		not for publication
	neuroendocrine tumors	NFPA	nonfluent progressive aphasia

NFT	no further treatment	NHE	sodium/hydrogen exchanger
NFTD	normal full-term delivery	NHEJ	nonhomologous end-joining
NFTE	not found this examination	NHGRI	National Human Genome Research Institute (NIH)
NFTs	neurofibrillary tangles		
	neurologic function tests	NHIS	National Health Interview Survey
NFTSD	normal full-term spontaneous delivery	NHL	nodular histiocytic lymphoma
			non-Hodgkin lymphomas
NFTT	nonorganic failure to thrive	nHL	normalized hearing level
NFV	nelfinavir (Viracept)	NHLBI	National Heart, Lung, and Blood Institute (NIH)
NFW	nursed fairly well		
NG	nanogram (ng) (10^{-9} gram)	NHLPP	hereditary neuropathy with liability for pressure palsy
	nasogastric		
	night guard	NHM	no heroic measures
	nitroglycerin	NHND	nonhemorrhagic neurological deficit
	no growth		
	norgestrel	NHO	notify house officer
ng	nanogram	NHP	Naval Hospital Pensacola
NGAL	neutrophil gelatinase-associated lipocalin		Nottingham Health Profile
			nursing home placement
NGB	neurogenic bladder	NHPs	natural health products
NGCs	nerve guidance conduits	NHPT	nine-hole peg test
NGF	nerve growth factor	NHS	National Health Service (UK)
n giv	not given		Newborn Hearing Screening (Program)
NGJ	nasogastro-jejunostomy		
NGM	norgestimate	NHSP	Newborn Hearing Screening Program
NGMAST	*Neisseria gonorrhoeae* multi-antigen sequence typing		
		NHT	neoadjuvant hormonal therapy
NGO	nongovernmental organization		nursing home transfer
NGOs	nongovernmental organizations	NHTR	nonhemolytic transfusion reaction
NGR	nasogastric (tube) replacement	NHTSA	National Highway Traffic Safety Administration
NGRI	not guilty by reason of insanity		
NGS	next-generation sequencing	NHW	nonhealing wound
NGSF	nothing grown so far	NI	neurological improvement
NGT	nasogastric tube		no improvement
	normal glucose tolerance		no information
NGTD	no growth to date		none indicated
NgTD	negative to date		not identified
NGU	nongonococcal urethritis		not isolated
NH	non-Hispanic		nutritional insufficiency
	normal-hearing	NIA	National Institute on Aging (NIH)
	nursing home		no information available
$-NH_2$	amine	NIAAA	National Institute on Alcohol Abuse and Alcoholism (NIH)
NH_4^+	ammonium		
NHA	no histologic abnormalities	NIACHO	National Integrated Accreditation for Healthcare Organizations
NHANES III	third National Health and Nutrition Examination Survey		
		NIADDK	National Institute of Arthritis, Diabetes, and Digestive and Kidney Diseases (NIH)
nHAp	hydroxyapatite nanocrystals		
NHB	Naval Hospital Bremerton		
	nonheart-beating (donor)	NIAID	National Institute of Allergy and Infectious Diseases (NIH)
NHBD	nonheart-beating donor		
NHC	neighborhood health center	NIAL	not in active labor
	neonatal hypocalcemia	NIAMS	National Institute of Arthritis and Musculoskeletal and Skin Diseases (NIH)
	nursing home care		
NH_3	ammonia		
NH_4Cl	ammonium chloride	NIA-RI	National Institute on Aging–Reagan Institute
NHCU	nursing home care unit		
NHD	nocturnal hemodialysis	NIBP	noninvasive blood pressure
	normal hair distribution	NIBPM	noninvasive blood pressure

N

	measurement	NIHD	noise-induced hearing damage
NIC	neonatal intensive care	NIHL	noise-induced hearing loss
	Nursing Intervention Classification	NIHSS	National Institutes of Health Stroke Scale
NICC	neonatal intensive care center		
	noninfectious chronic cystitis	NIID	neuronal intranuclear inclusion disease
NICE	National Institute for Clinical Excellence (United Kingdom)	NIL	not in labor
	new, interesting, and challenging experiences	NIM	nerve integrity monitor
		NIMAs	noninherited maternal antigens
NICHD	National Institute of Child Health and Human Development (NIH)	NIMH	National Institute of Mental Health (NIH)
NICMP	nonischemic cardiomyopathy	NIMHDIS	National Institute for Mental Health Diagnostic Interview Schedule (NIH)
NICO	neuralgia-inducing cavitational osteonecrosis		
	noninvasive cardiac output (monitor)	NIMR	National Institute of Medical Research (United Kingdom)
NicoE	National Intrepid Center of Excellence	NINDS	National Institute of Neurological Disorders and Stroke (NIH)
NICS	noninvasive carotid studies	NINR	National Institute for Nursing Research (NIH)
NICU	neonatal intensive care unit		
	neurosurgical intensive care unit	NINU	neuro intermediate nursing unit
	new infant care unit	NINVS	noninvasive neurovascular studies
NID	no identifiable disease	NIOPCs	no intraoperative complications
	not in distress	NIOSH	National Institute of Occupational Safety and Health (Centers for Disease Control and Prevention)
NIDA	National Institute of Drug Abuse (NIH)		
NIDA five	National Institute on Drug Abuse screen for cannabinoids, cocaine metabolite, amphetamine/ metham-phetamine, opiates, and phencyclidine	NIP	catnip
			National Immunization Program
			no infection present
			no inflammation present
		NIPAs	noninherited paternal antigens
NIDCD	National Institute of Deafness and other Communication Disorders (NIH)	NIPD	nocturnal intermittent peritoneal dialysis
		NIPPV	noninvasive positive-pressure ventilation
NIDCR	National Institute of Dental and Craniofacial Research (NIH)	NIPS	Neonatal Infant Pain Scale
NIDD	noninsulin-dependent diabetes	NIP/S	noninvasive programming stimulation
NIDDK	National Institute of Diabetes and Digestive and Kidney Diseases (NIH)	NIPSV	noninvasive pressure support ventilation
		NIR	near infrared
NIDDM	noninsulin-dependent diabetes mellitus		nitroprusside-induced relaxation
NIDR	National Institute of Dental Research (NIH)	NIRCA	nonisotopic RNase cleavage assay
		NIRS	near infrared spectroscopy
NIEHS	National Institute of Environmental Health Sciences (NIH)	NIS	Nationwide Inpatient Sample
			sodium iodide symporter (protein)
NIF	negative inspiratory force	NISH	nonradioactive *in situ* hybridization
	neutrophil inhibitory factor	NISS	New Injury Severity Score
	not in file	NISs	no-impact sports
NIFS	noninvasive flow studies	NIST	National Institute of Standards and Technology
NIG	NSAIA (nonsteroidal anti-inflamatory agent) induced gastropathy		
		NISV	nonionic surfactant vesicle
		NITD	neuroleptic-induced tardive dyskinesia'
NIGDM	non-insulin dependant gestational diabetes mellitus	Nitro	nitroglycerin (this is a dangerous abbreviation)
NIGMS	National Institute of General Medical Sciences (NIH)		sodium nitroprusside (this is a dangerous abbreviation)
NIH	National Institutes of Health		

N

NIV	noninvasive ventilation		(Nordiska Lakemedelsnamnden)
NIVLS	noninvasive vascular laboratory studies	NLNAC	National League for Nursing Accrediting Commission
NIVs	nutrient intake values	NLO	nasolacrimal occlusion
NJ	nasojejunal	NLP	natural language processing
NJT	nasojejunal tube		nodular liquifying panniculitis
NK	natural killer (cells)		no light perception
	not known	NLPHL	nodular lymphocyte-predominant
NK$_1$	neurokinin 1		Hodgkin lymphoma
NKA	no known allergies	NLS	neonatal lupus syndrome
nkat	nanokatal (nanomole/sec)	NLs	neuroimmunophilin ligands
NKB	no known basis	NLT	not later than
	not keeping baby		not less than
	neurokinin B	NLV	nelfinavir (Viracept)
NKC	nonketotic coma	NM	nanometer (nm) (10^{-9} meters)
NKD	no known diseases		Negro male
NKDA	no known drug allergies		neoplastic meningitis
NKFA	no known food allergies		neuromuscular
NKH	nonketotic hyperglycemia		neuronal microdysgenesis
NKHA	nonketotic hyperosmolar acidosis		nodular melanoma
NKHHC	nonketotic hyperglycemic-hyperosmolar coma		nonmalignant
			not measurable
NKHOC	nonketotic hyperosmolar coma		not measured
NKHS	nonketotic hyperosmolar syndrome		not mentioned
NKMA	no known medication (medical) allergies		nuclear medicine
			nurse manager
NKT	natural-killer T (cells)	N & M	nerves and muscles
NL	nasolacrimal		night and morning
	needle localization	NMB	neuromuscular blockade
	nonlatex	NMBA	neuromuscular blocking agent
	normal	NMBS	nuclear medicine bone scan
	normal libido	NMC	no malignant cells
nL	nanoliter (if nL was used in the clinical setting it would be dangerous as it could be seen or heard as mL)	NMD	Doctor of Naturopathic Medicine
			neuromaturational delay
			neuromuscular disorders
			neuronal migration disorders
NLB	needle liver biopsy		Normosol M and 5% Dextrose®
NLC	nocturnal leg cramps	NMDA	N-methyl-D-aspartate
NLC & C	normal libido, coitus, and climax	NMDP	National Marrow Donor Pool
NLD	nasolacrimal duct	NME	new molecular entity
	necrobiosis lipoidica diabeticorum	NMES	neuromuscular electrical stimulation
	no local doctor		
NLDO	nasolacrimal duct obstruction	NMF	neuromuscular facilitation
NLE	neonatal lupus erythematosus	NMH	neurally mediated hypotension
	nursing late entry	NMHH	no medical health history
NLEA	Nutrition Labeling and Education Act of 1990	NMI	no manifest improvement
			no mental illness
NLF	nasolabial fold		no middle initial
	nelfinavir (Viracept)		no more information
NLFGNR	nonlactose fermenting gram-negative rod		normal male infant
		NMIBC	non-muscle-invasive bladder cancer
NLM	National Library of Medicine		
	no limitation of motion	NMJ	neuromuscular junction
NLMC	nocturnal leg muscle cramp	NML	normal
NLN	National League for Nursing	NMKB	not married, keeping baby
	no longer needed	NMM	nodular malignant melanoma
	Nordic Council on Medicines	NMN	no middle name

NMNKB	not married, not keeping baby	NNR	not necessary to return
NMO	neuromyelitis optica (Devic syndrome)	NNRTI	non-nucleoside reverse transcriptase inhibitor
nmol	nanomole (one billionth [10^{-9}] of a mole)	NNS	neonatal screen (hematocrit, total bilirubin, and total protein)
NMOH	no medical ocular history		nicotine nasal spray
NMP	normal menstrual period		non-nutritive sucking
NMPPAS	non-resonant multiphoton photoacoustic spectroscopy		number needed to screen
		NNT	number needed to treat
NMR	nuclear magnetic resonance (same as magnetic resonance imaging)	NNTB	number needed to treat to benefit
		NNTB/ NNTH	number needed to treat, benefit-to-harm ratio
NMRS	nuclear magnetic resonance spectroscopy	NNTH	number needed to treat to harm
		NNU	net nitrogen utilization
NMRT (R)	Nuclear Medicine Radiologic Technologist (Registered)	NNWT	noncontact normothermic wound therapy
NMS	neonatal morphine solution neuroleptic malignant syndrome	NO	nasal oxygen nitric oxide
NMSC	nonmelanoma skin cancer		nitroglycerin ointment
NMSE	normalized mean square root		none obtained
NMSIDS	near-miss sudden infant death syndrome		nonobese number (no.)
NMT	nebulized mist treatment		nursing office
	no more than	NO_2	nitrogen dioxide
NMTB	neuromuscular transmission blockade	N_2O	nitrous oxide
		NOA	nonobstructive azoospermia
NMTCB	Nuclear Medicine Technology Certification Board	NOAA	National Oceanic and Atmospheric Administration
NMT(R)	Nuclear Medicine Technologist Registered	NOAE	nonoccupational asbestos exposures
NMU	nitrosomethylurea	NOAEL	no observed adverse effect level
NN	narrative notes	$N_2O:O_2$	nitrous oxide to oxygen ratio
	Navajo neuropathy	NOC	nonorgan-confined
	neonatal		Nursing Outcome Classification
	neural network	noc.	night
	normal nursery	noct	nocturnal
	nurses' notes	NOD	nonobese diabetic
N/N	negative/negative		notice of disagreement
NNB	normal newborn		notify of death
	number-needed-to-benefit	NOE	naso-orbitoethmoid
NNBC	node-negative breast cancer	NOED	no observed effect dose
NND	neonatal death	NOEL	no observable effect level
	number needed to detain	NOF	National Osteoporosis Foundation (treatment criteria)
NNDSS	National Notifiable Diseases Surveillance System		nonossifying fibroma
NNE	neonatal necrotizing enterocolitis	NOFT	nonorganic failure to thrive
NNH	number needed to harm	NOFTT	nonorganic failure to thrive
NNIS	National Nosocomial Infections Surveillance	NOGM	nonoxidative glucose metabolism
		NOH	neurogenic orthostatic hypotension
NNM	Nicolle-Novy-MacNeal (media)	NOI	nature of illness
NNL	no new laboratory (test orders)	NOK	next of kin
NNN	normal newborn nursery	NOL	not on label
NNO	no new orders	NOM	nonoperative management
NNP	Neonatal Nurse Practitioner		nonsuppurative otitis media
	non-nociceptive pain	NOMI	nonocclusive mesenteric infarction
N:NPK	grams of nitrogen to non-protein kilocalories	NOMID	neonatal-onset multisystem inflammatory disease

N

NOMS	not on my shift	near point
NO/N$_2$	nitric oxide; nitrogen	neuropathic pain
NONMEM	nonlinear mixed-effects model (modeling)	neurophysin
		neuropsychiatric
non pal	not palpable	neutrogenic precautions
NonPARs	Nonparticipating Physicians (Medicare)	newly presented
		nonpalpable
non-REM	nonrapid eye movement (sleep)	no pain
non rep	do not repeat	not performed
non-res	nonresident	not pregnant
NON VIZ	not visualized	not present
NOOB	not out of bed	nuclear pharmacist
NOP	not on patient	nuclear pharmacy
NOR	norethynodrel	nursed poorly
	normal	nurse practitioner
	nortriptyline	NPA	nasal pharyngeal airway
NOR-EPI	norepinephrine (Levophed)	nasopharyngeal aspirate
norm	normal	near point of accommodation
NOS	neonatal opium solution (diluted deodorized tincture of opium)	no previous admission
		npAIR	nonparaneoplastic autoimmune retinopathy
	new-onset seizures	
	nitric oxide synthase	NPAT	nonparoxysmal atrial tachycardia
	no organisms seen	
	not on staff	NPBC	node-positive breast cancer
	not otherwise specified	NPBCC	nonpigmented basal cell carcinoma
NOS3	nitric oxide synthase, type 3	NPC	nasopharyngeal carcinoma
NOSI	nitric oxide synthase inhibitors	near-point convergence
NOSIE	Nurse's Observation Scale (Schedule) for Inpatient Evaluation	Niemann-Pick disease Type C (sphingomyelin lipidosis)
		nodal premature contractions
NOSPECS	categories for classifying eye changes in Graves ophthalmopathy: **n**o signs or symptoms, **o**nly signs, **s**oft tissue involvement with symptoms and signs, **p**roptosis, **e**xtraocular muscle involvement, **c**orneal involvement, and **s**ight loss (visual acuity)	nonpatient contact
		nonproductive cough
		nonprotein calorie
		no prenatal care
		no previous complaint(s)
		NP-C	Nurse Practitioner, Certified
		NPCC	nonprotein carbohydrate calories
		NPCPAP	nasopharyngeal continuous positive airway pressure
NOT	nocturnal oxygen therapy	NPD	narcissistic personality disorder
NOTES	natural orifice transluminal endoscopic surgery	Niemann-Pick disease
		nonpolarized (contact) dermoscopy
NOTT	nocturnal oxygen therapy trial	nonprescription drugs
NOU	not on unit	no pathological diagnosis
NOV	Novartis	NPDB	Niemann-Pick disease type B
NoV	Norovirus	NPDEP	National Kidney Disease Education Program (guidelines on drug dosing)
NOV 70/30	human insulin, regular 30 units/mL with human insulin isophane suspension 70 units/mL (Novolin 70/30)	
		NPDL	nodular poorly differentiated lymphocytic
NOV L	human insulin zinc suspension (Novolin L)	NPDR	nonproliferative diabetic retinopathy
NOV N	human insulin isophane suspension (Novolin N)	NPDS	Neck Pain and Disability Scale
		NPE	neurogenic pulmonary edema
NOV R	human insulin regular (Novolin R)	neuropsychologic examination
NP	nasal polyps	no palpable enlargement
	nasal prongs	normal pelvic examination
	nasopharyngeal	NPEM	nocturnal penile erection

N

	monitoring
NPEV	new patient evaluation program
NPF	nasopharyngeal fiberscope
	no predisposing factor
N-PFMSO$_4$	nebulized preservative-free morphine sulfate (This is a dangerous abbreviation)
NPFS	nonpenetrating filtering surgery
NPG	nonpregnant
	normal-pressure glaucoma
NPH	isophane insulin (neutral protamine Hagedorn)
	no previous history
	normal-pressure hydrocephalus
NPhx	nasopharynx
NPI	National Provider Identifier
	Neuropsychiatric Inventory
	no present illness
	Nottingham Prognostic Index
NPIS	Numeric Pain Intensity Scale
NPIT	nonpalpable intraabdominal testis
NPJT	nonparoxysmal junctional tachycardia
NPL	insulin lispro protamine suspension
component	neural protamine lispro (insulin)
NPLSM	neoplasm
NPK	nonprotein kilocalories
NPM	nothing per mouth
NPN	nonprotein nitrogen
NPNC	no prenatal care
NPNT	nonpalpable, nontender
NPO	new patient orientation (this is a dangerous abbreviation as it will be read as nothing by mouth)
n.p.o.	nothing by mouth
NPOC	nonpurgeable organic carbon
NPOD	Neuropsychiatric Officer of the Day
NPP	nonphysician practitioner
	normal postpartum
	Nurse Practitioner, Psychiatric
NPPE	negative-pressure pulmonary edema
NPPI	nonpeptidic protease inhibitor
NPPNG	nonpenicillinase-producing *Neisseria gonorrhoeae*
NPPV	noninvasive positive-pressure ventilation
NPQ	Northwick Park (Neck Pain) Questionnaire
NPR	normal pulse rate
	nothing per rectum
NPRL	normal pupillary reaction to light
NPRM	Notice of Proposed Rulemaking
NPRS	numerical pain rating scale
NPS	nasopharyngoscopy
	National Pharmaceutical Stockpile
	neuropsychiatric symptoms

	new patient set-up
NPSA	nonphysician surgical assistant
NPSD	nonpotassium-sparing diuretics
NPSF	National Patient Safety Foundation
NPSG	National Patient Safety Goal
	nocturnal polysomnography
NPSLE	neuropsychiatric systemic lupus erythematosus
NPT	near-patient tests
	neopyrithiamin hydrochloride
	nocturnal penile tumescence
	no prior tracings
	normal pressure and temperature
NPU	net protein utilization
NPV	negative predictive value
	nothing per vagina
NPWT	negative pressure wound therapy
NPY	neuropeptide Y
NPZ	neuropsychologic text z
NQECN	nonqueratinizing epidermoid carcinoma
NQF	National Quality Forum
NQMI	non-Q wave myocardial infarction
NQR	not quite right (slang)
NQT	narrow QRS complex tachycardia
NQW	non-Q-wave
NQWMI	non-Q wave myocardial infarction
NR	do not repeat
	newly reformulated
	none reported
	nonreactive
	nonrebreathing
	nonresponder
	no refills
	no report
	no response
	no return
	normal range
	normal reaction
	not reached
	not reacting
	not remarkable
	not resolved
	number
NRAF	nonrheumatic atrial fibrillation
NRAS	neuroblastoma RAS viral (v-ras) oncogene homolog
NRB	Noninstitutional Review Board
	nonrebreather (oxygen mask)
NRBC	normal red blood cell
	nucleated red blood cell
NRBS	nonrebreathing system
NRC	National Research Council
	normal retinal correspondence
	Nuclear Regulatory Commission
NRCT	National Registry of Childhood Tumours (UK)
NREH	normal renin essential hypertension

N

NREM	nonrapid eye movement	NSA	National Security Agency
NREMS	nonrapid eye movement sleep		neck-shaft angle
NREMT-P	National Registry of Emergency Medical Technicians–Paramedic level		nonstandard appearance (slang)
			normal serum albumin (albumin, human)
NRF	normal renal function		no salt added
NRFHT	nonreasurring fetal heart rate		no significant abnormalities
NRI	nerve root involvement		number of signals averaged (radiology)
	nerve root irritation		
	no recent illnesses	NSAA	nonsteroidal antiandrogen
	norepinephrine reuptake inhibitor	NSABP	National Surgical Adjuvant Breast Project
NRL	natural rubber latex		
N-RLX	nonrelaxed	NSAD	no signs of acute disease
NRM	nonrebreathing mask	NSAIA	nonsteroidal anti-inflammatory agent
	no regular medicines		
	normal range of motion	NSAID	nonsteroidal anti-inflammatory drug
	normal retinal movement		
NRN	no return necessary	NSAP	nonspecific abdominal pain
NRNST	nonreassuring-nonstress test	NSBGP	nonspecific bowel gas pattern
NRO	neurology	NSC	neural stem cells
NROM	normal range of motion		no significant change
NRP	neonatal resuscitation program		nonservice-connected
	nonreassuring patterns		nuclear sclerotic cataract
NRPR	nonbreathing pressure relieving	NSCC	nonsmall cell carcinoma
NRR	net reproduction rate	NSCD	nonservice-connected disability
NRS	Neurobehavioral Rating Scale	NSCFPT	no significant change from previous tracing
	noninvasive respiratory support		
	Numerical Rating Scale	NSCIDRC	National Spinal Cord Injury Data Research Center
NRSs	nonrandomized studies		
NRSTS	non-rhabdomyosarcoma soft tissue sarcoma	NSCLC	nonsmall-cell–lung cancer
		NSCST	nipple stimulation contraction stress test
NRT	neural response telemetry (audiology testing)		
		NSD	nasal septal deviation
	neuromuscular reeducation techniques		nominal standard dose
			nonstructural deterioration
	nicotine-replacement therapy		normal spontaneous delivery
NRTI	nucleoside reverse transcriptase inhibitor		no significant disease (difference, defect, deviation)
NRTs	nitron radical traps	NSDA	nonsteroid dependent asthmatic
NS	nephrotic syndrome	NSDU	neonatal stepdown unit
	neurological signs	NSE	neuron-specific enolase
	neurosurgery		normal saline enema (0.9% sodium chloride)
	never-smokers		
	nipple stimulation	N s E	nausea without emesis
	nodular sclerosis	NSEACS	non-ST-elevation acute coronary syndromes
	no-show		
	nonsmoker	NSF	nephrogenic systemic fibrosis
	normal saline solution (0.9% sodium chloride solution)		no significant findings
		NSFTD	normal spontaneous full-term delivery
	normospermic		
	no sample	NSG	nursing
	not seen	NSGCT	nonseminomatous germ-cell tumors
	not significant	NSGCTT	nonseminomatous germ-cell tumor of the testis
	nuclear sclerosis		
	nursing service	NSGI	nonspecific genital infection
	NuStep	NSGT	nonseminomatous germ-cell tumor
	nutritive sucking	NSHC	no-self-harm contract
	nylon suture	NSHD	nodular sclerosing Hodgkin disease

N

NSHL	nonsyndromic hearing loss		nonstress test
NSI	needlestick injury		normal sphincter tone
	negative self-image		not sooner than
	no signs of infection		nutritional support team
	no signs of inflammation	NSTD	nonsexually transmitted disease
NSICU	neurosurgery intensive care unit	NSTE	non-ST segment elevation
NSILA	nonsuppressible insulin-like	nSTE-ACS	non-ST-elevation acute coronary
	activity		syndrome
NSIP	nonspecific interstitial pneumonia	NSTEMI	non-ST-segment elevation
NSLP	National School Lunch Program		myocardial infarction
NSLRP	nerve-sparing laparoscopic radical	NSTGCT	nonseminomatous testicular germ
	prostatectomy		cell tumor
NSM	neurogenic stunned myocardium	NSTI	necrotizing soft-tissue infection
NSMMVT	nonsustained monomorphic	NSTT	nonseminomatous testicular tumors
	ventricular tachycardia	NSU	neurosurgical unit
NSN	Neo-Synephrine		nonspecific urethritis
	nephrotoxic serum nephritis	NSV	nonspecific vaginitis
NSNSAIDs	nonselective nonsteroidal anti-	NSVD	nonstructural valve deterioration
	inflammatory drugs		normal spontaneous vaginal
NSO	Neosporin® ointment		delivery
NSOH	normal state of health	NSVT	nonsustained ventricular
NSOM	near field scanning optical		tachycardia
	microscope	NSX	neurosurgical examination
NSOP	no soft organs palpable	NSY	nursery
NSP	neck and shoulder pain	NT	nasotracheal
NSPs	needle and syringe exchange		next time
	programs		Nordic Track®
	nonstarch polysaccharides		normal temperature
NSPVT	nonsustained polymorphic		normotensive
	ventricular tachycardia		nortriptyline
NSR	nasoseptal repair		not tender
	nonspecific reaction		not tested
	normal sinus rhythm		nourishment taken
	not seen regularly		nuchal translucency
NSRP	nerve-sparing radical prostatectomy		numbness and tingling
NSS	nephron-sparing surgery		nursing technician
	neurological signs stable	N&T	nose and throat
	neuropathy symptom score		numbness and tingling
	normal size and shape	N Tachy	nodal tachycardia
	not statistically significant	NT-ANP	N-terminal atrial natriuretic peptide
	nutritional support service	NTBR	not to be resuscitated
	sodium chloride 0.9% (normal	NTC	neurotrauma center
	saline solution)	NTCS	no tumor cells seen
1/2 NSS	sodium chloride 0.45% (1/2 normal	NTD	negative to date
	saline solution)		neural-tube defects
NSSC	normal size, shape and consistency		nitroblue tetrazolium dye (test)
	(uterus)	NTE	neutral thermal environment
NSSI	nonsuicidal self-injury		not to exceed
NSSL	normal size, shape, and location	NTED	neonatal toxic-shock-syndrome-like
NSSNTFM	normal size shape nontender freely		exanthematous disease
	moveable (uterus)	NTF	neurotrophic factor
NSSP	normal size, shape, and position		normal throat flora
NSSTT	nonspecific ST and T-wave	NTG	nitroglycerin
NSST- TWCs	nonspecific ST-T wave changes		nontoxic goiter nontreatment group
NST	nonmyeloablative stem-cell		normal tension glaucoma
	transplant	NTGO	nitroglycerin ointment
	Nonsense Syllable Test	NTI	narrow therapeutic index

N

	no treatment indicated		new vessel
NTIS	National Technical Information Service (U.S. Department of Commerce)		next visit
			nonvenereal
			nonveteran
NTL	nectar-thick liquid (diet consistency)		normal value
			not vaccinated
	nortriptyline (Aventyl; Pamelor)		not verified
	no time limit	N&V	nausea and vomiting
NTLE	neocortical temporal-lobe epilepsy	NVA	near visual acuity
NTM	nocturnal tumescence monitor	NVAB	nonvalvular atrial fibrillation
	nontuberculous mycobacterium	NVAF	nonvalvular atrial fibrillation
NTMB	nontuberculous myobacteria	NVAS	numeric visual analog scale
NTMI	nontransmural myocardial infarction	NVB	Navelbine (vinorelbine tartrate)
			neurovascular bundle
NTND	not tender, not distended	NVBo	oral vinorelbine
NTP	narcotic treatment program	NVC	nailfold video capillaroscopy
	National Toxicology Program		neurovascular checks
	Nitropaste® (nitroglycerin ointment)	nvCJD	new-variant Creutzfeldt-Jakob disease
	nonthrombocytopenic preterm (infant)	NVD	nausea, vomiting, and diarrhea
			neck vein distention
	non-ThinPrep (slides)		neovascularization of the (optic) disc
	normal temperature and pressure		
	sodium nitroprusside		neurovesicle dysfunction
NTPD	nocturnal tidal peritoneal dialysis		normal vaginal delivery
NTPR	National Transplantation Pregnancy Registry		no venereal disease
			no venous distention
NT-proBNP	N-terminal pro-brain natriuretic peptide		nonvalvular disease
		NVDC	nausea, vomiting, diarrhea, and constipation
NTS	nasotracheal suction		
	nicotine transdermal system	NVDRS	National Violent Death Reporting System
	nontyphoidal salmonellae		
	nucleus tractus solitarii	NVE	native
NTSCI	nontraumatic spinal cord injury		native valve endocarditis
NTT	nasotracheal tube		neovascularization elsewhere
	near-total thyroidectomy	NVG	neovascular glaucoma
	nonthrombocytopenic term (infant)		neoviridogrisein
	nontreponemal test	NVI	neovascularization of the iris
NTTP	no tenderness to palpation	NVL	neurovascular laboratory
NTU	nephelometric turbidity units	NVLD	nonverbal learning disability
NTX	naltrexone (ReVia)	NVM	neovascular membrane
	neurotoxicity		noncompaction of the ventricular myocardium
Ntx	N-telopeptide		
NTZ	nitazoxanide (Alinia)	NVO	near vision only (glasses prescription)
NTZ Long-acting®	oxymetazoline nasal spray		
		NVOP	neurovascular orofacial pain (facial migraine)
NU	name unknown		
NUD	nonulcer dyspepsia	NVP	nausea and vomiting of pregnancy
NUG	necrotizing ulcerative gingivitis		nevirapine (Viramune)
nullip	nullipara	NVR	nonviolent restraint
NUN	nonurea nitrogen	NVS	neurological vital signs
nutr	nutrition		neurovascular status
NV	naked vision	NVSS	normal variant short stature
	nausea and vomiting	NW	naked weight
	near vision		nasal wash
	negative variation		normal weight
	neovascularization		not weighed
	neurovascular	NWB	nonweight bearing

NWBL	nonweight bearing, left
NWBR	nonweight bearing, right
NWC	number of words chosen
NWD	neuroleptic withdrawal
	normal well developed
NWS	New World screwworm
	(*Cochliomyia hominivorax*
	[Coquerel])
NWTS	National Wilms Tumor Study
	(rating scale)
NWTSG	National Wilms Tumor Study
	Group
Nx	nephrectomy
	next
NX211	liposomal lurtotecan
NXG	necrobiotic xanthogranuloma
NXY-059	disufenton sodium (Cerovive)
NYB	New York Blood Center
NYD	not yet diagnosed
NYHA	New York Heart Association
	(classification of heart disease)
NYST	nystagmus
NZ	enzyme

O	eye
	objective findings
	obvious
	occlusal
	often
	open
	oral
	ortho
	O sign; a patient whose mouth is
	open when unconscious (slang)
	other
	oxygen
	pint
	zero
°	degrees (as in 40°C; 40 degrees
	centigrade)
	hours (as in every 4°) ths is a
	dangerous abbreviation as it is
	read as a zero)
∅	zero (the handwritten ∅ has been
	mistaken for a 4, 6, and 9) (the ∅
	can be found with the symbols)
ō	negative
	no
	none
	pint
	without
O+	blood type O positive
	(O positive is preferred)
O−	blood type O negative
	(O negative is preferred)
Ⓞ	orally (by mouth)
$_1O_2$	singlet oxygen
O_2	both eyes
	oxygen
O_2^-	superoxide
O_3	ozone
O157	*Escherichia coli* O157
OA	occipital artery
	occipitoatlantal
	occiput anterior
	old age
	on admission
	on arrival
	ophthalmic artery
	oral airway
	oral alimentation
	osteoarthritis
	ovarian ablation
	Overeaters Anonymous
O/A	on or about
O & A	observation and assessment
	odontectomy and alveoloplasty

OAA	Old Age Assistance	OBD	obscure digestive bleeding
OAA/S	Observer's Assessment of Alertness/Sedation		optimal biologic dose
		OB-Del	obstetrics-delivered
OAB	overactive bladder	OBE	out-of-body experience
OAC	omeprazole, amoxicillin, and clarithromycin	OBE-CALP	placebo capsule or tablet
	oral anticoagulant(s)	OBF	ocular blood flow
	overaction	OBG	obstetrics and gynecology
OAD	obliterative airway disease	Ob-Gyn	obstetrics and gynecology
	obstructive airway disease	Obj	objective
	occlusive arterial disease	obl	oblique
	overall diameter	OB marg	obtuse marginal
OAE	otoacoustic emissions	OB-ND	obstetrics-not delivered
OAF	oral anal fistula	OBOR	obstetric operating room
	osteoclast activating factor	OBP	office blood pressure
OAG	open angle glaucoma	OBR	optimized background regimen
OAM	omeprazole, amoxicillin, and metronidazole	OBRR	obstetric recovery room
		OBS	observation
OAMER	over-active milk ejection reflex		observed
OA/OS	ovarian ablation/suppression		obstetrical service
OAP	old age pension		organic brain syndrome
	over-anxious patient	OBT	obtained
OAR	off-access ratio	OBTM	omeprazole, bismuth subcitrate, tetracycline, and metronidazole
	Ottawa Ankle Rules		
OARs	organs at risk (from radiation therapy)	OBUS	obstetrical ultrasound
		OBW	open bed warmer
OAS	Older Adult Services	OC	observed cases
	oral allergy syndrome		obstetrical conjugate
	organic anxiety syndrome		occlusal curvature (dental)
	outpatient assessment service		office call
	overall survival		on call
	Overt Aggression Scale		only child
OASDHI	Old Age, Survivors, Disability, and Health Insurance		open cholecystectomy
			open colectomy
OASI	Old Age and Survivors Insurance		open crib
OASIS	Outcomes and Assessment Information Set		optical chromatography
			oral care
OASO	overactive superior oblique		oral contraceptive
OASR	overactive superior rectus		osteocalcin
OASS	Overt Agitation Severity Scale		osteoclast
OAT	oligoasthenoteratozoospermia		ovarian cancer
	oral anticoagulant therapy		OxyContin (oxycodone)
	ornithine aminotransferase	O/C	off cord
OATP	organic anion-transporting polypeptide	O & C	onset and course
		OCA	oculocutaneous albinism
OATS	osteochondral autograft transfer system		open care area
			oral contraceptive agent
OAV	oculoauriculovertebral (dysplasia)	OCAD	occlusive carotid artery disease
OAW	oral airway	OCB	obstructive chronic bronchitis
OB	obese	OCBZ	oxcarbazepine(Trileptal)
	obesity	OCC	occasionally
	obstetrics		occipital
	occult blood		occlusal
	osteoblast		old chart called
OBA	office-based anesthesia	OCCC	open chest cardiac compression
	Office of Biotechnology Activities (NIH)		ovarian clear cell carcinoma
		occl	occlusion
OB-A	obstetrics-aborted	OCCM	open chest cardiac massage

OCC PR	open chest cardiopulmonary resuscitation	Δ OD 450	deviation of optical density at 450
OCC Th	occupational therapy	ODA	occipitodextra anterior
Occup Rx	occupational therapy		once-daily aminoglycoside
OCD	obsessive-compulsive disorder		osmotic driving agent
	osteochondritis dissecans	ODAC	Oncologic Drugs Advisory
OCE	outpatient code editor		Committee (of the US Food and
OCG	oral cholecystogram		Drug Administration)
OcHTN	ocular hypertension		on-demand analgesia computer
OCI	Obsessive-Compulsive Inventory	ODAT	one day at a time
	optic canal involvement	ODC	oral disease control
OCJ	osteochondral junction		ornithine decarboxylase
OCL®	oral colonic lavage		outpatient diagnostic center
OCME	Office of the Chief Medical	ODCH	ordinary diseases of childhood
	Examiner	ODCs	ozone-depleting chemicals
OCN	obsessive-compulsive neurosis	ODD	oculodentodigital (dysplasia)
	Oncology Certified Nurse		oppositional defiance disorder
OCNS	Obsessive-Compulsive Neurosis	OD'd	overdosed
	Scale	ODE	optic disc edema
O-CNV	occult choroidal neovascularization	ODECL	open-door expansile cervical
OCOR	on-call to operating room		laminoplasty
OCP	ocular cicatricial pemphigoid	ODed	overdosed
	oral contraceptive pills	ODI	Oswestry Disability Index
	ova, cysts, parasites		oxygen desaturation index
OCR	oculocephalic reflex	ODM	occlusion dose monitor
	optical character recognition		Operational Data Model
OCRL	oculocerebrorenal syndrome of		ophthalmodynamometry
	Lowe	ODMP	on-going data management plan
OCS	Obsessive-Compulsive Scale	ODN	optokinetic nystagmus
	Office of Child Services	ODP	occipitodextra posterior
	(government agency)		offspring of diabetic parents
	oral cancer screening	OD/P	right eye patched
11-OCS	11-oxycorticosteroid	ODQ	on direct questioning
OCT	octreotide (Sandostatin)	ODS	Office of Drug Safety (FDA)
	optical coherence tomograph		organized delivery system
	(tomography)		osmotic demyelination syndrome
	oral cavity tumors	ODSS	Office of Disability Support
	ornithine carbamyl transferase		Services
	oxytocin challenge test	ODSU	oncology day stay unit
OCU	observation care unit		One-Day Surgery Unit
OCVM	occult cerebrovascular	ODT	occipitodextra transerve
	malformations		optical Doppler tomography
OCX	oral cancer examination		orally disintegrating tablet
OD	Doctor of Optometry	ODTS	organic dust toxic syndrome
	Officer-of-the-Day	OE	on examination
	oligodendroglial		orthopedic examination
	once daily (this is a dangerous		otitis externa
	abbreviation as it is read as right	O-E	standard observed minus
	eye; use "once daily")		expected
	on duty	O&E	observation and examination
	optical density (radiology)	OEC	outer ear canal
	optic disc	OECD	Organization for Economic
	oral-duodenal		Cooperation and Development
	outdoor	OECs	olfactory ensheathing cells
	outside diameter	OEI	opioid escalation index
	ovarian dysgerminoma	O₂EI	oxygen extraction index
	overdose	OEL	occupational exposure level
	right eye	OENT	oral endotracheal tube
		OEP	Office of Emergency Preparedness

O

	oil of evening primrose (evening primrose oil)		ocular hypertension
OEPA	vincristine (Oncovin), etoposide, prednisone, and doxorubicin (Adriamycin)		on hand
			open-heart
			oral hygiene
			orthostatic hypotension
OER	oxygen extraction ratios		outside hospital
O₂ER	oxygen extraction ratio	−OH	hydroxyl
OERR	order entry/results-reports (Veterans Administration's physician computer order entry system)	17-OH	17-hydroxycorticosteroids
		OHA	oral hypoglycemic agents
		OHC	outer hair cell (in cochlea)
		OHCA	out-of-hospital cardiac arrest
OET	oral esophageal tube	OH Cbl	hydroxycobalamine
OETT	oral endotracheal tube	17-OHCS	17-hydroxycorticosteroids
OF	occipital-frontal	OHD	hydroxy vitamin D
	optic fundi		organic heart disease
	oral facial	25(OH)D	25-hydroxyvitamin D
	osteitis fibrosa	25(OH)D₃	25-hydroxyvitamin D (calcifediol, Calderol)
	outlet forceps (delivery)		
	ovarian function	OHF	old healed fracture
OFC	occipital-frontal circumference		Omsk hemorrhagic fever
	orbitofacial cleft		overhead frame
	osteitis fibrosa cystica	OHFA	hydroxy fatty acid
OFF	shoes off during weighing	OHFT	overhead frame and trapeze
OFFD	organ-failure-free days	OHG	oral hypoglycemic
OFG	orofacial granulomatosis	OHI	oral hygiene instructions
OFI	other febrile illness		other health impairment
OFLOX	ofloxacin (Floxin)	OHIAA	hydroxyindolacetic acid
OFLX	ofloxacin (Floxin)	OHL	oral hairy leukoplakia
OFM	open-face mask	7-OHMTX	7-hydroxymethotrexate
	oral focal mucinosis	OHNS	Otolaryngology, Head, and Neck Surgery (Dept.)
OFNE	oxygenated fluorocarbon nutrient emulsion		
		OHP	obese hypertensive patient
OFPF	optic fundi and peripheral fields		oxygen under hyperbaric pressure
OFR	oxygen-free radicals	17 OHP	17-hydroxyprogesterone
OFRs	ocular following responses	OHQOL	oral health-related quality of life
OFS	osteoplastic frontal sinusotomy	OHRP	Office for Human Research Protections (Department of Health Human Services)
OFTT	organic failure to thrive		
OG	Obstetrics-Gynecology		
	orogastric (feeding)		open-heart rehabilitation program
	outcome goal (long-term goal)	OHR-QOL	oral health-related quality of life
OGC	oculogyric crisis	OHRR	open-heart recovery room
OGCT	ovarian germ cell tumor	OHS	obesity hypoventilation syndrome
OGD	oesophagogastro-duodenoscopy (United Kingdom and other countries)		occupational health service
			ocular histoplasmosis syndrome
			ocular hypoperfusion syndrome
	Office of Generic Drugs (of the Food and Drug Administration)		open-heart surgery
			Oxford hip score
OGIB	obscure gastrointestinal bleeding	OHSS	ovarian hyperstimulation syndrome
OGNP	Obstetric-Gynecology Nurse Practitioner	OHT	ocular hypertension
			overhead trapeze
OGPA	oxygen generating portable equipment	OHTN	ocular hypertension
		OHTx	orthotopic heart transplantation
OGT	orogastric tube	OI	opportunistic infection
	Oxford Gene Technology (Oxford UK)		osteogenesis imperfecta
			otitis interna
OGTT	oral glucose tolerance test		ovulation induction
OH	occupational history		oxygen index
	ocular history	OIC	opioid-induced constipation

O

OICD	occupational irritant contact dermatitis	OLTP	online transaction processing
OIF	oil-immersion field	OLTx	orthotopic liver transplantation
OIG	Office of the Inspector General	OLV	one-lung ventilation
OIH	orthoiodohippurate	OLZ	olanzapine (Zyprexa)
OIHA	orthoiodohippuric acid	OM	every morning (this is a dangerous abbreviation)
OI&I	occupational injury and illness		obtuse marginal
OIM	optical immunoassay		ocular melanoma
OINT	ointment		oral motor
OIR	oxygen-induced retinopathy		oral mucositis
OIRDA	occipital intermittent rhythmical delta activity		organomegaly
			osteomalacia
OIS	ocular ischemic syndrome		osteomyelitis
	optical intrinsic signal (imaging)		otitis media
	optimum information size	O_2M	oxygen mask
OIs	opportunistic infections	OM_1	first obtuse marginal (branch)
OIT	ovarian immature teratoma	OM_2	second obtuse marginal (branch)
OIU	optical internal urethrotomy	OMA	older maternal age
OJ	orange juice (this is a dangerous abbreviation as it is read as OS, left eye)	OMAC	otitis media, acute, catarrhal
		OMAS	Olerud-Molander Ankle Score
			otitis media, acute, suppurating
	orthoplast jacket	OMB	obtuse marginal branch
OK	all right		Office of Management and Budget
	approved	OMB_1	first obtuse marginal branch (of the circumflex coronary artery)
	correct		
OKAN	optokinetic after nystagmus	OMB_2	second obtuse marginal branch (of the circumflex coronary artery)
OKC	odontogenic keratocyst		
	open kinetic chain	OMC	open mitral commissuortomy
OKN	optokinetic nystagmus		ostiomeatal complex
OKS	Oxford Knee Score	OMCA	otitis media, catarrhalis, acute
OKT	Ortho Kung T-cell, designation for a series of antigens	OMCC	otitis media, catarrhalis, chronic
		OMD	organic mental disorder
OL	left eye	OME	Office of Medical Examiner
	open label (study)		otitis media with effusion
OLA	occiput left anterior	7-OMEN	menogaril
	occipitolaevoanterior	OMFS	oral and maxillofacial surgery
OLAP	online analytical processing	OMG	ocular myasthenia gravis
OLB	open-liver biopsy	OMI	old myocardial infarct
	open-lung biopsy	OMIEI	oral medication induced esophageal injury
OLBPQ	Oswestry Low Back Pain Questionnaire		
		OMIF	oral maxillofacial
OLC	ouabain-like compound	OMP	oculomotor (third nerve) palsy
OLD	obstructive lung disease		open mediastinal biopsy
OLE	olive leaf extract	OMPA	otitis media, purulent, acute
OLED	optimal long exposure dose	OMPC	otitis media, purulent, chronic
OLF	ouabain-like factor	OMR	operative mortality rate
OLM	ocular larva migrans	OMS	oral morphine sulfate
	ophthalmic laser microendoscope		organic mental syndrome
OLNM	occult lymph node metastases		organic mood syndrome
OLP	oral lichen planus	OMSA	otitis media secretory (or suppurative) acute
OLR	optic labyrinthine righting		
	otology, laryngology, and rhinology	OMSC	otitis media secretory (or suppurative) chronic
OLRM	ordinary linear regression model	OMSS	order management scanning system
OLS	ordinary least squares	OMT	oral mucosal transudate
	ouabain-like substance		Osteopathic manipulative technique (treatment)
OLT	occipitolaevoposterior		
	orthotopic liver transplantation	OMVC	open mitral valve commissurotomy

O

OMVD	optimized microvessel density (analysis)	OOI	out of isolette
		OOL	onset of labor
OMVI	operating motor vehicle intoxicated	OOLR	ophthalmology, otology, laryngology, and rhinology
ON	every night (this is a dangerous abbreviation)	OOM	onset of menarche
	optic nerve	OOP	out of pelvis
	optic neurophathy		out of plaster
	oronasal		out on pass
	Ortho-Novum®	OOPD	Office of Orphan Product Development (FDA)
	osteonecrosis		
	overnight	OOPS	out of program status
ONB	olfactory neuroblastoma	OOR	out-of-range (values)
ONC	Orthopedic Nurse, Certified		out of room
	over-the-needle catheter	OORW	out of radiant warmer
	vincristine (Oncovin)	OOS	out of sequence
OND	Office of New Drugs (FDA)		out of specification (deviation from standard)
	ondansetron (Zofran)		
	other neurologic disorder(s)		out of splint
ONF	oronasal fistula		out of stock
ONH	optic nerve head	OOT	out of town
	optic nerve hypoplasia	OOW	out of wedlock
ONJ	osteonecrosis of the jaw		out of work
ONM	ocular neuromyotonia	OP	oblique presentation
ON-Q®	an automatic-continuous delivery local anesthetic pump and catheter		occiput posterior
			open
			operation
ONQI	Overall Nutritional Quality Index		organophosphorous
ON RR	overnight recovery room		oropharynx
ONS	Office for National Statistics (United Kingdom)		oscillatory potentials
			osteoporosis
ONSD	optic nerve sheath decompression		outpatient
ONSF	optic nerve sheath fenestration		overpressure
ONTD	open neural tube defect(s)	O&P	ova and parasites (stool examination)
ONTR	orders not to resuscitate		
OO	ophthalmic ointment	OPA	Office of the Public Advocate (guardians)
	oral order		
	out of		oral pharyngeal airway
o/o	on account of		outpatient anesthesia
O_2O_3	oxygen-ozone (mixture)	OPAC	opacity (opacification)
O&O	off and on	OPAT	outpatient parenteral antibiotic therapy
OOB	out of bed		
OOBL	out of bilirubin light	OPB	outpatient basis
OOBBRP	out of bed with bathroom privileges	OPC	operable pancreatic carcinoma
			oropharyngeal candidiasis
OOBTC	out of bed to chair		oropharynx cancer
OOBTT	out of bed to toilet		outpatient care
OOC	onset of contractions		outpatient catheterization
	out of cast		outpatient clinic
	out of control	OPCA	olivopontocerebellar atrophy
OO Con	out of control	OPCAB	off-pump coronary artery bypass (grafting)
OOD	outer orbital diameter		
	out of doors	op cit	in the work cited
OO-EMG	electromyographic recording of the orbicularis oculi muscles	OPCR	outpatient cardiac rehabilitation
		OPCs	oligodendrocyte precursor cells
OOF	out of facility		oligodendrocyte progenitor cells
OOH	out of hospital	OPCS-4	Classification of Surgical Operations and Procedures (4th revision)
OOH&NS	ophthalmology, otorhinolaryngology, and head and neck surgery		

OPCx — oligodendrocyte progenitor cells

OPD — oropharyngeal dysphagia
Orphan Products Development (office of)
outpatient department

O'p'-DDD — mitotane (Lysodren)

OPDRA — Office of Postmarketing Drug Risk Assessment (FDA) (name changed to Office of Drug Safety [ODS])

OPDUR — on-line prospective drug utilization review

OPE — oral peripheral examination
outpatient evaluation

OPEN — vincristine (Oncovin), prednisone, etoposide, and mitoxantrone (Novantrone)

OPERA — outpatient endometrial resection/ablation

OPG — ocular plethysmography
optic pathway glioma
orthopantomogram (dental)
osteoprotegerin

OPHTH — ophthalmic
Ophthalmology

OPIDP — organophosphate-induced delayed polyneuropathy

OPK — ovulation predictor kit

OPKA — opsonophagocytic killing assay

OPL — oral premalignant lesion
other party liability

OPLC — optimum performance liquid chromatography

OPLL — ossification of the posterior longitudinal ligament

OPM — occult primary malignancy
oral and pharyngeal mucositis

OPMD — oculopharyngeal muscular dystrophy

OPN — open partial nephrectomy
osteopontin

OPO — organ procurement organizations
overnight pulse oximetry

OPOC — oral pharynx, oral cavity

OPP — opposite

OPPG — oculopneumoplethysmography

OPPOS — opposition

OPPR — outpatient pulmonary rehabilitation

OPPS — Outpatient Prospective Payment System

OPQRST — onset, provocation, quality, radiation, severity, and time (an EMT mnemonic used in initial patient questioning)

OPRDU — outpatient renal dialysis unit

OPRT — orotate phosphoribosyl transferase

OPS — Objective Pain Scores
operations

orange palpebral spots
Orpington prognostic scale
orthogonal polarization spectral (imaging)
outpatient surgery
overnight polysomnography

OPSCC — oropharyngeal squamous cell carcinoma

OPSI — overwhelming postsplenectomy infection

OPSU — oblique partial sit-up
outpatient surgical unit

O PSY — open psychiatry

OPT — optimal pharmacological therapy
optimum
outpatient treatment

OPT c CA — Ohio pediatric tent with compressed air

OPT c O_2 — Ohio pediatric tent with oxygen

OPTN — Organ Procurement and Transplantation Network

OPT-NSC — outpatient treatment, nonservice-connected

OPT-SC — outpatient treatment, service-connected

OPTX — occult pneumothorax

OPV — oral polio vaccine
outpatient visit

OR — odds ratio
oil retention
oocyte retrievals
open reduction
operating room
Orthodox
own recognizance

ORA — occiput right anterior

ORB — order read back (orders taken verbally or by telephone from a physician)

ORC — outpatient rehabilitation centers

ORCH — orchiectomy

ORD — ordering
orderly

OREF — open reduction, external fixation

ORF — open reading frame

OR&F — open reduction and fixation

ORIF — open reduction internal fixation

ORL — oblique retinacular ligament
otorhinolaryngology (otology, rhinology and laryngology)

ORMF — open reduction metallic fixation

ORN — operating room nurse
osteoradionecrosis

ORO — olfactory recess opacity

OROS — ostomotic release oral system

ORP — occiput right posterior
open radical prostatectomy

ORR — objective response rate

O

	overall response rate	OSFT	outstretched fingertips
ORS	oculorespiratory syndrome	OSG	osteosonogram
	olfactory reference syndrome		(osteosonogrammetry)
	oral rehydration salts	OSH	open saphenous (vein) harvest
ORSA	oxacillin-resistant *Staphylococcus*		outside hospital
	aureus	OSHA	Occupational Safety & Health
ORT	oestrogen (estrogen)-replacement		Administration
	therapy (United Kingdom and	O sign	abdominal radiograph showing an
	elsewhere)		O-shaped configuration of the
	operating room technician		gastric band
	oral rehydration therapy		a patient whose mouth is open
	Registered Occupational Therapist		when unconscious (slang)
ORTHO	Orthopedics	OSM S	osmolarity serum
OR XI	oriented to time	OSM U	osmolarity urine
OR X2	oriented to time and place	OSN	off-service note
OR X3	oriented to time, place, and person	OSP	outside pass
OR X4	oriented to time, place, person, and	OS/P	left eye patched
	objects (watch, pen, book)	OSR	open septorhinoplasty
OS	left eye		open sigmoid resection
	mouth (this is a dangerous abbre-	OSS	osseous
	viation as it is read as left eye)		outside records
	occipitosacral		open-source software
	oligospermic		over-shoulder strap
	opening snap	OSSI	orthognathic surgery simulating
	open surgery		instrument
	ophthalmic solution (this is a	OSSN	ocular surface squamous neoplasia
	dangerous abbreviation as it is	OST	occipitosubtemporal
	read as left eye)		optimal sampling theory
	oral surgery		osteogenic sarcoma
	Osgood-Schlatter (disease)	OT	occiput transverse
	osmium		Occupational Therapist
	osteosarcoma		occupational therapy
	overall survival		old tuberculin
OSA	obstructive sleep apnea		on-treatment
	off-site anesthesia		oral transmucosal
	online sexual activities		orotracheal
	osteosarcoma		outlier threshold
OSA/HS	obstructive sleep apnea/ hypopnea		oxytocin (Pitocin)
	syndrome	O/T	oral temperature
OSAS	obstructive sleep apnea syndrome	OTA	Occupational Therapy Assistant
OSC	oral self-care		open to air
OSCAR	On-line Survey Certification and	OTC	occult tumor cell
	Reporting		ornithine transcarbamoylase
OSCC	oral squamous cell carcinoma		Orthopedic Technician, Certified
OSCE	Office of Surveillance and		over-the-counter (sold without
	Epidemiology (FDA)		prescription)
	Objective Structured Clinical		oxytetracycline
	Examination	OTCD	ornithine-transcarbamylase
OSD	one-stop dispensing (United		deficiency
	Kingdom)	OTD	onset-to-door (time)
	Osgood-Schlatter disease		optimal therapeutic dose
	overseas duty		organ tolerance dose
	overside drainage		out-the-door
OSE	Office of Surveillance and	OTE	(McMaster) Overall Treatment
	Epidemiology (FDA)		Evaluation
	ovarian surface epithelium		over-the-ear
OSESC	opening-snap ejection systolic click	OTFC	oral transmucosal fentanyl citrate
OSFM	oral saliva fertility monitoring		(Fentanyl Oralet; Actiq)

O

OTH	other	OX	oximeter
OTHS	occupational therapy home service	O×1	oriented to time
OTIS	Organization of Teratology Information Services	O×2	oriented to time and place
		O×3	oriented to time, place, and person
OTJ	on-the-job (injury; training)	O×4	oriented to time, place, person, and
OTO	one-time only		objects (watch, pen, book)
	otolaryngology	OXA	oxacillinase
	otology		oxaliplatin (Eloxatin)
OTPT	oral triphasic tablets (contraceptive)	OXC	oxcarbazepine (Trileptal)
		Oxi	oximeter (oximetry)
OTR	Occupational Therapist, Registered	Ox-LDL	oxidized low-density lipoprotein
OTRL	Occupational Therapist, Registered Licensed	OXLIPN	oxaliplatin-induced peripheral neuropathy
OT/RT	occupational therapy/recreational therapy	OXPHOS	oxidative phosphorylation
		OxPt	oxaliplatin (Eloxatin)
OTS	orotracheal suction	OXM	pulse oximeter
OTSCC	oral tongue squamous cell carcinoma	OXT	oxytocin (Pitocin)
		Oxy-5®	benzoyl peroxide
OTT	oral transit time	OxyIR®	oxycodone immediate release capsules
	orotracheal tube		
	overall treatment time	OXZ	oxazepam (Serax)
OTW	off-the-wall	OZ	optical zone
	over-the-wire (stent)		ounce
OU	each eye		
	observation unit		
OUES	oxygen uptake efficiency slope		
OULQ	outer upper left quadrant		
OU/P	both eyes patched		
OURQ	outer upper right quadrant		
OUS	obstetric ultrasound		
OV	office visit		
	ovary		
	ovum		
OVAL	ovalocytes		
OvCa	ovarian cancer		
OVD	occlusal vertical dimension		
	ophthalmic viscosurgical device		
OVF	Octopus® visual field		
OVLT	organum vasculosum of lamina terminalis		
OVR	Office of Vocational Rehabilitation		
OVS	obstructive voiding symptoms (syndrome)		
OW	once weekly (this is a dangerous abbreviation)		
	open wound		
	oral warts		
	outer wall		
	out of wedlock		
	ova weight		
	overweight		
O/W	oil in water (emulsion)		
	otherwise		
OWL	out of wedlock		
OWNK	out of wedlock, not keeping (baby)		
OWR	Osler-Weber-Rendu (disease)		
OWT	zero work tolerance		

O

P

P	Lasix (furoseminde) as in vitamin P (slang)
	para
	peripheral
	phosphorus
	pint
	plan
	Plasmodium
	poor
	posterior
	protein
	Protestant
	pulse
	pupil
P	statistical probability value
Ⓟ	pending
	posterior
p̄	after
/P	partial lower denture
P/	partial upper denture
P1	pilocarpine 1% ophthalmic solution
	postnatal day 1
	first phalanx
P₂	pulmonic second heart sound
P2	middle phalanx
	postnatal day 2
P3	distal phalanx
P20	Ocusert® P20
³²P	radioactive phosphorus
P40	Ocusert® P40
P53	tumor suppressive gene
PA	panic attack
	paranoid
	peanut allergy
	periapical (x-ray)
	pernicious anemia
	phenol alcohol
	physical activity
	Physician Assistant
	pineapple
	platelet aggregometry
	posterior-anterior (posteroanterior) (x-ray)
	premature adrenarche
	presents again
	primary aldosteronism
	prior approval
	professional association (similar to a corporation)
	Pseudomonas aeruginosa
	psychiatric aide
	psychoanalysis
	pulmonary artery

Pa	pascal
P&A	percussion and auscultation
	phenol and alcohol
	position and alignment
P₂ > A₂	pulmonic second heart sound greater than aortic second heart sound
PAA	pulmonary artery aneurysm
PAAA	para-anastomotic aneurysm of the aorta
PAAD	persistently and acutely disabled
PAB	posterior axillary boost
	prealbumin (transthyretin)
	premature atrial beat
	pulmonary artery banding
PABA	aminobenzoic acid (para-aminobenzoic acid)
PABC	pregnancy-associated breast cancer
PABD	preoperative autologous blood donation
PAC	cisplatin (Platinol), doxorubicin (Adriamycin), and cylcophosphamide
	phenacemide
	Physical Assessment Center
	Physician Assistant, Certified
	picture archiving communication (system)
	Port-a-cath®
	Preadmission Clinic
	premature atrial contraction
	prophylactic anticonvulsants
	pulmonary artery catheter
PA-C	Physician Assistant, Certified
PACATH	pulmonary artery catheter
PACE	population-adjusted clinical epidemiology
	Programs of All-Inclusive Care for the Elderly
PACG	primary angle-closure glaucoma
PACH	pipers to after coming head
PACI	partial anterior cerebral infarct
PACO₂	partial pressure (tension) of carbon dioxide, alveolar
PaCO₂	partial pressure (tension) of carbon dioxide, artery
PACS	picture archiving and communications systems
PACT	prism and alternate cover test
	Program of Assertive Community Treatment
PAC-V	cisplatin (Platinol), doxorubicin (Adriamycin), and cyclophosphamide
PACU	postanesthesia care unit
PAD	pelvic adhesive disease

	peripheral artery disease
	persistently and acutely disabled
	pharmacologic atrial defibrillator
	physician-assisted death
	preliminary anatomic diagnosis
	preoperative autologous donation
	primary affective disorder
	pulmonary artery diastolic
PADCAB	perfusion-assisted direct coronary artery bypass
PADP	pulmonary arterial diastolic pressure
	pulmonary artery diastolic pressure
PADS	Post Anesthesia Discharge Scoring System
PADT	primary androgen deprivation therapy
PAE	percutaneous angiographic embolization
	postanoxic encephalopathy
	postantibiotic effect
	pre-admission evaluation
	pre-anesthesia evaluation
	progressive assistive exercise
PAEDP	pulmonary artery and end-diastole pressure
PAEE	physical activity energy expenditure
PAEF	primary aortoenteric fistula
PAF	paroxysmal atrial fibrillation
	platelet-activating factor
	population attributable fraction
PA&F	percussion, auscultation, and fremitus
PAFE	postantifungal effect
PAFO	pissed and fell over (slang for drunk patient)
PAG	periaqueductal gray (also known as central gray)
PAGA	premature appropriate for gestational age
PAGCL	postarthroscopic glenohumeral chondrolysis
PAGE	polyacrylamide gel electrophoresis
PAH	para-aminohippurate
	partial abdominal hysterectomy
	phenylalanine hydroxylase
	polycyclic aromatic hydrocarbons
	polynuclear aromatic hydrocarbon
	predicted adult height
	primary adrenal hyperplasia
	pulmonary arterial hypertension
PAHO	Pan American Health Organization
PAI	penetrating abdominal injury
	plasminogen activator inhibitor

	platelet accumulation index
PAIDS	pediatric acquired immunodeficiency syndrome
PAIgG	platelet-associated immunoglobulin G
PAINAD	Pain Assessment (Tool) in Advanced Dementia
PAIR	Puncture, Aspiration, Injection, Reaspiration (technique)
PAIS	Psychological Adjustment to Illness Scale
PAIVMs	passive accessory intervertebral movements
PAIVS	pulmonary atresia with intact ventricular septum
PAK	p21-activated kinase
	pancreas and kidney
PAL	physical activity levels
	posterior axillary line
	posteroanterior and lateral
	pyothorax-associated lymphoma
PALA	N-phosphoacetate-L aspartate
Pa Line	pulmonary artery line
PALN	para-aortic lymph node
PALP	palpation
PALS	pediatric advanced life support
	periarterial lymphatic sheath
PAM	partial allosteric modulators
	Payment Accuracy Measurement
	potential acuity meter
	primary acquired melanosis
	primary amebic meningoencephalitis
	protein A mimetic
	pulmonary artery mean
2-PAM	pralidoxime (Protopam)
PAMP	pulmonary arterial (artery) mean pressure
PAN	pancreas
	pancreatic
	pancuronium (Pavulon)
	panobinostat
	panoral x-ray examination
	periodic alternating nystagmus
	polyacrylonitrile (filter)
	polyarteritis nodosa
	polyomavirus-associated nephropathy
pANCA	perinuclear antineutrophil cytoplasmic antibody
PANDAS	pediatric autoimmune neuropsychiatric disorders associated with streptococcal infections
PANENDO	panendoscopy
PANESS	physical and neurological examination for soft signs

P

pan-HER	pan-human EGF (epidermal growth factor) receptor	
PanIN-1	pancreatic intraepithelial neoplasm (low grade); there is a 1A and 1B	
PanIN-2	pancreatic intraepithelial neoplasm (moderate grade)	
PanIN-3	pancreatic intraepithelial neoplasm (high grade)	
PANP	pelvic autonomic nerve preservation	
PANSS	Positive and Negative Syndrome Scale	
PANSS-EC	Positive and Negative Symptoms of Schizophrenia-Excited Component	
PAO	peak acid output	
	peripheral arterial occlusion	
PAO_2	alveolar oxygen pressure (tension)	
PaO_2	arterial oxygen pressure (tension)	
PAOD	peripheral arterial occlusive disease	
PAOP	pulmonary artery occlusion pressure	
PAP	partial atretic plate	
	passive-aggressive personality	
	patient assistance program	
	peroxidase-anti-peroxidase	
	pokeweed antiviral protein	
	positive airway pressure	
	primary atypical pneumonia	
	prostatic acid phosphatase	
	pulmonary alveolar proteinosis	
	pulmonary artery pressure	
PAPAW	pushrim-activated power-assisted wheelchair	
PAPm	mean pulmonary artery pressure	
PAPP-A	pregnancy-associated plasma protein A	
PAPR	powered air purifying respirator	
PAPS	primary antiphospholipid syndrome	
Pap smear	Papanicolaou smear	
PA/PS	pulmonary atresia/pulmonary stenosis	
PAPVC	partial anomalous pulmonary venous connection	
PAPVR	partial anomalous pulmonary venous return	
PAQLQ	Pediatric Asthma Quality of Life Questionnaire	
PAR	parafin	
	parainfluenza (paramyxovirus) vaccine	
	parallel	
	participating (physician)	
	perennial allergic rhinitis	
	platelet aggregate ratio	
	population attributable risks	
	possible allergic reaction	

	postanesthetic recovery
	procedures, alternatives, and risks
	pulmonary arteriolar resistance
PAR1	pseudoautosomal region 1
PARA	number of pregnancies producing viable offspring
	paraplegic
	parathyroid
PARA 1	having borne one child
Paraflu	Parainfluenza
PARC	perennial allergic rhinoconjunctivitis
	pulmonary and activation-regulated chemokine
PAROM	passive assistance range of motion
PARP	polyadenosine ribose polymerase
PARQ	procedures, risks, alternatives and questions
PARR	plasma aldosterone/renin activity ratio
	postanesthesia recovery room
PARS	postanesthesia recovery score
PARs	participating physicians (Medicare)
PART	para-aortic radiotherapy
PARU	postanesthetic recovery unit
PAS	aminosalicylic acid (para-aminosalicylic acid)
	perinatal arterial stroke
	periodic acid-Schiff (reagent)
	peripheral anterior synechia
	physician-assisted suicide
	pneumatic antiembolic stocking
	postanesthesia score
	postanesthetic shivering
	premature auricular systole
	Professional Activities Study
	pulmonary artery stenosis
	pulmonary artery systolic
	pulsatile antiembolism system (stockings)
PA-S	Physician Assistant, Student
PASA	aminosalicylic acid (para-aminosalicylic acid)
	proximal articular set angle
PAS-ADD	Psychiatric Assessment Schedule for Adults with Developmental Disability
PASARR	Preadmission Screening Assessment and Annual Resident Review
PASAT	Paced Auditory Serial Addition Test
PA/S/D	pulmonary artery systolic/diastolic
PASE	pacing atrial stress echocardiography
	Physical Activity Scale for the Elderly
Pas Ex	passive exercise

PASG	pneumatic antishock garment		pyridostigmine bromide (Mestinon)
PASH	pseudoangiomatous stromal hyperplasia	Pb	lead phenobarbital
PASI	Psoriasis Area and Severity Index	p/b	postburn
PASI 75	at least 75% improvement in psoriasis area and severity index	P&B	pain and burning Papanicolaou and breast (examinations)
PASK	peripheral anterior stromal keratopathy		phenobarbital and belladonna
PASP	pulmonary artery systolic pressure	PBA	percutaneous bladder aspiration
PASS	Pain Anxiety Symptoms Scale		pseudobulbar affect
PASTA	partial articular supraspinatus tendon avulsion	PBAC	Pharmaceutical Benefits Advisory Committee
PAT	Paddington alcohol test	PBAL	protected bronchoalveolar lavage
	paroxysmal atrial tachycardia	PbB	whole blood lead
	passive alloimmune thrombocytopenia	PBC	point of basal convergence prebed care
	patella		primary biliary cirrhosis
	patient	PBCC	pigmented basal cell carcinoma
	percent acceleration time	PBD	percutaneous biliary drainage
	peripheral arterial tone		postburn day
	platelet aggregation test		proliferative breast disease
	preadmission testing	PBDE	poly brominated diphenyl ether (flame retardant)
	pregnancy at term		
	process analytical technology	PBDs	psychotic and behavioral disturbances
PATB	pes anserinus tendonitis/bursitis		
PATH	Physicians at Teaching Hospitals (Medicare Audit)	PBE	partial breech extraction population bioequivalence
	pituitary adrenotropic hormone		power building exercise
	pathology	PBF	peripheral blood film
PATP	preadmission testing program		placental blood flow
PATS	payment at time of service		pulmonary blood flow
PAU	penetrating aortic ulcer	PBFS	penile blood flow study
PAV	Pavulon (pancuronium bromide)	PBG	porphobilinogen
	pre-admission visit (hospice care initial home visit)		pressure breathing for G protection
PAVe	procarbazine, melphalan (Alkeran), and vinblastine (Velban)		pupillary block glaucoma
		PBGD	porphobilinogen deaminase
PAVF	pulmonary arteriovenous fistula	PBI	partial breast irradiation
PAVM	pulmonary arteriovenous malformation		protein-bound iodine
		PBK	pseudophakic bullous keratopathy
PAVNRT	paroxysmal atrial ventricular nodal re-entrant tachycardia	PBL	peripheral blood lymphocyte
PAWP	pulmonary artery wedge pressure		positive beam limitation (radiology)
PAX	periapical x-ray		primary breast lymphoma
PB	barometric pressure		primary brain lymphoma
	British Pharmacopeia		problem-based learning
	parafin bath	PBLC	premature birth live child
	peripheral blood	PB-LC-	particle beam liquid
	phenylbutyrate	EI-MS	chromatography-electron impact-
	piggyback		mass spectrometry
	powder board	PBM	pancreaticobiliary maljunction
	power building		peroneus brevis muscle
	premature beat		pharmacy benefit management (manager)
	Presbyterian		
	protein-bound	PBMA	polybutylmethacrylate
	Prussian blue	PBMC	peripheral blood mononuclear cell
	pudendal block	PBMNC	peripheral blood mononuclear cell
	pusher behavior		

P

PBMT	Perioperative Blood Management Technologist		psychiatric counselor
			pubococcygeus (muscle)
PBN	polymyxin B sulfate, bacitracin, and neomycin		pulmonary contusion
		p.c.	after meals
PB:ND	problem: nursing diagnosis	PCA	passive cutaneous anaphylaxis
PBNS	percutaneous bladder neck stabilization		patient care assistant (aide)
			patient-controlled analgesia
PBO	placebo		penicillamine (Cuprimine)
PBP	penicillin-binding protein		pill count adherence
	phantom breast pain		porous coated anatomic (joint replacement)
	protein-bound polysaccharide		
PBPC	peripheral blood progenitor cell		postcardiac arrest
PBPCT	peripheral blood progenitor cell transplantation		postciliary artery
			postconceptional age
PBPI	penile-brachial pulse index		posterior cerebral artery
PBPK	physiologically based pharmacokinetic		posterior communicating artery
			posterior cricoarytenoid (muscles)
PBPs	penicillin-binding proteins		procainamide
PBS	Pharmaceutical Benefit Scheme (lists all of the subsidized medicines available from the Australian Government)		procoagulation activity
			prostate cancer
		PCa	prostate cancer
		PCA3	prostate cancer gene 3
	phosphate-buffered saline	PCAC	Physical Care Assessment Center
	prune-belly syndrome	P-CAC	preparative continuous annular chromatography
PBSC	peripheral blood stem cells		
PBT	primary brain tumor	PCAD	posterior circulation arterial dissection
	proton beam therapy		
PBT$_4$	protein-bound thyroxine	PCASSO	patient-centered access to secure systems online
PbtO$_2$	brain tissue partial pressure of oxygen		
		PCB	pancuronium bromide
PBV	percutaneous balloon valvuloplasty		para cervical block
PBZ	phenoxybenzamine (Dibenzyline)		placebo
	phenylbutazone		postcoital bleeding
	pyribenzamine		prepared childbirth
ΦBZ	phenylbutazone		procarbazine (Matulane)
PC	after meals (*p.c.* preferred)		*Pseudomonas cepacia* bacteremia
	cisplatin (Platinol) and cyclophosphamide	PCBH	personal care boarding home
		PCBMN	palmar cutaneous branch of the median nerve
	packed cells		
	paclitaxel; carboplatin	PC-BPPV	posterior canal benign paroxysmal positional vertigo
	palliative care		
	pancreatic carcinoma	PCBs	polychlorinated biphenyls
	pathologic consultation	PCBUN	palmar cutaneous branch of the ulnar nerve
	patient condition		
	photocoagulation	PCC	patient care coordinator
	placebo-controlled (study)		petrous carotid canal
	platelet concentrate		pheochromocytoma
	Pneumocystis carinii		pneumatosis cystoides coli
	poor condition		poison control center
	politically correct		post coital contraception
	popliteal cyst		precipitated calcium carbonate
	posterior canals (vestibular)		progressive cardiac care
	posterior chamber	PCCC	pediatric critical care center
	prednicarbate	PCCI	penetrating craniocerebral injuries
	premature contractions	PCCM	primary care case management
	present complaint		pulmonary and critical care medicine
	productive cough		
	professional corporation	PCCP	percutaneous compression plate

P

PCCTC	Prostate Cancer Clinical Trials Consortium	PCL	pacing cycle length
			plasma cell leukemia
PCCU	postcoronary care unit		posterior chamber lens
PCD	pacer-cardioverter-defibrillator		posterior cruciate ligament
	paroxysmal cerebral dysrhythmia		proximal collateral ligament
	plasma cell dyscrasias	PCLD	polycystic liver disease
	polarized contact dermoscopy	PCLI	plasma cell labeling index
	postmortem cesarean delivery	PCLN	psychiatric consultation liaison nurse
	primary ciliary dyskinesia		
	programmed cell death	PCLR	paid claims loss ratio
PCDAI	Pediatric Crohn Disease Activity Index	PCLS	precision-cut lung slices
		PCM	paracoccidioidomycosis
PCE	physical capacities evaluation		pharmaceutical case management
	potentially compensable event		primary cutaneous melanoma
	pseudophakic corneal edema		protein-calorie malnutrition
PCE®	erythromycin particles in tablets		pubococcygeal muscle
PCEA	patient-controlled epidural analgesia	PC-MRI	phase-contrast magnetic resonance imaging
PCEAO	postcarotid endarterectomy airway obstruction	PCMX	chloroxylenol
		PCMZL	primary cutaneous marginal zone B-cell lymphoma
PCEC	purified chick embryo cell (culture)	PCN	penicillin
			percutaneous nephrostomy
PCECV	purified chick embryo cell vaccine		primary care nursing
PCF	pharyngeal conjunctival fever	PCNA	patient care nursing assistant
	postcancer fatigue		proliferating cell nuclear antigen
	posterior cervical fusion	PCNL	percutaneous nephrostolithotomy
PCFL	primary cutaneous follicular lymphoma	PCNs	posterior cervical nodes
		PCNSL	primary central nervous system lymphoma
PCFT	platelet complement fixation test		
PCG	phonocardiogram	PCNT	percutaneous nephrostomy tube
	plasma cell granuloma	PCO	patient complains of
	primary congenital glaucoma		polycystic ovary
	pubococcygeus (muscle)		posterior capsular opacification
PCGG	percutaneous coagulation of gasserian ganglion	PCO_2	partial pressure (tension) of carbon dioxide, artery
PCGLV	poorly contractile globular left ventricle	PCOD	polycystic ovarian disease
		PCOE	prescriber (physician) computer order entry
PCG/Ts	Primary Care Groups and Trusts		
PCH	paroxysmal cold hemoglobinuria	P COMM A	posterior communicating artery
	periocular capillary hemangioma		
	personal care home	PCOS	polycystic ovary syndrome
PCHI	permanent childhood hearing impairment	PCP	Palliative Care Program
			pancytopenia
PCHL	permanent childhood hearing loss		patient care plan
PC&HS	after meals and at bedtime		phencyclidine (phenylcyclohexyl piperidine)
PCI	percutaneous coronary intervention		
	pneumatosis cystoides intestinalis		Pneumocystis carinii (jirovecii) pneumonia
	prophylactic cranial irradiation		
PCINA	patient-controlled intranasal analgesia		primary care person
			primary care physician
PCIOL	posterior chamber intraocular lens		primary care provider
PC-IPAA	proctocolectomy and ileal pouch-anal anastomosis		prochlorperazine (Compazine)
			pulmonary capillary pressure
PC-IRV	pressure-controlled inverse-ratio ventilation	PCPC	Pediatric Cerebral Performance Category (Scale)
PCI-S	percutaneous coronary intervention with stenting	PCPs	personal care products
PCKD	polycystic kidney disease	PCR	patient care report

P

249

		PCXR	portable chest radiograph
	percutaneous coronary revascularization	PCZ	procarbazine (Matulane)
	polymerase chain reaction		prochlorperazine (Compazine)
	protein catabolic rate	PD	interpupillary distance
PCr	plasma creatinine		Paget disease
pCR	pathological complete response		pancreaticoduodenectomy
PCRA	pure red-cell aplasia		panic disorder
PCR/PSA	polymerase chain reaction analysis of prostate-specific antigen		Parkinson disease
PCS	patient care system		patient detected
	patient-controlled sedation		penile sclerosis
	personal care service		percutaneous drain
	photon correlation spectroscopy		peritoneal dialysis
	physical component summary		personality disorder
	portable cervical spine		pharmacodynamics
	portacaval shunt		pocket depth (dental)
	postconcussion syndrome		poorly differentiated
P c/s	primary cesarean section		post dates
PCSM	prostate cancer-specific mortality		postnatal day
PC-SPES	an herbal refined powder preparation of eight medicinal plants		postural drainage
			pressure dressing
			prism diopter
			probing depth (dental)
PCT	parasite-clearance time		progressive disease
	Patient Care Technician		pupillary distance
	percent	P/D	packs per day (cigarettes)
	perfusion computed tomography	2PD	two point discriminatory test
	photochemical treatment	^{103}Pd	palladium 103
	poker chip tool (for rating pain)	PDA	pancreatic ductal adenocarcinoma
	porphyria cutanea tarda		parenteral drug abuser
	postcoital test		patent ductus arteriosus
	posterior chest tube		pathological demand avoidance (syndrome)
	Primary Care Trust (United Kingdom)		personal digital assistant
			polymorphic delta activity (electroencephalograph)
	primary chemotherapy		
	procalcitonin		poorly differentiated adenocarcinoma
	progesterone challenge test		
PCTA	percutaneous transluminal angioplasty		posterior descending (coronary) artery
PCTS	patient-controlled transdermal system		property damage accident
PCU	palliative care unit	PDAC	pancreatic ductal adenocarcinoma
	primary care unit	PDAD	photodiode array detector
	progressive care unit	PDAF	platelet-derived angiogenesis factor
	protective care unit	PDAP	peritoneal dialysis-associated peritonitis
PCV	packed cell volume		
	polycythemia vera	PDB	preperitoneal distention balloon
	pressure-controlled ventilation	PDC	patient denies complaints
	procarbazine, lomustine (CCNU [Cee Nu]), and vincristine		poorly differentiated carcinoma
			private diagnostic clinic
PCV 7	pneumococcal 7-valent conjugate vaccine (Prevnar)		property damage collision (crash)
			proportion of days covered
PCV 23	pneumococcal vaccine polyvalent (Pneumovax 23; Pnu-Imune 23)		pyruvate dehydogenase complex
		PD&C	postural drainage and clapping
PCVC	percutaneous central venous catheter	PDCA	Plan-Do-Check-Act (process improvement)
PCWP	pulmonary capillary wedge pressure	PDD	cisplatin (Platinol)
			Parkinson disease cases with dementia
PCX	paracervical		

P

	percentage depth dose	PD/PV	postural drainage/percussion/vibration
	pervasive developmental disorder	PDQ	pretty damn quick (at once)
	premenstrual dysphoric disorder	PDQ-39	Parkinson Disease Questionnaire
	prescribed daily dose	PDQ-R	Personality Diagnostic Questionnaire-Revised
	primary degenerative dementia		
PDDNOS	pervasive developmental disorder, not otherwise specified	PDR	patients' dining room
PDDs	pervasive developmental disorders		*Physicians' Desk Reference*
PDE	paroxysmal dyspnea on exertion		point of decreasing response
	pulsed Doppler echocardiography		postdelivery room
PDE4	phosphodiesterase type 4		proliferative diabetic retinopathy
PDE5	phosphodiesterase type 5		prospective drug review
PDEGF	platelet-derived epidermal growth factor	PDRcVH	proliferative diabetic retinopathy with vitreous hemorrhage
PDEIs	phosphodiesterase inhibitors (Viagra, Levitra, and Cialis)	PDRM	preventable drug-related morbidity
		PDRP	proliferative diabetic retinopathy
PDF	Portable Document Format	PDRUL	palmar distal radioulnar ligament
PDFC	premature dead female child	PDS	pain dysfunction syndrome
PDGF	platelet-derived growth factor		persistent developmental stuttering
PDGXT	predischarge graded exercise test		pigment dispersion syndrome
PDH	past dental history		Pharmaceutical Development Section (NIH)
	pyruvate dehydrogenase		
PDI	Pain Disability Index		polydioxanone suture
	phasic detrusor instability		power Doppler sonography
	psychomotor developmental index		Progressive Deterioration Scale
PDIGC	patient dismissed in good condition	PDSA	Plan, Do, Study, and Act
PDL	periodontal ligament	PDSCC	poorly differentiated squamous cell carcinoma
	poorly differentiated lymphocytic		
	postures of daily living	PDSS	Postpartum Depression Screening Scale
	preferred drug list		
	progressively diffused leukoencephalopathy	PDT	percutaneous dilatational tracheostomy
	pulsed-dye laser		photodynamic therapy
PDL-D	poorly differentiated lymphocytic-diffuse		postdisaster trauma
		PDTC	pyrrolidine dithiocarbamate
PDL-N	poorly differentiated lymphocytic-nodular	PDU	PCR (polymerase chain reaction)-detectable units
PDM	primary dermal melanoma		pulsed Doppler ultrasonography
PDMC	premature dead male child	PDUFA	Prescription Drug User Fee Act (1992)
PD-MSCs	placenta-derived mesenchymal stem cells		
		PDUR	postdialysis urea rebound
PDN	Paget disease of the nipple		prospective drug utilization review
	painful diabetic neuropathy	PDW	platelet distribution width
	prednisone	PDWHF	platelet-derived wound healing factors
	private duty nurse		
	prosthetic disk nucleus	PDWI	proton-density-weighted image(s)
PDNE	poorly differentiated neuroendocrine (carcinoma)	PDX	pyridoxine (vitamin B_6)
		PDx	principal diagnosis
PDNV	postdischarge nausea and vomiting	pDXA	peripheral dual energy x-ray absorptiometry
PDOX	pegylated doxorubicin		
PDP	pachydermoperiostosis	PE	cisplatin (Platinol) and etoposide
	peak diastolic pressure		pedal edema
	prescription drug plan		pelvic examination
PD & P	postural drainage and percussion		pharyngoesophageal
PDPH	postdural puncture headache		phenytoin equivalent (150 mg of fosphenytoin sodium is equivalent to 100 mg of phenytoin sodium)
PDPM	peripapillary detachment in pathologic myopia		
PDPT	patient-delivered partner therapy		

P

	physical education (gym)	PEDs	performance-enhancing drugs
	physical examination		periodic epileptiform discharges
	physical exercise	Peds	pediatrics
	plasma exchange	PedsQL 4.0	Pediatric Quality of Life Inventory, version 4.0
	pleural effusion		
	pneumatic equalization	PEE	punctate epithelial erosion
	polyethylene	PEEK	polyetheretherketone
	preeclampsia	PEEP	positive end-expiratory pressure
	premature ejaculation	PEF	cisplatin (Platinol), epirubicin, and fluorouracil
	pressure equalization		
	pulmonary edema		peak expiratory flow
	pulmonary embolism	PEFR	peak expiratory flow rate
P₁E₁®	epinephrine 1%, pilocarpine 1% ophthalmic solution	PEFSR	partial expiratory flow static recoil curve
P&E	prep and enema	PEG	pegylated
PE24	Preemie Enfamil 24		percutaneous endoscopic gastrostomy
PEA	pelvic examination under anesthesia		pneumoencephalogram
	phenylethylamine		polyethylene glycol
	pre-emptive analgesia	PEG-ELS	polyethylene glycol and iso-osmolar electrolyte solution
	pulseless electrical activity		
Peanut	primitive neuroectodermal tumor (PNET) (slang)	PEGG	Parent Education and Guidance Group
PEARL	physiologic endometrial ablation/resection loop	PEG-J	percutaneous endoscopic gastrojejunostomy
	pupils equal accommodation, reactive to light	PEG-JET	percutaneous endoscopic gastrostomy with jejunal extension tube
	pupils equal and reactive to light		
PEARLA	pupils equal and react to light and accommodation	PEG-SOD	polyethylene glycol-conjugated superoxide dismutase (pegorgotein)
PEB	cisplatin, etoposide, and bleomycin		
PEC	pectoralis	PEH	paraesophageal hernia
	Physician Emergency Certificate (the 15 day hold certificate used in psychiatric hospitals)		postexercise hypotension
		PEI	cisplatin (Platinol), etoposide, and ifosfamide
	posterior exterior chain (of muscles)		percutaneous ethanol injection
			phosphate excretion index
	preeclampsia		physical efficiency index
	Psychiatric Emergency Clinic		polyethylenimine
	pulmonary ejection click	PEIT	percutaneous ethanol injection therapy
PECCE	planned extracapsular cataract extraction		
		PEITC	phenethyl isothiocyanate
PECHO	prostatic echogram	PEJ	percutaneous endoscopic jejunostomy
PECHR	peripheral exudative choroidal hemorrhagic retinopathy		
		PEK	punctate epithelial keratopathy
PECO₂	mixed expired carbon dioxide tension	PEL	pelvis
			permissible exposure limits
PED	paroxysmal exertion-induced dyskinesia		primary effusion lymphomas
			protein electrophoresis
	pediatrics	PELD	percutaneous endoscopic lumbar diskectomy
	pedicle		
	pigment epithelial detachments	PELE	postextubation laryngeal edema
PEDD	proton-electron dipole-dipole	PELOD	pediatric logistic organ dysfunction (score)
PEDF	pigment epithelial-derived factor		
PEDI	pediatric evaluation of disability inventory	PELV	pelvimetry
		PEM	prescription event monitoring
PEDI-DEG	pediatric deglycerolized red blood cells		protein-energy malnutrition
		PEMA	phenylethylmalonamide

PEMS	physical, emotional, mental, and safety	PERRRLA	pupils equal, round, regular, react to light and accommodation
	postexercise muscle soreness	PERS	personal emergency response systems
PEN	pancreatic endocrine neoplasm		
	parenteral and enteral nutrition	PERT	pancreatic enzyme replacement therapy
	penicillin		
	Pharmacy Equivalent Name		program evaluation and review technique
PENS	percutaneous electrical nerve stimulation	PERV	porcine endogenous retroviruses
	percutaneous epidural nerve stimulator	PER$_w$	pertussis, whole-cell antigens, vaccine
PEO	progressive external ophthalmoplegia	PES	paclitaxel-eluting stent
			polyethersulfone
PEP	patient education program		postextubation stridor
	pharmacologic erection program		preexcitation syndrome
	positive expiratory pressure		programmed electrical stimulation
	postexposure prophylaxis		pseudoexfoliation syndrome
	preejection period	PESA	percutaneous epididymal sperm aspiration
	primary endpoint		
	primer extension preamplification	peSPL	peak equivalent sound pressure level
	protein electrophoresis		
PEPD	paroxysmal extreme pain disorder	PET	poor exercise tolerance
PEP/ET	pre-ejection period/ ejection time		positron-emission tomography
PEPI	preejection period index		preeclamptic toxemia
PEPP	payment error prevention program		pressure equalizing tubes
			problem elicitation technique
PER	by	PETCT	positron emission tomography-computed tomography
	pediatric emergency room		
	pertussis (whooping cough) vaccine, antigens not otherwise unspecified	PEth	phosphatidyl ethanol
		PETN	pentaerythritol tetranitrate
		PEX	plasma exchange
	protein efficiency ratio		pseudoexfoliation (glaucoma)
PER$_a$	pertussis, acellular antigen(s), vaccine	PEx	physical examination
		PEX# 3	plasma exchange number three
PERC	perceptual	PEY	patient exposure years
	percutaneous	PF	patellofemoral
PERF	perfect		peak flow
	perforation		pemphigus foliaceus
Peri Care	perineum care		peripheral fields
PERIO	periodontal disease		Pharmacopeia Forum
	periodontitis		plantar flexion
Periop	perioperative		Pontiac fever
peri-pads	perineal pads		power factor
PERL	pupils equal, reactive to light		preservative free
PERLA	pupils equally reactive to light and accommodation		prostatic fluid
			pulmonary fibrosis
per os	by mouth (this is a dangerous abbreviation as it is read as left eye [OS])		push fluids
		Pf	*Plasmodium falciparum*
		PF3	platelet factor 3
PERP	perpetrator	PF4	platelet factor 4
PERR	pattern evoked retinal response	16PF	The Sixteen Personality Factors test
PERRL	pupils equal, round, and reactive to light		
		PFA	foscarnet (phosphonoformatic acid) (Foscavir)
PERRLA	pupils equal, round, reactive to light and accommodation		
			patellofemoral arthritis
PERR-LADC	pupils equal, round, reactive to light and accommodation directly and consensually		platelet function analysis
			psychological first aid
			pure free acid

P

PFAA	profunda femoris artery aneurysm	patient financial services
PFAPA	periodic fever, aphthous stomatitis, pharyngitis, and cervical adenitis	Physician Fee Schedule
		prefilled syringe
PFB	potential for breakdown	preservative-free solution (system)
	pseudofolliculitis barbae	primary fibromyalgia syndrome
PFC	patient-focused care	progression-free survival
	perfluorochemical	prolonged febrile seizure
	permanent flexure contracture	pulmonary function studies (study)
	persistent fetal circulation	PFSH	past, family, and social history (histories)
	prefrontal cortex	
	prolonged febrile convulsions	PFT	parafascicular thalamotomy
P̄ FEEDS	after feedings		pulmonary function test
PFFD	proximal femoral focal deficiency (defect)	PFTC	primary fallopian tube carcinoma
		PFU	plaque-forming unit
PFFFP	Pall filtered fresh frozen plasma	PFW	pHisoHex® face wash
PFG	patellofemoral grind	PFWB	Pall filtered whole blood
	percutaneous fluoroscopic gastrostomy		Psychological General Well-Being (index)
	proximal femur geometry	PFWT	pain-free walking time
	pulsed-field gradient	PG	paclitaxel and gemcitabine
PFGE	pulsed field gel electrophoresis		paged in hospital
PFH	progressive facial hemiatrophy (Parry-Romberg syndrome)		paregoric
			performance goal (short-term goal)
PfHRP-2	*Plasmodium falciparum* histidine-rich protein 2		phosphatidylglycerol
			picogram (pg) (10^{-12} gram)
PFHx	positive family history		pigmentary glaucoma
PFI	pill-free intervals		placental grade (biophysical profile)
	progression-free interval	
PFIC	progressive familial intrahepatic cholestasis		polygalacturonate
			practice guidelines
PFJ	patellofemoral joint		pregnant
PFJS	patellofemoral joint syndrome		propylene glycol
PFL	cisplatin (Platinol), fluorouracil, and leucovorin		prostaglandin
			pyoderma gangrenosum
	patellofemoral ligament	PGA	prostaglandin A
PFL+IFN	cisplatin (Platinol), fluorouracil, leucovorin, and interferon alfa 2b		**p**rothrombin time, **g**amma-glutamyl transpeptidase activity, and serum **a**polipoprotein AI concentration
PFM	peak flow meter	
	permanent first molars	PGAD	persistent genital arousal disorder
	porcelain fused to metal	PGB	pregabalin (Lyrica)
	primary fibromyalgia	PGBD	polyglucosan body disease
PFME	pelvic floor muscle exercise	PGCA	gutta-percha-filled canal area(s)
PFN	proximal femoral nail	PGCG	peripheral giant cell granuloma
PFO	patent foramen ovale	PGCH	postinfantile giant cell hepatitis
	pissed, fell over (slang for drunk patient)	PGCR	pharyngoglottal closure reflex
		PGCs	primordial germ cells
PFP	progression free probability	PGD	pelvic girdle dysfunction
	proinsulin fusion protein		preimplantation genetic diagnosis
PFPC	Pall filtered packed cells	3-PGDH	3-phosphoglyerate-dehdyrogenase
PFPS	patellofemoral pain syndrome	PGE	partial generalized epilepsy
PfSPZ	*Plasmodium falciparum* sporozoite		posterior gastroenterostomy
PFR	parotid flow rate		prostaglandin E
	peak flow rate		proximal gastric exclusion
	pelvic floor relaxation	PGE$_1$	alprostadil (prostaglandin E$_1$)
PFRC	plasma-free red cells	PGE$_2$	dinoprostone (prostaglandin E$_2$)
PFROM	pain-free range of motion	PGED	Practice Guideline for Eating Disorders
PFS	patellar femoral syndrome	

P

PGESM	Patient's Global Evaluation of Study Medication	Ph4	Phase IV (post marketing surveillance trials)
PGF	paternal grandfather	PHA	arterial pH
	placental growth factor		passive hemagglutinating
PGF$_{2\alpha}$	dinoprost (prostaglandin F$_{2\alpha}$)		paternal history of alcoholism
PGGF	paternal great-grandfather		peripheral hyperalimentation
PGGM	paternal great-grandmother		phenylalanine
PGH	pituitary growth hormones		phytohemagglutinin antigen
PGI	potassium, glucose, and insulin		postoperative holding area
PGI$_2$	epoprostenol (Prostacyclin)	PHAC	Public Health Agency of Canada
PGL	persistent generalized lymphadenopathy	PHACE	posterior fossa malformation, facial cavernous hemangioma, arterial anomalies, coarctation of the aorta/cardiac defects and eye abnormalities (syndrome)
	primary gastric lymphoma		
PGM	paternal grandmother		
	phosphoglucomutase		
PGP	paternal grandparent	PHACO	phacoemulsification
Pgp	P-glycoprotein	PHACO OD	phacoemulsification of the right eye
PGR	pulse-generated runoff		
PgR	progesterone receptor	PHACO OS	phacoemulsification of the left eye
P-graph	penile plethysmograph		
PGRN	Pharmacogenomics Research Network	PHAL	peripheral hyperalimentation
		PHAR	pharmacist
	progranulin		pharmacy
PGS	Persian Gulf syndrome		pharynx
	posterior glottic stenosis	Pharm	Pharmacy
	purple glove syndrome	PharmD	Doctor of Pharmacy
PGT	play-group therapy	PHb	pyridoxylated hemoglobin
PGTC	primary generalized tonic-clonic (seizures)	PHC	permissive hypercapnia
			posthospital care
P±GTC	partial seizures with or without generalized tonic-clonic seizures		primary health care
			primary hepatocellular carcinoma
pGTD	persistent gestational trophoblastic disease	PHCA	profound hypothermic cardiac arrest
		PHD	paroxysmal hypnogenic dyskinesia
PGTP	primary glaucoma triple procedure		Public Health Department
PG-TXL	poly (L-glutamic acid)-paclitaxel	PhD	Doctor of Philosophy
PGU	postgonococcal urethritis		phospholipase D
PGW	person gametocyte week	PHE	periodic health examination
PGx	pharmacogenomics	PHEN-FEN	phentermine and fenfluramine
PGY-1	postgraduate year one (first year resident)		
		phenobarb	phenobarbital
pH	hydrogen ion concentration	PHEO	pheochromocytoma
PH	past history	PHEP	progressive home exercise program
	personal history	PhEur	European Pharmacopoeia
	pinhole	PHF	paired helical filament
	poor health	PHG	portal hypertensive gastropathy
	profound hypothermia	PHH	paraesophageal hiatus hernia
	pubic hair		posthemorrhagic hydrocephalus
	public health		
	pulmonary hypertension	PHHI	persistent hyperinsulinemic hypoglycemia of infancy
P&H	physical and history		
Ph^1	Philadelphia chromosome	PHI	patient health information
Ph1	Phase I clinical trial (studies assess the safety of a drug or device)		personal health information
			phosphohexose isomerase
Ph2	Phase II clinical trial (studies test efficacy of a drug or device)		prehospital index
			protected health information
Ph3	Phase III clinical trial (studies involve randomized and blind testing in several hundred to several thousand patients)	PHIS	posthead injury syndrome
		PHL	permanent hearing loss
			Philadelphia (chromosome)

P

PHLIS	Public Health Laboratory Information System	PI	package insert
			pallidal index
PHLS	Public Health Laboratory Service (United Kingdom)		pancreatic insufficiency
			Pearl Index
PHM	partial hydatidiform mole		performance improvement
	preventative health maintenance		peripheral iridectomy
PHMB	polyhexamethylene biguanide		persistent illness
PHMD	polyhexamethylene (Baquacil, a pool cleaner)		physically impaired
			plaque index (dental)
PHN	postherpetic neuralgia		poison ivy
	Public Health Nurse		postincident
	Puritan® heated nebulizer		postinfection
PHNC	public health nurse coordinator		postinjury
PHNI	pinhole no improvement		premature infant
PHO	Physician/Hospital Organization		present illness
PHOB	phobic anxiety		principal investigator
PHONO	phonophoresis		protease inhibitor
PHOS	phosphatase		pulmonary infarction
	Phosphate		pulmonic insufficiency
	Phosphorous	Pi	infusion pressure (ultrafiltration circuit line pressure)
PHP	pooled human plasma		
	postheparin plasma	PI-3	parainfluenza 3 virus
	prepaid health plan	P & I	probe and irrigation
	pseudohypoparathyroidism	PIA	personal injury accident
	pyridoxalated hemoglobin polyoxyethylene conjugate		polysaccharide intercellular adhesine
PHPPO	Public Health Practice Program Office	PIAF	cisplatin (Platinol), recombinant interferon alpha 2B, doxorubicin (Adriamycin), and fluorouracil
PHPT	primary hyperparathyroidism		
PHPV	persistent hyperplastic primary vitreous	PIAT	Peabody Individual Achievement Test
PHQ-9	Patient Health Questionnaire (9-item depression scale)	PIB	partial ileal bypass
			professional information brochure
PHR	peak heart rate	PiB	Pittsburgh Compound B
	personal health record	PIBD	paucity of interlobular bile ducts
PhRMA	Pharmaceutical Research and Manufacturers of America	PIBF	progesterone-induced blocking factor
PHRN	Pre-Hospital Registered Nurse	PIC	penicillin-inhibitor combinations
PHS	partial hospitalization program		peripherally inserted catheter
	Prolene hernia system		personal injury collision (crash)
	US Public Health Service		polysaccharide-iron complex
PHT	phenytoin (Dilantin)		postintercourse
	portal hypertension	PICA	Porch Index of Communicative Ability
	posterior hyaloidal traction		
	postmenopausal hormone therapy		posterior inferior cerebellar artery
	primary hyperthyroidism		posterior inferior communicating artery
	pulmonary hypertension		
PHTC	pulmonary hypertensive crises	PICC	peripherally inserted central catheter
PHV	peak height velocity		
	pediatric health visit	PICHI	pulse-inversion contrast harmonic imaging
PHVA	pinhole visual acuity		
pHVA	plasma homovanillic acid	PICT	pancreatic islet cell transplantation
PHVD	posthemorrhagic ventricular dilatation	PICU	pediatric intensive care unit
			psychiatric intensive care unit
PHx	past history	PICVA	percutaneous in situ coronary venous arterialization
Phx	pharynx		
PHY	physician	PICVC	peripherally inserted central venous catheter
PhyO	physician's orders		

P

| PID | pelvic inflammatory disease | PIO₂ | partial pressure of inspired oxygen |

PID	pelvic inflammatory disease
	primary immunodeficiency
	prolapsed intervertebral disk
	proportional-integral-derivative (controller)
PIDD	primary immunodeficiency disease
PIE	pulmonary infiltration with eosinophilia
	pulmonary interstitial emphysema
PIEE	pulsed irrigation for enhanced evacuation
PIF	peak inspiratory flow
	powdered infant formula
PIFG	poor intrauterine fetal growth
PIFR	peak inspiratory flow rate
PIG	pertussis immune globulin
PIGD	postural instability and gait difficulty (disorder)
PIGI	pregnancy-induced glucose intolerance
PIGN	postinfectious glomerulonephritis
PIH	postinflammatory hyperpigmentation
	pregnancy-induced hypertension
	preventricular intraventricular hemorrhage
	prolactin-inhibiting hormone
PIIID	peripheral indwelling intermediate infusion device
PIIIP	aminoterminal type three procollagen propeptide
PIIS	posterior inferior iliac spine
PIL	patient information leaflet
	purpose in life
PILO	pilocarpine
PIM	potentially inappropriate medication
	Program Integrity Manual
	pulse-inversion mode (ultrasound)
PIMIA	potentiometric ionophore mediated immunoassay
PIMS	programmable implantable medication system
PIN	pain in the neck (no place for such a term in a written document)
	personal identification number
	population impact number
	posterior interosseous nerve
	prostatic intraepithelial neoplasia
	provider identification number
PIND	progressive intellectual and neurological deterioration
pINN	proposed International Nonproprietary Name
PINP	N-terminal propeptide of type I collagen
PINS	persons in need of supervision
PIO	pemoline (Cylert)

PIO₂	partial pressure of inspired oxygen
PIOK	poikilocytosis
PIOL	phakic intraocular lens
	primary intraocular lymphoma
PIOP	patient informed of policy
PIP	peak inspiratory pressure
	Performance in Practice
	postictal psychosis
	postinfusion phlebitis
	proximal interphalangeal (joint)
	pulmonary immaturity of prematurity
	pulmonary insufficiency of the premature
PIPB	performance index phonetic balance
PI-PB	performance intensity-phonemically balanced
PIPIDA	N-para-isopropyl-acetanilide-iminodiacetic acid
PIPJ	proximal interphalangeal joint
PIPP	Premature Infant Pain Profile
PIP/TZ	piperacillin-tazobactam (Zosyn)
PIQ	Performance Intelligence Quotient (part of Wechsler tests)
PIR	pirarubicin
PIS	pregnancy interruption service
PISA	phase invariant signature algorithm
	proximal isovelocity surface area
PIT	pancreatic islet transplantation
	patellar inhibition test
	peak isometric torque
	Pitocin (oxytocin)
	Pitressin (vasopressin) (this is a dangerous abbreviation as it can be taken for Pitocin)
	pituitary
	pulsed-inotrope therapy
PITA	pain in the ass (slang)
PITP	pseudo-idiopathic thrombocytopenic purpura
PITR	plasma iron turnover rate
PIV	peripheral intravenous
PIV-3	parainfluenza virus type 3
PIVD	protruded intervertebral disk
PIVH	periventricular-intraventricular hemorrhage
PIVKA	proteins induced in vitamin K absence
PIWT	partially impacted wisdom teeth
PIXI	Peripheral Instantaneous X-ray Imaging (dual-energy x-ray absorptiometry system)
PJ	procelin jacket (crown)
PJB	premature junctional beat
PJC	premature junctional contractions
PJI	prosthetic joint infection

P

PJIF	prosthetic joint implant failure	PLAP	placental alkaline phosphatase
PJP	pneumocystis jirovecii pneumonia	PLAT C	platelet concentration
PJRT	permanent form of junctional reciprocating tachycardia	PLAT P	platelet pheresis
		PLAX	parasternal long axis
PJS	peritoneojugular shunt	PLB	percutaneous liver biopsy
	Peutz-Jeghers syndrome		phospholamban
PJT	paroxysmal junctional tachycardia		placebo
PJVT	paroxysmal junctional-ventricular		posterolateral branch
	tachycardia		pursed-lip breathing
PK	penetrating keratoplasty	PLBF	posterolateral bone fusion
	pharmacokinetics	PLBO	placebo
	plasma potassium	PLC	peripheral lymphocyte count
	pyruvate kinase		permanent legal custodianship
PKB	prone knee bend		pityriasis lichenoides chronica
PKC	protein kinase C	PLCH	pulmonary Langerhans cell
PKD	paroxysmal kinesigenic dyskinesia		histiocytosis
	pharmacodynamics	PLD	partial lower denture
	polycystic kidney disease		pegylated liposomal doxorubicin
PKDL	post-kala-azar dermal leishmaniasis		(Doxil)
PKI	public key infrastructure		percutaneous laser diskectomy
PKMzeta	protein kinase Mzeta	PLDD	percutaneous laser disk
PKND	paroxysmal nonkinesigenic		decompression
	dyskinesia	PLE	polymorphic light eruption
	pyknodysostosis		*polypodium leucotomos* extract
PKP	penetrating keratoplasty		(natural fern extract)
PK/PD	pharmacokinetic/		protein-losing enteropathy
	pharmacodynamic	PLED	periodic lateralizing epileptiform
PKR	phased knee rehabilitation		discharge
PKS	Pallister Killian syndrome	PLEK	posterior lamellar endothelial
PK Test	Prausnitz-Küstner transfer test		keratoplasty
PKU	phenylketonuria	PLEVA	pityriasis lichenoides et
pk yrs	pack-years (smoking one pack of		varioliformis acuta
	cigarettes a day for one year is	PLF	prior level of function
	termed 1 pack-year of smoking,	PLFC	premature living female child
	thus 2 packs a day for 20 years	PLG	plague (*Yersinia pestis*) (*la Peste*)
	would be 40 pack-years)		vaccine
PL	light perception	PLH	paroxysmal localized hyperhidrosis
	palmaris longus	PLIF	posterior lumbar interbody fusion
	peroneus longus	PLIG	posterior lumbar interbody graft
	pharyngolaryngectomy	PLIL	partial laryngectomy with
	place		imbrication laryngoplasty
	placebo	PLK	posterior lamellar keratoplasty
	plantar	PLL	posterior longitudinal ligament
	plethoric (infant color)		prolymphocytic leukemia
	project leader	PLLA	poly-l-lactic acid (Sculptra)
	transpulmonary pressure	PLM	partial lateral meniscectomy
PLA	placebo		periodic leg movement
	Plasma-Lyte A		Plasma-Lyte M
	poly-L-lactic acid (Sculptra)		polarized-light microscope
	posterolateral (coronary) artery		precise lesion measuring (device)
	potentially lethal arrhythmia		product-line manager
	Product License Application	PLMC	premature living male child
	pulpolinguoaxial	PLMD	periodic limb movement disorder
PLAC	placenta	PLMS	periodic limb movements during
PLAD	proximal left anterior descending		sleep
	(artery)	PLMT	painful legs and moving toes
Plan B®	levonorgestrel (a progestogen		(syndrome)
	emergency contraceptive)		partial lateral meniscal tear

PLN	pelvic lymph node	Pm	*Plasmodium malariae*
	popliteal lymph node	PM$_{10}$	particulate matter less than 10
PLND	pelvic lymph node dissection		micrometers diameter
PLO	pluronic lecithin organogels	PMA	positive mental attitude
PLOF	previous level of functioning		post-menstrual age
PLOS	postoperative length of stay		premarket approval (application)
PLOSA	physiologic low stress angioplasty		(for medical devices)
PLP	partial laryngopharyngectomy		premenstrual asthma
	phantom limb pain		primary meningococcal arthritis
	protolipid protein		Prinzmetal angina
PLPH	postlumbar puncture headache		progress myoclonic ataxia
PLR	pupillary light reflex	PMAA	Premarket Approval Application
PLRT	postlumpectomy radiotherapy		(medical devices)
PLS	Papillon-Lefèvre syndrome	PMB	polymorphonuclear basophil
	phantom limb syndrome		(leukocytes)
	plastic surgery		polymyxin B
	point locator stimulator		postmenopausal bleeding
	Preschool Language Scale	PMC	posterior medial cortex
	primary lateral sclerosis		premature mitral closure
PLs	premalignant lesions		pseudomembranous colitis
PLSD	protected least significant	PMCP	para-monochlorophenol
	difference (statistical test)		perinatal mortality counseling
PLSO	posterior leafspring orthosis		program
PLST	progressively lowered stress	PMCT	perinatal mortality counseling team
	threshold		postmortem computed tomography
PLSURG	plastic surgery	PMCWR	post-mastectomy chest wall relapse
PLT	platelet	PMD	Pelizaeus-Merzbacher disease
PLTC	posterolateral-temporal cortex		pellucid marginal degeneration
PLT EST	platelet estimate		perceptual motor development
PLTF	plaintiff		persistent microvascular damage
PLTS	platelets		primary myocardial disease
PLUG	plug the lung until it grows		primidone (Mysoline)
PLV	partial left ventriculectomy		private medical doctor
	posterior left ventricular		progressive muscular dystrophy
PLX	plexus	PMDA	Pharmaceuticals and Medical
PLYO	plyometric		Devices Agency (Japan)
PLZF	promyelocytic leukemia zinc finger	PMDD	premenstrual dysphoric disorder
PM	afternoon	pMDI	pressurized metered-dose inhaler
	evening	PM/DM	polymyositis and dermatomyositis
	pacemaker	PME	pelvic muscle exercise
	papillary muscles		phosphomonoester(s)
	paraspinal mapping		polymorphonuclear esosinophil
	particulate matter		(leukocytes)
	petit mal		postmenopausal estrogen
	physical medicine		progressive myoclonus epilepsy
	pilomatricoma	PMEALS	after meals
	pneumomediastinum	PMEC	pseudomembranous enterocolitis
	poliomyelitis	PMED	particle mediated epidermal
	polymyositis		delivery (vaccination)
	poor metabolizers	PMF	peptide mass fingerprinting
	postmenopausal		primary myelofibrosis
	postmortem		progressive massive fibrosis
	presents mainly		pupils mid-position, fixed
	pretibial myxedema	PMH	past medical history
	primary motivation	PMHNP	Psychiatric Mental Health Nurse
	project manager		Practitioner
	prostatic massage	PMHx	past medical history
	pulpomesial	PMI	Pain Management Index

P

past medical illness
patient medication instructions
perioperative myocardial injury
plea of mental incompetence
point of maximal impulse
posterior myocardial infarction

PMID   PubMed Unique Identifier
(National Library of Medicine)

PML   polymorphonuclear leukocytes
posterior mitral leaflet
premature labor
progressive multifocal
leukoencephalopathy
promyelocytic leukemia

PMLCL   primary mediastinal large-cell
lymphoma

PMLD   Pelizaeus-Merzbacher-like disease

PMM   partial medial meniscectomy

PMMA   polymethyl methacrylate

PMMF   pectoralis major myocutaneous
flap

PMMT   partial medial meniscal tear

PMN   polymodal nociceptors
polymorphonuclear leukocyte
Premarket Notification (medical
devices)

PMNL   polymorphonuclear leukocyte

PMNN   polymorphonuclear neutrophil

PMNS   postmalarial neurological
syndrome

PMO   postmenopausal osteoporosis
probable medication overuse

pmol   picomole

PMP   pain management program
previous menstrual period
psychotropic medication plan

PMPA   tenofovir (Viread)

PMPM   per member, per month

PMPO   postmenopausal palpable ovary

PMPY   per member, per year

PMR   pacemaker rhythm
percutaneous revascularization
polymorphic reticulosis
polymyalgia rheumatica
premedication regimen
prior medical record
progressive muscle relaxation
proportional mortality ratios

PM&R   physical medicine and
rehabilitation

PMRT   postmastectomy radiotherapy

PMS   performance measurement system
periodic movements of sleep
poor miserable soul
postmarketing surveillance
postmenopausal syndrome
permanent metal stent(s)
premenstrual syndrome

psammomatous melanotic
schwannoma
pulse, motor, and sensory

PMSF   phenylmethylsulfonyl fluoride

PMT   pacemaker-mediated tachycardia
percutaneous mechanical
thrombectomy
pharmacomechanical
thrombectomy
photomultiplier tube (radiology)
point of maximum tenderness
premenstrual tension

PMTS   premenstrual tension syndrome

PMV   Passy-Muir valve
percutaneous mitral (balloon)
valvuloplasty
prolapse of mitral valve

PMW   pacemaker wires

PMX-B   polymyxin-B

PMX-HP   polymyxin-B hemoperfusion

PMZ   postmenopausal zest

PN   parenteral nutrition
peanut (when testing for an
allergy)
percussion note
percutaneous nephrosonogram
percutaneous nephrostomy
percutaneous nucleotomy
periarteritis nodosa
peripheral neuropathy
plexiform neurofibroma
pneumonia
polyarteritis nodosa
poorly nourished
positional nystagmus
postnasal
postnatal
practical nurse
premie nipple
primary nurse
progress note
pyelonephritis

P & N   pins and needles
psychiatry and neurology

PN$_2$ partial pressure of nitrogen

PNA   Pediatric Nurse Associate
peptide nucleic acid
pneumonia
polynitroxyl albumin

PNa   plasma sodium

PNAB   percutaneous needle aspiration
biopsy

PNAC   parenteral nutrition associated
cholestasis

PNAR   perennial nonallergic rhinitis

PNAS   prudent no added salt

PNB   percutaneous needle biopsy
popliteal nerve block

	premature newborn	PNS	partial nonprogressing stroke
	premature nodal beat		peripheral nerve stimulator
	prostate needle biopsy		peripheral nervous system
PNC	penicillin		practical nursing student
	peripheral nerve conduction		Pump N' Style (breast pump machine)
	postnecrotic cirrhosis		
	premature nodal contraction	PNSP	penicillin-nonsusceptible *Streptococcus pneumoniae*
	prenatal care		
	prenatal course	PNT	percutaneous nephrostomy tube
	Psychiatric Nurse Clinician		percutaneous neuromodulatory therapy
PNCV7	pneumococcal 7-valent conjugate vaccine (Prevnar)		
			pneumatic trabeculoplasty
PND	paroxysmal nocturnal dyspnea	pnthx	pneumothorax
	pelvic node dissection	PNTML	pudendal-nerve terminal motor latency
	postnasal drip		
	pregnancy, not delivered	PNU	pneumococcal (*Streptococcus pneumoniae*) vaccine, not otherwise specified
PNDS	Perioperative Nursing Data Set		
	postnasal drip syndrome		
PNE	peripheral neuroepithelioma		protein nitrogen units
	primary nocturnal enuresis	PNUcn-7	pneumococcal (*Streptococcus pneumoniae*) conjugate vaccine, 7-valent vaccine (Prevnar)
PNECs	predicted no effect concentrations		
PNES	psychogenic nonepileptic seizures		
PNET	primitive neuroectodermal tumors	PNUps23	pneumococcal (*Streptococcus pneumoniae*) polysaccharide, 23-valent vaccine (Pneumovax-23; Pnu-Imune-23)
PNET-MB	primitive neuroectodermal tumors-medulloblastoma		
PNEUMO	pneumothorax		
PNF	primary nonfunction		
	proprioceptive neuromuscular fasciculation (reaction)	PNV	postoperative nausea and vomiting
			prenatal vitamins
PNFA	progressive nonfluent aphasia	Pnx	pneumonectomy
PNH	paroxysmal nocturnal hemoglobinuria		pneumothorax
		PO	by mouth
	polynitroxyl-hemoglobin		phone order
	progressive nodular hyperplasia		postoperative
PNI	perineural invasion		*Plasmodium ovale*
	peripheral nerve injury		prophylactic oophorectomy
	Prognostic Nutrition Index		pulse oximetry
PNKD	paroxysmal nonkinesigenic dyskinesia		punctal occlusion
		Po	polonium
PNL	percutaneous nephrolithotomy	P/O	prosthetics and orthotics
	prenatal labs	P&O	parasites and ova
PNM	primary nodular melanoma		prosthetics and orthotics
PNMG	persistent neonatal myasthenia gravis	Po2	partial pressure (tension) of oxygen, artery
PNMT	phenylethanolamine-N-methyltransferase	PO4	phosphate
		POA	pancreatic oncofetal antigen
PNNP	Perinatal Nurse Practitioner		power of attorney
PNP	peak negative pressure		present on admission
	Pediatric Nurse Practitioner		present on arrival
	progressive nuclear palsy		primary optic atrophy
	purine nucleoside phosphorylase	POACH	prednisone, vincristine (Oncovin), doxorubicin (Adriamycin), cyclophosphamide, and cytarabine
PNQ	pyranonaphthoquinone		
PNR	person needed ride (minor ailment but called ambulance instead of taxi) (slang)		
		POAF	postoperative atrial fibrillation
	physician's nutritional recommendation	POAG	primary open-angle glaucoma
		POB	phenoxybenzamine (Dibenzyline)
PNRB	partial non-rebreather (oxygen mask)		place of birth
		POBA	plain old balloon angioplasty

P

POBC	primary operable breast cancer	POL	physician's office laboratory
POC	peri-operative chemotherapy		poliovirus vaccine, not otherwise specified
	plans of care		
	point-of-care		premature onset of labor
	position of comfort	POLS	postoperative length of stay
	postoperative care	POLY	polychromic erythrocytes
	product of conception		polymorphonuclear leukocyte
POCD	postoperative cognitive dysfunction	POLY-CHR	polychromatophilia
POCT	point-of-care testing (test)	POM	pain on motion
	point-of-care therapy		polyoximethylene
POD	pacing on demand		postoperative morbidity
	place of death		prescription-only medication
	Podiatry	POMA	Performance-Oriented Mobility Assessment
	polycystic ovarian disease		
	prevention of disability	POMC	pro-opiomelanocortin
	progression of disease	POMP	prednisone, vincristine (Oncovin), methotrexate, and mercaptopurine (Purinthol)
POD 1	postoperative day one		
PODs	patients' own drugs		
PODx	preoperative diagnosis	POMR	problem-oriented medical record
POE	patient-oriented evidence	POMS	Profile of Mood States
	point (portal, port) of entry	POMS-FI	Fatigue-Inertia Subscale of the Profile of Mood States
	position of ease		
	prone on elbows	PON	paraoxonase (genes)
	provider order entry		postoperative note
POEM	Patient-Oriented Evidence That Matters	PONI	postoperative narcotic infusion
		PONV	postoperative nausea and vomiting
POEMS	plasma cell dyscrasia with polyneuropathy, organomegaly, endocrinopathy, monoclonal protein (M-protein), and skin changes	POOH	postoperative open heart (surgery)
		POOL	premature onset of labor
		POP	pain on palpation
			persistent occipitoposterior
			persistent organic pollutants
POEx	postoperative exercise		plaster of paris
POF	physician's order form		popiliteal
	position of function		posterior oral pharynx
	premature ovarian failure	POp	postoperative
P of I	proof of illness	POPC	Pediatric Overall Performance Category (scale)
POG	Pediatric Oncology Group		
	Penthrane,® oxygen, and gas (nitrous oxide)	poplit	popliteal
		POPS	postoperative pain service
	products of gestation	POPs	persistent organic pollutants
POGO	percentage of glottic opening		progesterone-only pills (oral contraceptive)
POH	perillyl alcohol		
	personal oral hygiene	POPTA	passed out prior to arrival
	presumed ocular histoplasmosis	POR	physician of record
	progressive osseous heteroplasia		problem-oriented record
	prone on hands	PORN	pornography
POHA	preoperative holding area		progressive outer retinal necrosis
POHI	physically or otherwise health impaired	PORP	partial ossicular replacement prosthesis
POHS	by mouth, at bedtime	PORR	postoperative recovery room
	presumed ocular histoplasmosis syndrome	PORT	perioperative respiratory therapy
			portable
POI	Personal Orientation Inventory		portal film
	point of interest		postoperative radiotherapy
	postoperative ileus		postoperative respiratory therapy
	postoperative instructions		
POIB	place outpatient in inpatient bed	POS	parosteal osteosarcoma
POIK	poikilocytosis		partial-onset seizures

	physician's order sheet		plasmapheresis
	point-of-service		plaster of paris
	positive		poor person
PoS	plane of surgery		posterior pituitary
POSHPATE	**p**roblem, **o**nset, associated **s**ymptoms, previous **h**istory, **p**recipitating factors, **a**lleviating/ aggravation factors, **t**iming, an **e**tiology (prompts for taking history and chief complaint)		postpartum
			postprandial
			presenting part
			private patient
			prophylactics
			protoporphyria
POSL	pulse optically stimulated luminescence dosimeter (radiology)		proximal phalanx
			psychogenic polydipsia
			pulse pressure
poss	possible		push pills
post	posterior	P-P	probability-probability (plots)
	postmortem examination (autopsy)	P&P	pins and plaster
PostC	posterior chamber		policy and procedure
PostCap	posterior capsule	PIIIP	aminoterminal type three protocollegan propeptide
Post-M	urine specimen after prostate massage	PPIX	protoporphyrin nine
post op	postoperative	PPA	palpation, percussion, and auscultation
Post Sag D	posterior sagittal diameter		phenylpropanolamine
post tib	posterial tibial		phenylpyruvic acid
PostVD	posterior vitreous detachment		postpartum amenorrhea
POSYC	Pain Observation Scale for Young Children		Prescription Pricing Authority (United Kingdom)
POT	peak occupancy time		primary progressive aphasia
	plans of treatment	PP&A	palpation, percussion, and auscultation
	potassium		
	potential	PPAR	peroxisome-proliferator-activated receptor
	primary orthostatic tremor		
POTS	postural orthostatic tachycardia syndrome	PPAR$_g$	peroxisome-proliferator-activated receptor gamma
POU	placenta, ovaries, and uterus	PPARs	peroxisome proliferator-activated receptors
	point-of-use		
POV	postoperative vomiting	PPAS	postpolio atrophy syndrome
	primary outcome variable	PPB	parts per billion
	privately owned vehicle		pleuropulmonary blastoma
POVD	peripheral occlusive vascular disease		positive pressure breathing
			prostate puncture biopsy
POVH	postoperative ventral hernia	PPBE	postpartum breast engorgment
POW	Powassan (virus)	PPBS	postprandial blood sugar
	prisoner of war	PPBTL	postpartum bilateral tubal ligation
POWSBP	pulse oximetry waveform systolic blood pressure	PPC	plaster of paris cast
			positive product control
POX	proline oxidase		primary peritoneal carcinoma
	pulse oximeter (reading)		progressive patient care
PP	near point of accommodation	PPCD	posterior polymorphous corneal dystrophy
	pancreatic pseudocyst		
	paradoxical pulse	PPCF	plasma prothrombin conversion factor
	partial upper and lower dentures		
	pedal pulse	PPCM	peripartum cardiomyopathy
	per protocol	PPD	packs per day
	periodontal pockets		para-phenylenediamine (a dye)
	peripheral pulses		permanent partial disability (rating)
	pin prick		pinch-point density (histologic)
	pink puffer (emphysema)		posterior polymorphous dystrophy
	Planned Parenthood		

P

	postpartum day	Ppl	pleural pressure
	postpartum depression	PPLO	pleuropneumonia-like organisms
	probing pocket depth (dental)	PPLOV	painless progressive loss of vision
	purified protein derivative (of tuberculin)	PPM	parts per million
			permanent pacemaker
	pylorus-sparing pancreaticoduodenectomy		persistent pupillary membrane
			physician practice management
P & PD	percussion & postural drainage		polypropylene mesh
PPD-B	purified protein derivative, Battey	PPMA	postpoliomyelitis muscular atrophy
PPDR	preproliferative diabetic retinopathy	PPMS	primary progressive multiple sclerosis
PPD-S	purified protein derivative, standard		psychophysiologic musculoskeletal (reaction)
PPE	palmar-plantar erythrodysesthesia (syndrome)	PPMs	potentially pathogenic microorganisms
	personal protective equipment	PPN	peripheral parenteral nutrition
	professional performance evaluation		peripheral polyneuropathy
		PPNAD	primary pigmented nodular adrenocortical disease
	pruritic papular eruption		
PPES	palmar-plantar erythrodysesthesia syndrome	PPNG	penicillinase-producing *Neisseria gonorrhoeae*
	pedal pulses equal and strong	PPO	permanent punctal occlusion
PPF	pellagra preventive factor		preferred provider organization
	plasma protein fraction		pump-prime only
	propofol (Diprivan)	PPOB	postpartum obstetrics
PPG	photoplethysmography	PPP	patient prepped and positioned
	portal pressure gradients		pearly penile papules
	postprandial glucose		pedal pulse present
	pylorus-preserving gastrectomy		peripheral pulses palpable (present)
PPGI	psychophysiologic gastrointestinal (reaction)		plaque-type palmoplantar psoriasis
			platelet-poor plasma
PPGSS	papular-purpuric "glove and socks" syndrome		postpartum psychosis
			preferred practice patterns
PPH	postpartum hemorrhage		proportional pulse pressure (SBP minus DBP)/SBP
	primary postpartum hemorrhage		
	primary pulmonary hypertension		protamine paracoagulation phenomenon
	procedure for prolapse and hemorrhoids	PPPBL	peripheral pulses palpable both legs
PPHN	persistent pulmonary hypertension of the newborn	PPPD	pylorus-preserving pancreatoduodenectomy
PPHTN	portopulmonary hypertension	PPPG	postprandial plasma glucose
PPHx	previous psychiatric history	PPPM	Parents' Postoperative Pain Measure
PPIX	protoporphyrin nine		
PPI	patient package insert		per patient, per month
	permanent pacemaker insertion	PPPY	per patient, per year
	postpacing interval	PPQ	Postoperative Pain Questionnaire
	prepulse inhibition	PPR	patient progress record
	Present Pain Intensity	PPr	periodontal prophylactics
	proton-pump inhibitor	PPRC	Physician Payment Review Commission
	Psychopathic Personality Inventory		
PPIA	parental presence during induction of anesthesia	pPROM	premature rupture of the membranes before 37 weeks gestation
PPIVMs	passive physiological intervertebral movements		
PPJ	pure pancreatic juice	PPS	pentosan polysulfate (Elmiron)
PPK	population pharmacokinetics		peripheral pulmonary stenosis
PPL	pars plana lensectomy		per protocol set
	posterior parietal lobe		postpartum sterilization

P

	post-pericardiotomy syndrome		patient relations
	postperfusion syndrome		perennial rhinitis
	postpoliomyelitis syndrome		per rectum
	postpump syndrome		pityriasis rosea
	prospective payment system		preferred route
	pulses per second		premature
PPSE	postprandial symptom exacerbation		profile
PPSS	peripheral protein sparing solution		progressive resistance
PPT	parts-per-trillion		prolonged remission
	person, place, and time		prone
	Physical Performance Test		Protestant
	posterior pelvic tilt		Puerto Rican
	postpartum thyroiditis		pulmonic regurgitation
PPTg	pedunculopontine tegmental		pulse rate
	nucleus	P=R	pupils equal in size and reaction
PPTL	postpartum tubal ligation	P & R	pelvic and rectal
PPTR	pulsed photothermal radiometry		pulse and respiration
PPU	perforated peptic ulcer	PR-2	Bennett pressure ventilator
	postpartum unit	PRA	panel reactive antibodies (organ
	prone press-ups		transplants)
PPV	pars plana vitrectomy		percent reactive antibody
	patent processus vaginalis		plasma renin activity
	percutaneous polymethyl-	PRAFO	pressure relief ankle-foot orthosis
	methacrylate vertebroplasty	PRAMS	Pregnancy Risk Assessment
	phakomatosis pigmentovascularis		Monitoring System
	pneumococcal polysaccharide	PRAT	platelet radioactive antiglobulin test
	vaccine	PRBC	packed red blood cells
	positive predictive value	PRC	packed red cells
	positive-pressure ventilation		peer review committee
PPVI	percutaneous pulmonary valve		People's Republic of China
	implantation		perirolandic cortex
PPVT	Peabody Picture Vocabulary Test		proximal row carpectomy
PPVT-R	Peabody Picture Vocabulary Test-	PRC2	polycomb repressive complex 2
	Revised	PRCA	pure red cell aplasia
PPW	plantar puncture wound	PrCa	prostate cancer
	posterior pharyngeal wall	PRCC	papillary renal cell carcinoma
	premature P-wave	PRCT	partial rotator-cuff tear
PPX	paclitaxel poliglumex		prospective randomized controlled
	pramipexole dihydrochloride		trial
	(Mirapex)	PRD	paired reflex depression
	prophylaxis		polycystic renal disease
PPY	packs per year (cigarettes)	Prdx6	peroxiredoxin 6
PPYLL	potentially productive years of life	PRE	passive resistance exercises
	lost		progressive resistive exercise
PQ	pronator quadratus		proton relaxation enhancement
pQCT	peripheral quantitative computed	PREA	Pediatric Research Equity Act
	tomography		(2003)
PQOCN	Psychiatric Questionnaire	Pred	prednisone
	Obsessive-Compulsive Neurosis	PREG	Pregestimil® (infant formula)
PQoL	perceived quality of life	Pre-M	urine specimen before prostate
PQRI	Physician Quality Reporting		massage
	Initiative (Medicare)	PREMIE	premature infant
	Product Quality Research Initiative	Pre-O_2	preoxygenation
PR	far point of accommodation	pre-op	before surgery
	pack removal	prep	prepare for surgery
	panoramic radiography (dental)		preposition
	partial remission	PRERLA	pupils round, equal, react to light
	partial response		and accommodation

P

PRES	posterior reversible encephalopathy syndrome	PROG	prognathism
			prognosis
PRE-SAT	presaturation (radiology)		program
prev	prevent		progressive
	previous	PROM	passive range of motion
PRFD	percutaneous radio-frequency denervation		premature rupture of membranes
		ProMACE	prednisone, methotrexate, calcium leucovorin, doxorubicin (Adriamycin), cyclophospha- mide, and etoposide
PRFNB	percutaneous radio-frequency facet nerve block		
PrFP	pre-exposure prophylaxis		
PRG	phleborheogram	PROMM	passive range of motion machine
PRH	past relevant history	Promy	promyelocyte
	postocclusive reactive hyperemia	PRO MYELO	promyelocytes
	preretinal hemorrhage		
PRHO	preregistration house officer	PRON	pronation
PRI	Pain Rating Index	PROP	physiologic-reduced oxygen protocol
	Patient Review Instrument		
prim	primary	PROS	prostate
PRIMIP	primipara (1st pregnancy)		prosthesis
PRIND	prolonged ischemic neurological deficit	PROs	patient-reported outcomes
		PROT REL	protrusive relationship
PR interval	part of the electrocardio- graphic cycle from onset of atrial depolarization on onset of ventricular depolarization		
		prov	provisional
		PROVIMI	proteins, vitamins, and minerals
		PROX	proximal
PRIS	propofol-related infusion syndrome	PRP	panretinal photocoagulation
			patient recovery plan
PRISM	Pediatric Risk of Mortality Score		penicllinase-resistant penicillin
PRIT®	pretargeted radioimmunotherapy		penicillin-resistant pneumococci
PRK	photorefractive keratectomy		pityriasis rubra pilaris
PRL	prolactin		platelet-rich plasma
PRLA	pupils react to light and accommodation		polyribose ribitol phosphate
			poor progression of R wave in precordial leads
PRM	partial rebreathing mask		
	passive range of motion		progressive rubella panencephalitis
	phosphoribomutase	PrP	prion protein
	photoreceptor membrane	PrPc	cellular prion protein
	prematurely ruptured membrane	PRP-D	*Haemophilus influenzae,* type b diphtheria conjugate vaccine
	primidone (Mysoline)		
PRMF	preretinal macular fibrosis	PRPP	5-phosphoribosyl-1-pyrophosphate
PRMS	progressive relapsing multiple sclerosis	PRP-T	polysaccharide tetanus conjugate vaccine
PRM-SDX	pyrimethamine; sulfadoxine (Fansidar)	PRRE	pupils round, regular, and equal
		PRRERLA	pupils round, regular, equal; react to light and accommodation
PRN	plaque reduction neutralization		
p.r.n.	as occasion requires	PrRP	prolactin-releasing peptide
PRNS	phrenic repetitive nerve stimulation	PRRs	proportional reporting ratios
PRNT	plaque-reduction neutralization test	PRS	Pain Rating Scale
PRO	patient-reported outcomes		photon radiosurgery system
	Professional Review Organization		Pierre Robin syndrome
	proline		postradiation sarcoma
	pronation		pressure-redistribution surface
	protein		prolonged respiratory support
	prothrombin	PRSL	potential renal solute load
prob	probable	PRSP	penicillinase-resistant synthetic penicillins
PROCTO	procotoscopic		
	proctology		penicillin-resistant *Streptococcus pneumoniae*
ProF	Profile of Fatigue		

P

PRSs	positive rolandic spikes
PRST	Blood Pressure, Heart Rate, Sweating, and Tears (scale to assess analgesic needs)
PRT	pelvic radiation therapy
	protamine response test
PRTCA	percutaneous rotational transluminal coronary angioplasty
PRTH-C	prothrombin time control
PRU	Plavix reaction units
PRV	polycythemia rubra vera
PRVC	pressure-regulated, volume-control (ventilation)
PRVEP	pattern reversal visual evoked potentials
PRW	past relevant work
	polymerized ragweed
PRX	panoramic facial x-ray
PRZF	pyrazofurin
PS	paradoxic sleep
	paranoid schizophrenia
	pathologic stage
	patient's serum
	performance status
	peripheral smear
	physical status
	plastic surgery (surgeon)
	polysulfone (filter)
	posterior subcapsular (cataract type)
	posterior synechiae
	posterior synechiotomy
	pressure sore
	pressure support
	protective services
	Proteus syndrome
	pulmonary stenosis
	pyloric stenosis
	pyrimethamine; sulfadoxine (Fansidar)
	serum from pregnant women
P/S	polyunsaturated to saturated fatty acids ratio
P & S	pain and suffering
	paracentesis and suction
	permanent and stationary
PS I	healthy patient with localized pathological process
PS II	a patient with mild to moderate systemic disease
PS III	a patient with severe systemic disease limiting activity but not incapacitating
PS IV	a patient with incapacitating systemic disease
PS V	moribund patient not expected to live

	(These are American Society of Anesthesiologists' physical status patient classifications. Emergency operations are designated by "E" after the classification.)
PSA	polysubstance abuse
	power spectral analysis
	product selection allowed
	Program Support Assistant
	prostate-specific antigen
	Pseudomonas aeruginosa
PsA	psoriatic arthritis
PSAB	pretreatment prostate-specific antigen
PSAD	prostate-specific antigen density
PSADT	prostate-specific antigen doubling time
PSAG	*Pseudomonas aeruginosa*
PSAP	prostate specific acid phosphatase
PSARP	posterior sagittal anorectoplasty
PSAV	prostate-specific antigen velocity
PSBO	partial small bowel obstruction
PSC	Pediatric Symptom Checklist
	percutaneous suprapubic cystostomy
	posterior semicircular canal
	posterior subcapsular cataract
	primary sclerosing cholangitis
	pronation spring control
	pubosacrococcygeal (diameter)
	pulmonary sclerosing cholangitis
PSCA	prostate stem cell antigen
PSCC	posterior subcapsular cataract
PSC Cat	posterior subcapsular cataract
PSCH	peripheral stem cell harvest
PSCP	papillary serous carcinoma of the peritoneum
	posterior subcapsular precipitates
PSCT	peripheral stem cell transplant
PSCU	pediatric special care unit
PSD	partial sleep deprivation
	pattern standard deviation
	peritoneal surface disease
	pilonidal sinus disease
	poststroke depression
	power spectral density
	psychosomatic disease
PSDA	Patient Self-Determination Act
PSDS	palmar surface desensitization
PSE	photosensitive epilepsy
	portal systemic encephalopathy
	pseudoephedrine
PSF	point spread function (radiology)
	posterior spinal fusion
PSG	peak systolic gradient
	polysomnogram
	portosystemic gradient

P

PSGN	poststreptococcal glomerulonephritis		primary Sjögren syndrome progressive systemic sclerosis
PSH	past surgical history postspinal headache	PSSP	penicillin-sensitive *Streptococcus pneumoniae*
PSHx	past surgical history	PSSV	Pre-Study Site Visit
PSI	passenger space intrusion (motor vehicle accident)	PST	paroxysmal supraventricular tachycardia
	Patient Safety Indicator		patient self-testing
	Physiologic Stability Index		Patient Service Technician
	pounds per square inch		penicillin skin testing
	prostate seed implant		platelet survival time
	punctate subepithelial infiltrate		posterior sub-Tenon (capsule)
PSIC	pediatric surgical intensive care		postural stress test
PSIG	pounds per square inch gauge		preoperative systemic therapy
PSIS	posterior superior iliac spine	p-STAT3	phosphorylated signal transducer and activator of transcription 3
PSM	patient self-management		
	pharyngeal squeeze maneuver	PSTJ	posterior subtalar joint
	positive surgical margin	PSTT	placental site trophoblastic tumor
	presystolic murmur	PSU	pseudomonas (*P. aeruginosa*) vaccine
PSMA	personal self-maintenance activities		
	progressive spinal muscular atrophy	PSUD	psychoactive substance use disorder
	prostate-specific membrane antigen	PSUR	Periodic Safety Update Reporting (EMEA)
PSMF	protein-sparing modified fasting (Blackburn diet)	PSV	peak systolic velocity
PSM-R	Optimism-Pessimism Scale, revised		persistent sciatic vein(s)
PSMS	Physical Self Maintenance Scale		pressure supported ventilation
PSN	peripheral sensory neuropathy		Pre-Study (Site) Visit
PSNP	progressive supranuclear palsy	PSVT	paroxysmal supraventricular tachycardia
PSO	Patient Safety Officer		
	pelvic stabilization orthosis	PSW	psychiatric social worker
	physician supplemental order	PSWC	periodic sharp wave complexes (electroencephalograph)
	Polysporin ointment		
	proximal subungual onychomycosis	PSWF	positive sharp wave fibrillations (electromyograph)
pSO$_2$	arterial oxygen saturation	PSWQ	Penn State Worry Questionnaire
PSOC	Puget Sound Oncology Consortium	PSY	presexual youth
P/sore	pressure sore	PSYCH	Psychiatry
PSP	pancreatic spasmolytic peptide		psychologic
	phenolsulfonphthalein		psychology
	photostimulable phosphor	PsyD	psychological distress
	posthumous sperm procurement	PSZ	pseudoseizures
	progressive supranuclear palsy	PT	cisplatin (Platinol)
PSPDV	posterior superior pancreaticoduodenal vein		parathormone
			parathyroid
PSQI	Pittsburgh Sleep Quality Index		paroxysmal tachycardia
PSR	posthumous sperm retrieval		patch test
	Psychiatric Status Rating (scale)		patellar tendon
PSRA	pressure sore risk assessment		patient
PSRBOW	premature spontaneous rupture of bag of waters		phacotrabeculectomy
			phage type
PSReA	poststreptococcal reactive arthritis		Pharmacy Technician
PSRT	photostress recovery test		phenytoin (Dilantin)
PSS	painful shoulder syndrome		phototoxicity
	pediatric surgical service		Physical Therapist
	phenotypic-sensitivity scores		physical therapy
	physiologic saline solution (0.9% sodium chloride)		pine tar
			pint

P

	posterior tibial		plasma thromboplastin components
	Preferred Term		post-tetanic count
	preterm		premature tricuspid closure
	pronator teres		prior to conception
	prothrombin time		pseudotumor cerebri
Pt	platinum	PT-C	prothrombin time control
pt	patient	PTCA	percutaneous transluminal coronary angioplasty
	pint (1 pint US = 473 mL; 1 pint UK = 568 mL)	PTCDLF	pregnancy, term, complicated delivered, living female
pT	pathologic tumor (various lettered and numbered stages, such as pT1)	PTCDLM	pregnancy, term, complicated delivered, living male
P/T	pain and tenderness	PTCL	peripheral T-cell lymphoma
	piperacillin/tazobactam (Zosyn®)	PTCR	percutaneous transluminal coronary recanalization
	prior to		
pT0	No tumor	PTCRA	percutaneous transluminal coronary rotational atherectomy
P1/2T	pressure one-half time		
P&T	pain and tenderness	PTD	percutaneous transpedicular diskectomy
	paracentesis and tubing (of ears)		period to discharge
	peak and trough		permanent and total disability
	permanent and total		persistent trophoblastic disease
	Pharmacy and Therapeutics (Committee)		pharmacy to dose
			pharyngotracheal duct
PTA	pancreas transplant alone		preterm delivery
	patellar tendon autograft		prior to delivery
	percutaneous transluminal angioplasty	PTDM	post-transplant diabetes mellitus
	peritonsillar abscess	PTDP	permanent transvenous demand pacemaker
	Physical Therapist Assistant		
	plasma thromboplastin antecedent	PTE	post-traumatic epilepsy
	posterior tibial artery		pretibial edema
	post-traumatic amnesia		proximal tibial epiphysis
	pretreatment anxiety		pulmonary thromboembolectomy
	prior to admission		pulmonary thromboembolism
	prior to arrival	PTE-4®	trace metal elements injection (there is also a #5 and #6)
	pure-tone average		
PTAB	popliteal-tibial artery bypass	PTED	pulmonary thromboembolic disease
PTAF	pressure transducer airflow	PTER	percutaneous transluminal endomyocardial revascularization
PTAS	percutaneous transluminal angioplasty with stent placement		
PTB	patellar tendon bearing	PTF	patient transfer form
	potassium taurine bicarbonate		Patient Treatment File
	prior to birth		pentoxifylline (Trental)
	pulmonary tuberculosis		post-tetanic facilitation
PTBA	percutaneous transluminal balloon angioplasty	PTFE	polytetrafluoroethylene
		PTFJ	proximal tibiofibular joint
PTBD	percutaneous transhepatic biliary drain (drainage)	PTFL	posterior talofibular ligament
		PTG	parathyroid gland
PTBD-EF	percutaneous transhepatic biliary drainage—enteric feeding		photoplethysmogram
		PTGBD	percutaneous transhepatic gallbladder drainage
PTBS	post-traumatic brain syndrome		
PTB-SC-SP	patellar tendon bearing-supracondylar-suprapatellar	PTH	parathyroid hormone
			post-transfusion hepatitis
PTC	papillary thyroid carcinoma		prior to hospitalization
	patient to call	PTHC	percutaneous transhepatic cholangiography
	percutaneous transhepatic cholangiography		
	Pharmacy and Therapeutics Committee	PTHrP	parathyroid hormone-related protein

PTHS	post-traumatic hyperirritability syndrome	PTS	patellar tendon suspension Pediatric Trauma Score
PTI	pressure-time integral prior to induction		permanent threshold shift post-traumatic seizure(s)
PTJV	percutaneous transtracheal jet ventilation		post-thrombotic syndrome prior to surgery
PTK	pancreas-after-kidney (transplantation)	pts	patients
	photexpertic keratectomy	PTSD	post-traumatic stress disorder
	phototherapeutic keratectomy protein tyrosine kinase	PTSD-T	post-traumatic stress disorder related to the transplant
PTL	preterm labor	PTT	partial thromboplastin time
	pudding-thick liquid (diet consistency)		pharyngeal transit time platelet transfusion therapy
	Sodium Pentothal		posterior tibial tendon protein truncation testing
PTLD	post-transplantation lymphoproliferative disorder (disease)		pulse transit time
		PTT-C	partial thromboplastin time control
PTLR	percutaneous transmyocardial laser revascularization	PTTD	posterior tibial tendonitis dysfunction
PTM	patient monitored	PTTG	pituitary tumor transforming gene
	posterior trabecular meshwork	PTTW	patient tolerated traction well
	post-translational modification	PTU	pain treatment unit
PTMC	percutaneous transvenous mitral commissurotomy		pregnancy, term, uncomplicated propylthiouracil
PTMDF	pupils, tension, media, disc, and fundus	PTUCA	percutaneous transluminal ultrasonic coronary angioplasty
PTMR	percutaneous transmyocardial revascularization	PTUDLF	pregnancy, term, uncomplicated delivered, living female
PT-NANB	post-transfusion non-A, non-B (hepatitis C)	PTUDLM	pregnancy, term, uncomplicated delivered, living male
PTNB	preterm newborn	PTV	patient-triggered ventilation
pTNM	postsurgical resection-pathologic staging of cancer		planning target volume (radiation therapy)
PTNS	percutaneous tibial nerve stimulation		posterior tibial vein
		PTWTKG	patient's weight in kilograms
PTO	part-time occlusion (eye patch)	PTX	paclitaxel (Taxol)
	please turn over		parathyroidectomy
	proximal tubal obstruction		pelvic traction
P-to-P	point-to-point		pentoxifylline (Trental)
PTP	phonation threshold pressure		phototherapy
	planned treatment period		pneumothorax
	posterior tibial pulse	PTX3	pentraxin 3
	post-transfusion purpura	PTZ	pentylenetetrazol
	pretest clinical probability (score)		phenothiazine
PTPM	post-traumatic progressive myelopathy	PU	paws up (dead) (Veterinary slang) pelvic-ureteric
PTPN	peripheral (vein) total parenteral nutrition		pelviureteral peptic ulcer
PTR	paratesticular rhabdomyosarcoma		pregnancy urine
	patella tendon reflex	Pu	ultrafiltrate pressure (ultrafiltration circuit line pressure)
	patient test results		
	patient to return	P & U	Pharmacia & Upjohn Company
	prothrombin time ratio	PUA	pelvic (examination) under anesthesia
PT-R	prothrombin time ratio		
PTRA	percutaneous transluminal renal angioplasty	PUB	pubic
		PUBS	percutaneous umbilical blood sampling
PTR-MS	proton transfer reaction mass spectrometry		purple urine bag syndrome

PUC	pediatric urine collector		prenatal vitamins
PUD	partial upper denture		projectile vomiting
	peptic ulcer disease		pulmonary vein
	percutaneous ureteral dilatation	Pv	*Plasmodium vivax*
PUE	pyrexia of unknown etiology	P & V	peak and valley (this is a
PUF	pure ultrafiltration		dangerous abbreviation, use peak
PUFA	polyunsaturated fatty acids		and trough)
PUFFA	polyunsaturated free fatty acids		pyloroplasty and vagotomy
PUJ	pelviureteral junction	PVA	polyethylene vinyl acetate
pul.	pulmonary		polyvinyl alcohol
PULP	pulpotomy		Prinzmetal variant angina
Pulse A	pulse apical	PVAD	prolonged venous access devices
PULSE OX	pulse oximetry	PVAI	pulmonary vein antrum isolation
		PVAM	potential visual acuity meter
Pulse R	pulse radial	PVAN	polyomavirus-associated
PULSES	(physical profile) **p**hysical		nephropathy
	condition, **u**pper limb functions,	PVAR	pulmonary vein atrial reversal
	lower limb functions, **s**ensory	PVB	cisplatin, (Platinol) vinblastine, and
	components, **e**xcretory functions,		bleomycin
	and **s**upport factors		paravertebral block
PUN	papillary urothelial neoplasm		porcelain veneer bridge
	plasma urea nitrogen		premature ventricular beat
PUND	pregnancy, uterine, not delivered	PVC	paclitaxel, vinblastine, and cisplatin
PUNL	percutaneous ultrasonic		polyethylene vacuum cup
	nephrolithotripsy		polyvinyl chloride
PUNLMP	papillary urothelial neoplasm of		porcelain veneer crown
	low malignant potential		postvoiding cystogram
PUO	pyrexia of unknown origin		premature ventricular contraction
PUP	percutaneous ultrasonic		pulmonary venous congestion
	pyelolithotomy	PVCD	percutaneous vascular closure
	previously untreated patient		device
PU/PL	partial upper and lower dentures	Pvco₂	partial pressure (tension) of carbon
PUPPP	pruritic urticarial papules and		dioxide, vein
	plaque of pregnancy	PVD	patient very disturbed
PUR	postoperative urinary retention		peripheral vascular disease
PURA	pressure-ulcer risk assessment		posterior vitreous detachment
PUS	percutaneous ureteral stent		premature ventricular
	preoperative ultrasound		depolarization
PUU	Puumala hantavirus	PVDA	prednisone, vincristine,
PUUV	Puumala virus		daunorubicin, and asparaginase
PUV	posterior urethral valves	PVDF	polyvinylidene difluoride
PUVA	psoralen (methoxsalen) plus	PVE	perivenous encephalomyelitis
	ultraviolet light of A wavelength		portal vein embolization
	(treatment)		premature ventricular extrasystole
PUW	pick-up walker		prosthetic value endocarditis
PV	papillomavirus	P vera	polycythemia vera
	Parvovirus	PVF	peripheral visual field
	pemphigus vulgaris	PVFS	postviral fatigue syndrome
	percutaneous vertebroplasty	PVGM	perifoveolar vitreoglial membrane
	per vagina	PVH	periventricular hemorrhage
	pharmacovigilance		periventricular hyperintensity
	plasma volume		pulmonary vascular hypertension
	polio vaccine	PVI	pelvic venous incompetence
	polycythemia vera		penile-vaginal intercourse
	popliteal vein		peripheral vascular insufficiency
	portal vein		peritumoral vascular invasion
	postoperative vomiting		Pleth variability index
	postvoiding		portal-vein infusion

P

	protracted venous infusion		private
	pulmonary valve insufficiency		proximal vein thrombosis
	pulmonary vein isolation	PVTT	tumor thrombus in the portal vein
PVK	penicillin V potassium	PVV	persistent varicose veins
PVL	Panton-Valentine leukocidin	PVWMD	periventricular white matter disease
	peripheral vascular laboratory	PW	pacing wires
	periventricular leukomalacia		patient waiting
	prosthesis paravalvular leak		plantar wart
PVM	paraverteabral muscle		posterior wall
	proteins, vitamins, and minerals		pulse width
PVMS	paravertebral muscle spasms		puncture wound
PVN	peripheral venous nutrition	P/W	presented with
PVNS	pigmented villonodular synovitis	Pw	withdrawal pressure (ultrafiltration
PVO	peripheral vascular occlusion		circuit line pressure)
	portal vein occlusion	P&W	pressures and waves
	pulmonary venous occlusion	PWA	persons with AIDS
PVo	pulmonary valve opening		P-wave axis
Pvo$_2$	partial pressure (tension) of	PWACR	Prader-Willi/Angelman critical
	oxygen, vein		region
	peripheral vascular occlusive	P wave	part of the electrocardio-graphic
	disease		cycle representing atrial
PVOD	pulmonary vascular obstructive		depolarization
	disease	PWB	partial weight bearing
PVOS	Pediatric Voice Outcome Survey		physical well-being
PVP	cisplatin (Platinol) and etoposide		Positive Well-being (scale)
	(VePesid)		psychological well-being
	penicillin V potassium	PWBL	partial weight bearing, left
	peripheral venous pressure	PWBR	partial weight bearing, right
	Photoselective Vaporization of the	PWC	personal watercraft
	Prostate (procedure)		physical working capacity
	polyvinylpyrrolidone		powered wheelchair
	portal venous pressure	PWCA	personal watercraft accident
	posteroventral pallidotomy	PWD	patients with diabetes
P-VP-B	cisplatin (Platinol), etoposide		person(s) with a disability
	(VP-16), and bleomycin		powder
PVR	peripheral vascular resistance	PWE	people with epilepsy
	perspective volume rendering	PWI	pediatric walk-in clinic
	portal vein reconstruction		perfusion-weighted (magnetic
	postvoiding residual		resonance) imaging
	proliferative vitreoretinopathy		posterior wall infarct
	pulmonary valve replacement	PWLV	posterior wall of left ventricle
	pulmonary vascular resistance	PWM	pokeweed mitogens
	pulse-volume recording	PWMI	posterior wall myocardial
PVRI	pulmonary vascular resistance		infarction
	index	PWO	persistent withdrawal occlusion
PVRQOL	Pediatric Voice-Related Quality-of-		per written order
	Life	PWP	pulmonary wedge pressure
PVS	percussion, vibration and suction	PWS	partial-wave spectroscopy
	peripheral vascular surgery		plagiocephaly without synostosis
	peritoneovenous shunt		port-wine stain
	persistent vegetative state		Prader-Willi syndrome
	Plummer-Vinson syndrome	PWT	pad weight test(s)
	pubovaginal sling		posterior wall thickness
	pulmonic valve stenosis		primary writing tremor
PVT	paroxysmal ventricular tachycardia	PWTd	posterior wall thickness at end-
	physical volume test		diastole
	portal vein thrombosis	PWV	polistes wasp venom
	previous trouble		pulse-wave velocity

P

Px	physical exam
	pneumothorax
	prognosis
	prophylaxis
PXA	pleomorphic xanthoastrocytoma
PXAT	paroxysmal atrial tachycardia
PXE	pseudoxanthoma elasticum
PXF	pseudoexfoliation
PXL	paclitaxel (Taxol)
PXS	dental prophylaxis (cleaning)
PY	pack-years (see pk yrs)
	person-year
PYAR	person-years at risk
PYE	person-years of exposure
PYHx	packs per year history
PYLL	potential years of life lost
PYP	pyrophosphate
PYP®	technetium Tc 99m pyrophosphate kit
PZ	peripheral zone
PZA	pyrazinamide
	pyrazoloacridine (a drug class of sedative/hypnotics)
PZD	partial zona drilling
	partial zonal dissection
PZI	protamine zinc insulin
PZR	posterior zygomatic root

Q

Q	Q sign; a patient whose mouth is open with their tongue hanging out when unconscious (slang)
	quadriceps
q	every (care must be taken to make sure that the handwritten q is not seen as a 9)
QA	quality assurance
QAC	before every meal (this is a dangerous abbreviation)
QALE	quality-adjusted life expectancy
QALYs	quality-adjusted life years
QAM	every morning (this is a dangerous abbreviation because the Q can be read as a 9 becoming 9 AM)
QAPI	quality assessment and performance improvement
QAS	quality-adjusted survival
QATTP	quality-adjusted time to progression
QB	blood flow
QC	quad cane
	quality checks
	quality control
	quick catheter
QCA	quantitative coronary angiography
Q compound	Chinese cucumber
QCSW	Qualified Clinical Social Worker
QCT	quantitative computed tomography
QD	dialysate flow
	every day (this is a dangerous abbreviation as it is read as four times daily-QID; use "once daily")
	quinupristin and dalfopristin (Synercid)
QDA	quality data code
QDAM	once daily in the morning (this is a dangerous abbreviation)
QDAY	every day
QDNs	quantum dot nanocrystals
QDPM	once daily in the evening (This is a dangerous abbreviation)
QDS	United Kingdom abbreviation for four times a day
QDs	quantum dots
QE	quinidine effect
QED	every even day (this is a dangerous abbreviation as it will be read as four times daily-QID)
	quick and early diagnosis
QEE	quadriceps extension exercise

qEEG	quantitative electroencephalography
QEMG	quantitative electromyography
QF	quadriceps femoris (muscle)
QFB	Qu'mico Farmacéutico Bi-logo (Chemist Pharmacist Biologist; Pharmacist in Mexico)
QF-PCR	quantitative fluorescence polymerase chain reaction
QFV	Q fever (*Coxiella burnetii*) vaccine
QGS	quantitative gate SPECT (single photon emission computed tomography)
q4h	every four hours
q.h.	every hour
qhs	once daily at bedtime, each day (this is a dangerous abbreviation as it is read as every hour-QHR or four times daily-QID)
QIAD	Quantitative Inventory of Alcohol Disorders
QIC	qualified independent contractor
q.i.d.	four times daily
QIDM	four times daily with meals and at bedtime
QIG	quantitative immunoglobulins
QIMT	quantitative intima media thickness
QIO	Quality Improvement Organization
QIW	four times a week (this is a dangerous abbreviation)
QJ	quadriceps jerk
QKD interval	Korotkoff sounds
QL	quality of life
QLI	Quality of Life Index
QLF	quantitative light-induced fluorescence
QLS	quality of life score
QM	every morning (this is a dangerous abbreviation as it will not be understood)
Qmax	maximal flow rate
QMB	qualified Medicare beneficiary
QMI	Q-wave myocardial infarction
QMRP	qualified mental retardation professional
QMT	quantitative muscle testing
q.n.	every night (this is a dangerous abbreviation as it is read as every hour)
q.n.s.	quantity not sufficient
QOC	quality of care
qod	every other day (this is a dangerous abbreviation as it is read as every day or four times a day-QID)

qoh	every other hour (this is a dangerous abbreviation as it is read as every day or four times a day-QID)
qohs	every other day at bedtime (this is a dangerous abbreviation as it is read as every hour-QHR or four times daily-QID)
QOL	quality of life
QOLIE-31	quality of life in epilepsy
QOM	quality of motion
QON	every other night (this is a dangerous abbreviation)
QOPI	Quality Oncology Practice Initiative (of the American Society of Clinical Oncology)
qPCR	quantitative polymerase chain reaction
qpm	every evening (this is a dangerous abbreviation as it is seen as 9 pm)
QPOS	Quality Point of Service
QP/QS	ratio of pulmonary blood to systemic blood flow
qqh	every four hours (United Kingdom)
qqs	every four hours (United Kingdom)
QR	quiet room
QRC	qualitative radiocardiography
QRDR	quinolone resistance-determining region(s)
QRE	quality-related event
QRNG	quinolone-resistant *N. gonorrhoeae*
QRS	part of electrocardio-graphic wave representing ventricular depolarization
QS	every shift
	quadriceps set
	quadrilateral socket
	Quality Services (Department)
	sufficient quantity
qs ad	a sufficient quantity to make
QSAR	quantitative structure-activity relationship
QSART	quantitative sudomotor axon reflex testing
Q sign	a patient whose mouth is open with their tongue hanging out when unconscious (slang)
QS&L	quarters, subsistence, and laundry
Qs/Qt	intrapulmonary shunt fraction
QSP	physiological shunt fraction
QSRL	Q-switched ruby laser
QT	the time between the beginning of the QRS complex and the end of the T-wave

qt	quart (US, 1 quart = 2 pints = 946 mL; UK, 1 quart = 1,137 mL)
QTB	quadriceps tendon bearing
QTC	quantitative tip cultures
QTc	the QTc interval is the length of time it takes the electrical system in the heart to repolarize, adjusted for heart rate (normal 350-440 milliseconds)
QTL	quantitative trait locus
QTP	quetiapine fumarate (Seroquel)
Q-TWiST	quality-adjusted time without symptoms (of disease) and toxicity
QTY	quantity
QUAD	quadrant
	quadriceps
	quadriplegic
QU	quiet
QUART	quadrantectomy, axillary dissection, and radiotherapy
QUEST	Quality of Upper Extremity Skills Test
QUICKI	quantitative insulin sensitivity check index
QUM	Quality Use of Medicines (Australia)
QuMA	quantitative microsatellite analysis
QUS	quantitative (bone) ultrasound
QW	every week (this is a dangerous abbreviation)
	Q-wave
q2w	every 2 weeks (this is a dangerous abbreviation)
q4w	every 4 weeks (this is a dangerous abbreviation)
QWB	Quality of Well-Being (scale)
QWE	every weekend (this is a dangerous abbreviation)
QWK	once a week (this is a dangerous abbreviation)
Q4wk	every four weeks (this is a dangerous abbreviation)
QWMI	Q-wave myocardial infarction

R

R	radial
	ragweed
	rate
	ratio
	reacting
	rectal
	rectum
	regular
	regular insulin (it is dangerous to use abbreviations for insulin therapy)
	resistant
	respiration
	reticulocyte
	retinoscopy
	rifampicin [part of tuberculosis regimen, see RHZ(E/S)/HR]
	right (this a dangerous abbreviation; spell out "right" to avoid surgical errors)
	Ritalin (methylphenidate) as in vitamin R
	roentgen
	rub
r	recombinant
®	rectal (rectally, rectum)
	registered trademark
	right (this is a dangerous abbreviation; spell out "right" to avoid surgical errors)
−R	Rinne test, negative
+R	Rinne test, positive
R-2	rohypnol (Roofies) (slang)
R10	nonstress (fetal well-being) test score reactive by 10 score
R15	nonstress (fetal well-being) test score reactive by 15 score
RA	radial artery
	radiographic absorptiometry
	rales
	readmission
	Regulatory Affairs
	renal artery
	repeat action
	retinoic acid
	rheumatoid arthritis
	right arm
	right atrium
	right auricle
	room air
	rotational atherectomy
RAA	renin-angiotensin-aldosterone
	right atrial abnormality

right atrial appendage

RAAA   ruptured abdominal aortic aneurysm

RAAS   renin-angiotensin-aldosterone system

RAB   rabies vaccine, not otherwise specified
rice (rice cereal), applesauce, and banana (diet)

RAB$_{DEV}$ rabies vaccine, duck embryo culture

RAB$_{FRhL-2}$ rabies vaccine, diploid fetal-rhesus-lung-2 cell line

RABG   room air blood gas

RAB$_{HDCV}$ rabies vaccine, human diploid cell culture

RABig   rabies immune globulin

RAB$_{PCEC}$ rabies vaccine, purified chick embryo cell culture

RAC   Recombinant DNA Advisory Committee
right antecubital
right atrial catheter

RACCO   right anterior caudocranial oblique

RACT   recalcified whole-blood activated clotting time

RaCT   randomized active control trial

RACZ   a procedure of dissolving lumbar scar tissue (epidurolysis)

RAD   ionizing radiation unit
radical
radiology
rapid antigen detection
reactive airway disease
reactive attachment disorder
renal (tubule) assist device
right axis deviation

RADCA   right anterior descending coronary artery

RADE   reactive airway disease exacerbation

Rad Imp   radium implant

RADISH   rheumatoid arthritis diffuse idiopathic skeletal hyperostosis

RADS   ionizing radiation units
rapid assay delivery systems
reactive airway disease syndrome

RADT   rapid antigen detection testing

RAE   right atrial enlargement

RAEB   refractory anemia, erythroblastic

RAEB-T   refractory anemia with excess blasts in transition

RAF   rapid atrial fibrillation

RAFF   rectus abdominis free flap

RAFT   Rehabilitative Addicted Family Treatment

RAG   room air gas

RAGE   receptor of advanced glycation endproducts

RAH   right atrial hypertrophy

RAHB   right anterior hemiblock

rAHF   antihemophilic factor (recombinant)

RAI   radioactive iodine
Resident Assessment Instrument

RAID   radioimmunodetection

RAIT   radioimmunotherapy

RAIU   radioactive iodine uptake

RALP   robotic-assisted laparoscopic prostatectomy

RALT   routine admission laboratory tests

RAM   radioactive material
rapid alternating movements
rectus abdominis myocutaneous

RA/MAC   regional anesthesia with monitored anesthesia care

RAMBAs   retinoic acid metabolism blocking agents

RAMP®   Rapid Analyte Measurement Platform

RAN   resident's admission notes

R$_2$AN   second year resident's admission notes

RANKL   receptor activator of nuclear factor kB ligand

RANTES   regulated upon activation, normal T cell expressed and secreted

RANZCOG   Fellows of the Royal Australian and New Zealand College of Obstetricians and Gynaecologists

RANZCP   Fellows of the Royal Australian and New Zealand College of Psychiatrists

RAO   right anterior oblique

rAOM   recurrent acute otitis media

RAP   renal artery pseudoaneurysm
request for advance payment
right abdominal pain
right atrial pressure

RAPA   radial artery pseudoaneurysm

RAQ   right anterior quadrant

RAP   recurrent abdominal pain
request for anticipated payment
Resident Assessment Protocol (long-term care)

RAPD   random amplified polymorphic DNA
relative afferent pupillary defect

RAPs   Resident Assessment Protocols

RAR   right arm, reclining

RARs   retinoic acid receptors

RAS   recurrent aphthous stomatitis
renal artery stenosis
renal artery stenting

	renin-angiotensin system	RBON	retrobulbar optic neuritis
	reticular activating system	RBOW	rupture bag of water
	retinoic acid syndrome	RBP	recurrent bacterial pneumonia
	right arm, sitting		retinol-binding protein
RASE	rapid-acquisition spin echo	RBRVS	Recourse-Based Relative Value
RASO	right anterior superior oblique		Scale (Medicare)
r-ASRM	Revised American Society for	RBS	random blood sugar
score	Reproductive Medicine		redback spider
	(score/staging) (Infertility with	RBT	rational behavior therapy
	endometriosis staging)	RBV	read-back verbal (order)
RASS	Richmond Agitation-Sedation Scale		right brachial vein
RAST	radioallergosorbent test	RBVO	read-back verbal order
RAT	right anterior thigh		right brachial vein occlusion
RA test	test for rheumatoid factor	RBX	ruboxistaurin
RATG	rabbit antithymocyte globulin	RC	race
RATx	radiation therapy		radiocarpal (joint)
RAU	recurrent aphthous ulcers		Red Cross
RAV	repeated and verified (refers to		report called
	verbal orders)		Respiratory Care
RAVLT	Rey Auditory Verbal Learning Test		retention catheter
R(AW)	airway resistance		retrograde cystogram
RB	recumbent bike		retruded contact (position)
	relieved by		right coronary
	retinoblastoma		Roman Catholic
	retrobulbar		root canal
	right breast		rotator cuff
	right buttock	R/C	reclining chair
R & B	right and below	R & C	reasonable and customary
RBA	right basilar artery		(charges)
	right brachial artery	RCA	radiographic contrast agent
	risks, benefits, and alternatives		radionuclide cerebral angiogram
	(discussion with patient)		regional citrate anticoagulation
RBAV	read back and verified (refers to		right carotid artery
	verbal orders)		right coronary artery
RBB	right breast biopsy		rolling circle amplification
RBBB	right bundle branch block		root cause analysis
RBBX	right breast biopsy examination	RC/AL	residential care, assisted living
RBC	ranitidine bismuth citrate	RCB	residual cancer burden
	red blood cell (count)	RCBF	regional cerebral blood flow
RBCD	right border cardiac dullness	RCC	rape crisis center
RBCM	red blood cell mass		Rathke cleft cyst
RBC s/f	red blood cells spun filtration		resectable colon cancer
RBCV	red blood cell volume		renal cell carcinoma
RBD	REM (rapid eye movement sleep)		right cranial-caudal (mammogram
	behavior disorder		view)
	right border of dullness		Roman Catholic Church
	right brain-damaged	RCCA	right common carotid artery
RbDe	residue-based diagram editor	RCCT	randomized controlled clinical trial
RBE	relative biologic effectiveness	RCD	refractory coeliac disease
RBF	renal blood flow		relative cardiac dullness
RBG	random blood glucose	RCDAD	recurrent *Clostridium difficile*-
RBILD	respiratory bronchiolitis-associated		associated diarrhea
	interstitial lung disease	RCE	right carotid endarterectomy
RBL	Roche Biomedical Laboratory	RCF	Reiter complement fixation
RBO	read back order (orders taken	RCF®	enteral nutrition product
	verbally or by telephone from a	RCFA	right common femoral
	physician)		angioplasty

	right common femoral artery	RCVS	reversible cerebral vasoconstriction syndrome
RCFE	residential care facility for the elderly	RCX	ramus circumflexus
RCH	residential care home	RD	radial deviation
RCHF	right-sided congestive heart failure		Raynaud disease
R-CHOP	rituximab (Rituxan), cyclophosphamide, doxorubicin (hydroxydaunorubicin), vincristine (Oncovin), and prednisone		reaction of degeneration
			reading disability
			reflex decay
			Registered Dietitian
			renal disease
RCIN	radiographic-contrast-media-induced nephropathy		respiratory disease
			respiratory distress
RCIP	rape crisis intervention program		restricted duty
RCL	radial collateral ligament		retinal detachment
	range of comfortable loudness		Reye disease
RCM	radiographic contrast media		rhabdomyosarcoma
	restricted cardiomyopathy		right deltoid
	retinal capillary microaneurysm		ruptured disk
	right costal margin	RDA	recommended daily allowance
RCMAR	Resource Centers for Minority Aging Research (NIH)		Registered Dental Assistant
			representational difference analysis
RCN	radiocontrast-agent-induced nephrotoxicity	RDB	randomized double-blind (trial)
RCO	revoked court order	RDCS	Registered Diagnostic Cardiac Sonographer
RCOG	Royal College of Obstetricians and Gynaecologists	RDD	renal dose dopamine
			Rosai-Dorfman disease
RCOT	revoked court-ordered treatment	RDE	remote data entry
RCP	respiratory care plan		respiratory disturbance events
	retrograde cerebral perfusion	RDEA	right deviation of electrical axis
	Royal College of Physicians	RDEB	recessive dystrophic epidermolysis bullosa
RCPM	raven-colored progressive matrices		
RCPSC	Royal College of Physicians and Surgeons of Canada	RDG	right dorsogluteal
		RDH	Registered Dental Hygienist
RCPT	Registered Cardiopulmonary Technician	RDI	respiratory disturbance (distress) index
RCR	replication-competent retrovirus (assay)	RDIH	right direct inguinal hernia
		RDLBBB	rate-dependent left bundle branch block
	responsible conduct of research		
	rotator cuff repair	RDM	right deltoid muscle
RCRA	Resource Conservation Recovery Act (U.S. Environmental Protection Agency)	RDMS	Registered Diagnostic Medical Sonographer
		RDMs	reactive drug metabolites
RCRI	revised cardiac risk index	RDOD	retinal detachment, right eye
RCS	repeat cesarean section	RDOS	retinal detachment, left eye
	reticulum cell sarcoma	RDP	random donor platelets
	Royal College of Surgeons		right dorsoposterior
RCT	randomized clinical trial	RDPE	reticular degeneration of the pigment epithelium
	Registered Care Technologist		
	root canal therapy	RDQ	Roland Disability Questionnaire
	Rorschach Content Test	RDS	research diagnostic criteria
	rotator cuff tear		respiratory distress syndrome
RCU	respiratory care unit	RDT	rapid diagnostic test
RCV	red cell volume		regular dialysis (hemodialysis) treatment
	right colic vein		
RCVD	received	RDTD	referral, diagnosis, treatment, and discharge
RCVP	retrograde coronary vein perfusion		
	rituximab, cyclophosphamide, vincristine, and prednisolone	RDU	recreational drug use

RDVT	recurrent deep vein thrombosis		regression analysis
RDW	red (cell) distribution width		regular
RE	concerning	Reg block	regional block anesthesia
	Rasmussen encephalitis	regurg	regurgitation
	rectal examination	rehab	rehabilitation
	reflux esophagitis	REL	relative
	regarding		religion
	regional enteritis	RELE	resistive exercise, lower extremities
	reticuloendothelial	REM	rapid eye movement
	retinol equivalents		recent event memory
	right ear (this is a dangerous abbreviation as it can be read as right eye)		remarried
			remission
			roentgen equivalent unit
	right eye (this a dangerous abbreviation as it can be read as right ear)	REMI	remifentanil (Ultiva)
		REMS	rapid eye movement sleep
			Risk Evaluation and Mitigation Strategies
	rowing ergometer		
^{186}Re	rhenium 186	REO	respiratory and enteric orphan (viruses)
R & E	rest and exercise		
	round and equal	REP	rapid electrophoresis
R ↑ E	right upper extremity		repair
R ↓ E	right lower extremity		repeat
RE✓	recheck		report
READM	readmission	REP CK	rapid electrophoresis creatine kinase
REAL	Revised European American Lymphoma (classification)		
		REPL	recurrent early pregnancy loss
REALM	Rapid Estimation of Adult Literacy in Medicine	repol	repolarization
		REPS	repetitions
REC	gingival recession	REPT	Registered Evoked Potential Technologist
	rear-end collision		
	recommend	RER	renal excretion rate
	record	RER+	replication error positive
	recovery	RERA	respiratory effort-related arousal
	recreation	ReRT	reirradiation
	recur	RES	recurrent erosion syndrome
RECA	right external carotid artery		resection
RECIST	Response Evaluation Criteria in Solid Tumors (guidelines)		resident
			reticuloendothelial system
	CR = complete response	RESC	resuscitation
	PR = partial response	RESP	respirations
	PD = progressive disease		respiratory
	SD = stable disease	REST	restoration
RECT	rectum		restriction of environmental stimulation therapy
REDA	Registered Eating Disorders Associate		
		RET	resistance exercise training
REDs	reproductive endocrine diseases		retention
reds	red blood cells		reticulocyte
RED SUBS	reducing substances		retina
REE	resting energy expenditure		retired
RE-ED	re-education		return
R-EEG	resting electroencephalogram		right esotropia
REEGT	Registered Electroencephalogram Technologist	ret detach	retinal detachment
		retic	reticulocyte
REF	referred	RETRO	retrograde
	refused	RETRX	retractions
	renal erythropoietic factor	REUE	resistive exercise, upper extremities
ref→	refer to	REV	reverse
REG	radioencephalogram		review

R

	revolutions		request for payment
	room eye view		request for proposal
RF	radiofrequency		right frontoposterior
	reduction fixation	RFS	rapid frozen section
	refill; refilled (prescriptions)		recurrence-free survival
	renal failure		refeeding syndrome
	respiratory failure		Reflux Finding Score
	restricted fluids		relapse-free survival
	rheumatic fever	RFT	radiofrequency treatment
	rheumatoid factor		respiratory function test
	ring finger		right frontotransverse
	right foot		routine fever therapy
	risk factor	RFTA	radiofrequency thermal ablation
	radiofrequency	RFTC	radiofrequency thermocoagulation
R/F	retroflexed	RFUT	radioactive fibrinogen uptake
R&F	radiographic and fluoroscopic	RFV	reason for visit
RF6	rejection-free survival at 6 months		right femoral vein
RFA	radiofrequency ablation	RFVTR	radiofrequency volumetric tissue
	right femoral artery		reduction
	right forearm	RG	regurgitated (infant feeding)
	right frontoanterior		right (upper outer) gluteus
rFVIIa	recombinant activated coagulation	R/G	red/green
	factor VII (NovoSeven)	RGA	right gastroepiploic artery
RFB	retained foreign body	rGBM	recurrent glioblastoma
	radial flow chromatography	RGCSE	refractory generalized convulsive
	residual functional capacity		status epilepticus
RFC	reduced folate carrier	RGEA	right gastroepiploic artery
RFCA	radiofrequency catheter ablation	RGM	rapidly growing *Mycobacteria*
RFD	residue-free diet		recurrent glioblastoma multiforme
RFDT	Reach in Four Directions Test		right gluteus medius
RFE	return flow enema	RGO	reciprocating gait orthosis
RFFF	radial forearm free flap	RGP	retrograde pyelogram (also RPG)
	(reconstruction of pharyngeal		rigid gas-permeable (contact lens)
	defect)	Rh	Rhesus factor in blood
RFFIT	rapid fluorescent focus inhibition	RH	radical hysterectomy
	test		reduced haloperidol
rFVIII FS	antihemophilic factor		relative humidity
	(recombinant), formulated with		rest home
	sucrose (Kogenate)		retinal hemorrhage
RFg	visual fields by Goldmann-type		right hand
	perimeter		right hemisphere
rFGF-2	recombinant fibroblast growth		right hyperphoria
	factor-2		room humidifier
RFI	request for information	Rh	rhodium
RFID	radio frequency identification	Rh+	Rhesus positive
RFIPC	Rating Form of IBD (inflammatory	Rh−	Rhesus negative
	bowel disease) Patient Concerns	RHA	rheumatoid arthritis (therapeutic)
RFL	radionuclide functional		vaccine
	lymphoscintigraphy		right hepatic artery
	right frontolateral	rHA	recombinant human albumin
RFLF	retained fetal lung fluid	RHABDO	rhabdomyolysis
RFLP·	restriction fragment length	rhAPC	recombinant human activated
	polymorphism (patterns)		protein C
RFM	rifampin (Rifadin)	RHB	raise head of bed
RFOV	reconstruction field of view		right heart border
	(radiology)	RH/BSO	radial hysterectomy and bilateral
RFP	Renal function panel (see page		salpingo-oophorectomy
	356)	RHC	respiration has ceased

	right heart catheterization	RHZ(E/S)/	a tuberculosis treatment
	right hemicolectomy	HR	regimen consisting of rifampicin,
	routine health care		isoniazid, pyrazinamide,
	rural health clinic		ethambutol, streptomycin,
rhCRP	recombinant human c-reactive		isoniazid, and rifampicin (also
	protein		see 2EHRZ/6HE)
RHD	radial head dislocation	RI	ramus intermedius (coronary
	relative hepatic dullness		artery)
	rheumatic heart disease		refractive index
	right-hand dominant		Registered Indian (Canada)
rh-DNase	dornase alfa (Pulmozyme)		regular insulin (it is dangerous to
rhEPO	recombinant human erythropoietin		use abbreviations for insulin
RHF	rheumatic fever vaccine		therapy)
	right heart failure		relapse incidence
RHG	right-hand grip		renal insufficiency
rhGAA	recombinant human lysosomal acid		respiratory illness
	alpha-glucosidase		retroillumination
rhGH	recombinant human growth		rooming in
	hormone	RIA	radioimmunoassay
r-hGH(m)	mammalian-cell–derived		reversible ischemic attack
	recombinant human growth	RIAC	rapid inflation, asymmetrical
	hormone (Serostim)		compression (device)
RHH	right homonymous hemianopsia	RIAO	right inferior anterior oblique
RHI	regular human insulin (it is	RIAT	radioimmune antiglobulin test
	dangerous to use abbreviations	RIBA	recombinant immunoblot assay
	for insulin therapy)	RIBC	residual infiltrating breast cancer
RHIA	Registered Health Information	RIC	reduced intensity conditioning
	Administrator		right iliac crest
RHINO	rhinoplasty		right internal carotid (artery)
RHIOs	regional health information	RICA	right internal carotid artery
	organizations	RICE	rest, ice, compression, and
RHIT	Registered Health Information		elevation
	Technician	RICM	right intercostal margin
RHIZ	rhizotomy	RICS	right intercostal space
RHL	right hemisphere lesions	RICU	respiratory intensive care unit
	right heptic lobe	RID	radial immunodiffusion
RhIg	Rhesus (blood Factor) immune		ruptured intervertebral disk
	globulin (RhoGAM)	RIDL	Release of Insects with a Dominant
rhm	roentgens per hour at one meter		Lethal (mutations)
RHO	right heel off	RIE	radiation induced emesis
Rho(D)	immune globulin to an Rh-negative		reactive ion etching
	woman		rocket immunoelectrophoresis
RhoGAM®	Rh$_O$ (D) immune globulin	RIF	rifampin
RHP	resting head pressure		right iliac fossa
rhPDGF	recombinant human platelet-		right index finger
	derived growth factor		rigid internal fixation
RHR	resting heart rate	RIFLE	Risk, Injury, Failure, Loss of
RHS	right-hand side		kidney function, End-stage
RHT	regional hyperthermia		kidney disease (classification)
	right hypertropia	RIG	rabies immune globulin
rHuEPO	recombinant human erythropoietin	RIGS	radioimmunoguided surgery
rHuKGF	recombinant human keratinocyte	RIH	right inguinal hernia
	growth factor (Palifermin)	RIHP	renal interstitial hydrostatic
Rhupus	coexistence of rheumatoid arthritis		pressure
	and systemic lupus	RIJ	right internal jugular
	erythematosus	RIJV	right internal jugular vein
RHV	right hepatic vein	RIMA	reversible inhibitor of monoamine
RHW	radiant heat warmer		oxidase-type A

	right internal mammary anastamosis	RLC	Registered Lactation Consultant
			residual lung capacity
	right internal mammary artery	RLD	Referenced Listed Drug (FDA)
RIN	radiocontrast-induced nephropathy		related living donor
RIND	reversible ischemic neurologic defect		remaining life expectancy
			right lateral decubitus
rINN	recommended International Nonproprietary Name		ruptured lumbar disk
		RLDP	right lateral decubital position
RINV	radiation-induced nausea and vomiting	RLE	right lower extremity
		RLF	retrolental fibroplasia
RIO	right inferior oblique (muscle)		right lateral femoral
RIOJ	recurrent intrahepatic obstructive jaundice	RLFP	Remaining Lifetime Fracture Probability
R-IOL	remove intraocular lens	RLG	right lateral gaze
RIP	radioimmunoprecipitin test	RLGS	restriction landmark genomic scanning
	rapid infusion pump		
	respiratory inductance plethysmograph	RLH	reactive lymphoid hyperplasia
		RLL	right liver lobe
	rhythmic inhibitory pattern		right lower lid
RIPA	ristocetin-induced platelet agglutination		right lower lobe
		RLN	recurrent laryngeal nerve
RIPV	right inferior pulmonary vein		regional lymph node(s)
RIR	right inferior rectus	RLND	regional lymph node dissection
RIS	radioimmunoscintigraphy	RLQ	right lower quadrant
	responding to internal stimuli	RLQD	right lower quadrant defect
	risperidone (Risperdal)	RLR	right lateral rectus
RISA	radioactive iodinated serum albumin	RLRTD	recurrent lower respiratory tract disease
RiskMAP	Risk Minimization Action Plan (FDA)	RLS	radial line scans
			resonance light scattering
RISO	right inferior superior oblique		restless legs syndrome
RISS	regular insulin sliding scale		Ringer lactate solution
RIST	radioimmunosorbent test		stammerer who has difficulty in enunciating R, L, and S
RIT	radioimmunotherapy		
	ritonavir (Norvir)	RLSB	right lower scapular border
	Rorschach Inkblot Test		right lower sternal border
RITA	right internal thoracic artery	RLT	right lateral thigh
RITE	receiver-in-the-ear	RLTCS	repeat low transverse cesarean section
RIVD	ruptured intervertebral disk		
RIX	radiation-induced xerostomia	RLUs	relative light units
RJ	radial jerk (reflex)	RLWD	routine laboratory work done
	right jugular	RLX	raloxifene (Evista)
RK	radial keratotomy		right lower extremity
	right kidney	RM	radical mastectomy
RKS	renal kidney stone		repetitions maximum
RKT	Registered Kinesiotherapist		respiratory movement
RL	right lateral		risk manager (management)
	right leg		risk model
	right lower		room
	right lung	R&M	routine and microscopic
	Ringer lactate	1-RM	single repetition maximum lift
	rotation left	RMA	reduction in metabolic activity
R → L	right to left		refused medical assistance
RLA	right lower arm		Registered Medical Assistant
RLB	right lateral bending		right mentoanterior
	right lateral border		Rivermead motor assessment
		RMB	right main bronchus
RLBCD	right lower border of cardiac dullness	RMBPC	Revise Memory and Behavior Problems Checklist

RMCA	right main coronary artery
	right middle cerebral artery
RMCAT	right middle cerebral artery thrombosis
RMCL	right midclavicular line
RMD	recommended maintenance dose
	restrictive myocardial disease
	rippling muscle disease
	risk management database
RMDQ	Roland and Morris disability questionnaire
RME	rapid maxillary expansion
	reasonable maximum exposure
	relative measurement error
	resting metabolic expenditure
	right mediolateral episiotomy
RMEE	right middle ear exploration
rMET	recombinant methioninase
RMF	respiratory muscle fatigue
	right middle finger
RMGIC	resin-modified glass ionomer cement (dental)
RMI	Rivermead Mobility Index
RMK #1	remark number 1
RML	right mediolateral
	right middle lobe
RMLE	right mediolateral episiotomy
RMLO	right medial-lateral oblique (mammogram view)
RMMA	rhythmic masticatory muscle activity
RMO	responsible medical officer
rMOG	recombinant myelin oligodendrocyte glycoprotein
RMP	right mentoposterior
	risk management program
RMR	resting metabolic rate
	right medial rectus
	root mean square residue
RMRM	right modified radical mastectomy
RMS	red-man syndrome
	Rehabilitation Medicine Service
	repetitive motion syndrome
	rhabdomyosarcoma
	Rocky Mountain spotted fever vaccine
	root-mean-square
RMS®	rectal morphine sulfate (suppository)
RMSB	right middle sternal border
RMSE	root-mean-square error
RMSF	Rocky Mountain spotted fever
RMT	Registered Music Therapist
	respiratory muscle training
	right mentotransverse
RMV	respiratory minute volume
RMW	respiratory muscle weakness
RN	radiation necrosis

	Registered Nurse
	right nostril (nare)
Rn	radon
R/N	renew
RNA	radionuclide angiography
	Restorative Nursing Assistant
	ribonucleic acid
	routine nursing assistance
RNAi	deoxyribonucleic acid interference
RN,BC	Registered Nurse, Board Certified (many clinical specialties)
RNC	Registered Nurse, Certified
RNCD	Registered Nurse, Chemical Dependency
RNCNA	Registered Nurse Certified in Nursing Administration
RNCNAA	Registered Nurse Certified in Nursing Administration Advanced
RNCS	Registered Nurse Certified Specialist
RND	radical neck dissection
RNEF	resting (radio-) nuclide ejection fraction
RNF	regular nursing floor
RNFA	registered nurse first assistant
RNFL	retinal nerve fiber layer
RNFLT	retinal nerve fiber layer thickness
RNI	reactive nitrogen intermediates
	rubella nonimmune
RNLP	Registered Nurse, license pending
RNP	Registered Nurse Practitioner
	restorative nursing program
	ribonucleoprotein
RNS	recurrent nephrotic syndrome
	replacement normal saline (0.9% sodium chloride)
RNST	reactive nonstress test
RNUD	recurrent nonulcer dyspepsia
RNV	radionucleotide ventriculogram
RNY	Roux-en-Y (gastric bypass surgery)
RO	reality orientation
	relative odds
	report of
	reverse osmosis
	routine order(s)
	Russian Orthodox
R/O	rule out
ROA	radiographic osteoarthritis
	right occiput anterior
ROAC	repeated oral doses of activated charcoal
ROAD	reversible obstructive airway disease
ROBE	routine operative breast endoscopy
ROBO	run over by owner (Veterinary slang)
ROC	receiver operating characteristic

	record of contact	ROSC	restoration of spontaneous circulation
	resident on call		
	residual organic carbon	ROSS	review of signs and symptoms
ROCF	Rey-Osterrieth complex figure	ROT	remedial occupational therapy
ROD	rapid opioid detoxification		right occipital transverse
	renal osteodystrophy		rotator
RODA	rapid opiate detoxification under anesthesia	ROU	recurrent oral ulcer
		ROUL	rouleaux (rouleau)
ROE	report of event	ROW	rest of (the) week
	right otitis externa	RP	radial pulse
ROF	review of outside films		radical prostatectomy
ROG	rogletimide		radiopharmaceutical
ROH	rubbing alcohol		Raynaud phenomenon
ROI	region of interest (radiology)		rectal pressure
	release of information		Registered Pharmacist
	request old information		responsible party
ROIDS	hemorrhoids		resting position
ROIH	right oblique inguinal hernia		restorative proctocolectomy
ROJM	range of joint motion		retinitis pigmentosa
ROL	right occipitolateral		retrograde pyelogram
ROLC	roentgenologically occult lung cancer		retropubic prostatectomy
			root plane
ROLL	radioguided occult lesion localization	RPA	radial photon absorptiometry
			recursive partitioning analysis
ROM	range of motion		Registered Physician's Assistant
	rifampicin 600 mg, ofloxacin 400 mg, and minocycline 100 mg		repolarization alternans
			restenosis postangioplasty
	right otitis media		retinitis punctata albescens
	rolling-over maneuver		ribonuclease protection assay
	rupture of membranes		right pulmonary artery
ROMA	representative oligonucleotide microarray analysis	RPAC	Registered Physician's Assistant Certified
Romb	Romberg	RPC	root planing and curettage
ROMCP	range of motion complete and painfree	RPCDBM	randomized, placebo-controlled, double-blind, multinational (study)
ROMI	rule out myocardial infarction		
ROMSA	right otitis media, suppurative, acute	RPCF	Reiter protein complement fixation
		RPD	removable partial denture
ROMSC	right otitis media, suppurative, chronic	RPDB	Registered Persons Database (Canada)
ROMWNL	range of motion within normal limits	RPE	rating of perceived exertion
			retinal pigment epithelium
RON	radiation optic neuropathy	RPED	retinal pigment epithelium detachment
RONTD	risk of neural tube defect		
ROP	retinopathy of prematurity	RPEP	rabies postexposure prophylaxis
	right occiput posterior		right pre-ejection period
Ropi	ropivacaine (Naropin)	RPF	regional progression-free
ROPS	roll-over protection structures		relaxed pelvic floor
ROR	the French acronym for measles-mumps-rubella vaccine		renal plasma flow
			retroperitoneal fibrosis
	retinoid-related orphan receptor	RPFT	Registered Pulmonary Function Technologist
	reporting odds ratio		
R or L	right or left	RPG	retrograde percutaneous gastrostomy
ROS	review of systems		
	rod outer segments		retrograde pyelogram
	rule out sepsis	RPGN	rapidly progressive glomerulonephritis
ROSA	rank-order stability analysis		

RPH	retroperitoneal hemorrhage	
RPh	Registered Pharmacist	
RPHA	reverse passive hemagglutination	
RPI	resting pressure index	
	reticulocyte production index	
RPICA	right posterior internal carotid artery	
RPICCE	round pupil intracapsular cataract extraction	
RPL	retroperitoneal lymphadenectomy	
RPLC	reversed-phase liquid chromatography	
RPLND	retroperitoneal lymph node dissection	
RPLS	reversible posterior leukoencephalopathy syndrome	
RPM/L	respirations per minute per liter	
RPN	renal papillary necrosis	
	resident's progress notes	
R₂PN	second year resident's progress notes	
RPO	right posterior oblique	
RPP	radical perineal prostatectomy	
	rate-pressure product	
	retropubic prostatectomy	
RPPS	retropatellar pain syndrome	
RPR	rapid plasma reagin (test for syphilis)	
	Reiter protein reagin	
rPS	residual pluripotent stem (cells)	
RPS	rhabdoid predisposition syndrome	
RPSGT	Registered Polysomnography Technologist	
RPSO	right posterior superior oblique	
RPT	Registered Physical Therapist	
RPTA	Registered Physical Therapist Assistant	
RPU	retropubic urethropexy	
RPV	right portal vein	
	right pulmonary vein	
RQ	respiratory quotient	
RQLQ	Respiratory Quality of Life Questionnaire	
RR	rate ratio(s)	
	recovery room	
	red reflex (normal eye reflex)	
	regular rate	
	regular respirations	
	relative risk	
	respiratory rate	
	response rate	
	retinal reflex	
	rotation right	
R/R	rales-rhonchi	
R&R	rate and rhythm	
	recent and remote	
	recession and resection	
	resect and recess (muscle surgery)	

	rest and recuperation	
	remove and replace	
RRA	radioreceptor assay	
	Registered Record Administrator (for newer title, see RHIA)	
	right radial artery	
	right renal artery	
RRAM	rapid rhythmic alternating movements	
RRC	cohort relative risk	
RRCT, no(m)	regular rate, clear tones, no murmurs	
RRD	removable rigid dressing	
	rhegmatogenous retinal detachment	
RRE	round, regular, and equal (pupils)	
RRED®	Rapid Rare Event Detection	
RREF	resting radionuclide ejection fraction	
RRI	renal resistive index	
RR-IOL	remove and replace intraocular lens	
RRM	reduced renal mass	
	right radial mastectomy	
	risk-reducing mastectomy	
RRMS	relapsing-remitting multiple sclerosis	
RRNA	Resident Registered Nurse Anesthetist	
rRNA	ribosomal ribonucleic acid	
RRND	right radical neck dissection	
RROM	resistive range of motion	
R rot	right rotation	
RRP	radical retropubic prostatectomy	
	recurrent respiratory papillomatosis	
RRR	recovery room routine	
	regular rhythm and rate	
	relative risk reduction	
RRRN	round, regular, and react normally	
RRRₛM	regular rate and rhythm without murmur	
RRS	rapid response system	
RRSO	risk-reducing salpingo-oophorectomy	
RRT	Registered Respiratory Therapist	
RRU	rapid reintegration unit	
RRVO	repair relaxed vaginal outlet	
RRVS	recovery room vital signs	
RRV-TV	rhesus rotavirus tetravalent (vaccine)	
RRW	rales, rhonchi or wheezes	
RS	Raynaud syndrome	
	rectal swab	
	recurrent seizures	
	Reed-Sternberg (cell)	
	Reiter syndrome	
	remote sensing	
	reschedule	
	restart	

	Rett syndrome	RSP	rapid straight pacing
	Reye syndrome		respirable suspended particles
	rhythm strip		restriction site polymophism
	right side		right sacroposterior
	Ringer solution	RS3PE	remitting seronegative symmetrical
	rumination syndrome		synovitis with pitting edema
R/S	reschedule	RSPV	right superior pulmomary vein
	rest stress	RSR	regular sinus rhythm
	rupture spontaneous		relative survival rate
R & S	restraint and seclusion		right superior rectus
R/S I	resuscitation status one (full	RSRI	renal:systemic renin index
	resuscitative effort)	RSS	Ramsey Sedation Scale
R/S II	resuscitation status two (no code,		reduced space symbologies
	therapeutic measures only)		representative sample sectioned
R/S III	resuscitation status three (no code,		Russell-Silver syndrome
	comfort measures only)	RSSE	Russian spring-summer
RSA	radiostereometric analysis		encephalitis
	recurrent spontaneous abortion	RST	rapid simple tests
	right sacrum anterior		rapid Streptococcal test
	right subclavian artery		right sacrum transverse
	Roentgen stereometric analysis	RSTs	Rodney Smith tubes
RSAPE	remitting seronegative arthritis with	RSV	respiratory syncytial virus
	pitting edema		right subclavian vein
RSB	right sternal border	RSVC	right superior vena cava
RSBI	rapid shallow breathing index	RSV$_{IGIV}$	respiratory syncytial virus immune
RSBQ	Rett Syndrome Behavior		globulin, intravenous
	Questionnaire	RSV$_{mab}$	respiratory syncytial virus
RSC	right subclavian (artery) (vein)		monoclonal antibody,
RScA	right scapuloanterior		intramuscular (palivizumab;
RSCL	Rotterdam Symptom Check List		Synagis)
RScP	right scapuloposterior	RSVP	rapid serial visual presentation
RSCS	respiratory system compliance	RSW	right-sided weakness
	score	RT	radiation therapy
rscu-PA	recombinant, single-chain,		Radiologic Technologist
	urokinase-type plasminogen		recreational therapy
	activator		rectal temperature
RSD	reflex sympathetic dystrophy		renal transplant
	relative standard deviation		repetition time
RSDS	reflex-sympathetic dystrophy		resistance training
	syndrome		Respiratory Therapist
RSE	rattlesnake envenomation		reverse transcriptase
	reactive subdural effusion		right
	refractory status epilepticus		right thigh
	right sternal edge		room temperature
RSI	rapid sequence intubation	R/t	related to
	Reflux Symptom Index	RTA	ready to administer
	repetitive strain (stress) injury		renal tubular acidosis
R-SICU	respiratory-surgical intensive care		road traffic accident
	unit	t-RA	tretinoin (*trans*-retinoic acid)
RSL	renal solute load	RTAE	right atrial enlargement
RSLR	reverse straight leg raise	RTAH	right anterior hemiblock
RSM	remote study monitoring	RTAT	right anterior thigh
RSNI	round spermatid nuclear injection	RTB	return to baseline
RSO	right salpingooophorectomy	RTC	Readiness to Change
	right superior oblique		(questionnaire)
rS$_{02}$	regional oxygen saturation		return to clinic
RSOC	regular source of care		round the clock
RSOP	right superior oblique palsy	RTCA	ribavirin

RTD	return to doctor		Rubinstein-Taybi syndrome
RT3D	real-time three-dimensional (echocardiography)	RTT	Respiratory Therapy Technician
		RTU	ready to use
RTER	return to emergency room	RT₃U	resin triiodothyronine uptake
rt.↑ext.	right upper extremity	RTUS	realtime ultrasound
RTF	ready-to-feed	RTV	ritonavir (Norvir)
	return to flow		rotavirus vaccine, not otherwise specified
RTFS	return to flying status		
RTH	right total hip (arthroplasty)	RTVrr	rotavirus vaccine, rhesus reassortant
RTI	reproductive tract infection		
	respiratory tract infection	RTW	return to ward
	reverse transcriptase inhibitor		return to work
	road traffic injuries		Richard Turner Warwick (urethroplasty)
RTIS	response to internal stimuli		
RTK	rhabdoid tumor of the kidney	RTWD	return to work determination
	right total knee (arthroplasty)	RTX	resiniferatoxin
RTKs	receptor tyrosine kinases	RTx	radiation therapy
RTL	reactive to light		renal transplantation
	right temporal lobectomy	RU	residual urine
RTLF	respiratory-tract lining fluids		resin uptake
RTM	regression to the mean		retrograde ureterogram
	routine medical care		returns demonstration (patient demonstrates an understanding)
RTMCI	real-time myocardial contrast perfusion imaging		
			right upper
RTMD	right mid-deltoid		routine urinalysis
rTMS	repetitive transcranial magnetic stimulation	R&U	radius and ulna
		RU 486	mifepristone (Mifeprex)
RTN	renal tubular necrosis	RUA	right upper arm
RTNM	retreatment staging of cancer		routine urine analysis
RTO	return to office	RUB	rubella virus vaccine
RTOG	Radiation Therapy Oncology Group	RUE	right upper extremity
		RUG	resource utilization group
RTP	renal transplant patient		retrograde urethrogram
	return to pharmacy	RUI	recurring urinary infections
	return-to-play	RUL	right upper lid
rtPA	alteplase (recombinant tissue-type plasminogen activator) (Activase)		right upper lobe
		RUOQ	right upper outer quadrant
		rupt.	ruptured
RT-PCR	reverse transcription polymerase chain reaction	RUQ	right upper quadrant
		RUQD	right upper quadrant defect
RT-PEPC	rituximab and thalidomide and prednisone, etoposide, procarbazine, and cyclophosphamide	RURTI	recurrent upper respiratory tract infection
		RUS	resonant ultrasound spectroscopy
		RUSB	right upper scapular border
RTPJ	right temporoparietal junction		right upper sternal border
RTR	renal transplant recipient(s)	RUT	rapid urease test
	return to room	RUTF	ready-to-use therapeutic food
RT (R)	Radiologic Technologist (Registered)	RUTI	recurring urinary tract infections
		RUV	residual urine volume
RTRR	return to recovery room	RUX	right upper extremity
RTS	radial tunnel syndrome	RV	rectovaginal
	raised toilet seat		residual volume
	real-time scan		respiratory volume
	Resolve Through Sharing		retinal vasculitis
	return to school		return visit
	return to sender		rhinovirus
	Revised Trauma Score		right ventricle
	Rothmund-Thomson syndrome		rubella vaccine

RVA	rabies vaccine, adsorbed	RVVC	recurrent vulvovaginal candidiasis
	right ventricular apex	RVVT	Russell viper venom time
	right vertebral artery	RW	radiant warmer
RVAD	right ventricular assist device		ragweed
RVCD	right ventricular conduction deficit		red welt
RVD	reference vessel diameter		respite worker
	regulatory volume decrease		rolling walker
	relative vertebral density	R/W	return to work
	renal vascular disease	RWIs	recreational water illnesses
	right ventricular dysfunction	RWM	regional wall motion
RVDP	right ventricular diastolic pressure	RWMA	regional wall motion abnormalities
RVE	right ventricular enlargement	RWP	ragweed pollen
RVEDP	right ventricular end-diastolic pressure	RWS	ragweed sensitivity
		RWT	relative wall thickness
RVEDV	right ventricular end-diastolic volume	Rx	drug
			medication
RVEF	right ventricular ejection fraction		pharmacy
RVET	right ventricular ejection time		prescription
RVF	Rift Valley fever		radiotherapy
	right ventricular function		take
	right visual field		therapy
RVG	radionuclide ventriculography		treatment
	Radio VisioGraphy	RXN	reaction
	right ventrogluteal	RXRs	retinoid X receptors
RVH	renovascular hypertension	RXT	radiation therapy
	right ventricular hypertrophy		right exotropia
RVHT	renovascular hypertension	RYGBP	Roux-en-Y gastric bypass (surgery)
RVI	right ventricle infarction		
RVIDd	right ventricle internal dimension diastole		
RVL	right vastus lateralis		
RVO	relaxed vaginal outlet		
	retinal vein occlusion		
	right ventricular outflow		
	right ventricular overactivity		
RVOT	right ventricular outflow tract		
RVOTH	right ventricular outflow tract hypertrophy		
RVOTO	right ventricular outflow tract obstruction		
RVP	right ventricular pressure		
RVPA	right ventricle-pulmonary artery (shunt)		
RVR	rapid ventricular response		
	renal vascular resistance		
	right ventricular rhythm		
RVS	routine vital signs		
RVSP	right ventricular systolic pressure		
rVSV	recombinant vesicular stomatitis virus		
RVSW	right ventricular stroke work		
RVSWI	right ventricular stroke work index		
RVT	recurrent ventricular tachycardia		
	renal vein thrombosis		
RV/TLC	residual volume to total lung capacity ratio		
RVU	relative-value units		
RVV	rubella vaccine virus		

S

S   sacral
second (s)
sensitive
serum
single
sister
son
South (as in the location 2S would
   be second floor, South wing)
sponge
Staphylococcus
streptomycin [part of tuberculosis
   regimen as in RHZ(E/S)/HR]
subjective findings
suicide
suction
sulfur
supervision
surgery
susceptible
/S/   signature
s̄   without (sin in Latin) (this is a
   dangerous abbreviation)
S'   shoulder
S_1 first heart sound
$S^{-1}...S^{-4}$ suicide risk classifications
S_2 second heart sound
S_3 third heart sound (ventricular
   filling gallop)
S_4 fourth heart sound (atrial gallop)
$S_1...S_5$ sacral vertebra or nerves
   1 through 5
SI..SIV symbols for the first to fourth heart
   sounds
SA   sacroanterior
salicylic acid
semen analysis
Sexoholics Anonymous
sexual activity
sinoatrial
skeletal abnormalities
sleep apnea
slow acetylator
Spanish American
spinal anesthesia
Staphylococcus aureus
subarachnoid
substance abuse
suicide alert
suicide attempt
surface area
surgical assistant
sustained action
Sa   Saturday

S/A   same as
   sugar and acetone
S&A   sugar and acetone
SAA   same as above
   serum amyloid A
   splenic artery aneurysm
   Stokes-Adams attacks
   synthetic amino acids
SAAG serum-ascites albumin gradient
SAANDs selective apoptotic antineoplastic
   drugs
SAARDs slow-acting antirheumatic drugs
SAB   serum albumin
   sinoatrial block
   Spanish-American Black
   spontaneous abortion
   Staphylococcus aureus bacteremia
   subarachnoid bleed
   subarachnoid block
SABA short-acting beta-2 agonist
SABR screening auditory brainstem
   response
SABs side air bags
SAC   safe abortion care
   school-age children
   segmental antigen challenge
   serial abdominal closure
   serum aminoglycoside
    concentration
   short arm cast
   substance abuse counselor
SACC short arm cylinder cast
SACD subacute combined degeneration
SACH solid ankle, cushioned heel
SACT sinoatrial conduction time
SAD   schizoaffective disorder
   seasonal affective disorder
   Self-Assessment Depression (scale)
   social anxiety disorder
   source-axis distance
   subacromial decompression
   subacute dialysis
   sugar and acetone determination
   superior axis deviation
SADBE squaric acid dibutyl ester
SADD Students Against Drunk Driving
SADL simulated activities of daily living
SADR suspected adverse drug reaction
SADRs serious adverse drug reactions
SADS Schedule for Affective Disorders
   and Schizophrenia
   sudden arrhythmic death syndrome
SADs severe autoimmune diseases
SADS-C Schedule for Affective Disorders
   And Schizophrenia – Change
   Version
SAE   sepsis-associated encephalopathy
   serious adverse event

short above elbow (cast)
splenic angioembolization

SAECG — signal-averaged electrocardiogram

SAEI — small artery elasticity index

SAEKG — signal-averaged electrocardiogram

SAESU — Substance Abuse valuating Screen Unit

SAF — Self-Analysis Form
self-articulating femoral
Spanish-American female
subcutaneous abdominal fat

SAFA — surgical atrial fibrillation ablation

SAFE — surgery, antibiotics, facial cleanliness, and environmental change (a trachoma control program)

SAFHS — sonic accelerated fracture healing system

SAG — sodium antimony gluconate

SAGAM — Scientific Advisory Group on Antimicrobials (EMEA)

Sag D — sagittal diameter

SAGE — serial analysis of gene expression

SAH — selective amygdalohippocampectomy
subarachnoid hemorrhage
systemic arterial hypertension

SAHA — suberoylanilide hydroxamic acid (vorinostat [Zolinza])

SAHS — sleep apnea/hypopnea (hypersomnolence) syndrome

SAI — self-administered injectable
Sodium Amytal® interview

SAL — salicylate
salmeterol (Serevent)
Salmonella
sensory acuity level
sterility assurance level

SAL 12 — sequential analysis of 12 chemistry constituents (see page 356)

SALAC — subacute lack of asthma control

SALAD — sound-alike, look-alike drug(s) (names)

SALK — surgical arthroscopy, left knee

SALS — sporadic amyotrophic lateral sclerosis

SAM — methylprednisolone sodium succinate (Solu-Medrol), aminophylline, and metaproterenol (Metaprel)
selective antimicrobial modulation
self-administered medication
severe acute malnutrition
short arc motion
sleep apnea monitor
Spanish-American male
systolic anterior motion

SAME — syndrome of arthralgias, myalgias, and edema

SAMe — *S*-adenosylmethionine (ademetionine)

SAMHSA — Substance Abuse and Mental Health Services Administration

SAMI — Substance Abuse, Mental Illness (program)

SAMPLE — symptoms/signs, allergies, medications, past medical history, last oral intake, and events prior to arrival (an EMT mnemonic used in initial patient questioning)

SAMS — spinal arteriovenous metameric syndrome (Cobb syndrome; juvenile type spinal arteriovenous malformation)

SAMU — Service d'Aide Médicale Urgente (French prehospital emergency system)

SAN — side-arm nebulizer
sinoatrial node
slept all night

SANC — short-arm navicular cast

SANDO — sensory ataxic neuropathy, dysarthria, and ophthalmoparesis

SANE — Sexual Assault Nurse Examiner

sang — sanguinous

SANS — Schedule (Scale) for the Assessment of Negative Symptoms
sympathetic autonomic nervous system

SAO — small airway obstruction
Southeast Asian ovalocytosis
superior anterior oblique

SaO$_2$ — arterial oxygen percent saturation

SAP — Sample Accountability Program
serum alkaline phosphate
serum amyloid P
standard automated perimetry
sporadic adenomatous polyps
statistical analysis plan

SAPAS — Standardized Assessment of Personality—Abbreviated Scale

SAPD — self-administration of psychotropic drugs

SAPH — saphenous

SAPHO — synovitis, acne, pustulosis, hyperostosis, and osteomyelitis (syndrome)

SAPS — Scale for the Assessment of Positive Symptoms
short-arm plaster splint
Simplified Acute Physiology Score

SAPs — shock-absorbing pylons

SAPS II	Simplified Acute Physiology Score version II	SAST	slide agglutination serotyping
SAPTA	stent-assisted percutaneous transluminal angioplasty	SAT	methylprednisolone sodium succinate (Solu-Medrol), aminophylline, and terbutaline
SAQ	saquinavir (Invirase)		saturated
	Sexual Adjustment Questionnaire		saturation
	short-arc quadriceps		Saturday
SAQ/r	saquinavir and ritonavir		self-administered therapy
SAR	seasonal allergic rhinitis		Senior Apperception Test
	Senior Assistant Resident		speech awareness threshold
	sexual attitudes reassessment		spontaneous awakening trial
	specific absorption rate (radiology)		subacute thyroiditis
	structural activity relationships		subcutaneous adipose tissue
	subacute rehabilitation (center)	SATC	substance abuse treatment clinic
SARA	sexually acquired reactive arthritis	SATL	surgical Achilles tendon lengthening
	SQUID (superconducting quantum interference device) array for reproductive assessment	SATP	substance abuse treatment program
		SATS	refers to oxygen saturation levels
	system for anesthetic and respiratory administration analysis	SATU	substance abuse treatment unit
		SAV	supra-annular valve
		SaV	sapovirus
SARAN	senior admitting resident's admission note	SAVD	spontaneous assisted vaginal delivery
SARC	seasonal allergic rhinoconjunctivitis	SAXS	small-angle X-ray scattering
SARK	surgical arthroscopy, right knee	SB	safety belt
SARM	*Staphylococcus aureus* resistant methicillin (French)		sandbag
			scleral buckling
SARMs	selective androgen receptor modulators		seat belt
			seen by
S Arrh	sinus arrhythmia		Sengstaken-Blakemore (tube)
SARS	severe acute respiratory syndrome		shave biopsy
SARS-CoV	severe acute respiratory syndrome-associated coronavirus		sick boy
			side bend
SART	sexual assault response team		side bending
	standard acid reflux test		sinus bradycardia
SAS	saline, agent, and saline		slide board
	scalenus anticus syndrome		small bowel
	Sedation-Agitation Scale		sodium bicarbonate
	see assessment sheet		spina bifida
	Self-rating Anxiety Scale		sponge bath
	short-arm splint		stand-by
	Simpson-Angus Scale		Stanford-Binet (test)
	sleep apnea syndrome		sternal border
	Social Adjustment Scale		stillbirth
	Specific Activity Scale		stillborn
	statistical applications software		stone basketing
	subarachnoid space		Swiss ball
	subaxial subluxation	Sb	antimony
	sulfasalazine (Azulfidine)	SB+	wearing seat belt
	synthetic absorbable sutures	SB−	not wearing seat belt
SASA	Sex Abuse Survivors Anonymous	SBA	serum bactericidal activity
SASH	saline, agent, saline, and heparin		standby angioplasty
SASP	sulfasalazine (salicylazo-sulfapyridine; Azulfidine)		standby assistant (assistance)
			Summary Basis of Approval
SASS	Social Adaptation Self-Evaluation Scale	SBAC	small bowel adenocarcinoma
		SBAR	Situation, Background, Assessment, and Recommendation (communication strategies)
SASSAD	six area, six sign atopic dermatitis (severity score)		

SBB	stereotactic breast biopsy	SBT	serum bactericidal titers
SBBO	small-bowel bacterial overgrowth		small bowel transplantation
SBC	sensory binocular cooperation		special baby Travesol
	single base cane		spontaneous breathing trial
	standard bicarbonate	SBTB	sinus breakthrough beat
	strict bed confinement	SBTs	spontaneous breathing trials
	superficial bladder cancer	SBTT	small bowel transit time
SBD	sleep-related breathing disorder	SBV	single binocular vision
	straight bag drainage	SBW	seat belts worn
SBE	saturated base excess	SBX	symphysis, buttocks, and xiphoid
	self-breast examination	SC	schizophrenia
	short below-elbow (cast)		Schwann cell
	shortness of breath on exertion		self-care
	subacute bacterial endocarditis		serum creatinine
SBF	splanchnic blood flow		service connected
SBFT	small bowel follow through		sick call
SBG	stand-by guard		sickle cell
SBGM	self blood-glucose monitoring		small (blood pressure) cuff
SBH	State Board of Health		Snellen chart
SBI	silicone (gel-containing) breast		spinal cord
	implants		sport cord
	something bad inside (undiagnosed		sternoclavicular
	cancer etc. discovered during		subclavian
	surgery) (Veterinary slang)		subclavian catheter
	systemic bacterial infection		subcutaneous (this is a dangerous
SBJ	skin, bones, and joints		abbreviation as it can be read as
SBK	spinnbarkeit		SL [sublingual]. Use subcut or
SBL	sponge blood loss		spell it out.)
sBLA	supplemental Biologic License		succinylcholine
	Application		sugar-coated (tablets)
SB-LM	Stanford-Binet Intelligence Test-		sulfur colloid
	Form LM		supportive care
SBM	stone basket manipulation		surveillance cultures
SBMA	spinobulbar muscular atrophy		systolic click
	(Kennedy disease)	s̄c	without correction (without
SBO	small bowel obstruction		glasses)
	specified bovine offals	S&C	sclerae and conjunctivae
SBOD	scleral buckle, right eye	SCA	sickle cell anemia
SBOE	surgical blood order equation		spinocerebellar ataxia
SBOH	State Board of Health		subclavian artery
SBOM	soybean oil meal		subcutaneous abdominal (block)
SBOS	scleral buckle, left eye		sudden cardiac arrest
SBP	school breakfast program		superior cerebellar artery
	scleral buckling procedure	SCa	serum calcium
	small bowel phytobezoars	ScA	*Scedosporium apiospermum*
	spontaneous bacterial peritonitis	SCA1	spinocerebellar ataxia type 1
	systolic blood pressure	SCA7	spinocerebellar ataxia type 7
SBQC	small-based quad cane	SCAD	segmental colitis associated with
SBR	sluggish blood return		diverticula
	strict bed rest		short chain acyl-coenzyme A
SBRN	sensory branch of the radial nerve		dehydrogenase
SBRT	stereotactic body radiation therapy		spontaneous cervical artery
SBS	serum blood sugar		dissection
	shaken baby syndrome	SCAN	suspected child abuse and neglect
	short (small) bowel syndrome	SCAP	scapula; scapulae; scapular
	sick-building syndrome		stem cell apheresis
	side-by-side	SCARMD	severe childhood autosomal
	small bowel series		recessive muscular dystrophy

SCARs	severe cutaneous adverse reactions		subclinical hypothyroidism
SCAT	sheep cell agglutination titer	SCh	succinylcholine chloride
	sickle cell anemia test	SCHF	subcondylar humerus fracture
SCB	stereotactic-guided core biopsy	SCHIP	State Children's Health Insurance
	strictly confined to bed		Program
SCBC	small cell bronchogenic carcinoma	SCHISTO	schistocytes
SCBE	single-contrast barium enema	SCHIZ	schizocytes
SCBF	spinal cord blood flow		schizophrenia
SCC	semicircular canals	SCHLP	supracricord hemilaryngopharyn-
	short course chemotherapy (for		gectomy
	tuberculosis)	SCHNC	squamous cell head and neck
	sickle cell crisis		cancer
	small cell carcinoma	SCI	silent cerebral infarct
	spinal cord compression		specific COX-2 inhibitor
	squamous cell carcinoma		spinal cord ischemia
SCCA	semi-closed circle absorber		spinal cord injury
	squamous cell carcinoma antigen		subcoma insulin
SCCa	squamous cell carcinoma	SCID	severe combined
SCCB	small cell cancer of the bladder		immunodeficiency disorders
SCCE	squamous cell carcinoma of the		(disease)
	esophagus		structured clinical interview for
SCCHN	squamous cell carcinoma of the		DSM-III-R
	head and neck	SCII	Strong-Campbell Interest Inventory
SCCI	subcutaneous continuous infusion	SCIP	Screening and Crisis Intervention
SCCOT	squamous cell carcinoma of the		Program
	oral tongue		Surgical Care Improvement Project
SCC/T	squamous sell carcinoma of the	SCIPP	sacrococcygeal to inferior pubic
	oral tongue		point
SCD	sequential compression device	SCIT	single-chain immunotoxin
	service connected disability		subcutaneous immunotherapy
	sickle cell disease	SCIU	spinal cord injury unit
	spinal cord disease	SCIV	subclavian intravenous
	subacute combined degeneration	SCI-WORA	spinal cord injury without
	sudden cardiac death		radiologic abnormalities
ScDA	scapulodextra anterior	SCJ	squamocolumnar junction
SCDM	soybean-casein digest medium		sternoclavicular joint
ScDP	scapulodextra posterior	sCJD	sporadic Creutzfeldt-Jakob
SCE	sister chromatid exchange		disease
	soft cooked egg	SCL	skin conductance level
	specialized columnar epithelium		symptom checklist
	spinal cord ependymoma	SCL-90	Symptoms Checklist—90 items
SCEMIA	self-contained enzymatic	ScLA	scapulolaeva anterior
	membrane immunoassay	SCLAX	subcostal long axis
SCEP	somatosensory cortical evoked	SCLC	small cell lung cancer
	potential	SCLD	sickle cell lung disease
SCF	slow coronary flow	SCLE	subacute cutaneous lupus
	special care formula		erythematosis
	stem cell factor	ScLP	scapulolaeva posterior
	supra ciliochoroidal fluid	SCLS	systemic capillary leak syndrome
SCFA	short-chain fatty acid	SCLs	soft contact lenses
SCFE	slipped capital femoral epiphysis		synthetic combinatorial libraries
SCFGT	Southern California Figure Ground	SCLV	supraclavicular
	Test	SCM	scalene muscle
SCG	seismocardiography		sensation, circulation, and motion
	serum Chemogram		split cord malformation
	sodium cromoglycate		spondylitic caudal myelopathy
	substitute care giver		sternocleidomastoid
SCH	schistosomiasis (*Schistosoma* sp.)		supraclavicular muscle
	vaccine		

SCMD	senile choroidal macular degeneration
SCMV	serogroup C meningococcal vaccine
SCN	severe congenital neutropenia
	special care nursery
	suprachiasmatic nucleus (nuclei)
SCNB	stereotactic core-needle biopsy
SCNs	subepidermal calcified nodules
SCNT	somatic-cell nuclear transfer
S/CO	signal-to-cut-off (ratios)
SCOB	Schedule-Controlled Operant Behavior
SCOH	services to children in their own homes
SCOP	scopolamine
SCOPE	arthroscopy
SCP	Scale for Contraversive Pushing
	secondary care provider
	sodium cellulose phosphate
	standardized care plan
SCPF	stem cell proliferation factor
S-CPK	serum creatine phosphokinase
SCPP	spinal cord perfusion pressure
SCQ	social communication questionnaire
SCR	silicon controlled rectifier (radiology)
	special care room (seclusion room)
	spondylitic caudal radioculopathy
	standard care regimen
	stem cell rescue
SCr	serum creatinine
sCR	soluble complement receptor
SCRIPT	prescription
SC/RP	scaling and root planing
SC-RNV	subcutaneous radionuclide venography
SCRT	sequential chemoradiation therapy
SCS	spinal cord stimulation
	splatter control shield
	stem cell support
	strain counterstrain (physical therapy)
	suspected catheter sepsis
SCSAX	subcostal short axis
SCSIT	Southern California Sensory Integration Tests
SCSVT	Southern California Space Visualization Test
SCT	Secondary Care Trust (United Kingdom)
	Sertoli cell tumor
	sex chromatin test
	sickle cell trait
	spiral computed tomography
	stem cell transplant
	sugar-coated tablet

SCTX	static cervical traction
SCU	self-care unit
	special care unit
	stroke care unit
SCUCP	small cell undifferentiated carcinoma of the prostate
SCUF	slow continuous ultrafiltration
SCUT	schizophrenia, chronic undifferentiated type
SCV	subclavian vein
	subcutaneous vaginal (block)
$ScvO_2$	central venous oxygen saturation
SCY	scytonemin
SD	scleroderma
	senile dementia
	sensory deficit
	severe deficit
	septal defect
	severely disabled
	sexual dysfunction
	shallow distance (aquatic therapy)
	shoulder disarticulation
	single dose
	skin dose
	sleep deprived
	solvent-detergent
	somatic dysfunction
	spasmodic dysphonia
	speech discrimination
	spontaneous delivery
	stable disease
	standard deviation
	standard diet
	step-down
	sterile dressing
	straight drainage
	streptozocin and doxorubicin
	sudden death
	surgical drain
S & D	seen and discussed
	stomach and duodenum
S/D	sharp/dull
	static/dynamic (balance)
	systolic-diastolic ratio
SDA	sacrodextra anterior
	same day admission
	serotonin/dopamine antagonist
	Seventh-Day Adventist
	steroid-dependent asthmatic
SDAC	single-dose activated charcoal
SDAT	senile dementia of Alzheimer type
SDB	Sabouraud dextrose broth
	self-destructive behavior
	sleep disordered breathing
	subdural bleeding
SDBP	seated diastolic blood pressure
	standing diastolic blood pressure
	supine diastolic blood pressure

SDC	serum digoxin concentration		somatropin deficiency syndrome
	serum drug concentration		Speech Discrimination Score
	Sleep Disorders Center		standard deviation score
	sodium deoxycholate		sudden death syndrome
SD&C	suction, dilation, and curettage		Symptom Distress Scale
SDD	selective digestive (tract)	SDSMs	standard deviation surface meshes
	decontamination	SDSO	same day surgery overnight
	sterile dry dressing	SDS-PAGE	sodium dodecyl sulfate –
	subantimicrobial dose doxycycline		polyacrylamide gel
	(dental; Periostat)		electrophoresis
SDDT	selective decontamination of the	SDT	sacrodextra transversa
	digestive tract		self-determination theory
SDE	subdural empyema		speech detection threshold
SDES	symptomatic diffuse esophageal	SDTM	Study Data Tabulation Model
	spasm	SDU	step-down unit
SDF	sexual dysfunction	SDUE	somatic dysfunction upper
	stromal-cell-derived factor		extremity
SDH	spinal detrusor hyperreflexia	SDV	single-dose vial
	subdural hematoma	SDX/PYR	sulfadoxine; pyrimethamine
SDHD	succinate dehydrogenase complex		(Fansidar)
	subunit D	SE	saline enema (0.9% sodium
SDI	Sandimmune (cyclosporine)		chloride)
	State Disability Insurance		self-examination
SDII	sudden death in infancy		side effect
SDL	serum digoxin level		sleep efficiency
	serum drug level		soft exudates
	speech discrimination loss		special education
SDLE	sex-difference in life expectancy		spin echo
	somatic dysfunction lower		staff escort
	extremity		standard error
SDM	soft drusen maculopathy		Starr-Edwards (valve, pacemaker)
	standard deviation of the mean		status epilepticus
	systolic-diastolic murmur		surgical excision
S/D/M	systolic, diastolic, mean	Se	selenium
SDMC	safety and data monitoring	S/E	suicidal and eloper
	committee	S & E	seen and examined
SD/N	signal-difference-to-noise ratio	SEA	sheep erythrocyte agglutination
SDNN	standard deviation of normal-to-		(test)
	normal beats		side-entry (venous) access
SD-NVP	single-dose nevirapine (Viramune)		Southeast Asia
SDO	surgical diagnostic oncology		Staphylococcal enterotoxin A
SD-OCT	spectral domain optical coherence		subdural electrode array
	tomography		synaptic electronic activation
SDP	sacrodextra posterior	SEAR	Southeast Asia refugee
	single donor platelets	SEB	Staphylococcus enterotoxin B
	solvent-detergent plasma		surrogate end-point biomarker
	stomach, duodenum, and pancreas	SEC	second
SDPTG	second derivative of		secondary
	photoplethysmogram		secretary
SDR	selective dorsal rhizotomy		size exclusion chromatography
	short-duration response		spontaneous echo contrast
	spatial dispersion of repolarization		steric exclusion chromatography
	standard deviation rate	SECG	scalp electrocardiogram
SDS	same day surgery	SECL	seclusion
	Self-Rating Depression Scale	SECPR	standard external cardiopulmonary
	Sheehan Disability Scale		resuscitation
	Shwachman-Diamond Syndrome	SE-CPT	single-electrode current perception
	sodium dodecyl sulfate		threshold

SED	sedimentation		sertraline (Zoloft)
	serious emotional disturbances		side effects records
	skin erythema dose		signal enhancement ratio
	socially and emotionally disturbed		surgical emergency room
	spondyloepiphyseal dysplasia	SERA-	technetium-99m
SeDBP	seated diastolic blood pressure	TEK	hexametazime
SEDDS	self-emulsifying drug-delivery	SERF	Severity of Exacerbation and Risk
	system		Factors
SED-NET	severely emotional disturbed -	Serial 7's	a mental status examination
	network		(starting with a 100, count
sed rt	sedimentation rate		backward by 7's)
SEEG	stereoelectroencephalographic	SER-IV	supination external rotation, type 4
SEER	Surveillance, Epidemiology, and		fracture
	End Results (program)	SERM	selective estrogen-receptor
SEF	spectral edge frequency		modulator
	(anesthesia-depth monitor)	SERO-	serosanguineous
SEG	segment	SANG	
	sonoencephalogram	SERP-	Skin Exposure Reduction
SEGRA	selective glucocorticoid-receptor	ACWA	Paste Against Chemical Warfare
	agonist		Agents
segs	segmented neutrophils	SERs	somatosensory evoked responses
SEH	spinal epidural hematomas	SES	sick euthyroid syndrome
	subependymal hemorrhage		sirolimus-eluting stents
SEI	subepithelial (comeal) infiltrate		socioeconomic status
SELDI	surface enhanced laser		standard electrolyte solution
	desorption/ionization	SeSBP	seated systolic blood pressure
SELDI-	surface enhanced laser desorption/	SET	signal extraction technology
TOF MS	ionization-time of flight mass		skin end-point titration
	spectrometry		social environmental therapy
SELEX	systematic evolution of ligands by		systolic ejection time
	exponential enrichment	SEV	sevoflurane (Ultane)
SELFVD	sterile elective low forceps vaginal	SEVO	Sevoflurane (Ultane)
	delivery	SEWB	social and emotional well-being
SEM	scanning electron microscopy	SEWHO	shoulder-elbow-wrist-hand orthosis
	semen	SF	salt-free
	slow eye movement		saturated fat
	standard error of mean		scarlet fever
	systolic ejection murmur		seizure frequency
SEMD	spondyloepimetaphyseal dysplasias		seminal fluid
sEMG	surface electromyography		skull fracture
SEMI	subendocardial myocardial		small finger
	infarction		soft feces
SEN	spray each nostril		sound field
SENS	sensitivity		spinal fluid
	sensorium		starch-free
SEOC	serous epithelial ovarian carcinoma		stone-free
SEP	multiple sclerosis (French)		sugar-free
	separate		symptom-free
	separation		synovial fluid
	serum electrophoresis	S&F	slip and fall
	somatosensory evoked potential		soft and flat
	syringe exchange program		store and forward
	systolic ejection period	SF-6	sulfahexafluoride
SEPS	subdural evacuation port system	SF 36	36-item short form health survey
	subfascial endoscopic perforator	SFA	saturated fatty acids
	surgery		superficial femoral artery
SEQ	sequela	SFB	single frequency bioimpedance
SER	scanning equalization radiography	SFC	spinal fluid count

	subarachnoid fluid collection
SFD	scaphoid fossa depression
	small for dates
SFDA	Chinese State Food and Drug Administration
SFE	supercritical fluid extraction
SFEMG	single-fiber electromyography
SFH	schizophrenia family history
SFJ	saphenofemoral junction
SFM	scanning force microscopy
	simple facemask
SF-MPQ	Short-Form, McGill Pain questionnaire
SFN	sulforaphane
SFNM	subfoveal neovascular membranes
SFOV	scan field of view (radiology)
SFP	simulated fluorescence process
	simultaneous foveal perception
	spinal fluid pressure
SFPT	standard fixation preference test
SFRT	stereotactic fractionated radiotherapy
SFS	split function studies
SFT	solitary fibrous tumor
SFTR	sagittal, frontal, transverse, rotation
SFTS	stenosing flexor tenosynovitis
SFTs	solitary fibrous tumors
SFUP	surgical follow-up
SFV	Semliki Forest virus
	simian foamy viruses
	superficial femoral vein
SFW	shell fragment wound
SFWB	social/family well-being
SFWD	symptom-free walking distance
SG	salivary gland
	scrotography
	serum glucose
	side glide
	skin graft
	specific gravity
	Swan-Ganz (catheter)
S/G	swallow/gag
SGA	small for gestational age
	subjective global assessment (dietary history and physical examination)
	substantial gainful activity (employment)
SGAR	spectral gradient acoustic reflectometry
SGAs	second-generation antihistamines
	second-generation antipsychotics
SGB	Swiss gym ball
SGC	Swan-Ganz catheter
SGCNB	stereotactic guided core-needle biopsy
SGD	salivary gland dysfunction
	specific granule deficiency

	specific growth delay
	speech generating device
	straight gravity drainage
	sweat gland density
SGE	significant glandular enlargement
SGHL	superior glenohumeral ligament
s̄ gl	without correction (without glasses)
SGM	serum glucose monitoring
SGNFD	sweat gland nerve fiber density
SGOT	serum glutamic oxalo-acetic transaminase (same as AST)
SGP	Schering-Plough Corporation
SGPT	serum glutamate pyruvate transaminase (same as ALT)
SGRQ-A	St. George's Respiratory Questionnaire translated into American English
SGS	second-generation sulfonylurea
	subglottic stenosis
sGS	surgical Gleason score
SGTCS	secondarily generalized tonic-clonic seizures
SH	sclerosing hemangioma
	self-help
	serum hepatitis
	sexual harassment
	short
	shoulder
	shower
	social history
	sulfhydryl (group)
	surgical history
	systemic hypertension
	thiol (-SH)
–SH	thiol
S&H	speech and hearing
	suicidal and homicidal
S/H	suicidal/homicidal ideation
SH2	sarc homology region 2
SHA	super-heated aerosol
SHAFT	shopping, housework, accounting (bills), food preparation, and transportation (driving); (instrumental activities of daily living)
SHAL	standard hyperalimentation
SHAS	supravalvular hypertrophic aortic stenosis
S Hb	sickle hemoglobin screen
SHBG	sex hormone-binding globulin
sHBO$_2$T	systemic hyperbaric oxygen therapy
SHC	subsequent hospital care
SHCP	spastic hemiparetic cerebral palsy
SHE	sexual health education
SHEENT	skin, head, eyes, ears, nose, and throat
SHF	systolic heart failure

SHG	shigellosis (*Shigella* sp.) vaccine		Standard Industrial Classification
	sonohysterography	SICD	sudden infant crib death
SHGT	somatic-cell human gene therapy	SICOG	Southern Italy Cooperative
SHI	Self-Harm Inventory		Oncology Group
	standard heparin infusion	SICT	selective intracoronary
Shig	*Shigella*		thrombolysis
SHIV	simian-human immunodeficiency	SICU	surgical intensive care unit
	virus	SID	source to image distance
SHL	sudden hearing loss		(radiology)
	supraglottic horizontal		strong ion difference
	laryngectomy	*SID*	once daily (used in veterinary
SHLD	shoulder		medicine)
SHMB	severe hypersensitivity to mosquito	SIDA	French and Spanish abbreviation
	bites		for AIDS
SHO	Senior House Officer		stable isotope dilution assay
SHOX	<u>S</u>hort stature <u>HO</u>meobo<u>X</u> (gene)	SIDAM	structured interview for the
SHP	secondary hypertension, pulmonary		diagnosis of dementia of
SHPT	secondary hyperparathyroidism		Alzheimer type
SHR	scapulohumeral rhythm	SIDAM-A	structured interview for the
SHRC	shortened, held, resisted		diagnosis of dementia of the
	contraction		Alzheimer type, multi-infarct
S-HRV	short-term heart rate variability		dementia, and dementias of other
SHS	second-hand smoke		etiology according to ICD-10
	sliding hip screw		and DSM-III-R
	student health service	SIDD	syndrome of isolated diastolic
SHV	short hepatic vein		dysfunction
	sulfhydryl variant	SIDERO	siderocyte
SHx	social history	SIDFF	superimposed dorsiflexion of foot
SI	International System of Units	SIDS	sudden infant death syndrome
	sacroiliac	SIEA	superficial inferior epigastric artery
	sagittal index	SIEDy	Structured Interview on Erectile
	sector iridectomy		Dysfunction
	self-inflicted	SIEP	serum immunoelectrophoresis
	sensory integration	*SIG*	let it be marked (appears on
	seriously ill		prescription before directions
	sexual intercourse		for patient)
	signal intensity		sigmoidoscopy
	small intestine	SIGECAPS	**S**leep changes, **I**nterest (loss),
	strict isolation		**G**uilt (worthlessness), **E**nergy
	stress incontinence		(lack), **C**oncentration (difficulty),
	stroke index		**A**ppetite (weight loss),
	suicidal ideation		**P**sychomotor (anxiety or
Si	silicon		lethargic), **S**uicidal (death
S & I	suction and irrigation		preoccupation); (SIG-E-CAPS, a
	support and interpretation		mnemonic for depression
SIA	small intestinal atresia		indicators)
SIADH	syndrome of inappropriate	Signal 99	patient in cardiac or respiratory
	antidiuretic hormone secretion		distress
SIAT	supervised intermittent ambulatory	sign(s)	see ABCD, ACHES, M, O, Q,
	treatment		STR, and VS
SIB	self-inflating bulb	SI/HI	suicidal/homicidal ideations
	self-injurious behavior	SIJ	sacroiliac joint
SIBC	serum iron-binding capacity	SIJS	sacroiliac joint syndrome
SIBO	small intestinal bacterial	SIL	seriously ill list
	overgrowth		sister-in-law
sibs	siblings		squamous intraepithelial lesion
SIC	self-intermittent catherization	SILFVD	sterile indicated low forceps
	squamous intraepithelial cells		vaginal delivery

SILS	single-incision laparoscopic surgery	SIT BAL	sitting balance
SILT	sensation intact to light touch	SIT TOL	sitting tolerance
SILV	simultaneous independent lung ventilation	SIUP	single intrauterine pregnancy
		SIV	self-inflicted violence
SIM	selective ion monitoring		simian immunodeficiency virus
	Similac®	SIVB	self-inflicted violent behavior
	simulation	SIVD	subcortical ischemic vascular dementia (disease)
	surface-induced mineralization		
SIMCU	surgical intermediate care unit	SIVP	slow intravenous push
Sim c Fe	Similac with iron®	SIW	self-inflicted wound
SIMS	secondary ion mass spectroscopy	SJ	surgical jejunostomy
SIMV	synchronized intermittent mandatory ventilation	SJC	swollen joint count
		SJCRH	St. Jude Children's Research Hospital (preferred abbreviation "St. Jude")
SIN	salpingitis isthmica nodose		
SIOD	Schimke immuno-osseous dysplasia		
		SJM	St. Jude Medical (heart valve prosthesis)
SIP	Sickness Impact Profile		
	spontaneous intestinal perforation	S-JRA	systemic juvenile rheumatoid arthritis
	stroke in progression		
	subcutaneously implanted ports	SJS	Schwartz-Jampel syndrome
	sympathetically independent pain		Stevens-Johnson syndrome
SIQ	sick in quarters		Swyer-James syndrome
SIQ-JR	Suicidal Ideation Questionnaire-Junior	S_{jv02}	jugular venous oxygen saturation
		SK	seborrheic keratosis
SIR	standardized incidence rate (ratio)		senile keratosis
siRNA	small interfering ribonucleic acid		solar keratosis
SIRGE	A drug-waste collection and recycling system used in the European Union		streptokinase
		S & K	single and keeping (baby)
		SKAO	supracondylar knee-ankle orthosis
SIRPIDs	stimulus-induced rhythmic, periodic, or ictal discharges	SKAs	skills, knowledge, and abilities (ratings)
SIRS	systemic inflammatory response syndrome	SKB	SmithKline Beecham
		SKC	single knee to chest
SIRT	selective internal radiation therapy	SKINT	skinfold thickness
SIS	saline infusion sonohysterography	SK-SD	streptokinase streptodornase
	sister	SKTC	single-knee to chest (stretch)
	small intestinal submucosa	SKU	stock keeping unit (related to product identification)
	Surgical Infection Stratification (system)		
		SKY	spectral karyotyping
SISI	Short Increment Sensitivity Index	SL	scapholunate
SISS	severe invasion streptococcal syndrome		secondary leukemia
			sensation level
SIT	serum inhibitory titers		sentinel lymphadenectomy
	silicon-intensified target		serious list
	Slossen Intelligence Test		shortleg
	specific immunotherapy (allergy)		side-lying
	sperm immobilization test		staging laparoscopy
	structured interrupted therapy		slight
	supraspinatus, infraspinatus, teres (insertions)		sublingual
		S/L	slit lamp (examination)
	surgical intensive therapy	SLA	sacrolaeva anterior
SITA	standard infertility treatment algorithm		sex and love addictions
			slide latex agglutination
	Swedish Interactive Thresholding Algorithm		The Satisfaction with Life Areas
		SLAA	Sex and Love Addicts Anonymous
SITA-SAP	Swedish Interactive Threshold Algorithm-standard automated perimetry	SLAC	scapholunate advanced collapse
		SLat	time to onset of sleep
		SLAM	Systemic Lupus Activity Measure

SLAP	serum leucine amino-peptidase	SLOS	Smith-Lemli-Opitz syndrome
	superior labral anteroposterior (shoulder lesion)	SLP	scanning laser polarimeter single-limb progression
SLB	short leg brace surgical lung biopsy		Speech Language Pathologist speech language pathology
SLBB	single-living baby boy		superficial lamina propria
SLBG	single-living baby girl	SLPI	secretory leukocyte protease inhibitor
SLC	short leg cast		
SLCC	short leg cylinder cast	SLPMS	short-leg posterior-molded splint
SLCG	sulfolithocholyglycine	SLR	straight-leg raising
SLCT	Sertoli-Leydig cell tumor	SLRS	stereotactic linac radiosurgery
SLD	seizure-line discharges	SLRT	straight-leg raising tenderness
	semantic linked data		straight-leg raising test
	specific language disorder	SLS	second-look sonography
	stealth liposomal doxorubicin		short leg splint
	sum of longest diameters		shrinking lungs syndrome
SLE	slit-lamp examination		single leg stance
	St. Louis encephalitis		single limb support
	systemic lupus erythematosus	SLT	sacrolaeva transversa
SLeA	sialyl Lewis a (antigen)		scanning laser tomography
SLEDAI	Systemic Lupus Erythematosus Disease Activity Index		selective laser trabeculoplasty single lung transplantation
SLEX	slit-lamp examination (biomicroscopy)		smokeless tobacco Speech Language Therapist (therapy)
SLex	sialyl Lewis x (antigen)		spontaneous labor at term
SLFVD	sterile low forceps vaginal delivery		swing light test
SLGXT	symptom-limited graded exercise test	SLT-I	Shiga-like toxin I
SLI	severe limb ischemia	SLTA	severe life-threatening asthma
	specific language impairment		standard language test for aphasia
SLIT	sublingual immunotherapy	SLTEC	Shiga-like toxin-producing
SLK	superior limbic keratoconjunctivitis		*Escherichia coli*
SLL	second-look laparotomy	sl. tr.	slight trace
	small lymphocytic lymphoma	SLUD	salivation, lacrimation, urination, and defecation
SLMFVD	sterile low midforceps vaginal delivery	SLUDGE	**s**alivation, **l**acrimation, **u**rination, **d**iarrhea, **g**astrointestinal upset, and **e**mesis (signs and symptoms of cholinergic excess)
SLMMS	slightly more marked since		
SLMP	since last menstrual period		
S-LMP	serous tumor(s) of low malignant potential	SLV	since last visit
SLN	sentinel lymph node(s)	SLVD	systolic left ventricular dysfunction
	superior laryngeal nerve		
SLNB	sentinel lymph node biopsy	SLWB	severely low birth weight
SLND	sentinel lymph node detection	SLWC	short leg walking cast
SLNM	sentinel lymph node mapping	SM	sadomasochism
SLNTG	sublingual nitroglycerin		service mark (such as The Pause that Refreshes)
SLNWBC	short leg nonweight-bearing cast		setup margin (for radiotherapy)
SLNWC	short leg nonwalking cast		skim milk
SLO	scanning laser ophthalmoscope (ophthalmoscopy)		small sports medicine
	second-look operation		Stairmaster®
	shark liver oil		streptomycin
	Smith-Lemli-Opitz (syndrome)		syringomyelia
	streptolysin O		systolic motion
SLOA	short leave of absence		systolic murmur
SLOM	serous left otitis media	[153]Sm	samarium 153
SLONM	sporadic late-onset nemaline myopathy	SMA	severe malarial anemia

	smallpox vaccine, not otherwise specified	SMIDS	suppertime mixed insulin and daytime sulfonylureas
	smooth muscle antibody	SMILE	safety, monitoring, intervention, length of stay and evaluation
	spinal muscular atrophy		sustained maximal inspiratory lung exercises
	superior mesenteric artery	
SMA-II	spinal muscular atrophy type II	SMIs	self-management interventions
SMA-6	simultaneous multichannel autoanalyzer (page 356)	SMIT	standard mycological identification techniques
SMA-7	See page 356	SMMVT	sustained monomorphic ventricular tachycardia
SMA-12	See page 356	SMN	second malignant neoplasia
SMA-18	See page 356		subsequent malignant neoplasms
SMA-23	See page 356	SMO	Senior Medical Officer
SMAC	sequential multiple analyzer computer		site management organization(s)
SMAE	spontaneous movement in all extremities		slip made out
		SMON	subacute myelo-opticoneuropathy
SMAO	superior mesenteric artery occlusion	SMORs	standardized mortality odds ratios
SMAR	self-medication administration record	SMP	safety management plan
			self-management program
SMAS	superficial musculoaponeurotic system (graft; flat)		sympathetic maintained plan
		SmPC	Summary of Product Characteristics (European Union)
	superior mesenteric artery syndrome	
SMAST	Short Michigan Alcoholism Screening Test	SMPN	sensorimotor polyneuropathy
SMAvac	smallpox (vaccinia virus) vaccine	SMQs	Standardized MedDRA (Medical Dictionary for Regulatory Activities) Queries
SMB	simulated moving bed (chromatography)	SMR	senior medical resident
SMBG	self-monitoring blood glucose		skeletal muscle relaxant
SMBP	self-measured blood pressure		sleeping metabolic rate
SMC	skeletal myxoid chondrosarcoma		standardized mortality ratio
	special mouth care		submucous resection
SMCA	sorbitol MacConkey agar	SMRR	submucous resection and rhinoplasty
SMCD	senile macular chorio-retinal degeneration	SMS	scalded mouth syndrome
SMCs	smooth muscle cells		senior medical student
SMD	senile macular degeneration		Smith-Magenis syndrome
	standardized mean difference		somatostatin (Zecnil)
SMDA	Safe Medical Defice Act		stiff-man syndrome
SME	significant medical event	SMSA	standard metropolitan statistical area
	surgical mediastinal exploration	
SMEI	severe myoclonic epilepsy in infancy	SMT	smooth muscle tumors
			sputum methylation testing
SMF	streptozocin, mitomycin, and fluorouracil		standard medical therapy
			study management team
SMFA	sodium monofluoroacetate	SMV	stentless mitral valve
SMFP	sodium monofluorophosphate		submentovertical
SMFT	surgical margins free of tumor		superior mesenteric vein
SMFVD	sterile midforceps vaginal delivery	SMVT	sustained monomorphic ventricular tachycardia
SMG	submandibular gland	SMX-TMP	sulfamethoxazole and trimethoprim (SMZ-TMP)
SMH	state mental hospital	
SMI	sensory motor integration (group)	SMZL	splenic marginal-zone lymphoma
	serious mental illness	SN	sciatic notch
	severely mentally impaired		see note
	service mix index		sinus node
	small volume infusion	
	suggested minimum increment	

	staff nurse	SNHL	sensorineural hearing loss
	student nurse	SNIP	silver nitrate immunoperoxidase
	suprasternal notch		strict no information in paper
	superior nasal	SNIPPV	synchronized nasal intermittent
Sn	tin		positive-pressure ventilation
sN	sentinel lymph node	SNIPS	single nucleotide polymorphism
S/N	signal to noise ratio		(SNP)
SNA	specimen not available	SNK	Student-Newman-Keuls (test)
	Student Nursing Assistant	SNM	sentinel (lymph) node mapping
	sympathetic nerve activity		serotoninergic neuroenteric
SNa	serum sodium		modulators
SNAC	scaphoid nonunion advanced		student nurse midwife
	collapse	SnMp	tin-mesoporphyrin
SNAE	sustained pain-free and *no adverse*	SNOMED	Systematized Nomenclature of
	events		Medicine
SNAP	scheduled nursing activities	SNOMED	Systemized Nomenclature of
	program	CT	Medicine, Clinical Terms
	Score for Neonatal Acute	SNOMED	Systemized Nomenclature of
	Physiology	RT	Medicine, Reference
	sensory nerve action potential		Terminology
	Swanson, Nolan, and Pelham	SNOOP	Systematic Nursing Observation of
	(rating scale)		Psychopathology
SNAP-25	synaptosome-associated protein	SNOs	S-nitrosothiols
	25 kilodaltons	SNP	simple neonatal procedure
SNAP-PE	Score for Neonatal Acute		single nucleotide polymorphism
	Physiology-Perinatal Extension		sodium nitroprusside (Nipride)
SNARC	Spatial-Numerical Association of	SNP-LP	single nucleotide polymorphisms –
	Response Codes		linkage disequilibrium
SNaRI	serotonin noradrenergic reuptake	SNPs	single nucleotide polymorphisms
	inhibitor	SN-PSG	split-night polysomnograms
SNASA	Salford Needs Assessment	SNR	signal-to-noise ratio (radiology)
	Schedule for Adolescents	SNr	substantia nigra reticularis
SNAT	suspected nonaccidental trauma	SNRB	selective nerve root block
SNB	scalene node biopsy	SNRI	selective noradrenergic reuptake
	sentinel (lymph) node biopsy		inhibitor
SNBx	sentinel node biopsy		serotonin norepinephrine reuptake
SNC	skilled nursing care		inhibitor
SNc	substantia nigra compacta	SNRT	sinus node recovery time
SNCV	sensory nerve conduction velocity	SNS	sacral nerve stimulation
SND	selective neck dissection		sterile normal saline (0.9% sodium
	single needle device		chloride, sterile)
	sinus node dysfunction		Strategic National Stockpile
	striatonigral degeneration		Supplemental Nursing System (for
	sympathetic nerve discharge		nursing mothers)
SNDA	Supplemental New Drug		sympathetic nervous system
	Application	SNSA	sympathetic nervous system
SNE	subacute necrotizing		activity
	encephalomyelopathy	SNT	sinuses, nose, and throat
SNEP	student nurse extern program		soft, non-tender
SnET2	tin ethyl etiopurpurin		suppan nail technique
SNF	Simon nitinol filter	SNU	skilled nursing unit
	skilled nursing facility	SNUB	super neurotransmitter uptake
SnF$_2$	stannous fluoride		blocker
SNF/MR	skilled nursing facility for the	SNV	Sin Nombre virus
	mentally retarded		skilled nursing visit
SNGFR	single nephron glomerular filtration		spleen necrosis virus
	rate	SO	second opinion
SNGP	supranuclear gaze palsy		Service Officer

	sex offender		surgical officer of the day
	shoulder orthosis	SODA	Severity of Dyspepsia Assessment
	significant other	SODAS	spheriodal oral drug absorption
	special observation		system
	sphincter of Oddi	SOE	source of embolism
	standing orders	SOFA	sepsis-related organ failure
	suboccipital		assessment
	suggestive of		Sequential Organ Failure
	superior oblique		Assessment (score)
	supraoptic	SOFAS	Social and Occupational
	supraorbital		Functioning Assessment Scale
	sutures out	SOG	suggestive of good
	sympathetic ophthalmia	SOGS	South Oaks Gambling Screen
S/O	suggestive of	SOH	sexually oriented hallucinations
S-O	salpingo-oophorectomy	SoHx	social history
S&O	salpingo-oophorectomy	SOI	slipped on ice
SO_2	sulfur dioxide		sudden overwhelming infection
SO_3	sulfite		surgical orthotopic implantation
SO_4	sulfate		(implant)
SOA	serum opsonic activity		syrup of ipecac
	shortness of air	S-OIV	swine-origin influenza A virus
	spinal opioid analgesia		(also known as H1N1)
	supraorbital artery	SOL	solution
	swelling of ankles		space occupying lesion
SOAA	signed out against advice	SOL I	special observations level one
SOAM	sutures out in the morning		(there are also SOL II and
SOAMA	signed out against medical advice		SOL III)
SOAP	subjective, objective, assessment,	SOM	secretory otitis media
	and plans		serous otitis media
SOAPIE	subjective, objective, assessment,		somatization
	plan, implementation,	SOMI	sterno-occipital mandibular
	(intervention), and evaluation		immobilizer
SOAPIER	subjective, objective, assessment,	SONICC	second-order nonlinear (optical)
	plan, intervention, evaluation,		imaging of chiral crystals
	and revision	SONK	spontaneous osteonecrosis of the
SOB	see order book		knee
	shortness of breath (this	Sono	sonogram
	abbreviation has caused	SONP	solid organs not palpable
	problems)	SOO	site of origin
	side of bed	SOOL	spontaneous onset of labor
SOBE	short of breath on exertion	SOP	standard operating procedure
SOBOE	short of breath on exertion	SOPM	sutures out in afternoon (or
SOC	see old chart		evening)
	socialization	SOR	sign own release
	stages of change		strength of recommendation
	standard of care	SORA	stable on room air
	start of care	SORL1	sortilin-related receptor 1 (gene)
	state of consciousness	SOS	if there is need
	synovial osteochondromatosis		may be repeated once if urgently
	system organ class		required (Latin: *si opus sit*)
S & OC	signed and on chart (e.g. permit)		sacrament of the sick
SOCMOB	standing on corner minding own		self-obtained smear
	business (when inexplicable		Signs of Suicide (prevention
	injured) (slang)		program)
SOCs	System Organ Classes		speed of sound
SOD	sinovenous occlusive disease		suicidal observation status
	sphincter of Oddi dysfunction	SOSOB	sit on side of bed
	superoxide dismutase	SOSs	standardized order sets

SOT	solid organ transplant	sclerosing pancreatocholangitis
	something other than	single-point cane
	stream of thought	statistical process control
SOTP	Sex-Offender Treatment Provider	Summary of Product
SOVS	self-obtained vaginal swabs	Characteristics
SOW	Scope of Work	suprapubic catheter
SOZ	seizure onset zone	SPCA	serum prothrombin conversion
SOZT	superior oblique Z-tenotomy		accelerator (factor VII)
SP	sacrum to pubis	SPCT	simultaneous prism and cover test
	sequential pulse	SPD	schizotypal personality disorder
	serum protein		subcorneal pustular dermatosis
	shoulder press		Supply, Processing, and
	silent period (related to		Distribution (department)
	electromyographic responses)		suprapubic drainage
	spastic dysphonia	SP-D	surfactant protein D
	speech	SPDT	sono-photo dynamic therapy
	Speech Pathologist	SPE	saw palmetto extract
	spinal		septic pulmonary embolism
	spouse		serum protein electrophoresis
	stand and pivot		solid-phase extraction
	stand pivot		superficial punctate erosions
	status post	SPEB	streptococcal pyrogenic exotoxins B
	Streptococcus pneumoniae	SPEC	specimen
	sulfadoxine; pyrimethamine		streptococcal pyrogenic exotoxins C
	(Fansidar)	Spec Ed	special education
	supplementary prescribing	SPECT	single-photon emission computed
	systolic pressure		tomography
sp	species	SPEEP	spontaneous positive end-
S/P	status post		expiratory pressure
	suprapubic	SPEP	serum protein electrophoresis
SP 1	suicide precautions number 1	SPET	single-photon emission tomography
SP 2	suicide precautions number 2	SPF	semipermeable film
SPA	albumin human (formerly known		S-phase fraction
	as salt-poor albumin)		split products of fibrin
	scintillation proximity assay		sun protective factor
	serum prothrombin activity	sp fl	spinal fluid
	sheep pulmonary adenomatosis	SPG	scrotopenogram
	single photon absorptiometry		sphenopalatine ganglion
	Speech Pathology and Audiology	SpG	specific gravity
	spontaneous platelet aggregation	SP GR	specific gravity
	stimulation produced analgesia	SPH	severely and profoundly
	student physician's assistant		handicapped
	subperiosteal abscess		sighs per hour
	suprapubic aspiration		spherocytes
SpA	spondyloarthropathy	SPHERO	spherocytes
SP-A	surfactant-specific protein A	SPHM	Safe Patient Handling and
SPAC	satisfactory postanesthesia course		Movement
SPAG	small-particle aerosol generator	SPI	speech processor interface
SPAMM	spatial modulation of		surgical peripheral iridectomy
	magnetization	SPIA	solid phase immunoabsor-bent
SPAP	State Pharmacy Assistance		assay
	Program	SPID	sum of pain intensity difference
SPARC	suprapubic sling operation	SPIDER	steady-state projection imaging
SPBE	saw palmetto berry extract		with dynamic echo-train readout
SPBI	serum protein bound iodine	SPIF	spontaneous peak inspiratory force
SPBT	suprapubic bladder tap	SPIFE	serum protein and immunofixation
SPC	saturated phosphatidylcholine		electrophoresis (system)
	second primary cancer	S-PIN	Steinmann pin

SPINK1	serine protease inhibitor Kazal type 1	SPRAS	Sheehan Patient Rated Anxiety Scale
SPIO	superparamagnetic iron oxide	SP-RIA	solid-phase radioimmunoassay
SPK	simultaneous pancreas-kidney (transplant)	SPR-MS	surface plasmon resonance mass spectrometry
	single parent keeping (baby)	SPROM	spontaneous premature rupture of membrane
	superficial punctate keratitis		
SPKT	simultaneous pancreas-kidney transplantation	SPS	shoulder pain and stiffness
			simple partial seizure
SPL	sound pressure level		sodium polyethanol sulfonate
	superior parietal lobule		sodium polystyrene sulfonate (Kayexalate; SPS®)
SPL®	Staphylococcal Phage Lysate		
SPLATTT	split anterior tibial tendon transfer		status post surgery
SPM	scanning probe microscopy		stiff-person syndrome
	second primary malignancy		systemic progressive sclerosis
	spontaneous pneumomediastinum	SPSU	straight partial sit-up
SPM96	statistical parametric mapping 96	SPT	second primary tumors
SPMA	spinal progressive muscle atrophy		skin prick test
sPMA	supplemental premarket approval application (FDA)		standing pivot transfer
			supportive periodontal therapy
SPMD	scapuloperoneal muscular dystrophy		suprapubic tenderness
			suprapubic tube
SPMDs	semipermeable membrane devices		surgical preparation time (start surgical preparation to incision)
SPME	solid-phase microextraction	SP TAP	spinal tap
SPMI	severely and persistently mentally ill	SPTL	spontaneous preterm labor
			subcutaneous panniculitis-like T-cell lymphoma
SPMS	secondary progressive multiple sclerosis		
		SPTs	second primary tumors
SPMSQ	Short Portable Mental Status Questionnaire		single-patient trials
		SP TUBE	suprapubic tube
SPN	solitary pulmonary nodule	SPTX	static pelvic traction
	student practical nurse	SPU	short procedure unit
	superficial peroneal nerve	SPVC	Shelhigh porcine pulmonic value conduits
SPn	Streptococcus pneumoniae		
SPNK	single parent not keeping (baby)	SPVR	systemic peripheral vascular resistance
SPNP	solid pseudopapillary neoplasm of the pancreas		
		SPX	smallpox vaccine, not otherwise specified
SPO	status postoperative		
	superior posterior oblique	SPx	spontaneous pneumothorax
SpO₂	oxygen saturation by pulse oximeter	SPXᵥ	smallpox vaccine (vaccinia virus)
		SQ	sleep quality
spont	spontaneous		status quo
SponVe	spontaneous ventilation		subcutaneous (this is a dangerous abbreviation, use subcut)
SPOREs	Specialized Programs of Research Excellence (National Cancer Institute)		
		Sq CCa	squamous cell carcinoma
		SQE	subcutaneous emphysema
SPP	Sexuality Preference Profile	SQM	square meter(s)
	single presentation phenotype	SQUID	superconducting quantum interference device
	skin perfusion pressure		
	super packed platelets	SQV	saquinavir (Fortovose; Invirase)
	suprapubic prostatectomy		Site Qualification Visit
spp	species	SR	screen
SPQ	Schizotypal Personality Questionnaire		sedimentation rate
			see report
SPR	scan projection radiograph (radiology)		senior resident
			service record
	surface plasmon resonance		side rails

S

	sinus rhythm
	slow release
	smooth-rough
	social recreation
	standard risks
	stretch reflex
	superior rectus
	suppression ratio
	sustained release
	sustained response
	suture removal
	system review
S/R	strong/regular (pulse)
S&R	seclusion and restraint
	smooth and rough
^{89}Sr	strontium 89
SRA	serotonin release assay
	steroid-resistant asthma
	surface replacement arthroplasty
SRAN	surgical resident admission note
SRBC	sheep red blood cells
	sickle red blood cells
SRBD	sleep-related breathing disorders
SRBOW	spontaneous rupture of bag of waters
SRC	sclerodermal renal crisis
SRCC	sarcomatoid renal cell carcinoma
SRCS	Division of Surveillance, Research, and Communication Support (FDA)
SRD	service-related disability
	smallest real difference
	sodium-restricted diet
SRE	sex and relationships education
	skeletal related event
SREs	skeletal related events
SRF	somatotropin releasing factor
	subretinal fluid
SRF-A	slow-releasing factor of anaphylaxis
SRGVHD	steroid-resistant graft-versus-host disease
SRH	self-rated health
	signs of recent hemorrhage
SRI	serotonin reuptake inhibitor
SRIB	severe recurrent intestinal bleeding
SRICU	surgical respiratory intensive care unit
SRIF	somatotropin-release inhibiting factor (somatostatin; Zecnil)
SRK	smooth-rod Kaneda (implant)
SRL	sirolimus (Rapamune)
SRM	spontaneous rupture of membranes
SRMD	stress-related mucosal damage
SRMS	sustained-release morphine sulfate
SRMs	specified risk materials
SR/NE	sinus rhythm, no ectopy

SRNV	subretinal neovascularization
SRNVM	subretinal neovascular membrane
SRO	sagittal ramus osteotomy
	single room occupancy
	smallest region of overlap
	sustained-release oral
SROA	sports-related osteoarthritis
SROCPI	Self-Rating Obsessive-Compulsive Personality Inventory
SROM	self range of motion
	serous right otitis media
	spontaneous rupture of membrane
SRP	scaling and root planing (dental)
	septorhinoplasty
	stapes replacement prosthesis
SRQ-20	self-reporting questionnaire of 20 questions (mental health)
SRR	surgical recovery room
SRRS	social readjustment rating scale
SRS	Silver-Russell syndrome
	somatostatin receptor scintigraphy
s̄RS	without redness or swelling
SRS-A	slow-reacting substance of anaphylaxis
SRSV	small round structured viruses
SRT	sedimentation rate test
	sleep-related tumescence
	speech reception threshold
	speech recognition threshold
	stereotactic radiotherapy
	surfactant replacement therapy
	sustained release theophylline
SRU	side rails up
SRUS	solitary rectal ulcer syndrome
SRVC	subcutaneous reservoir and ventricular catheter
SRx	spectacle refraction
SR ↑ X2	both siderails up
SS	half (this is a dangerous abbreviation as it is not understood or read as sliding scale)
	sacral sulcus
	sacrosciatic
	saline soak (sodium chloride 0.9%)
	saline solution (0.9% sodium chloride)
	saliva sample
	salt sensitivity (sensitive)
	salt substitute
	serotonin syndrome
	serum sickness
	Sézary syndrome
	short stay
	sickle cell
	single-session (treatment)
	single-strength (as compared to double-strength)
	Sjögren syndrome

	sliding scale (this is a dangerous abbreviation as it is not understood or read as one half)	SSCr	stainless steel crown
		SSCU	surgical special care unit
		SSCVD	sterile spontaneous controlled vaginal delivery
	slip sent		
	Social Security	SSD	schizophrenia-spectrum disorders
	social service		serosanguineous drainage
	somatostatin (Zecnil)		sickle cell disease
	stainless steel		silver sulfadiazine (Silvadene)
	steady state		skin-to-stone distance
	step stool		Social Security disability
	subaortic stenosis		source to skin distance
	susceptible		surface shaded display (radiology)
	suprasciatic (notch)	SSDI	Social Security death index
	Sweet syndrome		Social Security disability income
	symmetrical strength		Social Security disability insurance
S/S	Saturday and Sunday	ss DNA	single-stranded desoxyribonucleic acid
	signs and symptoms		
	sprain/strain	SSDs	schizophrenia spectrum disorders
S2S	skin-to-skin (infant and mother)	SSE	saline solution enema (0.9% sodium chloride)
SS#	Social Security number		
S & S	shower and shampoo		skin self-examination
	signs and symptoms		soapsuds enema
	sitting and supine		sterile speculum exam
	sling and swathe		subacute spongiform encephalopathy
	soft and smooth (prostate)		
	support and stimulation		systemic side effects
	swish and spit	SSEH	spontaneous spinal epidural hematoma
	swish and swallow		
SSA	sagittal split advancement	SSEPs	somatosensory evoked potentials
	salicylsalicylic acid (salsalate)	SSF	subscapular skinfold
	Sjögren syndrome antigen A	SSFP	steady-state free precession
	Social Security Administration	SSG	sodium stibogluconate
	specific surface area		sublabial salivary gland
	Subjective Symptoms Assessment (profile)	SSHL	sudden sensorineural hearing loss
		SSI	sliding scale insulin
	sulfasalicylic acid (test)		Social Skills Inventory
SSADH	succinic semialdehyde dehydrogenase		sub-shock insulin
			superior sector iridectomy
SSAs	standard sedative agents		Supplemental Security Income
SSBP	sitting systolic blood pressure		surgical site infection
SSC	sign symptom complex	SSI-CCM	synthetic sentence identification with contralateral competing message
	silver sulfadiazine and chlorhexidine		
		SSI-ICM	synthetic sentence identification with ipsilateral competing message
	Similac® and special care		
	sliding scale coverage		
	Special Services for Children	SSKI	saturated solution of potassium iodide
	spermatogonial stem cell		
	stainless steel crown	SSL	second stage of labor
	standard straight cane		selective sentinel lymphadenectomy
SSc	systemic sclerosis (scleroderma)		
SSCA	single shoulder contrast arthrography		subtotal supraglottic laryngectomy
		SSLF	sacrospinous ligament fixation
SSCM	Society of Critical Care Medicine (guidelines for the sustained use of sedatives and analgesics)	SSLPs	Sure Start Local Programmes (UK)
		SSLR	seated straight leg raise
		SSM	short stay medical
SSCP	single-stranded conformational polymorphism		skin-sparing mastectomy
			skin surface microscopy
	substernal chest pain		

S

	superficial spreading melanoma
SSN	severely subnormal
	Social Security number
SSNB	suprascapular nerve block
SSO	second surgical opinion
	sequence-specific oligonucleotide
	short stay observation (unit)
	Spanish speaking only
SSOP	Second Surgical Opinion Program
	sequence-specific oligonucleotide probe
SSP	sequence-specific primer
	short stay procedure (unit)
	superior spermatic plexus
	supragingival scaling and prophylaxis (dental)
SSPA	staphylococcal-slime polysaccharide antigens
SSPE	subacute sclerosing panencephalitis
SSPG	steady-state plasma glucose
SSPH	System of Social Protection in Health (Mexico)
SSPL	saturation sound pressure level
SSPU	surgical short procedure unit
SSQ	Staring Speel Questionnaire
SSR	Sleep Self-Reporting
	substernal retractions
	sympathetic skin response
SSRFC	surrounding subretinal fluid cuff
SSRI	selective serotonin reuptake inhibitor
ssRNA	single-stranded deoxyribonucleic acid
SSRO	sagittal split ramus osteotomy (dental)
SSRP	subgingival scaling and root planing (dental)
SSRs	simple sequence repeats
SSS	layer upon layer
	scalded skin syndrome
	Scandinavian Stroke Scale
	Sepsis Severity Score
	Severity Scoring System (Dart Snakebite)
	short stay service (unit)
	sick sinus syndrome
	skin and skin structures
	Spanish-speaking sometimes
	sphincter-saving surgery
	spontaneous saliva swallowing
	Stanford Sleepiness Scale
	Steiner silver stain
	sterile saline soak
	subclavian steal syndrome
SSSB	sagittal split setback
SSSDW	significant sharp, spike, or delta waves
SSSE	self-sustained status epilepticus

SSSIs	skin and skin structure infections
SSSS	staphylococcal scalded skin syndrome
SSSs	small short spikes (encephalography)
SST	sagittal sinus thrombosis
	Simple Shoulder Test
	somatostatin (Zecnil)
SSTI	skin and soft tissue infection(s)
SSU	short stay unit
SSX	sulfisoxazole acetyl
S/SX	signs/symptoms
SSYC	Salmonella, Shigella, Yersinia, Campylobacter (*bacteria*)
ST	esotropic
	sacrum transverse
	Schiotz tonometry
	Schirmer Test (dry-eye test)
	scleral thickness
	shock therapy
	sinus tachycardia
	skin tear
	skin test
	slight trace
	slow-twitch
	smokeless tobacco
	soft tissue
	sore throat
	spasmodic torticollis
	speech therapist
	speech therapy
	sphincter tone
	split thickness
	spondee threshold
	station (obstetrics)
	stomach
	stone (1 stone = 6.35 kg or 14 pounds)
	straight
	strength training
	stress testing
	stretcher
	subtotal
	Surgical Technologist
	survival time
	synapse time
S/T	short term
S & T	sulfamethoxazole and trimethoprim (SMZ-TMP or SMX-TMP)
STA	second trimester abortion
	spike-triggered averaging
	staphylococcus vaccine, not otherwise specified
	superficial temporal artery
STA$_{aur}$	*Staphylococcus aureus* vaccine
stab.	polymorphonuclear leukocytes (white blood cells, in nonmature form)

STAI	State-Trait Anxiety Inventory	STG	short-term goals
STAI-I	State-Trait-Anxiety Index—I		split-thickness graft
STA-MCA	superficial temporary artery-middle cerebral artery (anastomosis; bypass)		superior temporal gyri
		STH	soft tissue hemorrhage
			soil-transmitted helminths
STAPES	stapedectomy		somatotrophic hormone
staph	*Staphylococcus aureus*		subtotal hysterectomy
STA_{SPL}	staphylococcus vaccine, bacteriophage lysate		supplemental thyroid hormone

STAI State-Trait Anxiety Inventory
STAI-I State-Trait-Anxiety Index—I
STA-MCA superficial temporary artery-middle cerebral artery (anastomosis; bypass)
STAPES stapedectomy
staph *Staphylococcus aureus*
STA$_{SPL}$ staphylococcus vaccine, bacteriophage lysate
STAT immediately (or as defined by the institution)
signal transducers and activators of transcription
STAT3 signal transducer and activator of transcription 3
STATINS HMG-CoA reductase inhibitors
STAXI State-Trait Anger Expression Inventory
STB SoluTab (a tablet that dissolves in the mouth for quicker absorption)
stillborn
STBAL standing balance
ST BY stand by
STC serum theophylline concentration
slow-transit constipation
soft tissue calcification
special treatment center
stimulate to cry
stroke treatment center
subtotal colectomy
sugar tongue cast
ST CLK station clerk
STD sexually transmitted disease(s)
short-term disability
skin test dose
skin to tumor distance
sodium tetradecyl sulfate
STD TF standard tube feeding
STE steps to enter
ST-segment elevation
STEAM stimulated-echo acquisition mode
STEC shiga toxin-producing *Escherichia coli*
STEM scanning transmission electron microscopic
STEMI ST-segment elevation myocardial infarction
Stereo steropsis
STEPS The System for Thalidomide Educating and Prescribing Safety
STET single photon emission tomography
submaximal treadmill exercise test
STETH stethoscope
STF slip, trip, and fall (injuries)
special tube feeding
standard tube feeding
sTfR soluble transferring receptor

STG short-term goals
split-thickness graft
superior temporal gyri
STH soft tissue hemorrhage
soil-transmitted helminths
somatotrophic hormone
subtotal hysterectomy
supplemental thyroid hormone
STHB said to have been
STI sexually transmitted infection
signal transduction inhibitor((s)
soft tissue injury
structured treatment interruption(s)
sum total impression
systolic time interval
STI-571 imatinib mesylate (Gleevec)
STILLB stillborn
STIM stimulation
STIR short TI (tau) inversion recovery
STIs sexually transmitted infections
systolic time intervals
STJ scapulothoracic joint
subtalar joint
STK streptokinase
STL sent to laboratory
serum theophylline level
STLE St. Louis encephalitis
STLI subtotal lymphoid irradiation
STLOM swelling, tenderness, and limitation of motion
STLV simian T-lymphotrophic viruses
STM scanning tunneling microscope
short-term memory
soft tissue mobilization
sternocleidomastoideus
streptomycin
STMS Short Test of Mental Status
STMT Seat Movement
STN subtalar neutral
subthalamic nucleus
STNI subtotal nodal irradiation
STNM surgical evaluative staging of cancer
STNR symmetrical tonic neck reflex
S to sensitive to
STO$_2$ microvascular oxygen saturation
STOP sensitive, timely, and organized programs (battered spouses)
STORCH syphilis, toxoplasmosis, other agents, rubella, cytomegalovirus, and herpes (maternal infections)
STP short-term plans
sodium thiopental
step training progression
STPD standard temperature and pressure—dry
STPI State-Trait Personality Inventory
STPS Short-Term Performance Status

S

STPT	second-trimester pregnancy termination	STV 0	short-term variability-absent
STR	scotopic threshold response	STV inter	short-term variability-intermittent
	short tandem repeat	STX	stricture
	short-termm rehabilitation	Stx EIA	Shiga toxin enzyme immunoassay
	signs of a stroke (ask patient to smile; talk [speak a simple sentence]; raise both arms)	STZ	streptozocin (Zanosar)
		SU	sensory urgency
			Somogyi units
	sister		stasis ulcer
	small tandem repeat		stroke unit
	stretcher		sulfonylurea
	strength		supine
	systolic time ratio	Su	Sunday
Strab	strabismus	S/U	set up
STRAWB	strawberry		shoulder/umbilicus
strep	streptococcus	S&U	supine and upright
	streptomycin	SUA	serum uric acid
STRICU	shock/trauma/respiratory intensive care unit		single umbilical artery
		SUB	Skene urethra and Bartholin glands
Str Post MI	strictly posterior myocardial infarction	Subcu	subcutaneous
		SUBCUT	subcutaneous
STS	serologic test for syphilis	Subepi M Inj	subepicardial myocardial injury
	short-term survivors		
	sit-to-stand	SUB-I	sub-investigator
	slide thin slab	SUBL	sublingual
	sodium tetradecyl sulfate	SUB-MAND	submandibular
	sodium thiosulfate		
	soft tissue sarcoma	sub q	subcutaneous (this is a dangerous abbreviation since the q is mistaken for every, when a number follows)
	soft tissue swelling		
	somatostatin (Zecnil)		
	standard threshold shift (audiology)		
	staurosporine	SUCC	succinylcholine
	superior temporal sulcus	SUCT	suction
	Surgical Technology Student	SUD	substance use disorder(s)
ST-SDDI	short-term sequential digital dermoscopy imaging		sudden unexpected death
		SuDBP	supine diastolic blood pressure
STSG	split thickness skin graft	SUDEP	sudden unexpected (unexplained) death in epilepsy
STSS	streptococcal-induced toxic shock syndrome		
		SUDI	sudden unexpected death in infancy
STS-SPT	simple two-step swallowing provocation test		
		SUDS	Subjective Unit of Distress (Disturbance) (Discomfort) Scale
STT	scaphoid-trapezium-trapezoid (scaphotrapeziotrapezoid; joint of the thumb)		
			sudden unexplained death syndrome
	serial thrombin time	SUF	symptomatic uterine fibroids
	skin temperature test	SUI	stress urinary incontinence
	soft tissue tumor		suicide
	subtotal thyroidectomy	SUID	sudden unexplained infant death
STT#1	Schirmer tear test one	SUIOS	Simplified Urinary Incontinence Outcome Score
STT#2	Schirmer tear test two		
STTA	sub-Tenon triamcinolone acetonide (injection)	SULF-PRIM	sulfamethoxazole and trimethoprim
		SUMO	small ubiquitin-like modifier
STTb	basal Schirmer tear test	SUN	serum urea nitrogen
STTOL	standing tolerance	SUNCT	short-lasting unilateral neuralgiform headache attacks with conjunctival injection and tearing
STU	shock trauma unit		
	surgical trauma unit		
STV	short-term variability	SUNDS	sudden unexplained nocturnal death syndrome
STV+	short-term variability-present		

SUO	syncope of unknown origin		*Streptococcus viridans* endocarditis
SUP	stress ulcer prophylaxis		subcortical vascular encephalopathy
	superior		supraventricular ectopy
	supervision	SV&E	suicidal, violent, and eloper
	supination	SVG	saphenous vein graft
	supinator	SVH	subjective visual horizontal (test)
	symptomatic uterine prolapse	SVI	seminal vesicle invasion
SUPAC	Scale-Up and Post Approval		stroke volume index
	Change	S VISC	serum viscosity
supp	suppository	SVL	severe visual loss
SUPRV	supervision	SVM	support vector machines
SUR	suramin (Metaret)	SVN	small volume nebulizer
	surgery	SVO	small vessel occlusion
	surgical	SVO$_2$	mixed venous oxygen saturation
Surgi	Surgigator	SVOO	systemic ventricular outflow
SUSARs	suspected and unsuspected serious		obstruction
	adverse reactions	SVP	spontaneous venous pulse
susp	suspension		synovial volar phalangeal
SUUD	sudden unexpected, unexplained	SVPB	supraventricular premature beat
	death	SVPC	supraventricular premature
SUV	standard uptake variable		contraction
SUVs	standard uptake values	SV/PP	stroke volume/pulse pressure
SUX	succinylcholine	SVR	superficial venous reflux
	suction		supraventricular rhythm
SUZI	subzonal insertion		sustained virological response
SV	scimitar vein		systemic vascular resistance
	seminal vesical	SVRI	systemic vascular resistance index
	severe	SVSR	supervisor
	sigmoid volvulus	SVT	splanchnic vein thrombosis
	single ventricle		superficial vein thrombosis
	single vessel		superficial venous thrombophlebitis
	snake venom		supraventricular tachycardia
	stroke volume		symptom validity test(s)
	subclavian vein	SVV	stroke volume variance
Sv	sievert (radiation unit)	SVVD	spontaneous vertex vaginal delivery
SV40	simian virus 40	SVZ	subventricular zone
SVA	small volume admixture	SW	sandwich
	supraventricular arrhythmia		sea water
SVAB	stereotactic vacuum-assisted biopsy		seriously wounded
SVAS	supravalvular aortic stenosis		shallow walk (aquatic therapy)
SVB	saphenous vein bypass		short wave
SVBG	saphenous vein bypass graft		Social Worker
SVC	service connected		stab wound
	slow vital capacity		standard walker
	subclavian vein compression		sterile water
	superior vena cava		swallowing reflex
SVCO	superior vena cava obstruction	S&W	soap and water
SVC-RPA	superior vena cava and right	S/W	somewhat
	pulmonary artery (shunt)	SWA	slow-wave activity
SVCS	superior vena cava syndrome		(electroencephalographic)
SVD	singular value decomposition		Social Work Associate
	(analysis)	SWAN	statewide adoption network
	single-vessel disease	SWAP	short-wavelength automated
	small vessel disease		perimetry
	spontaneous vaginal delivery	SWAT	skin wound assessment and
	structural valve deterioration		treatment
	(dysfunction)	SWB	social well-being
SVE	sterile vaginal examination		subjective well-being

	swing bed
SWD	short wave diathermy
Sweet Milk	propofol (Diprivan) (slang)
SWer	Social Worker
SWFI	sterile water for injection
SWG	standard wire gauge
SWI	sterile water for injection
	surgical wound infection
S&WI	skin and wound isolation
SWL	shock wave lithotripsy
SWMA	segmental wall-motion abnormalities
SWME	Semmes-Weinstein monofilament examination
SWO	superficial white onychomycosis
SWOG	Southwest Oncology Group
SWOT	strengths, weaknesses, opportunities, threats (analysis)
SWP	small whirlpool
	southwest Pacific
SWR	surface wrinkling retinopathy
	surgical waiting room
SWS	sheltered workshop
	slow-wave sleep
	social work service
	student ward secretary
	Sturge-Weber syndrome
SWSD	shift-work sleep disorder
SWT	stab wound of the throat
	shuttle-walk test
SWU	septic work-up
SWW	static wall walk (aquatic therapy)
Sx	signs
	surgery
	symptom
SXA	single-energy x-ray absorptiometry
SXR	skull x-ray
SYN	synovial
SYN-D	synthadotin
SYN Fl	synovial fluid
SYPH	syphilis
SYR	syrup
SYS BP	systolic blood pressure
SZ	schizophrenic
	seizure
	suction
SZN	streptozocin (Zanosar)

T	inverted T wave
	tablespoon (15 mL) (this is a dangerous abbreviation)
	taenia
	teach (taught)
	temperature
	tender
	tension
	tesla (unit of magnetic flux density in radiology)
	testicles
	testosterone
	thoracic
	thymidine
	Toxoplasma
	trace
	transcribed
	Tuesday
	tympanic
t	teaspoon (5 mL) (this is a dangerous abbreviation)
T+	increase intraocular tension
T−	decreased intraocular tension
2,4,5-T	2,4,5-trichlorophenoxyacetic acid
T°	temperature
$T_{1/2}$	half-life
T_1	tricuspid first sound
T_2	tricuspid second sound
T-2	dactinomycin, doxorubicin, vincristine, and cyclophosphamide
T_3	triiodothyronine (liothyronine; Cytomel)
T3	transurethral thermo-ablation therapy (Targis)
	Tylenol with codeine 30 mg (this is a dangerous abbreviation)
$T_{3/4}$ind	triiodothyronine to thyroxine index
T_4	levothyroxine sodium (synthroid)
	thyroxine
T4	CD4 (helper-inducer cells)
T-7	free thyroxine factor
T-10	methotrexate, calcium leucovorin rescue, doxorubicin, cisplatin, bleomycin, cyclophosphamide, and dactinomycin
T-20	enfuvirtide (Fuzeon)
$T_1...T_{12}$	thoracic nerve 1 through 12
	thoracic vertebra 1 through 12
TA	Takayasu arteritis
	teaching assistant
	temperature axillary
	temporal arteritis
	temporal artery

S

tendon Achilles
therapeutic abortion
therapeutic activity
tibialis anterior (muscle)
tracheal aspirate
traffic accident
transversus abdominus (muscle)
tricuspid atresia
truncus arteriosus

Ta tonometry applanation
T&A tonsillectomy and adenoidectomy
tonsils and adenoids
T(A) axillary temperature
TA1 thymosin alpha-1
TA-55 stapling device
TAA Therapeutic Activities Aide
thoracic aortic aneurysm
total ankle arthroplasty
transverse aortic arch
triamcinolone acetonide
tumor-associated antigen (antibodies)
TAAA thoracoabdominal aortic aneursym
TAB tablet
therapeutic abortion
threatened abortion
total androgen blockade
triple antibiotic (bacitracin, neomycin, and polymyxin (this is a dangerous abbreviation)
TABO triple antibiotic ointment (bacitracin, neomycin, and polymyxin)
TAC docetaxel (Taxotere), doxorubicin (Adriamycin), and cyclophosphamide
tacrolimus (Prograf, also TRL)
tetracaine, Adrenalin® and cocaine
total arterial compliance
tibial artery catheter
total abdominal colectomy
total allergen content
triamicinolone cream
trigeminal autonomic cephalgias
TACC thoracic aortic cross-clamping
TACE transarterial chemoembolization
transcatheter arterial chemoembolization
Tachy tachycardia
TACI total anterior cerebral infarct
tac-MRA timed arterial compression magnetic resonance angiography
TACO transfusion-associated circulatory overload
TACT tuned aperture computed tomography
TAD thoracic asphyxiant dystrophy
transverse abdominal diameter

TADAC therapeutic abortion, dilation, aspiration, and curettage
TADC tumor-associated dendritic cells
TAE transcatheter arterial embolization
TAF tissue angiogenesis factor
TAFI thrombin-activatable fibrinolysis inhibitor
TAG triacylglycerol
tumor-associated glycoprotein
TAGA term, appropriate for gestational age
term, average gestational age
TA-GVHD transfusion-associated graft-versus-host disease
TAH total abdominal hysterectomy
total artificial heart
TAHBSO total abdominal hysterectomy, bilateral salpingo-oophorectomy
TAHL thick ascending limb of Henle loop
TAI thoracic aortic injury
T Air air puff tonometry
TAKE Targeting Abnormal Kinetic Effects
TAL tendon Achilles lengthening
total arm length
T ALCON Alcon® tonometry
T-ALL T-cell acute lymphoblastic leukemia
TALP total alkaline phosphatase
TAML therapy-related acute myelogenous leukemia
t-AML therapy-related acute myeloid leukemia
TAM tamoxifen (Novaldex)
teenage mother
total active motion
tumor-associated macrophages
TAN treatment-as-needed
Treatment Authorization Number
tropical ataxic neuropathy
TANF Temporary Assistance for Needy Families
TANI total axial (lymph) node irradiation
TAO thromboangitis obliterans
thyroid-associated ophthalmopathy
triple antibiotic ointment (neomycin, polymyxin b sulfates, and bacitracin zinc [Neosporin ointment])
troleandomycin
TAP tone and positioning
tonometry by applanation
transabdominal preperitoneal (laparoscopic hernia repair)
transesophageal atrial paced
transversus abdominis plant (block)
trypsinogen activation peptide
tumor-activated prodrug
TAPES Trinity Amputation and Prosthesis Experience Scales

TAPP	transabdominal preperitoneal polypropylene (mesh-plasty)		tuberculosis
		TBA	to be absorbed
T APPL	applanation tonometry		to be added
TAPVC	total anomalous pulmonary venous connection		to be administered
			to be admitted
			to be announced
TAPVD	total anomalous pulmonary venous drainage		to be arranged
			to be assessed
TAPVR	total anomalous pulmonary venous return		thyroid biochemical abnormalities
			total body (surface) area
TAR	thoracic aortic rupture	TBAGA	term birth appropriate for gestational age
	thrombocytopenia with absent radius		
		T-bar	tracheotomy bar (a device used in respiratory therapy)
	tissue-air ratio		
	total ankle replacement	TBARS	thiobarbituric acid reactive substances
	total anorectal reconstruction		
	treatment administration record	TBB	transbronchial biopsy
	treatment authorization request	TBBL	transblepharoplasty brow lift
TARA	total articular replacement arthroplasty	TBC	to be cancelled
			total-blood cholesterol
TART	tenderness, asymmetry, restricted motion, and tissue texture changes		total-body clearance
			tuberculosis
		TBD	to be determined
	tumorectomy and radiotherapy	TBE	tick-borne encephalitis
TAS	therapeutic activities specialist		timed-barium esophagogram
	Thrombolytic Assessment System		time to bacterial eradication
	transabdominal sutures		to be evaluated
	turning against self	TBE$_e$	tick-borne encephalitis, eastern subtype (Far eastern encephalitis, Russian spring-summer e., Taiga e.) vaccine
	typical absence seizures		
TASS	toxic anterior segment syndrome		
TAT	tandem autotransplants		
	tell a tale	T-berg	Trendelenburg (position)
	tetanus antitoxin	TBEV	tick-borne encephalitis virus
	thematic apperception test	TBE$_w$	tick-bone encephalitis, western subtype (Central European encephalitis) vaccine
	thrombin-antithrombin III complex		
	'til all taken		
	tired all the time	TBF	total-body fat
	total adipose tissue	TBG	thyroxine-binding globulin
	transactivator of transcription	TBI	tick-borne illness(es)
	transfusion-associated transmission		to be infused
	transplant-associated thrombocytopenia		toothbrushing instruction
			total-body irradiation
	turnaround time		traumatic brain injury
	tyrosine aminotransferase	T bili	total bilirubin
TATT	tired all the time	TBK	total-body potassium
TAU	tumescence activity units	tbl	tablespoon (15 mL)
TAUC	target area under the curve	TBLB	transbronchial lung biopsy
	time-averaged urea concentration	TBLC	term birth, living child
TAUSA	thrombolysis and angioplasty in unstable angina	TBLF	term birth, living female
		TBLI	term birth, living infant
TAX	cefotaxime (Claforan)	TBLM	term birth, living male
	paclitaxel (Taxol)	TBLN	tuberculous lymphadenitis
TB	Tapes for the Blind	TBM	tracheobronchomalacia
	terrible burning		tuberculous meningitis
	thought broadcasting		tubule basement membrane
	toothbrush	TBMg	total-body magnesium
	total base	TBN	total-body nitrogen
	total bilirubin	TBNA	transbronchial needle aspiration
	total body		

	treated but not admitted
TBNa	total-body sodium
TBO	toluidine blue O
TBOCS	Tale-Brown Obsessive-Compulsive Scale
TBP	thyroxine-binding protein
	toe blood pressure
	total-body phosphorus
	total-body protein
	tuberculous peritonitis
TBPA	thyroxine-binding prealbumin
TBPM	time-based prospective memory
TBR	total-bed rest
TBRF	tick-borne relapsing fever
TBS	tablespoon (15 mL)(this is a dangerous abbreviation)
	tachycardia-bradycardia syndrome
	The Bethesda System (reporting cervical and vagina cytology)
	total-serum bilirubin
	Townes-Brocks syndrome
TBSA	total-body surface area
	total-burn surface area
tbsp	tablespoon (15 mL)
TBT	tolbutamide test
	tracheal bronchial toilet
	transbronchoscopic balloon tipped
TBUT	tear break-up time (dry-eye test)
TBV	thiotepa, bleomycin, and vinblastine
	total-blood volume
	transluminal balloon valvuloplasty
TBW	total-body water
TBZ	tetrabenazine (Xenazine)
	thiabendazole (Mintezol)
TC	paclitaxel (Taxol) and cisplatin
	tactile cues
	tai chi (exercise program)
	talocrural (joint)
	team conference
	telephone call
	terminal cancer
	testicular cancer
	thioguanine and cytarabine
	thoracic circumference
	throat culture
	tinea capitis
	tissue culture
	tolonium chloride
	tonic-clonic
	tonsillar coblation
	total cholesterol
	total communication
	to (the) chest
	tracheal collar
	trauma center
	true conjugate
	tubocurarine

Tc	technetium
T/C	telephone call
	ticarcillin-clavulanic acid (Timentin)
	to consider
3TC	lamivudine (Epivir)
TC7	Interceed®
T&C	turn and cough
	type and crossmatch
T&C#3	Tylenol with 30 mg codeine
TCA	thioguanine and cytarabine
	tissue concentrations of antibiotic(s)
	trichloroacetic acid
	tricuspid atresia
	tricyclic antidepressant
	tumor chemosensitivity assay
	tumor clonogenic assays
TCABG	triple coronary artery bypass graft
TCAD	transplant-related coronary-artery disease
	tricyclic antidepressant
TCAR	tiazofurin
TCB	to call back
	tumor cell burden
TcB	transcutaneous bilirubin
TCBS	thiosulfate-citrate-bile salt-sucrose (agar)
TCC	tobacco cessation counseling
	total cost of care
	transitional cell carcinoma
	2,3,5-triphenyl tetrazolium chloride
TCCa	transitional cell carcinoma
TCCB	transitional cell carcinoma of bladder
TC/CL	ticarcillin-clavulanate (Timentin)
$TcCO_2$	transcutaneous carbon dioxide
TCD	T-cell depleted
	transcerebellar diameter
	transcranial Doppler (ultrasonography)
	transverse cardiac diameter
	transcystic duct
TcdA	*Clostridium difficile* toxin A
TcdB	*Clostridium difficile* toxin B
TAB	tablet
TCDB	turn, cough, and deep breath
TCDD	tetrachlorodibenzo-p-dioxin (dioxin)
	threshold contrast detail detectability (radiology)
^{99m}Tc DTPA	technetium Tc 99m pentetate
TCE	tetrachloroethylene
	total-colon examination
	toxicity composite endpoint
	transcatheter embolotherapy
T cell	small lymphocyte

TCES	transcranial electrical stimulation		topical corticosteroid
TCF	docetaxel, (Taxotere) cisplatin, and fluorouracil		Treacher Collins syndrome
		99mTcSC	technetium Tc 99m sulfur colloid
TCFA	thin cap fibroatheroma	TCT	thyrocalcitonin
99mTcGHA	technetium Tc 99m gluceptate		tincture
TCH	paclitaxel (Taxol), carboplatin, and trastuzumab (Herceptin)		transcatheter therapy
			triple combination tablet (abacavir, lamivudine, and zidovudine) (Trizivir)
	total cost of hospitalization		
	turn, cough, hyperventilate		
99mTc-HAS	technetium Tc 99m-labeled human serum albumin	TCU	transitional care unit
		TCVA	thromboembolic cerebral vascular accident
TCHRs	traditional Chinese herbal remedies		
TCI	target-control infusion	TCW	telephone caseworker
	to come in	TD	Takayasu disease
	transcutaneous immunization		tardive dyskinesia
TCID	tissue culture infective dose		temporary disability
TCIE	transient cerebral ischemic episode		terminal device
TCIT	therapeutic crisis intervention training		test dose
			tetanus-diphtheria toxoids (pediatric use)
TCL	tibial collateral ligament		
	transverse carpal ligament		tidal volume
TCM	tissue culture media		tolerance dose
	traditional Chinese medicine		tone decay
	transcutaneous (oxygen) monitor		total disability
99mTc-MAA	technetium Tc 99m albumin microaggregated		transdermal
			transverse diameter
tcMEP	transcranial motor-evoked potential		travelers' diarrhea
TCMH	tumor-direct cell-mediated hypersensitivity		treatment discontinued
		Td	tetanus-diphtheria toxoids (adult type)
TCMS	transcranial cortical magnetic stimulation		
		T1D	type 1 diabetes (mellitus); (This is a dangerous abbreviation as it will be read as "three times daily" [TID]. Use DM1
TCMZ	trichlormethiazide (Naqua)		
TCN	tetracycline		
	triciribine phosphate (tricyclic nucleoside)		
		T2D	type 2 diabetes mellitus
TCNS	transcutaneous nerve stimulator	TDAC	tumor-derived activated cell (cultures)
TCNU	tauromustine		
TcO2	transcutaneous oxygen pressure	Tdap	tetanus toxoid, reduced diphtheria toxoid, and acellular pertussis vaccine, absorbed (BOOSTRIX and ADACEL). It is meant to be used as *booster* shots for older children, adolescents, and adults.
TcO4−	pertechnetate		
TCOM	transcutaneous oxygen monitor		
T Con	temporary conservatorship		
TCP	thrombocytopenia		
	transcutaneous pacing		
	tranylcypromine (Parnate)	TDB	total daily basal (insulin dose)
	tricalcium phosphate	tDCS	transcranial direct current stimulation
	tumor control probability		
TCPC	total cavopulmonary connection	TDD	telephone device for the deaf
TcPCO2	transcutaneous carbon dioxide		thoracic duct drainage
TCPL	time-cycled, pressure-limited (ventilation)		total daily dose
		TDE	total daily energy (requirement)
TcPO2	transcutaneous oxygen	TDF	tenofovir disoproxil fumarate (Virend)
99mTcPYP	technetium Tc 99m pyrophosphate		
TCR	T-cell receptor		testis determining factor
TCRE	transcervical resection of the endometrium		total-dietary fiber
			tumor dose fractionation
TCRFTA	temperature-controlled radiofrequency tissue ablation	TDI	time-delay integration (radiology)
			tissue Doppler imaging
TCS	tonic-clonic seizure		tolerable daily intake

	toluene diisocyanate		testosterone/estrogen (ratio)
	total daily insulin		trunk-to-extremity skinfold
TDIs	therapist-directed interventions		thickness (index)
TDK	tardive diskinesia	T&E	testing and evaluation
TDL	thoracic duct lymph		training and evaluation
TDLN	tumor-draining lymph nodes		trial and error
TDM	therapeutic drug monitoring	TEA	thoracic epidural analgesia
T1DM	type 1 diabetes mellitus (this is a		thromboendarterectomy
	dangerous abbreviation as it will		Time and Extent Application (FDA)
	be read as "three times daily		total elbow arthroplasty
	with meals" [TIDM]. Use DM1		transluminal extraction
T2DM	type 2 diabetes mellitus		atherectomy
TDMAC	tridodecylmethyl ammonium	TEAE	treatment-emergent adverse event
	chloride	TEAP	transesophageal atrial pacing
TD-MALS	time-dependent, multiangle (static)	TEB	thoracic electrical bioimpedance
	light scattering	TEBG	testosterone-estradiol binding
TDN	totally digestible nutrients		globulin
	transdermal nitroglycerin	TeBG	testeosterone binding globulin
TDNTG	transdermal nitroglycerin	TeBIDA	technetium 99m trimethyl 1-
TDNWB	touchdown nonweightbearing		bromo-imono diacetic acid
TdP	torsades de pointes	TEC	thromboembolic complication
TDPDS	temporomandibular disorder pain		thymic epithelial cancer(s)
	dysfunction syndrome		total eosinophil count
TDPWB	touchdown partial weight-bearing		toxic *Escherichia coli*
TDR	total disk replacement		transient erythroblastopenia of
	transmural dispersion of		childhood
	repolarization		transluminal extraction-
TdR	thymidine		endarterectomy catheter
TDS	Teacher Drool Scale		transpapillary endoscopic
	traveler's diarrhea syndrome		cholecystostomy
TDS	three times a day (United		triethyl citrate
	Kingdom)	T&EC	trauma and emergency center
TDT	tentative discharge tomorrow	TECA	titrated extract of *Centella asiatica*
	transmission disequilibrium test	TECAB	totally endoscopic (off-pump)
	Trieger Dot Test		coronary artery bypass grafting
	tumor doubling time	Tech	technician
TdT	terminal deoxynucleotidyl	TED	thromboembolic disease
	transferase		thyroid eye disease
TDW	target dry weight		tobacco, ETOH (alcohol), and
TDWB	touch down weight bearing		drugs
TDx®	fluorescence polarization	T/E/D	tobacco, ETOH (alchol), and drugs
	immunoassay	TEDS	thromboembolic disease stockings
TE	echo time		transesophageal echo-Doppler
	tennis elbow		system
	terminal extension		Treatment Episode Data Set
	therapeutic equivalence	TEE	total energy expended
	therapeutic exercise		transnasal endoscopic
	tissue engineering		ethmoidectomy
	tooth extraction		transesophageal echocardiography
	toxoplasmic encephalitis	TEEU	transesophageal endoscopic
	trace elements (chromium, copper,		ultrasound
	iodine, manganese, selenium,	TEF	tracheoesophageal fistula
	molybdenum and zinc)	TEG	thromboelastogram
	tracheoesophageal		(thromboelastography)
	transesophageal echocardiography	TEH	theophylline, ephedrine, and
	transrectal electroejaculation		hydroxyzine
*t*E	total expiratory time	TEI	therapeutic equivalence interchange
T/E	testosterone to epitestosterone ratio		total episode of illness

	transesophageal imaging		treadmill exercise test
TEL	telemetry	TETE	too early to evaluate
	telephone	TETig	tetanus immune globulin
tele	telemetry	TEU	token economy unit
TEM	temozolomide (Temodar)		transesophageal ultrasound
	transanal endoscopic microsurgery	TEV	talipes equinovarus (deformity)
	transmission electron microscopy		venous thromboembolism (French
TEMI	transient episodes of myocardial		and Spanish abbreviation)
	ischemia	TEVAP	transurethral electrovaporization of
TEMP	temperature		the prostate
	temporal	TEVAR	thoracic endovascular aneurysm
	temporary		repair
TEN	tension (intraocular pressure)	TF	tactile fremitus
	toxic epidermal necrolysis		tail flick (reflex)
TEN®	Total Enteral Nutrition		tetralogy of Fallot
TENS	transcutaneous electrical nerve		Thomsen-Friedenreich (antigen)
	stimulation		tibiofemoral
TEOAE	transient evoked otoacoustic		to follow
	emission (test)		transfer (patient)
TEP	total endoprosthesis		trigger finger
	total extraperitoneal (laparoscopic		tube feeding
	hernia repair)	TFA	topical fluoride application
	tracheoesophageal puncture		trans fatty acids
	tubal ectopic pregnancy		trifluoroacetic acid
TEQ	toxic equivalents	TFB	trifascicular block
TER	terlipressin	TFBC	The Family Birthing Center
	total elbow replacement	TFC	thoracic fluid content
	total energy requirement		time to following commands
	transnasal endoscopic resection	TFCC	triangular fibrocartilage complex
	transurethral electroresection	TFESI	transforaminal epidural steroid
TERB	terbutaline		injection
TERC	Test of Early Reading	TFF	tangential flow filtration
	Comprehension		trefoil factor family (peptides)
TERM	full-term	TF-Fe	transferrin-bound iron
	terminal	TFI	total fluid intake
TERT	human telomerase reverse		treatment-free interval
	transcriptase (also hTRT)	TFL	tensor fasciae latae
	tertiary		transnasal fiberoptic laryngoscopy
	total end-range time		trimetrexate, fluorouracil, and
TES	therapeutic electrical stimulation		leucovorin
	thoracic endometriosis syndrome		trunk-forward lean
	thoracic endoscopic	TFM	transverse friction massage
	sympathectomy	TFN	trochanteric fixation nail
	transcorneal electrical stimulation	TFO	triplex-forming oligonucleotide
	treatment emergent symptoms	TFOs	triplex-forming oligonucleotides
TESA	testicular sperm aspiration	TFPI	tissue-factor pathway inhibitor
TESE	testicular sperm extraction	TFR	total fertility rate
TESI	thoracic epidural steroid injection	TFSI	transforaminal (epidural) steroid
TESS	Toronto Extremity Salvage Score		injection
	Toxic Exposure Surveillance	TFT	thin-film transistor
	System		Thought Field Therapy
	treatment emergent signs and		thumb-finding test
	symptoms		trifluridine (trifluorothymidine)
	Treatment Emergent Symptom	TFTs	thyroid function tests
	Scale	TFV	tenofovir (Viread)
TEST	testosterone	T25FW	timed 25-foot walk
TET	transcranial electrostimulation	TG	total gym
	therapy		triglycerides

Tg	thyroglobulin
6-TG	thioguanine
TGA	Therapeutic Goods Administration (Australia)
	third-generation antidepressant
	transient global amnesia
	transposition of the great arteries
TGAR	total graft area rejected
TGB	tiagabine (Gabatril)
TGC	tight glucose control
TGCE	temperature gradient capillary electrophoresis
TGCT	tenosynovial giant-cell tumor
	testicular germ cell tumor(s)
TGD	thyroglossal duct
	tumor growth delay
TGDC	thyroglossal duct cyst
TGE	transmissible gastroenteritis
TGFA	triglyceride fatty acid
TGF	transforming growth factor
TGF-β	transforming growth factor-beta
TGGE	temperature-gradient gel electrophoresis
TGN	trans-Golgi network
	trochanteric gamma nail
TGR	tenderness, guarding, and rigidity
TGS	tincture of green soap
TGs	triglycerides
TGT	thromboplastin generation test
TGTL	total glottic transverse laryngectomy
TGV	thoracic gas volume
	transposition of great vessels
TGXT	thallium-graded exercise test
TGZ	troglitazone (Rezulin)
TH	thrill
	thyroid hormone
	total hysterectomy
Th	thorium
	Thursday
T&H	type and hold
TH1	T helper cell, type 1
TH2	T helper cell, type 2
THA	tacrine (tetrahydroacridine; Cognex)
	total hip arthroplasty
	transient hemispheric attack
THAA	thyroid hormone autoantibodies
	tubular hypoplasia aortic arch
THAL	thalassemia
	thalidomide (Thalomid)
THAT	Toronto Hospital Alertness Test
THBI	thyroid hormone binding index
THBR	thyroid hormone-binding ratio
THAM®	tromethamine
THBO$_2$	topical hyperbaric oxygen
THC	tetrahydrocannabinol (dronabinol)
	thigh circumference
	transhepatic cholangiogram
THCT	triple-phase helical computer tomography
TH-CULT	throat culture
tHcy	total homocysteine
THDC	tunnelled hemodialysis catheter
THE	total-head excursion
	transhepatic embolization
Ther Ex	therapeutic exercise
THF	thymic humoral factor
THG	tetrahydrogestrinone
THg	total mercury
THI	transient hypogamma-globinemia of infancy
THKAFO	trunk-hip-knee-ankle-foot orthosis
THKAFO-LU	lockable joints using trunk-hip-knee-ankle-foot orthosis
THL	transvaginal hydrolaparoscopy
THLAA	tubular hypoplasia left aortic arch
THM	take-home methadone
THMs	trihalomethanes
THP	take home packs
	topical hemostatic powder
	total hip prosthesis
	transhepatic portography
	trihexyphenidyl (Artane)
THR	target heart rate
	thrombin receptor
	total hip replacement
	training heart rate
THRL	total hip replacement, left
THRR	total hip replacement, right
	transient hyperemic response ratio
THS	Tolosa-Hunt syndrome
THTV	therapeutic home trial visit
THV	therapeutic home visit
THz	terahertz (a unit of electromagnetic wave frequency equal to one trillion hertz [10^{12} hertz])
TI	inversion time (radiology)
	terminal ileus
	thallium imaging
	therapeutic index
	thought insertion
	time following inversion pulse (radiology)
	transischial
	transverse diameter of inlet
	tricuspid incompetence
	tricuspid insufficiency
TI4	therapeutic interchange for ...
TIA	transient ischemic attack
TIB	tibia
	time in bed (polysomnography related)
TIBC	total iron-binding capacity
tib-fib	tibia and fibula

TIBI-CaP	Total Illness Burden Index for Prostate Cancer
TIBS	transillumination breast spectroscopy
TIC	paclitaxel (Taxol), ifosfamide, and cisplain
	total ion chromatograms
	trypsin-inhibitor capacity
	tubal intraepithelial carcinoma
TICOSMO	**t**rauma, **i**nfection, **c**hemical/drug exposure, **o**rgan systems, **s**tress, **m**usculoskeletal, and **o**ther (prompts used during history taking for possible etiologies of problems)
TICS	diverticulosis
TICU	thoracic intensive care unit
	transplant intensive care unit
	trauma intensive care unit
t.i.d.	three times a day
TIDM	three times daily with meals
TIE	transient ischemic episode
TIF	tracheal intubation fiberscope
TIG	tetanus immune globulin
TIH	tumor-inducing hypercalcemia
TKI	tyrosine kinase inhibitor
TIL	tumor-infiltrating lymphocytes
%tile	percentile
TIMI	Thrombolysis in Myocardial Infarction (studies)
TIMP	tissue inhibitor of metalloproteinase
TIMP-2	Tissue inhibitors of metallo-proteinase 2
TIN	Taxpayer Identification Number
	testicular intraepithelial neoplasia
	three times a night (this is a dangerous abbreviation)
	tubulointerstitial nephritis
tinct	tincture
TIND	Treatment Investigational New Drug (application)
TINEM	there is no evidence of malignancy
TIP	toxic interstitial pneumonitis
	tube in place
	tubularized incised plate (urethroplasty)
TIP & P	tube in place and patent
TIPS	transvenous intrahepatic portosystemic shunt (stent-shunt)
TIPSS	transjugular intrahepatic portosystemic shunt (stent)
TIPU	tubularized-incised plate urethroplasty
TIRDA	temporal intermittent rhythmic delta activity (electroencephalograph)

TIRFM	total-internal reflection fluorescence microscopy
TIS	tumor *in situ*
TISS	Therapeutic Intervention Scoring System
TIT	*Treponema (pallidum)* immobilization test
	triiodothyronine (liothyronine)
TIUP	term intrauterine pregnancy
TIV	trivalent inactivated influenza vaccine
TIVA	total intravenous anethesia
TIVC	thoracic inferior vena cava
+tive	positive
TIW	three times a week (this is a dangerous abbreviation)
TJ	tendon jerk
	tight junction
	triceps jerk
TJA	total joint arthroplasty
TJC	tender joint count
	The Joint Commission (formerly JCAHO, the Joint Commission on Accreditation of Healthcare Organizations)
TJN	tongue jaw neck (dissection)
	twin-jet nebulizer
TJR	total joint replacement
TK	thymidine kinase
	toxicokinetics
TKA	total knee arthroplasty
	tyrosine kinase activity
TKD	tokodynamometer
TKE	terminal knee extension
TKIC	true knot in cord
TKNO	to keep needle open
TKP	thermokeratoplasty
	total knee prosthesis
TKO	to keep (vein; intravenous line) open
TKR	total knee replacement
TKRL	total knee replacement, left
TKRR	total knee replacement, right
TKVO	to keep vein open
TL	team leader
	thermoluminescence
	thoracolumbar
	total laryngectomy
	transverse line
	trial leave
	tubal ligation
T/L	terminal latency
Tl	thallium
TLA	translumbar arteriogram (aortogram)
	transverse ligament of atlas
TLAC	triple lumen Arrow catheter
TL BLT	tubal ligation, bilateral

TLC	tender loving care		Tibetan Medicine
	therapeutic lifestyle changes		trabecular meshwork
	thin layer chromatography		Trach (tracheostomy) mask
	titanium linear cutter		trademark (unregistered)
	T-lymphocyte choriocarcinoma		transcendental meditation
	total lift chair		transformed migraine
	total lung capacity		transmetatarsal
	total lymphocyte count		treadmill
	transitional living center		tropical medicine
	triple lumen catheter		tumor
TLD	thermoluminescent dosimeter		tympanic membrane
TLDA	temporal lobe delta activity	T & M	type and crossmatch
	(electroencephalograph)	TMA	thrombotic microangiopathy
TLE	temporal lobe epilepsy		tissue microarray
TLE-HS	temporal lobe epilepsy-		trained medication aid
	hippocampal sclerosis		transcription mediated
TLESI	transforaminal lumbar epidural		amplification
	steroid injection		transmetatarsal amputation
TLFB	timeline follow back (interview)		trimethylamine
T-LGLL	T-cell large granular lymphocyte	T/MA	tracheostomy mask
	leukemia	TMAS	Taylor Manifest Anxiety Scale
TLH	total laparoscopic hysterectomy	TMAs	tissue microarrays
TLI	total lymphoid irradiation	TMA-uria	trimethylaminuria
	translaryngeal intubation	T_{max}	temperature maximum
TLIF	transforaminal lumbar interbody	t_{max}	time of occurrence for maximum
	fusion		(peak) drug concentration
TLK	thermal laser keratoplasty	TMB	tetramethylberizidine
TLM	thalidomide (Thalomid)		therapeutic back massage
	torn lateral meniscus		transient monocular blindness
	transoral laser microsurgery		trimethoxybenzoates
TLNB	term living newborn	TMC	transmural colitis
TLOA	temporary leave of absence		Transtheoretical Model of Change
TLOVR	time to loss of virologic response		trapeziometacarpal
TLP	transitional living program		triamcinolone
TLR	target-lesion revascularization	TMCA	trimethylcolchicinic acid
	tonic labyrinthine reflex	TMCC	temporal mandibular cervical chain
TLR9	Toll-like receptor 9		(of muscles)
TLRs	Toll-like receptors	TMCN	triamcinolone
TLS	tumor lysis syndrome	TMD	temporomandibular dysfunction
TLSO	thoracic lumbar sacral orthosis		(disorder)
TLSP	trypsin-like serine protease		transient myeloproliferative
TLSSO	thoracolumbosacral spinal orthosis		disorder
TLT	tonsillectomy		treating physician
TLTBI	treatment of latent tuberculosis	t-MDS	therapy-related myelodysplastic
	infection		syndrome
TLUS	the time elapsed from ingestion of	TME	thermolysin-like
	the first dose of medication to		metalloendopeptidase
	passage of the last unformed		total mesorectal excision
	stool	TMET	treadmill exercise test
TLV	threshold limit value	TMEV	Theiler murine encephalomyelitis
	total lung volume		virus
TLVAB	transient left-ventricular apical	TMG	trimegestone
	ballooning	TMH	trainable mentally handicapped
TM	temperature by mouth	TMI	threatened myocardial infarction
	tetrathiomolybdate		transmandibular implant
	thalassemia major		transmural infarct
	Thayer-Martin (culture)	T>MIC	time above minimum inhibitory
	thyromegaly		concentration

T

TMJ	temporomandibular joint		Tru-Cut® needle biopsy
TMJD	temporomandibular joint dysfunction	TNBC	triple-negative breast cancer(s)
		TNBP	transurethral needle biopsy of prostate
TMJS	temporomandibular joint syndrome		
TML	tongue midline	TNCC	Trauma Nursing Course Certified
	treadmill	TND	term, normal delivery
TMLR	transmyocardial laser revascularization	TNDM	transient neonatal diabetes mellitus
		TNF	tumor necrosis factor
TMM	torn medial meniscus	TNF-bp	tumor necrosis factor binding protein
	total muscle mass		
Tmm	McKay-Marg tension	TNG	nitroglycerin
TMNG	toxic multinodular goiter		toxic nodular goiter
TMO	transcaruncular medial orbitotomy	TNI	total nodal irradiation
TMP	thallium myocardial perfusion	TnI	troponin I
	transmembrane pressure	TNKase®	tenecteplase
	trimethoprim	TNM	primary tumor, regional lymph nodes, and distant metastasis (used with subscripts for the staging of cancer)
TMP/SMZ	trimethoprim and sulfamethoxazole (correct name is sulfamethoxazole and trimethoprin; SMZ-TMP)		
		t-NNT	threshold number needed to treat
TMR	targeted motor reinnervation	TNP	test not performed
	temporary medication refill		time to neurologic progression
	tissue-maximum ratio		transdermal nicotine patch
	trainable mentally retarded	TNR	tonic neck reflex
	transmyocardial revascularization	TNS	transcutaneous nerve stimulation (stimulator)
	transverse digital microradiography		
TMS	transcranial magnetic stimulation		transient neurologic symptoms
TMSI	Task Management Strategy Index		Trauma Nurse Specialist
TMST	treadmill stress test		Tullie-Niebörg syndrome
TMT	tarsometatarsal	TNT	thiotepa, mitoxantrone (Novantrone), and paclitaxel (Taxol)
	teratoma with malignant transformation		
	treadmill test		treating to new targets
	tympanic membrane thermometer		triamcinolone and nystatin
TMTC	too many to count	TnT	troponin T
TMTX	trimetrexate (Neutrexin)	TNTC	too numerous to count
TMUGS	Tumor Marker Utility Grading Scale	TNU	tobacco nonuser
		TNY	trichomonas and yeast
TMVL	transient monocular visual loss	TO	old tuberculin
TMX	tamoxifen (Novaldex)		telephone order
TMZ	temazepam (Restoril)		throughout
	temozolomide (Temodar)		time off
TN	normal intraocular tension		tincture of opium (warning: this is NOT paregoric)
	team nursing		
	temperature normal		total obstruction
	tree nut		transfer out
	trigeminal neuralgia	T(O)	oral temperature
	triple negative	T/O	throughout
T&N	tension and nervousness		time out
	tingling and numbness	T&O	tandem and ovoid (insertion)
TNA	total nutrient admixture		tubes and ovaries
tNAA	total N-acetylaspartate	TOA	time of arrival
TNAs	transient neurological attacks		tubo-ovarian abscess
TNAB	transthoracic needle biopsy	TOAA	to affected areas
TNB	term newborn	TOAST	Trial of Org 10172 (danaparoid sodium) in Acute Stroke Treatment (criteria for nonpostoperative strokes)
	transnasal butorphanol		
	transrectal needle biopsy (of the prostate)		

TOB	tobacco	TOS	intraocular pressure of the left eye
	tobramycin		thoracic outlet syndrome
TOC	table of contents		Type of Service
	test-of-cure (post-therapy visit)	TOT	tip-of-the-tongue
	total occlusal convergence		transobturator tape
	total organic carbon	TOT BILI	total bilirubin
TOCE	transcatheter oily chemoembolization	TOTM	trioctyltrimellitate
		TOV	telephone order verified
TOCO	tocodynamometer		trial of void
TOD	intraocular pressure of the right eye	TOW	time off work
	target organ damage	TOWL	Test of Written Language
	target-organ disease	TOX	toxoplasmosis (*Toxoplasma gondii*) vaccine
	time of death		
	time of departure	TOXO	toxoplasmosis
	tubal occlusion device	TP	teaching physician
TOE	transoesophageal echocardiography (United Kingdom and other countries)		temperature and pressure
			temporoparietal
			tender point
TOF	tetralogy of Fallot		therapeutic pass
	time of flight (radiology)		ThinPrep Pap (test)
	total of four		thought process
	train-of-four		thrombophlebitis
TOFMS	time-of-flight mass spectrometry		thymidine phosphorylase
TOGV	transposition of the great vessels		time to progression
TOH	throughout hospitalization		Todd paralysis
TOI	Trial Outcome Index		toe pressure
TOL	tolerate		toilet paper
	tolerated		total protein
	trial of labor		"T" piece
TOLAC	trial of labor after cesarean section		transverse process
TOLD	Test of Language Development		treating physician
TOM	therapeutic outcomes monitoring		trigger point
	tomorrow	T:P	trough-to-peak ratio
	transcutaneous oxygen monitor	T & P	temperature and pulse
ToM	theory-of-mind		turn and position
Tomo	tomography	TPA	alteplase, recombinant (tissue plasminogen activator) (Activase)
TON	tonight		
	traumatic optic neuropathy		temporary portacaval anastomosis
TOP	termination of pregnancy		third-party administrator
	Topografov (virus)		tissue polypeptide antigen
	topotecan (Hycamtin)		total parenteral alimentation
TOP-8	Treatment Outcome PTSD (post-traumatic stress disorder) (scale)	TPAL	term infant(s), premature infant(s), abortion(s), living children
TOPO	topotecan (Hycamtin)	TPB	Theory of Planned Behavior
TOPO 1	topoisermerase	TPC	target plasma concentration
TOPPS	trans-obturator polypropylene sling		tender-point count
TOPS	Take Off Pounds Sensibly		total patient care
TOPV	trivalent oral polio vaccine		total plate count
TOR	toremifene (Faneston)		total proctocolectomy
TORB	telephone order read back		touch preparation cytology
TORC	Test of Reading Comprehension		treatment of physician's choice
TORCH	toxoplasmosis, others (other viruses known to attack the fetus), rubella, cytomegalovirus, and herpes simplex (maternal viral infections)	TPC + IP AA	total proctocolectomy with ileal J-pouch with pouch-anal anastomosis
		TPD	treatable protocol depth
			tropical pancreatic diabetes
TORP	total ossicular replacement prosthesis		typhoid vaccine, not otherwise specified

T

TPD$_a$	typhoid vaccine, attenuated live (oral Ty21a strain)
TPD$_{AKD}$	typhoid vaccine, acetone-killed and dried (U.S. military)
TPD$_{HP}$	typhoid vaccine, heat and phenol inactivated, dried
TPD$_{VI}$	typhoid vaccine, *Vi* capsular polysaccharide
TPE	therapeutic plasma exchange
	total placental estrogens
	total protective environment
T-penia	thrombocytopenia
TPF	docetaxel (Taxotere), cisplatin (Platinol), and fluorouracil
	trained participating father
TPG	translesional pressure gradients
	transpulmonary gradient
TPH	the patient has . . .
	thromboembolic pulmonary hypertension
	trained participating husband
TPHA	*Treponema pallidum* hemagglutination
T PHOS	triple phosphate crystals
TPI	*Treponema pallidum* immobilization
	triose phosphate isomerase
TPIT	trigger point injection therapy
t$_{pk}$	time to peak
TPL	thromboplastin
T plasty	tympanoplasty
TPLO	tibial plateau leveling osteotomy (Veterinary)
TPLSM	two-photon laser-scanning microscope
TPM	temporary pacemaker
	topiramate (Topamax)
TPMT	thiopurine methyltransferase
TPN	total parenteral nutrition
TPO	thrombopoietin
	thyroid peroxidase
	thyroperoxidase
	trial prescription order
TPOAb	thyroid peroxidase antibodies
TPP	thiamine pyrophosphate
TpP	thrombus precursor protein
TP & P	time, place, and person
TPPN	total peripheral parenteral nutrition
TPPS	Toddler-Preschooler Postoperative Pain Scale
TPPV	trans pars plana vitrectomy
TPR	temperature
	temperature, pulse, and respiration
	termination of parental rights
	tissue-phantom ratio
	total peripheral resistance
TPRI	total peripheral resistance index
T PROT	total protein

TPS	tender point score
	typhus (*rickettsiae* sp.) vaccine
tPSA	total prostate-specific antigen
TPT	thermal perception threshold
	time to peak tension
	topotecan (Hycamtin)
	transpyloric tube
	treadmill performance test
*t*PTEF	time to peak tidal expiratory flow
TPU	tropical phagedenic ulcer
T-putty	Theraputty
TPV	tipranavir (Aptivus)
TPVA	tibioperoneal vessel angioplasty
TPVR	total peripheral vascular resistance
TPV/r	tipranavir (Aptivus) and ritonavir (Norvir)
TPZ	tirapazamine
TQD	target quit date
TQM	total quality management
TR	repetition time (radiology)
	therapeutic recreation
	time to repeat
	time to repetition (radiology)
	tincture
	to return
	trace
	transfusion reaction
	transplant recipients
	trapezius
	treatment
	tremor
	tricuspid regurgitation
	tumor registry
T(R)	rectal temperature
T & R	taking and retaining
	tenderness and rebound
	treated and released
	turn and reposition
TRA	therapeutic recreation associate
	to run at
	trastuzumab (Herceptin; also TRAS and H)
	traumatic rupture of the aorta
	tumor regression antigen
TRAb	thyrotropin-receptor antibody
TRAC	traction
TRACE	time-resolved amplified cryptate emission
TRACH	tracheal
	tracheostomy
TRAEs	treatment-related adverse events
TRAFO	tone-reducing ankle/foot orthosis
TRAIL	tumor-necrosis-factor-related apoptosis-inducing ligand
TRALI	transfusion-associated lung injury
TRAM	transverse rectus abdominis myocutaneous (flap)

transverse rectus abdominum muscle

Treatment Response Assessment Method

TRAMP transversus and rectus abdominis musculo-peritoneal (flap)

TRANCE tumor necrosis factor–related activation-induced cytokine

TRANS transfers

Trans D transverse diameter

TRANS Rx transfusion reaction

TRAP tartrate-resistant (leukocyte) acid phophatase

Telomeric Repeat Amplification Protocol

thrombospondin-related anonymous protein

total radical-trapping antioxidant parameter

trapezium

trapezius muscle

twin-reversed arterial perfusion

TRAS transplant renal artery stenosis

trastuzumab (Herceptin)

TRB return to baseline

TRBC total red blood cells

TRC tanned red cells

TRCB transretinal choroidal biopsy

TRD tongue-retaining device

total-retinal detachment

traction retinal detachment

treatment-related death

treatment-resistant depression

TRD-F treatment-related discontinuation-failure

TRDN transient respiratory distress of the newborn

TREC T-cell receptor-rearrangement excision circles

Tren Trendelenburg

TRF terminal restriction fragment

TrgEMG triggered electromyographic (stimulation)

TRH protirelin (thyrotropin-releasing hormone) (Relefact TRH®; Thypinone®)

TRI transient radicular irritation

trimester

TriA tricuspid atresia

T₃RIA triiodothyronine level by radioimmunoassay

TRIAC triiodothyroacetic acid

TRIAM triamcinolone

TRIC trachoma inclusion conjunctivitis

TRICH *Trichomonas*

TRICKS time-resolved imaging contrast kinetics

TRIG triglycerides

TRISS Trauma Related Injury Severity Score

Trk tropomyosin-related kinase

TRL tacrolimus (Prograf, also TAC)

TR-LSC time-resolved liquid scintillation counting

TRM transplant-related mortality

treatment-related mortality

TRM-SMX trimethoprim-sulfamethoxazole (correct name is sulfamethoxazole and trimethoprim; SMZ-TMP; SMX-TMP)

tRNA transfer ribonucleic acid

TRNBP transrectal needle biopsy prostate

TRND Trendelenburg (position)

TRNG tetracycline-resistant *Neisseria gonorrhoeae*

TRO to return to office

troponin

TROFO trofosfamide

TROM torque range of motion

total range of motion

TrOOP true out-of-pocket costs

TRP tubular reabsorption of phosphate

TRP-1 tyrosine-related protein-1

TRPS trichorhinophalangeal syndrome (types I, II, and III)

TrPs trigger points

TRPT transplant

TRR tumor response rate

TRS Therapeutic Recreation Specialist

the real symptom

time-resolved spectroscopy

tremor rating scale

TRT tangential radiation therapy

testosterone replacement therapy

thermoradiotherapy

thoracic radiation therapy

tinnitus retraining therapy

treatment-related toxicity

TR/TE time to repetition and time to echo in spin (echo sequence of magnetic resonance imaging)

T₃RU triiodothyronine resin uptake

TRUS transrectal ultrasonography

TRUSP transrectal ultrasonography of the prostate

TRUST toluidine red unheated serum test

TRZ triazolam (Halcion)

TS Tay-Sachs (disease)

telomerase

temperature sensitive

test solution

thoracic spine

throat swab

thymidylate synthase

timed samplings

	toe signs
	Tourette syndrome
	transsexual
	Trauma Score
	tricuspid stenosis
	triple strength
	tuberous sclerosis
	Turner syndrome
T/S	trimethoprim/sulfamethoxazole (correct name is sulfamethoxazole and trimethoprin)
T&S	type and screen
Ts	Schiotz tension
	T suppressor cell
TSAb	thyroid stimulating antibodies
TSA	toluenesulfonic acid
	total shoulder arthroplasty
	trichostatin A
	tryptone soya (blood) agar
	tumor-specific antigen
	type-specific antibody
	tyramine signal amplification
TSAR®	tape surrounded Appli-rulers
TSAS	Total Severity Assessment Score
TSAT	transferrin saturation
TSB	total serum bilirubin
	trypticase soy broth
TSBB	transtracheal selective bronchial brushing
TSC	technetium sulfur colloid
	theophylline serum concentration
	total symptom complex
	tuberous sclerosis complex
T-score	number of standard deviations from the average bone mineral density (BMD) of a 25-30 year old woman
TSD	target to skin distance
	Tay-Sachs disease
	total sleep deprivation
	T-(tumor) stage downstaging
TSDP	tapered steroid dosing package
TSE	targeted systemic exposure
	testicular self-examination
	total skin examination
	transmissible spongiform encephalopathy
	turbo spin-echo (magnetic resonance imaging)
TSEBT	total skin electron beam therapy
T set	tracheotomy set
TSF	tricep skin fold (thickness)
TSGA	term, small gestational age
TSGs	tumor suppressor genes
TSH	thyroid-stimulating hormone
TSH-RH	thyrotropin-releasing hormone
TSI	thyroid stimulating immunoglobulin

	tobramycin solution for inhalation (TOBI®)
TSIs	thymidylate synthase inhibitors
T-skull	trauma skull
TSM	two-spotted spider mite
T-SMBP	telemetric data transmission self-measured blood pressure
TSNAs	tobacco-specific nitrosamines
tsp	teaspoon (5 mL)
TSP	thrombospondin
	total serum protein
	tropical spastic paraparesis
TSPA	thiotepa
TSPE	thymidylate synthetase protein expression
TSperm	total number of sperm per ejaculate
T-spine	thoracic spine
TSR	total shoulder replacement
TSS	thumb spica splint
	total serum solids
	total symptom scores
	toxic shock syndrome
	transsphenoidal surgery
	treatment-satisfaction status (score)
	tumor score system
TSST	toxic shock syndrome toxin
TST	titmus stereocuity test
	total sleep time
	trans-scrotal testosterone
	treadmill stress test
	tuberculin skin test(s)
TSTA	tumor-specific transplantation antigens
TSTM	too small to measure
TT	targeted therapy
	testicular torsion
	Test Tape®
	tetanus toxoid
	thiotepa (Thioplex)
	thoracostomy tube
	thrombin time
	thrombolytic therapy
	thymol turbidity
	tilt table
	tilt testing
	tonometry
	total thyroidectomy
	transit time
	transtracheal
	treponemal test
	triceps thickness
	tuberculin tested
	tuberculoid leprosy
	twitch tension
	tympanic temperature
	tympanostomy tube
T-T	time-to-time
T/T	trace of ____/trace of ____

T&T	tobramycin and ticarcillin	TTOD	tetanus toxoid outdated
	touch and tone	TTOP	time to objective progression
	tympantomy and tube (insertion)	TTOT	transtracheal oxygen therapy
TT4	total thyroxine	TTP	tender to palpation
TTA	total toe arthroplasty		tender to pressure
	transtracheal aspiration		thrombotic thrombocytopenic
	trauma team activation		purpura
TTAT	toe touch as tolerated		time to pregnancy
	traumatic thoracic aortic		time to tumor progression
	transaction		time-to-progression
TTB	time-to-boundary	TTP/HUS	thrombotic thrombocytopenic
	transfer-tub bench		purpura and hemolytic-uremic
TTC	transtracheal catheter		syndrome
TTD	tarsal tunnel decompression	TTR	time in (to) therapeutic range
	temporary total disability		transthyretin
	total tumor dose		triceps tendon reflex
	transverse thoracic diameter	TTS	tarsal tunnel syndrome
	trichothiodystrophy		temporary threshold shift
TTDE	touch-tone data entry		through the skin
	transthoracic color Doppler		Toddler Temperament Scale
	echocardiography		transdermal therapeutic system
TTDM	thallim threadmill		transfusion therapy service
TTDP	time-to-disease progression		transtympanic steroids
TTE	time-to-event	TTs	tympanostomy tubes
	transthoracic echocardiography	TTT	tilt-table test
	trial terminated early		time to treatment termination
t test	Student's t-test		tolbutamide tolerance test
TTF	time-to-treatment failure		total tourniquet time
	tumor treatment fields		transpupillary thermotherapy
TTF-1	thyroid transcription factor-1		turn-to-turn transfusion
tTg	tissue transglutaminase	TTTG	tibial tuberosity to trochlear groove
TTGE	timed-temperature gradient		(distance)
	electrophoresis	TTTS	twin-twin transfusion syndrome
TTH	table-top height	TTUTD	tetanus toxoid up-to-date
	tension-type headache	TTV	Torque-TenoVirus
TTI	Teflon tube insertion		total tumor volume
	total time to intubate		transfusion-transmitted virus
	transfer to intermediate	TTVIs	transfusion-transmitted viral
	tympanostomy tube insertion		infections
TTII	thyrotropin-binding inhibitory	TTVP	temporary transvenous pacemaker
	immunoglobulins	TTWB	touch-toe weight bearing
TTJV	transtracheal jet ventilation	TTX	tetrodotoxin (a neurotoxin)
TTM	total tumor mass	TTx	thrombolytic therapy
	transtelephonic monitoring	TU	Todd units
	transtheoretical model		transrectal ultrasound
	trichotillomania		transurethral
TTMV	Torque-TenoMiniVirus		tuberculin units
TTN	time to normalization		tumor
	transient tachypnea of the newborn	Tu	Tuesday
TTNA	transthoracic needle aspiration	1-TU	1 tuberculin unit
TTNB	transient tachypnea of the newborn	5-TU	5 tuberculin units
TTND	time to nondetectable	250-TU	250 tuberculin units
TTO	tea tree oil	TUB	tuberculosis vaccine, not BCG
	time trade-off	tubal	tubal ligation
	to take out		tubal pregnancy
	transfer to open	TUBB3	class III beta-tubulin
	transtracheal oxygen	TUBS	traumatic, unidirectional instability
	triple tibial osteotomy (Veterinary)		and Bankart lesion

TUD	take as directed (this is a dangerous abbreviation as it may be read as TID [three times daily] or not understood)	T/V	touch-verbal
		TVC	triple voiding cystogram
			true vocal cord
		TVc	tricuspid valve closure
TUDS	temporary ureteral drainage system	TVD	triple vessel disease
TUE	transurethral extraction	TVDALV	triple vessel disease with an abnormal left ventricle
TUF	total ultrafiltration		
TUG	timed Up and GO (test)	TVF	tactile vocal fremitus
	total urinary gonadotropin		target vessel failure
TUIBN	transurethral incision of bladder neck		true vocal fold
		TVH	total vaginal hysterectomy
TUIP	transurethral incision of the prostate	TVI	time velocity integral
		TVN	tonic vibration response
TUL	tularemia (*Francisella tularensis*) vaccine	TVP	deep vein thrombosis (French and Spanish abbreviation)
TULIP®	transurethral ultrasound-guided laser-induced prostatectomy (system)		tensor veli palatini (muscle)
			transvenous pacemaker
			transvesicle prostatectomy
TULIPS	touch-up and loop incorporated primers (an alternative PCR technique)	TVR	target vessel revascularization (rate)
			tricuspid valve replacement
TUMT	transurethral microwave thermotherapy	TVRSS	total vasomotor rhinitis symptom score
TUN	total urinary nitrogen	TVS	transvaginal sonography
TUNA	transurethral needle ablation		transvenous system
TUNEL	terminal deoxynucleotidyl transferase-mediated dUTP-biotin nick-end labeling		trigemino-vascular system
		TVSC	transvaginal sector scan
		TVT	tension-free vaginal tape
TUPAC	tobacco use prevention and cessation		transvaginal taping
			transvaginal tension-free
TUPR	transurethral prostatic resection	TVT-O	tension-free vaginal tape-obturator
TUR	transurethral resection	TVU	total volume of urine
T₃UR	triiodothyronine uptake ratio		transvaginal ultrasonography
TURB	transurethral resection of the bladder	TVUS	transvaginal ultrasonography
		TW	talked with
	turbidity		tapwater
TURBN	transurethral resection bladder neck		test weight
TURBT	transurethral resection bladder tumor		thought withdrawal
			Trophermyma whippleii
TURP	transurethral resection of prostate		T-wave
TURV	transurethral resection valves	T1WI	T1 weighted image (magnetic resonance imaging term for short repetition time and short echo time)
TURVN	transurethral resection of vesical neck		
TUTL	transuterine tubal lavage		
TUU	transureteroureterostomy	T2WI	T2 weighted image (magnetic resonance imaging term for long repetition time and long echo time)
TUV	transurethral valve		
TUVP	transurethral vaporization of the prostate		
TV	television	T25W	timed 25-foot Walk
	temporary visit	TW2	Tanner-Whitehouse mark 2 (bone-age assessment)
	thyroid volume		
	tidal volume	5TW	five times a week (this is a dangerous abbreviation)
	tonic vergence		
	transvenous	TWA	time-weighted average
	trial visit		total wrist arthroplasty
	Trichomonas vaginalis		T-wave alternans
	tricuspid valve	TWAR	*Chlamydia pneumoniae*

T

T-wave	part of the electrocardiographic cycle, representing a portion of ventricular repolarization	TYVM	thank you very much
		TZ	temozolomide (Temodar) transition zone
TWB	total weight bearing	TZCS	time-zone change syndrome
TWD	total white and differential count	TZD	thiazolidinedione
TWE	tapwater enema	TZDs	thiazolidinediones
TWEAK	tumor necrosis factor-like weak inducer of apoptosis	TZM	temozolomide (Temodar)
TWETC	tapwater enema 'til clear		
TWG	total weight gain		
TWH	transitional wall hyperplasia		
TWHW ok	toe walking and heel walking all right		
TWI	tooth-wear index T-wave inversion		
TWiST	time without symptoms of progression or toxicity		
TWOC	trial without catheter		
TWP	twin pregnancy		
TWR	total wrist replacement two-week rule (referrals)		
TWSTRS	Toronto Western Spasmodic Torticollis Rating Scale		
TWT	timed walking test		
TWWD	tap water wet dressing		
Tx	therapist therapy traction transcription transfer transfuse transplant transplantation treatment tympanostomy		
T & X	type and crossmatch		
TXA₂	thromboxane A₂		
TXB₂	thromboxane B₂		
TXE	Timoptic-XE®		
TXL	paclitaxel (Taxol) (this is a dangerous abbreviation as it can be read as TXT)		
TXM	type and crossmatch		
TXP	transplant		
TXS	type and screen		
TXT	docetaxel (Taxotere) (this is a dangerous abbreviation as it can be read as TXL)		
TY	tympanic		
T & Y	trichomonas and yeast		
TYCO #3	Tylenol with 30 mg of codeine (#1=7.5 mg, #2=15 mg and #4=60 mg of codeine present)		
Tyl	Tylenol (acetaminophen) tyloma (callus)		
TYMP	tympanogram		
Tyr	tyrosinase		

T

U

U	Ultralente Insulin® (it is dangerous to use abbreviations for insulin therapy)
	units (this is the most dangerous abbreviation—spell out "unit")
	unknown
	upper
	uranium
	urine
Ⓤ	Kosher
U/1	1 finger breadth below umbilicus
1/U	1 finger over umbilicus
U/	at umbilicus
24U	24-hour urine (collection)
U100	100 units per milliliters
UA	umbilical artery
	unauthorized absence
	uncertain about
	unstable angina
	upper airway
	upper arm
	uric acid
	urinalysis
	uterine activity
UABD	upper airway bronchodilation
UAC	umbilical artery catheter
	under active
	upper airway congestion
UA/C	uric acid to creatinine (ratio)
UAD	upper airway disease
	use as directed
UADE	unanticipated adverse device event
UADT	upper aerodigestive tract
UAE	urinary albumin excretion
	uterine artery embolization
UACEs	unplanned acute care encounters
UAER	urinary albumin excretion rate
UAI	unprotected anal intercourse
UAL	umbilical artery line
	up *ad lib*
UA&M	urinalysis and microscopy
UANC	uncomplicated antenatal confinement
UA/ NSTEMI	unstable angina and non-ST-segment elevation myocardial infarction
UAO	upper airway obstruction
UAP	upper abdominal pain
UAPD	Union of American Physicians and Dentists
UAPF	upon arrival patient found
UAPs	unlicensed assistive personnel
U-ARM	upper arm
UARS	upper airway resistance syndrome

UAS	upstream activating sequence
UASA	upper airway sleep apnea
UASQ	Unstable Angina Symptoms Questionnaire
UAT	up as tolerated
UAVC	univentricular atrioventricular connection
UB	upper body
UBAs	urethral bulking agents
UBC	unicameral bone cyst
	University of British Columbia (brace)
UBD	universal blood donor
UBE	upper body ergometer
UBF	unknown black female
	uterine blood flow
UBI	ultraviolet blood irradiation
UBM	unknown black male
UBO	unidentified bright object
UBT	^{13}C-urea breath test
	uterine balloon therapy
UBW	usual body weight
UC	ulcerative colitis
	umbilical cord
	unchanged
	unconscious
	Unit clerk
	United Church of Christ
	urea clearance
	urinary catheter
	urine culture
	usual care
	uterine contraction
	urothelial carcinoma
U&C	urethral and cervical
	usual and customary
UCABG	urgent coronary artery bypass graft (surgery)
UCAD	unstable coronary artery disease
UCB	umbilical cord blood
	unconjugated bilirubin (indirect)
	Unicorn Campbell Boy (orthotics)
UCBT	umbilical cord-blood transplantation
	unrelated cord-blood transplant
UCCL	ulnocarpal collateral ligament
UCD	urine collection device
	usual childhood diseases
UCE	urea cycle enzymopathy
UCF	unexplained chronic fatigue
UCG	urinary chorionic gonadotropins
UCHD	usual childhood diseases
UCHI	usual childhood illnesses
UCHS	uncontrolled hemorrhagic shock
UCI	urethral catheter in
	usual childhood illnesses
UCL	ulnar collateral ligament

	uncomfortable loudness level	UE	ultrasound elastography
UCLA	University of California, Los Angeles (activity score)		under elbow
			undetermined etiology
UCLP	unilateral cleft lip and palate		upper extremity
UCN	urocortin	U & E	urea and electrolytes (see page 356)
UCN-01	7-hydroxystaurosporin		
UCO	urethral catheter out	UEBW	ultrasound estimated bladder weight
UCP	umbilical cord prolapse		
	uncoupling protein	UEC	uterine endometrial carcinoma
	United Cerebral Palsy	UEDs	unilateral epileptiform discharges
	urethral closure pressure	UEDVT	upper extremities deep venous thrombosis
UCPs	urine collection pads		
UCR	unconditioned reflex	UES	undifferentiated embryonal sarcoma
	unconditioned response		
	usual, customary, and reasonable (fees)		upper esophageal sphincter
		UESEP	upper extremity somatosensory evoked potential
UCP-3	uncoupling protein −3		
UCRE	urine creatinine	UESP	upper esophageal sphincter pressure
UCRP	universal coagulation reference plasma		
		UF	ultrafiltration
UCS	unconscious		until finished
UC&S	urine culture and sensitivity	UFC	urinary free cortisol
UCTD	undifferentiated connective tissue disease	UFF	unusual facial features
		UFFI	urea formaldehyde foam insulation
UCVA	uncorrected visual acuity	UFH	unfractionated heparin
UCX	urine culture	UFN	until further notice
UD	as directed (this is a dangerous abbreviation as it may not be understood)	UFO	unflagged order
			unidentified foreign object
		UFOV	useful field of view
	ugly duckling (sign) (pigmented moles)	UFR	ultrafiltration rate
		UFS	urofacial syndrome
	ulnar deviation	UFT	uracil and tegafur
	ultrasonic dissection	UFV	ultrafiltration volume
	unit dose	UG	until gone
	urethral dilatation		urinary glucose
	urethral discharge		urogenital
	urodynamics	UGA	under general anesthesia
	uterine distension		urogenital atrophy
u.d.	as directed (this is a dangerous abbreviation as it may not be understood)	UGB	upper-gastrointestinal-tract bleeding
		UGCR	ultrasound-guided compression repair
UDC	uninhibited detrusor (muscle) capacity		
		UGDP	University Group Diabetes Project
	usual diseases of childhood	UGFS	ultrasound-guided foam sclerotherapy
UDCA	ursodeoxycholic acid (Ursodiol)		
UDI	Urogenital Distress Inventory	UGH	uveitis, glaucoma, and hyphema (syndrome)
UDN	updraft nebulizer		
UDO	undetermined origin	UGI	upper gastrointestinal series
UDP	unassisted diastolic pressure	UGIB	upper gastrointestinal bleeding
UDPGT	uridinediphospho-glucuronyl transferase	UGIE	upper gastrointestinal endoscopy
		UGIH	upper gastrointestinal hemorrhage
UDS	uncomplicated diverticulitis of the sigmoid	UGIS	upper gastrointestinal series
		UGIT	upper gastrointestinal tract
	unconditioned stimulus	UGI	upper gastrointestinal
	urodynamic study(ies)	w/SBFT	(series) with small bowel follow through
	urine drug screen		
UDT	undescended testicle(s)	UGK	urine, glucose, and ketones
UDU	uniformity of dosage units	UGP	urinary gonadotropin peptide

UGT1A1	uridine diphosphate glucuronosyltransferase	U & L	upper and lower
UGTI	ultrasound-guided thrombin injection	ULBW	ultra low birth weight (between 501 and 750 g)
UGVA	ultrasound-guided vascular access	ULD	Unverricht-Lundborg disease
UH	umbilical hernia	ULDT	ultra low-dose therapy
	unfavorable history	ULL	ulnolunate ligament
	University Hospital	ULLE	upper lid, left eye
UHBI	upper hemibody irradiation	ULMCA	unprotected left main coronary artery
UHDDS	Uniform Hospital Discharge Data Set	ULMS	uterine leiomyosarcomas
		ULN	upper limits of normal
UHDRS	Unified Huntington Disease Rating Scale	ULOD	ultra-late-onset disease
		ULPA	ultra-low particulate air
UHDs	ulcer-healing drugs	ULQ	upper left quadrant
UHMWPE	ultra-high molecular weight polyethylene	ULRE	upper lid, right eye
		ULSB	upper left sternal border
UHP	University Health Plan	ULTT1	upper limb tension test 1 (median nerve)
UHPLC	ultra-high-performance liquid chromatography	ULTT2a	upper limb tension test 2a (medial nerve)
UI	urinary incontinence		
UIB	Unemployment Insurance Benefits	ULTT2b	upper limb tension test 2b (radial nerve)
UIBC	unbound iron binding capacity		
	unsaturated iron binding capacity	ULTT3	upper limb tension test 3 (ulnar nerve)
UID	once daily (this is a dangerous abbreviation, spell out "once daily")		
		ULYTES	electrolytes, urine
		UM	unmarried
UIEP	urine (urinary) immunoelectrophoresis		utilization management
		Umb A Line	umbilical artery line
UIP	usual interstitial pneumonitis (pneumonia)	Umb V Line	umbilical venous line
UIQ	upper inner quadrant	umb ven	umbilical vein
UITN	Urinary Incontinence Treatment Network	UMCD	uremic medullary cystic disease
		UMLS	Unified Medical Language System
UJ	universal joint (syndrome)	UMN	upper motor neuron (disease)
UK	United Kingdom	UN	undernourished
	unknown		urinary nitrogen
	urine potassium	UNA	urinary nitrogen appearance
	urokinase	UNa	urine sodium
UKA	unicompartmental knee arthroplasty	unacc	unaccompanied
		UNC	uncrossed
UK IC	urokinase intracoronary	UNDEL	undelivered
UKE	unknown etiology	UNDP	United Nations Development Program
UKNDS	United Kingdom Neurological Disability Score		
		UNE	ulnar neuropathy at the elbow
UKO	unknown origin		urinary norepinephrine
UKOSS	United Kingdom Obstetric Surveillance System	ung	ointment
		UNHS	universal newborn hearing screening
UKR	unicompartmental knee replacement		
		unilat	unilateral
UL	Unit Leader	UNK	unknown
	upper left	UNL	upper normal levels
	upper lid	UNOS	United Network for Organ Sharing
	upper limb	UN/P	unpatched eye
	upper lobe	UN/P OD	unpatched right eye
U/L	units per liter (this is a dangerous abbreviation since a handwritten U can be mistaken for a zero)	UN/P OS	unpatched left eye
		UNS	universal neonatal screening
	upper and lower		unsatisfactory

UNSAT	unsatisfactory	UR AC	uric acid
uNTx	urinary N-telopeptide	URAS	unilateral renal artery stenosis
UO	under observation	URD	undifferentiated respiratory disease
	undetermined origin		unrelated donor
	ureteral orifice		upper respiratory disease
	urinary output	URE	Uniform Rules of Evidence
UONx	unilateral optic nerve transection	URG	urgent
UOP	urinary output	URI	upper respiratory infection
UOQ	upper outer quadrant	URIC A	uric acid
UORBC	uncrossmatched type-O packed red	url	unrelated
	blood cells	UR&M	urinalysis, routine and microscopic
UOS	upper oesophageal sphincter	URO	urology
	(United Kingdom and other	UROB	urobilinogen
	countries)	UroCa	urothelial cancer
Uosm	urinary osmolality	UROD	ultra-rapid opiate detoxification
✓ up	check up		[under anesthesia]
UP	unipolar	UROL	Urologist
	ureteropelvic		urology
U/P	urine to plasma (creatinine)	URQ	upper right quadrant
UP3	uvulopalatopharyngoplasty	URR	urea reduction ratio
UPC	unknown primary carcinoma	URS	ureterorenoscopy
UPD	uniparental disomy	URSB	upper right sternal border
UPDRS	Unified Parkinson Disease Rating	URT	upper respiratory tract
	Scale		uterine resting tone
UPEP	urine protein electrophoresis	URTI	upper respiratory tract infection
UPG	uroporphyrinogen	US	ultrasonography
UPIN	unique physician (provided)		ultrasound
	identification number		unit secretary
UPJ	ureteropelvic junction		United States of America
UPJO	ureteropelvic junction obstruction	USA	unit services assistant
UPLIF	unilateral posterior lumbar		United States Army
	interbody fusion		United States of America
UPN	unique patient number		unstable angina
UPNC	uncomplicated postnatal course	USAF	United States Air Force
UPO	metastatic carcinoma of unknown	USAISR	United States Army Institute of
	primary origin		Surgical Research
UPOR	usual place of residence	USAMRIID	United States Army Medical
UPP	urethral pressure profile		Research Institute of Infectious
	urethral pressure profilometry		Diseases
	uvulopalatoplasty	USAN	United States Adopted Names
UPPP	uvulopalatopharyngoplasty	USAP	unstable angina pectoris
U/P ratio	urine to plasma ratio	USB	upper sternal border
UPS	ubiquitin-dependent proteasomal	USC	uterine serous carcinoma
	system	USCB	ultrasound-guided core biopsy
	ubiquitin-proteasome system	U-SCOPE	ureteroscopy
UPSC	uterine papillary serous carcinoma	USCVD	unsterile controlled vaginal
UPSIT	University of Pennsylvania Smell		delivery
	Identification Test	USD	urethral stricture disease
UPT	uptake	USDA	United States Department of
	urine pregnancy test		Agriculture
UR	unrelated	USED-	ureterosigmoidostomy,
	upper respiratory	CARP	small bowel fistula, extra
	upper right		chloride, diarrhea, carbonic
	urinary retention		anhydrase inhibitors, adrenal
	utilization review		insufficiency, renal tubular
URA	unilateral renal agenesis		acidosis, and pancreatic fistula
URAC	Utilization Review Accreditation		(common causes of nonanion
	Commission		gap metabolic acidosis)

U

USEIR	United States Eye Injury Registry	
USG	ultrasmall gold (particles)	
	ultrasonography	
	urine specific gravity	
USH	United Services for Handicapped	
	usual state of health	
USI	urinary stress incontinence	
USLS	uterosacral ligaments suspension	
	uterosacral ligaments	
USL	uterosacral ligament	
USM	ultrasonic mist	
USMC	United States Marine Corps	
USMLE	United States Medical Licensing Examination	
USN	ultrasonic nebulizer	
	United States Navy	
USO	unilateral salpingo-oophorectomy	
USOGH	usual state of good health	
USOH	usual state of health	
USP	unassisted systolic pressure	
	United States Pharmacopeia	
USPHS	United States Public Health Service	
USPSTF	United States Preventive Services Task Force	
USS	Upshaw-Schulman syndrome	
USUCVD	unsterile uncontrolled vaginal delivery	
USVMD	urine specimen volume measuring device	
UT	upper thoracic	
UTA	unable to assess	
	urinary tract anomaly	
UTC	undifferentiated thyroid carcinoma	
	urinary tract calculi	
UtCa	uterine cancer	
UTD	unable to determine	
	up to date	
ut dict	as directed	
UTF	usual throat flora	
UTI	urinary tract infection	
UTL	ulnotriquetral ligament	
	unable to locate	
	useful therapeutic life	
UTM	urinary-tract malformations	
UTMDACC	University of Texas M.D. Anderson Cancer Center	
UTO	unable to obtain	
	upper tibial osteotomy	
	uterus, tubes, and ovaries	
UTP	uridine triphosphate	
UTR	untranslated region	
UTS	ulnar tunnel syndrome	
	ultrasound	
UTUC	upper-tract urothelial carcinoma	
U/U−	uterine fundus at umbilicus (usually modified as number of finger breadths below)	

U/U+	uterine fundus at umbilicus (usually modified as number of finger breadths above)
UUD	uncontrolled unsterile delivery
UUI	urge urinary incontinence
UUN	urinary urea nitrogen
UUTI	uncomplicated urinary tract infections
UV	ultraviolet
	umbilical vein
	ureterovesical
	urine volume
UVA	ultraviolet A light
	ureterovesical angle
UVB	ultraviolet B light
UVBI	ultraviolet blood irradiation
UVC	umbilical vein catheter
	ultraviolet C light
UVEB	unifocal ventricular ectopic beat
UVGI	ultraviolet germicidal irradiation
UVH	univentricular heart
UVIB	ultraviolet irradiation of blood
UVJ	ureterovesical junction
UVL	ultraviolet light
	umbilical venous line
UVR	ultraviolet radiation
UVT	unsustained ventricular tachycardia
UV-VIS	ultraviolet-visible (spectrometer)
U/WB	unit of whole blood
UW	unilateral weakness
UWF	unknown white female
UWM	unknown white male
	unwed mother
UXO	unexploded ordnance

U

V

V five
gas volume
minute volume
vaccinated
vagina
Valium (diazepam); as in vitamin V (slang)
vein
ventricular
verb
verbal
vertebral
very
veteran
Viagra (sildenafil citrate) as in "vitamin V"
viral
vision
vitamin
volume (with any number, such as V20)
vomiting

$\dot{V}$ ventilation (L/min)

+V positive vertical divergence

V1 fifth cranial nerve, ophthalmic division

V2 fifth cranial nerve, maxillary division

V3 fifth cranial nerve, mandibular division

3V 3-vessel (cord)

V_1 to V_6 precordial chest leads

VA vacuum aspiration
valproic acid
ventriculoatrial
venous access
venous aneurysms
verbal autopsy
vertebral artery
Veterans Administration
visual acuity

V_A alveolar gas volume

V&A vagotomy and antrectomy

VAAESS Vaccine-Associated Adverse Events Surveillance System (Canada)

VAB vacuum-assisted biopsy
variable atrial blockage
vinblastine, dactinomycin (actinomycin D), bleomycin

VABS Vineland Adaptive Behavior Scales

VAC etoposide (VePesid), cytarabine (ara-C), and carboplatin
vacuum-assisted closure (dressings)
ventriculoarterial conduction
vincristine, dactinomycin (actinomycin D), and cyclophosphamide
vincristine, doxorubicin (Adriamycin), and cyclophosphamide

VA cc distance visual acuity with correction

VA ccl near visual acuity with correction

VACE *Vitex agnus-castus* extract (Chaste tree berry extract)

VAC EXT vacuum extractor

VAC/IE vincristine, doxorubicin (Adriamycin), cyclophosphamide, ifosfamide, and etoposide

VAC_{ig} vaccinia immune globulin

VACIME vincristine, doxorubicin (Adriamycin), cyclophosphamide, ifosfamide, mesna, and etoposide

VACO Veterans Administration Central Office

VACTERL vertebral, anal, cardiac, tracheal, esophageal, renal, and limb anomalies

VAD vascular (venous) access device
ventricular assist device
vertebral artery dissection
Veterans Administration Domiciliary
vincristine, doxorubicin (Adriamycin), and dexamethasone

VaD vascular dementia

VADCS ventricular atrial distal coronary sinus

VADRIAC vincristine, doxorubicin (Adriamycin), and cyclophosphamide

VAE venous air embolism

VAERS Vaccine Adverse Events Reporting System

VAFD vascular access flush device

VAG vagina

VAG HYST vaginal hysterectomy

VAH Veterans Administration Hospital

VAHBE ventricular atrial His bundle electrocardiogram

VAHRA ventricular atrial height right atrium

VAHS virus-associated hemophagocytic syndrome

VAI vertebral artery injury
Voluntary Action Indicated (FDA)

VAIN vaginal intraepithelial neoplasia

VALE visual acuity, left eye

VALI ventilator-associated lung injury

VAMC	Veterans Affairs Medical Center		virtual bronchoscopy
VAMP®	venous-arterial management	VB₁	first voided bladder specimen
	protection system	VB₂	second midstream bladder
VAMS	Visual Analogue Mood Scale		specimen
VAN	vanilla	VB₃	third voided urine specimen
VANCO/P	vancomycin-peak	VBAC	vaginal birth after cesarean
VANCO/T	vancomycin-trough	VBAI	vertebrobasilar artery insufficiency
VAOD	visual acuity, right eye	VBAP	vincristine, carmustine (BiCNU),
VAOS	visual acuity, left eye		doxorubicin (Adriamycin), and
VA OS LP	visual acuity, left eye,		prednisone
with P	left perception with projection	VBC	vinblastine, bleomycin, and
VAP	venous access port		cisplatin
	ventilator-associated pneumonia	VBDS	vanishing bile duct syndrome
	vincristine, asparaginase, and	VBG	venous blood gas
	prednisone		vertical banded gastroplasty
VAPCS	ventricular atrial proximal coronary	VBGP	vertical banded gastroplasty
	sinus	VBI	vertebrobasilar insufficiency
VAPP	vaccine-associated paralytic	VBICAD	vertebrobasilar intracranial
	poliomyelitis		atheromatous disease
VAR	variant	VBL	vinblastine (Velban)
	varicella (chickenpox) (*varicella*	VBM	vinblastine, bleomycin, and
	zoster virus) vaccine (Varivax)		methotrexate
VARE	visual acuity, right eye		voxel-based morphometry
VARig	varicella-zoster immune globulin	VBP	vinblastine, bleomycin, and
VAS	vasectomy		cisplatin
	vascular	VBR	ventricular brain ratio
	vibroacoustic stimulator	VBS	vertebral-basilar system
	Visual Analogue Scale (Score)		videofluoroscopic barium swallow
VASC	Visual-Auditory Screen Test for		(evaluation)
	Children	VC	color vision
VA sc	distance visual acuity without		etoposide (VePesid) and
	correction		carboplatin
VA scl	near visual acuity without		pulmonary capillary blood volume
	correction		vena cava
VASO	Veteran's Administration Service		verbal cues
	Officer		vincristine (Oncovin)
VASPI	Visual Analogue Self Assessment		virtual colonoscopy
	Scales For Pain Intensity		vital capacity
VAS RAD	vascular radiology		vocal cords
VAT	ventilatory anaerobic threshold		volume control
	ventricular activation time		voluntary cough
	vertebral artery test	Vc	bortezomib (Velcade)
	video-assist thoracoscopy	3VC	3-vessel cord
	visceral adipose tissue	V&C	vertical and centric (a bite)
VATER	vertebral, anal, tracheal,	VCA	vasoconstrictor assay
	esophageal, and renal anomalies	VCAM	vascular cell adhesion molecule
VATH	vinblastine, doxorubicin	VCAP	vincristine, cyclophosphamide,
	(Adriamycin), thiotepa, and		doxorubicin (Adriamycin), and
	fluoxymesterone (Halotestin)		prednisone
VATS	video assisted thoracic surgery	Vcc	vision with correction
VAVD	vacuum-assisted vaginal delivery	VCCA	velocity common carotid artery
	vacuum-assisted venous drainage	VCD	vocal cord dysfunction
VAX-D	vertebral axial decompression	VCDR	vertical cup-to-disc ratio
VB	vaginal bleeding	VCE	vaginal cervical endocervical
	Van Buren (catheter)		(smear)
	venous blood	VCF	Vaginal Contraception Film™
	vinblastine (Velban)		vertebral compression fracture(s)
	vinblastine and bleomycin	VCFS	velo-cardio-facial syndrome

V

VCG	vectorcardiography	VDO	varus derotational osteotomy
	voiding cystogram	VD or M	venous distention or masses
VCI	vascular cognitive impairment	VDP	vinblastine, dacarbazine, and
	vocal cord injuries		cisplatin (Platinol)
	volume contrast imaging	VDPCA	variable-dose patient-controlled
vCJD	variant Creutzfeldt-Jakob disease		analgesia
VCO	ventilator CPAP oxyhood	VDPV	vaccine-derived poliovirus
V_{CO_2}	carbon dioxide output	VDR	vitamin D receptor (gene)
VCP	vocal cord palsy	VDRF	ventilator dependent respiratory
VCPR	veterinarian-client-patient		failure
	relationship	VDRL	Venereal Disease Research
VCR	video cassette recorder		Laboratory (test for syphilis)
	vincristine sulfate (Oncovin)	VDRO	varus derotational osteotomy
VCSEL	vertical cavity surface emitting	VDRR	vitamin D-resistant rickets
	laser	VDRS	Verdun Depression Rating Scale
VCT	venous clotting time	VDS	vasodepressor syncope
	volumetric computed tomography		Verbal Descriptor Scale
	voluntary counselling and testing		venereal disease—syphilis
VCTS	vitreal corneal touch syndrome		vindesine (Eldisine)
VCU	voiding cystourethrogram	VDT	vibration detection threshold
VCUG	vesicoureterogram		video display terminal
	voiding cystourethrogram		visual display terminal
VCV	varicella virus		volume doubling time
	volume-control ventilation	VD/VT	dead space to tidal volume ratio
VD	vaginal delivery	VD/VT phy	dead space physiologic to tidal
	venereal disease		volume
	vessel disease	VE	vaginal examination
	viral diarrhea		ventricular ectopy
	voided		vertex
	voiding diary		Vietnam era
	volume of distribution		virtual endoscopy
V_D	deadspace volume		visual examination
V_d	volume of distribution		vitamin E
V&D	vomiting and diarrhea		vocational evaluation
1-VD	one-vessel disease	V_E	minute volume (expired)
VDA	vascular disrupting agent	+VE	positive
	venous digital angiogram	–VE	negative
	visual discriminatory acuity	V/E	violence and eloper
VDAC	vaginal delivery after cesarean	VEA	ventricular ectopic activity
VDAC1	voltage dependent anion channel		viscoelastic agent
	type 1	VEB	ventricular ectopic beat
VDC	vincristine, doxorubicin, and	VEC	vecuronium (Norcuron)
	cyclophosphamide		velocity-encoded cine
VDD	atrial synchronous ventricular	VECG	vector electrocardiogram
	inhibited pacing	VED	vacuum erection device
VDDR I	vitamin D dependency rickets		vacuum extraction delivery
	type I		ventricular ectopic depolarization
VDDR II	vitamin D dependency rickets		vitamin E deficiency
	type II	VEE	Venezuelan equine encephalitis
VDE	vasodilatory edema	VEE_a	Venezuelan equine encephalitis
VDEPT	virus-directed enzyme prodrug		vaccine, attenuated live
	therapy	VEE_I	Venezuelan equine encephalitis
VDG	venereal disease–gonorrhea		vaccine, inactivated
Vdg	voiding	VEEG	video-electroencephalography
VDH	valvular disease of the heart	VEEV	Venezuelan equine encephalitis
VDJ	variable diversity joining		virus
VDL	vasodepressor lipid	VEF	visually evoked field
	visual detection level	VEG	vegetation (bacterial)

V

VEGF	vascular endothelial growth factor	VFR	visiting friends and relatives (possible contacts for communicable diseases)
VeIP	vinblastine (Velban), ifosfamide, and cisplatin (Platinol)		
VEMP	vestibular evoked myogenic potentials	VFRN	Volu-feed regular nipple
		VFSS	videofluoroscopic swallowing study
VE-MRI	velocity-encoded magnetic resonance imaging	VFT	venous filling time
VENC	velocity encoding value (radiology)		ventricular fibrillation threshold
VENT	ventilation	VFVT	very fast ventricular tachycardia
	ventilator	VG	vein graft
	ventral		ventricular gallop
	ventricular		ventrogluteal
VEP	visual evoked potential		very good
VEPTR	vertical expandable prosthetic titanium rib	V&G	vagotomy and gastroenterotomy
		VGAD	vein of Galen aneurysmal dilatation
VER	ventricular escape rhythm		
	visual evoked responses	VGAM	vein of Galen aneurysmal malformation
VERDICT	Veterans Evidence-based Research Dissemination Implementation Center		
		VGB	vigabatrin (Sabril)
		VGE	viral gastroenteritis
VERP	ventricular effective refractory period	VGH	very good health
		VGKC	voltage-gated potassium channel
VERT	velocity-enhanced resistance training	VGM	vein graft myringoplasty
		VGPO	volume-guaranteed pressure option
VES	ventricular extrasystoles	VH	vaginal hysterectomy
	video-endoscopic surgery		Veterans Hospital
	vitamin E succinate		viral hepatitis
	Vulnerable Elders Survey (UK)		visual hallucinations
VESS	video endoscopic swallowing study		vitreous hemorrhage
			von Herrick (grading system)
VET	veteran	VH I	very narrow anterior chamber angles
	Veterinarian		
	veterinary	VH II	moderately narrow anterior chamber angles
VF	left leg (electrode)		
	ventricular fibrillation	VH III	moderately wide open anterior chamber angles
	vertical float (aquatic therapy)		
	videofluoroscopic	VH IV	wide open anterior chamber angles
	virologic failure		
	visual field	VHA	Veterans Health Administration
	vocal fremitus		Voluntary Hospitals of America
VFC	Vaccines for Children (program)	VHC	valved-holding chamber
VFCB	vertical flow clean bench	VHD	valvular heart disease
VFD	ventilator-free days		vascular hemostatis device
	visual fields	VHF	viral hemorrhagic fever
VFFC	visual fields full to confrontation	VHI	Voice Handicap Index
VFI	viable female infant	VHL	von Hippel-Lindau disease (complex)
	visual fields intact		
	Visual Functioning index	VHP	vaporized hydrogen peroxide
V. Fib	ventricular fibrillation	VI	six
VFL	vinflunine		velocity index
VFMI	vocal fold motion impairment		volume index
VFP	vertical float progression (aquatic therapy)	VIA	visual inspection (of the cervix) with 4% acetic acid
	vitreous fluorophotometry	via	by way of
	vocal fold paralysis	vib	vibration
VFPN	Volu-feed premie nipple	VIBS	Victim's Information Bureau Service
VFQ-25	National Eye Institute 25-item Visual Function Questionnaire		
		VICA	velocity internal carotid artery

VIU	visual internal urethrotomy	VICH	International Cooperation on Harmonization of Technical Requirements for Registration of Veterinary Products
VIZ	namely		
V-J	ventriculo-jugular (shunt)		
VKA	vitamin K antagonists		
VKC	vernal keratoconjunctivitis	VICP	Vaccine Injury Compensation Program
VKDB	vitamin K deficiency bleeding		
VKH	Vogt-Koyanagi-Harada disease	Vi CPs	typhoid Vi (capsular) polysaccharide vaccine (Typhim Vi)
VKORC1	vitamin K epoxide reductase complex, subunit 1 (gene)		
VL	left arm (electrode)	VID	videodensitometry
	vial	VIG	vaccinia immune globulin
	viral load		vinblastine, ifosfamide, and gallium nitrate
	visceral leishmaniasis (kala-azar)		
VLA	very-late antigen	VIGRT	volumetrically image-guided radiotherapy
VLAD	variable life-adjusted display		
VLAP	vaporization laser ablation of the prostate	VIH	human immunodeficiency virus (Spanish and French abbreviation)
VLBW	very low birth weight (less than 1500 g)	VILI	visual inspection (of the cervix) with Lugol's iodine
VLBWPN	very low birth weight preterm neonate	VIMS	visually induced motion sickness
VLCAD	very-long-chain acyl coenzyme A dehydrogenase	VIN	vibration-induced nystagmus vulvar intraepithelial neoplasm
VLCD	very low calorie diet	VIP	etopside (VePesid), ifosfamide, and cisplatin (Platinol)
VLCFA	very-long-chain fatty acids		
VLDL	very-low-density lipoprotein		vasoactive intestinal peptide
VLE	vision left eye		vasoactive intracorporeal pharmacotherapy
VLED	very-low-energy diet		
VLH	ventrolateral nucleus of the hypothalamus		Vattikuti Institute prostatectomy very important patient
VLK	vascularized limbal keratitis		vinblastine, ifosfamide, and cisplatin (Platinol)
VLL	vastus lateralis longus		
VLM	visceral larva migrans		voluntary interruption of pregnancy
VLP	virus-like particle	VIPN	vincristine-induced peripheral neuropathy
VLPFC	ventrolateral prefrontal cortex		
VLPP	Valsalva lead-point pressure	VIPomas	vasoactive intestinal peptide-secreting tumors
VLR	vastus lateralis release		
VLUs	venous leg ulcers	VIQ	Verbal Intelligence Quotient (part of Wechsler tests)
VM	venous malformation		
	ventilated mask	VIS	Vaccine Information Statement
	ventimask		Visual Impairment Service
	Venturi mask	VISA	vancomycin-intermediate-resistant *Staphylococcus aureus*
	vestibular membrane		
	voice mail	VISC	vitreous infusion suction cutter
VM 26	teniposide (Vumon)	VISI	Vaccine Identification Standards Initiative
VMA	vanillylmandelic acid		
Vmail	voicemail		volar intercalated segmental instability
VMATs	Veterinary Medical Assistance Teams		
		VISN	Veterans Integrated Service Networks
VMCP	vincristine, melphalan, cyclophosphamide, and prednisone		
		VISs	Vaccine Information Statements
		VIT	venom immunotherapy
VMD	Doctor of Veterinary Medicine (DVM)		vital
			vitamin
	vertical maxillary deficiency		vitreous
VME	vertical maxillary excess	Vitamin	see individual letters such as B, D, G, H, K, P, R, V, etc.
VMH	ventromedial hypothalamus		
VMI	vendor-managed inventory	VIT CAP	vital capacity

V

	viable male infant	VP-16	etoposide (VePesid)
	visual motor integration	VPA	valproic acid
VMO	vaccinia melanoma oncolysate		ventricular premature activation
	vastus medialis oblique		vigorous physical activity
VMR	vasomotor rhinitis	V-Pad	sanitary napkin
VMS	vanilla milkshake	VPB	ventricular premature beat
VMTS	Vitreomacular-traction syndrome	VPC	ventricular premature contractions
VMU	vertebral motion unit		
VN	vestibular neuritis	VPD	ventricular premature depolarization
	visiting nurse		
VNA	Visiting Nurses' Association	VPDC	ventricular premature depolarization contraction
VNB	vinorelbine (Navelbine)		
VNC	vesicle neck contracture	VPDF	vegetable protein diet plus fiber
VNG	videonystagmograph	VPDs	ventricular premature depolarizations
VNS	vagal nerve stimulation (stimulator)		
VNTR	variable number of tandem repeats	VPI	velopharyngeal incompetence
VO	verbal order		velopharyngeal insufficiency
	visual observation	VPL	ventro-posterolateral
V_2O_5	vanadium pentoxide	VPLN	vaccine-primed lymph node (cells)
VO_2	oxygen consumption	VPLS	ventilation-perfusion lung scan
VOC	vaso-occlusive crisis	VPM	venous pressure module
VOCA	voice-output communication aid	VPR	virtual patient record
VOCAB	vocabulary		volume pressure response
VOCOR	vaso-occlusive crisis	Vpr	viral protein R
	void on-call to operating room	VPS	valvular pulmonic stenosis
VOCs	volatile organic compounds		ventriculoperitoneal shunt
VOCTOR	void on-call to operating room	VPT	vascularized patellar tendon
VOD	veno-occlusive disease		vibration perception threshold
	vision right eye	VQ	ventilation perfusion
VOE	vascular occlusive episode	VQM	voice quality measurements
VO_2I	oxygen consumption index	VR	right arm (electrode) valve replacement
VOL	Valuation of Life		
	volume		venous resistance
	voluntary		ventricular rhythm
VOM	vomited		verbal reprimand
VOO	continuous ventricular asynchronous pacing		violent restraint
			vocational rehabilitation
VOOD	vesico-outlet obstructive disease		volume rendered (radiology)
VOR	vestibulo-ocular reflex	$V_3R\cdot\cdot V_6R$	right sided precordial leads
VORB	verbal order read back	VRA	visual reinforcement audiometry
VOR/VSR	vestibulo-ocular and vestibulospinal reflexes		visual response audiometry
		VRB	vinorelbine (Navelbine)
VOS	vision left eye	VRC	vocational rehabilitation counselor
VOSS	visual observation shivering score	VRE	vancomycin-resistant enterococci
VOT	Visual Organization Test		vision right eye
VOU	vision both eyes	VREF	vancomycin-resistant *Enterococcus faecium*
VOV	verbal order verified		
VP	etoposide (VePesid) and cisplatin (Platinol)	VRI	viral respiratory infection
		VRL	ventral root, lumbar
	vagal paraganglioma		vinorelbine (Navelbine)
	variegate porphyria	VRP	vocational rehabilitation program
	venipuncture	VRS	vestibulospinal reflex
	venous pressure		viral rhinosinusitis
	ventriculoperitoneal	VRSA	vancomycin-resistant *Staphylococcus aureus*
	visual perception		
	voiding pressure	VRT	variance of resident time
V & P	vagotomy and pyloroplasty		ventral root, thoracic
	ventilation and perfusion		vertical radiation topography

V

	visual restoration therapy	VTEC	verotoxin-producing *Escherichia coli*
	Visual Retention Test		
	vocational rehabilitation therapy	VTED	venous thromboembolic disease
VRTA	Vocational Rehabilitation Therapy Assistant	Vteff/kg	tidal volume effective/kilogram
		Vti	tidal volume inhaled
VRU	ventilator rehabilitation unit	VT-NS	ventricular tachycardia nonsustained
VS	vagal stimulation		
	vegetative state	VTOP	voluntary termination of pregnancy
	versus (*vs*)	VTP	voluntary termination of pregnancy
	very sensitive	VTS	Volunteer Transport Service
	vestibular schwannomas	VT-S	ventricular tachycardia sustained
	visit	VTSRS	Verdun Target Symptom Rating Scale
	visited		
	vital signs (temperature, pulse, and respiration)	VT/VF	ventricular tachycardia/fibrillation
		VTX	vertex
	volume support	VU	venous ulcer
VSA	variant surface antigens		vesicoureteral (reflux)
VSADP	vocational skills assessment and development program	V/U	verbalizes understanding
		VUC	voided-urine cytology
VSBE	very short below elbow (cast)	VUD-BMT	volunteer unrelated-donor bone marrow transplantation
VSCC	vertical semicircular canal		
VSD	Vaccine Safety Datalink	VUJ	vesico ureteral junction
	ventricular septal defect	VUR	vesicoureteric reflux
	vesicosphincter dyssynergia	VV	vaccina virus
VSGP	vertical supranuclear gaze palsy		varicose veins
VSI	visual motor integration		verruca vulgaris
VSLI	vincristine sulfate liposomal injection		vulvar vestibulitis
		V-V	ventriculovenous (shunt)
VSMC	vascular smooth muscle cell	V&V	vulva and vagina
VSN	visuospatial neglect	V/V	volume to volume ratio
	vital signs normal	VVB	venovenous bypass
VSO	vertical subcondylar oblique	VVC	vulvovaginal candidiasis
VSOK	vital signs normal	VVD	vaginal vertex delivery
VSP	vertical stabilization program	VVETP	Vietnam Veterans Evaluation and Treatment Program
VSQOL	Vital Signs Quality of Life		
VSR	venous stasis retinopathy	VVFR	vesicovaginal fistula repair
	ventricular septal rupture	VVI	vector velocity imaging
VSS	variable spot scanning		venous valvular insufficiency
	visual sexual stimulation		ventricular demand pacing
	vital signs stable	V/VI	grade 5 on a 6 grade basis
V$_{ss}$	apparent volume of distribution	VVI-40	ventricular backup pacing at 40/minute
VSSAF	vital signs stable, afebrile		
VST	visual search task	VVIR	ventricular demand inhibited pacemaker (V = chamber paced-ventricle, V = chamber sensed-ventricle, I = response to sensing-inhibited, R = programmability–rate modulation)
VSTM	visual short-term memory		
VSULA	vaccination scar, upper left arm		
VSV	vesicular stomatitis virus		
VT	validation therapy		
	ventricular tachycardia		
V$_t$	tidal volume		
VTA	vascular targeting agents	VVL	varicose veins ligation
	ventral tegmentum area		verruca vulgaris of the larynx
v. tach.	ventricular tachycardia	VVOR	visual-vestibulo-ocular-reflex
VTBI	volume to be infused	VVR	ventricular response rate
VTD	bortezomib (Velcade), thalidomide and dexamethasone	VVS	vasovagal syncope
			vulvar vestibulitis syndrome
VTE	venous thromboembolic events	VVs	varicose veins
	venous thromboembolism	VVT	ventricular synchronous pacing
Vte	tidal volume exhaled	VW	vessel wall

V

VWD	ventral wall defect
vWD	von Willebrand disease
VWF	vibration-induced white finger (syndrome)
vWF	von Willebrand factor
VWFS	visual word-form system
VWM	ventricular wall motion
	visual working memory
V_x	vaccination
	vitrectomy
V-XT	V-pattern exotropia
VY	surgical replacement flap
VZ	varicella zoster
VZIG	varicella zoster immune globulin
VZV	varicella zoster virus (Varivax)

V

W

W	tungsten
	wash
	watts
	wearing glasses
	Wednesday
	week
	weight
	well
	West (as in the location e.g. 2W, is second floor, West wing)
	white
	widowed
	wife
	with
	work
w/	with
W-1	insignificant (allergies)
W-3	minimal (allergies)
W-5	moderate (allergies)
W-7	moderate-severe (allergies)
W-9	severe (allergies)
W-10	Interagency Transfer Form
W 22	Central Institute for the Deaf 22 Word List
WA	when awake
	while awake
	White American
	wide awake
	with assistance
W-A	Wyeth-Ayerst Laboratories
W & A	weakness and atrophy
W or A	weakness or atrophy
WAC	wholesale acquisition cost
WACH	wedge adjustable cushioned heel
WAD	whiplash-associated disorder(s)
WADA	World Anti-Doping Agency
WAF	weakness, atrophy, and fasciculation
	white adult female
WAGR	Wilm tumor, aniridia, genitourinary malformations, and mental retardation (syndrome)
WAIS	Wechsler Adult Intelligence Scale
WAIS-R	Wechsler Adult Intelligence Scale-Revised
WAL	Wyeth-Ayerst Laboratories
WALK	weight-activated locking knee (prosthesis)
WAM	white adult male
WAP	wandering atrial pacemaker
WAPRT	whole-abdominopelvic radiation therapy
WARI	wheezing associated respiratory infection

WAS	whiplash-associated disorders	WCA	work capacity assessment
	Wiskott-Aldrich syndrome	WCB	Workers' Compensation Board
WASI	Wechsler Abbreviated Scale of	WCBP	women of child-bearing potential
	Intelligence	WCC	well-child care
WASO	wakefulness after sleep onset		white cell count
WASP	Wiskott-Aldrich syndrome protein	WCE	white coat effect
WASS	Wasserman test		wireless capsule endoscopy
WAT	word association test		work capacity evaluation
WAZ	weight-for-age Z scores	WCH	white coat hypertension
WB	waist belt	WCHE	well-child health examination
	weight bearing	WC/LC	warm compresses and lid scrubs
	well baby	WCM	whole cow's milk
	Western blot	W/cm^2	watts per square centimeter
	whole blood	WCS	work capacity specialist
WBACT	whole-blood activated clotting time	WCST	Wisconsin Card Sorting Test
WBAT	weight bearing as tolerated	WCT	wide-complex tachycardia
WBC	weight bearing with crutches	WCV	within-subject coefficient of
	well baby clinic		variation
	white blood cell (count)	WCVs	well-child visits
WBCT	whole-blood clotting time	WD	ward
WBD	weeks by dates (for gestational		well developed
	age)		well differentiated
WBDOs	waterborne disease and outbreaks		wet dressing
WBE	weeks by examination (for		Wilson disease
	gestational age)		word
	whole-body extract		working distance
WBGD	whole-body glucose disposal		wound
WBH	weight-based heparin (dosing)	W/D	warm and dry
	whole-body hyperthermia		withdrawal
WBI	whole-bowel irrigation	W → D	wet to dry
W Bld	whole blood	W4D	Worth four-dot (test for fusion)
WBN	wellborn nursery	WDCC	well-developed collateral
WBNAA	whole-brain N-acetylaspartate		circulation
WBOS	wide base of support	WDEIA	wheat-dependent, exercise-induced
WBPTT	whole-blood partial thromboplastin		anaphylaxis
	time	WDF	white divorced female
WBQ	web-based questionnaires	WDHA	watery diarrhea, hypokalemia, and
WBQC	wide-base quad cane		achlorhydria
WBR	whole-body radiation	WDHH	watery diarrhea, hypokalemia, and
WBRT	whole-brain radiotherapy		hypochlorhydria
WBS	weeks by size (for gestational age)	WDL	within defined limits
	whole body scan	WDLL	well-differentiated lymphocytic
	Williams-Beuren syndrome		lymphoma
WBTF	Waring Blender tube feeding	WDM	white divorced male
WBTT	weight bearing to tolerance	WDP	within defined parameters
WBUS	weeks by ultrasound	WDR	weighed dietary records
WBV	whole blood volume	WDS	word discrimination score
WC	waist circumference	WDTC	well-differentiated thyroid cancer
	ward clerk	WDWG	well dressed, well groomed
	ward confinement	WDWN-	well-developed, well-
	warm compress	AAF	nourished African-American
	wet compresses		female
	wheelchair	WDWN-	well-developed,
	when called	BM	well-nourished black male
	white count	WDWN-	well-developed,
	whooping cough	WF	well-nourished white female
	will call	WDXRF	wavelength-dispersive x-ray
	workers' compensation		fluorescence

W

WE	weekend	WHO	World Health Organization
	Wernicke encephalopathy		wrist-hand orthosis
	wide excision	WHOART	World Health Organization
W/E	weekend		Adverse Reaction Terms
WEBINO	wall-eyed bilateral internuclear		(Terminology)
	ophthalmoplegia	WHOL	worst headache of (his/her) life
WE-D	withdrawal-emergent dyskinesia		(describes the most common
WE-DESS	water excitation double-echo		characteristic of subarachnoid
	steady state (magnetic resonance		hemorrhage)
	imaging)	WHOQOL-	World Health
WEE	Western equine encephalitis	100	Organization Quality of Life
WEMINO	wall-eyed monocular internuclear		100-Item (instrument)
	ophthalmoplegia	WHP	whirlpool
WEP	weekend pass	WHPB	whirlpool bath
WESR	Westergren erythrocyte	WHpR	waist-to-hip ratio
	sedimentation rate	WHR	ratio of waist to hip circumference
	Wintrobe erythrocyte sedimentation	WHS	Wolf-Hirschhorn syndrome
	rate	WHSS	well-healed surgical scar
WEUP	willful exposure to unwanted	WHV	woodchuck hepatitis virus
	pregnancy	WHVP	wedged hepatic venous pressure
WF	well flexed	WH/WD	withholding/withdrawal (of life
	wet film		support)
	white female	WHZ	wheezes
W/F	weakness and fatigue	WI	ventricular demand pacing
WFB	wooden foreign body		walk-in
WFE	Williams flexion exercises	W/I	within
W FEEDS	with feedings	W+I	work and interest
WFH	white-faced hornet	WIA	wounded in action
WFI	water for injection	WIC	Women, Infants, and Children
WFL	within full limits		(program)
	within functional limits	WID	widow
WFLC	white female living child		widower
WFNS	World Federation of Neurosurgical	WIED	walk-in emergency department
	Societies (grade or scale)	WIP	work in progess
WF-O	will follow in office	WIQ	Walking Impairment Questionnaire
WFR	wheel-and-flare reaction	WIR	with in reach (call light)
WG	Wegener granulomatosis	WIS	Ward Incapacity Scale
WGA	week gestational age		Wister Institute
	wheat germ agglutinin	WISC	Wechsler Intelligence Scale for
	whole genome amplification		Children
WGL	wire-guide localization	WISC-R	Wechsler Intelligence Scale for
WH	walking heel (cast)		Children-Revised
	well healed	WISN	warfarin-induced skin necrosis
	well hydrated	WIT	warm ischemia time
	work hardening (physical therapy)		water-induced thermotherapy
WHA	warmed humidified air	WK	week
WHAS	Women's Health Assessment Scale		work
WHI	Women's Health Initiative	WKHL	Weck hem-o-lock (suture clip)
WHIM	Worts, Hypogammaglobulinamia,	WKI	Wakefield Inventory
	Infections, and Myelokathexis	WKS	Wernicke-Korsakoff Syndrome
	(syndrome)	WL	waiting list
WHIS	War Head-Injury Score		Warning Letter (FDA)
whites	white blood cells		wave length
WHNP	Women's Healthcare Nurse		weight loss
	Practitioner	WLE	white light endoscopy
WHNR	well-healed, no residuals		wide local excision
WHNS	well-healed, no sequelae	WLI	weight-length index
	well-healed, nonsymptomatic	WLM	working level months

W

WLQ	Work Limitation Questionnaire		written order
WLS	weight-loss surgery	W/O	water-in-oil (emulsion)
	wet lung syndrome		without
WLST	withdrawal of life-sustaining therapy	WOB	work of breathing
		WOCF	worst observation carried forward
WLT	waterload test	WOCN	Wound, Ostomy and Continence
WM	Waldenstrom macroglobulinemia		Nurses (Society)-formerly known
	wall motion		as the International Association
	warm, moist		for Enterostomal Therapy (IEAT)
	weight maintenance	WOMAC	Western Ontario and McMaster
	Western medicine		Universities Osteoarthritis
	wet mount		Index
	white male	WOP	without pain
	white matter	W or A	weakness or atrophy
	whole milk	WORD	Wechsler objective reading
	working memory		dimensions
WMA	wall motion abnormality	WORLD/	a test used in mental
WMD	warm moist dressings (sterile)	DLROW	status examinations
	weapons of mass destruction		(patient is asked to spell WORLD
	weighted mean differences		backwards)
WME	well-male examination	WP	wedge pressure
WMF	white married female		whirlpool
WMFT	Wolf Motor Function Test	WPAI	Work Productivity and Activity
WMH	white matter hyperintensities		Impairment (Questionnaire)
WMH-CIDI	World Mental Health Composite	WPBT	whirlpool, body temperature
	International Diagnostic	WPCs	washed packed cells
	Interview	WPFM	Wright peak flow meter
WMI	wall motion index	WPOA	wearing patch on arrival
	weighted mean index	WPP	Wechsler Preschool and Primary
WML	white matter lesions (cerebral)		Scale of Intelligence
WMLC	white male living child	WPPSI	Wechsler Preschool and Primary
WMM	white married male		Scale of Intelligence
WMP	warm moist packs (unsterile)	WPPSI-R	WPPSI revised
	weight management program	WPR	written progress report
WMS	watermelon stomach (gastric antral	WPS	Worker Protection Standard
	vascular ectasia)	WPV	wild poliovirus
	Wechsler Memory Scale		within-person variability
	Wilson-Mikity syndrome		workplace violence
WMSI	wall-motion score index	WPW	Wolff-Parkinson-White
WMT	Word Memory Test		(syndrome)
WMTS	wireless medical telemetry service	WR	Wassermann reaction
WMX	whirlpool, massage, and exercise		word recognition
WN	well nourished		wrist
WND	wound	WRA	with-the-rule astigmatism
WNE	West Nile encephalitis	WRAIR	Walter Reed Army Institute of
WNF	well-nourished female		Research
	West Nile fever	WRAMC	Walter Reed Army Medical Center
WNL	within normal limits	WRARU	Walter Reed AFRIMS (Armed
WNL x 4	upper and lower extremities within		Forces Research Institute of
	normal limits		Medical Sciences) Research Unit
WNLS	weighted nonlinear least squares	WRAT	Wide Range Achievement Test
WNM	well-nourished male	WRAT-R	The Wide Range Achievement
WNND	West Nile neuroinvasive disease		Test, Revised
WNR	within normal range	WRBC	washed red blood cells
WNt^{50}	Wagner-Nelson time 50 hours	WRC	washed red (blood) cells
WNV	West Nile virus	WRF	worsening renal function
WO	weeks old	WRIOT	Wide Range Interest-Opinion Test
	wide open		(for career planning)

W

WRL	World Reference Laboratory for Foot-and-Mouth Disease (Institute for Animal Health, Survey, United Kingdom)		wheeled walker
		4WW	four-wheel walker
		WWI	World War One
		WWII	World War Two
WRN	Werner syndrome protein	W/W	weight-to-weight ratio
WRT	weekly radiation therapy	W → W	wet-to-wet
	with respect (regards) to	WWAC	walk with aid of cane
WRUED	work-related upper-extremity disorder	WW Brd	whole wheat bread
		WWE	well-woman examination
WS	Waardenburg syndrome (classified into four subtypes, WS1-WS4)	WWidF	white widowed female
		WWidM	white widowed male
	walking speed	WWP	warm and well perfused
	ward secretary	WWTP	wastewater treatment plant
	watt seconds	WWW	World Wide Web
	Werner syndrome	WYOU	women years of usage
	West syndrome		
	Williams syndrome		
	work simplification		
	work simulation		
	work status		
W&S	wound and skin		
WSCP	Williams Syndrome Cognitive Profile		
WSEP	Williams syndrome, early puberty		
WSepF	white separated female		
WSepM	white separated male		
WSF	white single female		
WSLP	Williams syndrome, late puberty		
WSM	white single male		
WSO	white superficial onychomycosis		
WSOC	water-soluble organic compounds		
WSP	wearable speech processor Wolbachia surface protein		
WSW	women who have sex with women		
WST	Wheelchair Skills Test Wheelchair Skills Training		
WSTP	Wheelchair Skills Training Program		
WT	wait times		
	walking tank		
	walking training		
	weight (wt)		
	wild type		
	Wilms tumor		
	wisdom teeth		
0WT	zero work tolerance		
WTC	World Trade Center		
W-T-D	wet to dry		
WTE	wean to extubate		
WTP	willingness to pay		
WTS	whole tomography slice		
WU	Wunsch units		
W/U	work-up		
WV	whispered voice wound vacuum		
W/V	weight-to-volume ratio		
WW	watchful waiting Weight Watchers		

X

X   break
           capecitabine (Xeloda) (This is a
              dangerous abbreviation)
           cross
           crossmatch
           exophoria for distance
           Ecstasy (methylenedioxy-
              methamphetamine; MDMA)
           extra
           female sex chromosome
           start of anesthesia
           ten
           times
           xylocaine
$\bar{x}$ except
           mean
X'   exophoria at 33 cm
X^2 chi-square
X+#   xyphoid plus number of
              fingerbreadths
X3   orientation as to time, place and
              person
3X   three times
X-ALD   X-linked adrenoleukodystrophy
XBT   xylose breath test
XC   excretory cystogram
XCCL   crossed-coupled-cavity-laser
           exaggerated craniocaudal lateral
XCF   aortic cross clamp off
XCI   X-chromosome inactivation
XCO   aortic cross clamp on
XD   times daily
           xanthoma dissemination
X&D   examination and diagnosis
X2d   times two days
XDP   xeroderma pigmentosum
XDR   extensively drug-resistant
              (tuberculosis)
XDR-TB   extensively drug-resistant
              tuberculosis
XE   capecitabine (Xeloda)
Xe   xenon
^{133}Xe xenon, isotope of mass 133
XeCl   xenon chloride
XeCT   xenon-enhanced computed
              tomography
X-ed   crossed
XELIRI   capecitabine (Xeloda) and
              irinotecan
XELOX   capecitabine (Xeloda) and
              oxaliplatin (Eloxatin)
XEM   xonics electron mammography
XES   x-ray energy spectrometer
XFER   transfer

XFS   exfoliation syndrome
XGP   xanthogranulomatous
              pyelonephritis
XI   eleven
XII   twelve
XIAP   X-linked inhibitor of apoptosis
XIP   x-ray in plaster
XKO   not knocked out
XL   extended release (once a day oral
              solid dosage form)
           extra large
           forty
XLA   X-linked infantile
              agammaglobulinemia
X-leg   cross leg
XLFDP   cross-linked fibrin degradation
              products
XLH   X-linked hypophos-phatemia
XLHED   X-linked hypohidrotic ectodermal
              dysplasia
XLIF   extreme lateral interbody fusion
XLJR   X-linked juvenile retinoschisis
XLMR   X-linked mental retardation
XLOA   X-linked optic atrophy
XLP   X-linked proliferative (syndrome)
XLRS   X-linked retinoschisis
XM   crossmatch
X-mat.   crossmatch
XMG   mammogram
XML   extensible markup language
XMM   xeromammography
XMR   magnetic resonance and X-rays
XMRV   xenotropic murine leukemia virus-
              related virus
XMT   cross matched
XNA   xenoreactive natural antibodies
XOM   extraocular movements
XOP   x-ray out of plaster
XP   xeroderma pigmentosum
XR   extended release
           x-ray
XRF   x-ray fluorescence
XRT   radiation therapy
XS   excessive
X-SCID   X-linked severe combined
              immunodeficiency
XS-LIM   exceeds limits of procedure
X-STOP   an interspinous process
              decompression system
XT   exotropia
           extract
           extracted
X(T')   intermittent exotropia at 33 cm
X(T)   intermittent exotropia
XTLE   extratemporal-lobe epilepsy
XU   excretory urogram
XULN   times upper limit of normal
XV   fifteen

X

3X/WK	three times a week
XX	normal female sex chromosome type
	twenty
XX/XY	sex karyotypes
XXX	thirty
XY	normal male sex chromosome type
XYL	xylose
XYLO	lidocaine (Xylocaine)
XZT	zolazepam and tiletamine

X

Y

Y	male sex chromosome
	year
	yellow
	Yes
Y90	yttrium 90
YAC	yeast artificial chromosome
YACs	yeast artificial chromosomes
YACP	young adult chronic patient
YADH	yeast alcohol dehydrogenase
YAG	yttrium aluminum garnet (laser)
YAS	youth action section (police)
Yb	ytterbium
YBOCS	Yale-Brown Obsessive-Compulsive Scale
Yel	yellow
YEPQ	Yale Eating Patterns Questionnaire
YF	yellow fever
YFH	yellow-faced hornet
YFI	yellow fever immunization
YFV	yellow-fever virus
YHL	years of healthy life
YJV	yellow jacket venom
Y2K	year 2,000
YLC	youngest living child
YLD	years of life with disability
YLL	years of life lost
YLS	years of life saved
YMC	young male Caucasian
YMRS	Young Mania Rating Scale
Y/N	yes/no
YO	years old
YOB	year of birth
YOD	year of death
YORA	younger-onset rheumatoid arthritis
YPC	YAG (yttrium aluminum garnet) posterior capsulotomy
YPLL	years of potential life lost before age 65
yr	year
YRBSS	Youth Risk Behavior Surveillance System
YRI	Yoruba from Ibadan, Nigeria (populations included in HapMap - see HapMap)
yrs	years
YSC	yolk sac carcinoma
5YSR	5-year survival rate(s)
YTD	year to date
YTDY	yesterday

Z

Z	impedance
	pyrazinamide [part of tuberculosis regimen, see RHZ(E/S)/HR]
ZA	zoledronic acid (Zometa)
ZAL	zaleplon (Sonata)
ZAP	zoster-associated pain
ZD	Zenker diverticulum
	zinc-deficient
ZDV	zidovudine (Retrovir)
Z-E	Zollinger-Ellison (syndrome)
ZEEP	zero end-expiratory pressure
ZES	Zollinger-Ellison syndrome
Z-ESR	zeta erythrocyte sedimentation rate
ZIFT	zygote intrafallopian (tube) transfer
ZIG	zoster serum immune globulin
ZIP	zoster immune plasma
ZLR	likelihood ratio Z-scores
ZMC	zygomatic
	zygomatic maxillary compound (complex)
Zn	zinc
ZnO	zinc oxide
ZnOE	zinc oxide and eugenol
ZnPc	zinc phthalocyanine
ZnPP	zinc protoporphyrin
ZNS	zolmitriptan nasal spray (Zomig)
	zonisamide (Zonegran)
$ZnSO_4$	zinc sulfate
ZOI	zone of inhibition
ZOL	zoledronic acid (Zometa, Reclast)
ZOOM	Guarana
ZOT	zonula occludens toxin
ZPC	zero point of charge
	zopiclone
z-Plasty	surgical relaxation of contracture
ZPO	zinc peroxide
ZPP	zinc protoporphyrin
ZPS	Zubrod performance status
ZPT	zinc pyrithione
ZSB	zero stools since birth
ZSR	zeta sedimentation rate
ZSRDS	Zung Self-Rating Depression Scale

Z

Additions, Corrections, and Suggestions are Welcomed

Please send them via any means shown below:

Neil M Davis
2049 Stout Drive, B-3
Warminster PA 18974-3861

FAX 888 333 4915 or 215 442 7432
Email med@neilmdavis.com
Secure website www.medabbrev.com

Thank you for your help in the past.

Have You Used the Internet Version of This Book?

- It is instantaneously searchable for the meanings of abbreviations
- It is reverse searchable (search for all the abbreviations containing a particular word)
- Each week, about 20 new entries are added

See the preface (page vii) for access instructions. A one-year, single-user access is included in the purchase price of the book. Also one-year subscriptions (no book) are available for purchase (see page 417).

WiFi-Enabled Devices

At no extra cost, WiFi-enabled devices can access the Internet version where it can be added as a home-page icon or bookmarked.

computer	iPhone®	iPad®	iPod Touch®	BlackBerry®	DROID™	Windows® Mobile	Palm®

Multi-User Site Licenses are Available

Medical facilities can substitute their own "Do Not Use" list of dangerous abbreviations for the one present. The ability also exists to list abbreviations that are unique to your region and/or organization which would normally not appear in any national list. These lists would be controlled by the facility or company. A no-cost, 3-week trial and pricing information are available by calling 888 333 1862 or 215 442 7430 or via an e-mail request to ev@neilmdavis.com

Chapter 7
Symbols and Greek Letters

Symbols

↑	above	↑↑	extensor
	alive		extensor response (positive Babinsky)
	elevated		testes undescended
	greater than		
	high	‖	parallel
	improved		parallel bars
	increase		
	rising	√	check
	up		flexion
	upper		
↑g	increasing	√'d	checked
↓	dead	√'ing	checking
	decrease		
	depressed	#	fracture
	diminished		number
	down		pound
	falling		weight
	lower		
	lowered	∴	therefore
	normal plantar reflex	∵	because
	restricted		
↓g	decreasing	Δ scan	delta scan (computed tomography scan)
→	causes to		
	greater than	+	plus
	progressing		positive
	results in		present
	showed		
	to	−	absent
	to the right		minus
	transfer to		negative
	yields		
←	less than	/	extend
	resulted from		extended
	to the left		slash mark signifying per, and, over, as a blood pressure of 160 over 100, or with (this is a dangerous symbol as it is mistaken for a one)
↔	same as		
	stable		
	to and from		
	unchanging	±	either positive or negative
			no definite cause
↓↓	flexor		plus or minus
	plantar response (Babinski)		very slight trace
	testes descended		

351

>   greater than (can be confused with <, use "greater than")
   left ear-bone conduction threshold

≥   greater than or equal to

<   caused by
   less than (can be confused with >, use "less than")
   right ear-bone conduction threshold

≤   less than or equal to
≮   not less than
≯   not more than
   above
∨   diastolic blood pressure
   increased

   below
   systolic blood pressure
≠   not equal to
≅   approximately equal to

=   equal
   equal to

′   feet
   minutes (as in 30′)

″   inches
   seconds

~   about
   approximately
   difference
≈   approximately equal to

≡   identical

×   left ear-air conduction threshold
   ten

]   left ear-masked bone conduction threshold

[right ear-masked bone conduction

△   right ear-masked air conduction threshold
   change

○   threshold
   reversible
?   question
   questionable
—   not tested
Ø   no
   none
   without

   zero
⊙   start of an operation
⊗   end of anesthesia
@   at
   one
   two
♂   male
♀   female
   gay
   lesbian

■   deceased male
●   deceased female
□   living male
   left ear-masked air conduction threshold
○   living female
   respiration
   right ear-air conduction threshold
◇   sex unknown

(□)   adopted living male
*   birth
†   dead
   death

♀   standing

○—<   recumbent position

♀   sitting position

♥   heart

Greek Letters

A α	alpha
β B	beta
Γ γ	gamma
Δ δ	anion gap
	change
	delta
	delta gap
	prism diopter
	temperature
	trimester
E ε	epsilon
Z ζ	zeta
H η	eta
Θ θ	negative
	theta
I ι	iota
K κ	kappa

\#

Λ λ	lambda		Υ υ	upsilon
M μ	micro		Φ φ	phenyl
	mu			phi
				thyroid
N ν	nu		X χ	chi
Ξ ξ	xi		Ψ ψ	psi
O o	omicron			psychiatric
Π π	pi		Ω ω	omega
P ρ	rho			ohm
Σ σ	sigma			
	sum of			
	summary			
T τ	tau			

Miscellaneous

L M   liver, kidneys, and spleen negative,
K O   no masses, or tenderness
S T

Additions, Corrections, and Suggestions are Welcomed

Please send them via any means shown below:

Neil M Davis
2049 Stout Drive, B-3
Warminster PA 18974-3861

FAX 888 333 4915 or 215 442 7432
Email med@neilmdavis.com
Secure website www.medabbrev.com

Thank you for your help in the past.

Have You Used the Internet Version of This Book?

- It is instantaneously searchable for the meanings of abbreviations
- It is reverse searchable (search for all the abbreviations containing a particular word)
- Each week, about 20 new entries are added

See the preface (page vii) for access instructions. A one-year, single-user access is included in the purchase price of the book. Also one-year subscriptions (no book) are available for purchase (see page 417).

WiFi-Enabled Devices

At no extra cost, WiFi-enabled devices can access the Internet version where it can be added as a home-page icon or bookmarked.

computer	iPhone®	iPad®	iPod Touch®	BlackBerry®	DROID™	Windows® Mobile	Palm®

Multi-User Site Licenses are Available

Medical facilities can substitute their own "Do Not Use" list of dangerous abbreviations for the one present. The ability also exists to list abbreviations that are unique to your region and/or organization which would normally not appear in any national list. These lists would be controlled by the facility or company. A no-cost, 3-week trial and pricing information are available by calling 888 333 1862 or 215 442 7430 or via an e-mail request to ev@neilmdavis.com

Chapter 8

Tables, Lists, and Conversions

Numbers and letters for teeth

Two adult numbering systems and a deciduous system are shown. The adult systems are shown as numbers, whereas deciduous teeth are lettered. The system commonly used in the U.S. is 1 to 32 (shown in bold face type).

1 (18)	upper right 3rd molar
2 (17) (A)	upper right 2nd molar
3 (16) (B)	upper right 1st molar
4 (15)	upper right 2nd bicuspid
5 (14)	upper right 1st bicuspid
6 (13) (C)	upper right canine (eyetooth)
7 (12) (D)	upper right lateral incisor
8 (11) (E)	upper right central incisor
9 (21) (F)	upper left central incisor
10 (22) (G)	upper left lateral incisor
11 (23) (H)	upper left canine
12 (24)	upper left 1st bicuspid
13 (25)	upper left 2nd bicuspid
14 (26) (I)	upper left 1st molar
15 (27) (J)	upper left 2nd molar
16 (28)	upper left 3rd molar
17 (38)	lower left 3rd molar
18 (37) (K)	lower left 2nd molar
19 (36) (L)	lower left 1st molar
20 (35)	lower left 2nd bicuspid
21 (34)	lower left 1st bicuspid
22 (33) (M)	lower left canine
23 (32) (N)	lower left lateral incisor
24 (31) (O)	lower left central incisor
25 (41) (P)	lower right central incisor
26 (42) (Q)	lower right lateral incisor
27 (43) (R)	lower right canine
28 (44)	lower right 1st bicuspid
29 (45)	lower right 2nd bicuspid
30 (46) (S)	lower right 1st molar
31 (47) (T)	lower right 2nd molar
32 (48)	lower right 3rd molar

UPPER   UPPER

	1	**2**	**3**	**4**	**5**	**6**	**7**	**8**	**9**	**10**	**11**	**12**	**13**	**14**	**15**	**16**
	18	17	16	15	14	13	12	11	21	22	23	24	25	26	27	28
		A	B			C	D	E	F	G	H			I	J	

Right ———————————————————————————— **Left**

		T	S			R	Q	P	O	N	M			L	K	
	48	47	46	45	44	43	42	41	31	32	33	34	35	36	37	38
	32	**31**	**30**	**29**	**28**	**27**	**26**	**25**	**24**	**23**	**22**	**21**	**20**	**19**	**18**	**17**

LOWER   LOWER

\#

Laboratory Test Panels*

	CI CO₂ K Na	BUN Ca Creat Gluc	Alb Alk P AST(SGOT) ALT(SGPT) T Bili TP	ANA ESR RF Ur Ac	Calc LDL HDL T Chol Trig VLDL	Alb Phos	HAAb, IgM Ab HbcAb, IgM Ab HbsAG HCAb
Lytes (electrolyte panel)	X						
BMP (basic metabolic panel) or MBP, MPB	X	X					
CMP (comprehensive metabolic panel)	X	X	X				
HFP (hepatic function panel)			X plus D Bili				
AP (arthritis panel)				X			
LP (lipid Panel)					X		
RFP (renal function panel)	X	X				X	
AHP (acute hepatitis panel)							X

*These can vary from institution to institution and from year to year

Abbreviation Key

Ab–antibody
Alb–albumin
Alk P–alkaline phosphate
ALT (SGPT)–alanine aminotransferase
   (serum glutamate pyruvate)
ANA–antinuclear antibody
AST (SGOT)–aspartate–aminotransferase
   (serum glutamate oxaloacetic transaminase)
BUN–blood urea nitrogen
Ca–calcium
Calc LDL–calculated low-density lipoprotein
LDL–low density lipoprotein

CI–chloride
CO₂–carbon dioxide
Creat–creatinine
D Bili–direct bilirubin
ESR–erythrocyte sedimentation rate
Gluc–glucose
HAAb–hepatitis A antibody
HBcAb–hepatitis B core antibody
HBsAg–hepatitis B surface antigen
HCAb–hepatitis C antibody
HDL–high–density lipoprotein

IgM–immunoglobulin M
K–potassium
Na–sodium
Phos–phosphate
RF–rheumatoid factor
T Bili–total bilirubin
T Chol–total cholesterol
TP–total protein
Trig–triglycerides
Ur Ac–uric acid
VLDI–very low-density lipoprotein

#

See text for meaning of the abbreviations shown

Complete Blood Count

$$10,000 \genfrac{}{}{0pt}{}{11.7}{36.5} \quad \genfrac{}{}{0pt}{}{\text{50S, 25B, 35L, 5M 2N, 3E}}{\genfrac{}{}{0pt}{}{83/29/30}{290,00}}$$

$$\text{WBC} \genfrac{}{}{0pt}{}{\text{HgB}}{\text{HCT}} \quad \genfrac{}{}{0pt}{}{\text{Segs/Bands/Lymphs/Monos/Basos/Eos}}{\genfrac{}{}{0pt}{}{\text{MCV-MCH-MCHC}}{\text{platelet count}}}$$

Electrolyte Panel

142	99	sodium	chloride
4.7	25	potassium	carbon dioxide

Blood Gases

7.4/80/48/98/25   pH/PO$_2$/PCO$_2$/% O$_2$ saturation/bicarbonate

Obstetrical shorthand

$$\frac{2\ \text{cm} | 80\%}{-2\ \text{Vtx}} \quad 2\ \text{cm} = \text{dilation of cervix}$$

80% = degree of cer-   Vtx = vertex; presen-
   vix effacement   tation of fetus,
                                (breech = Br)

−2 = station; distance
    above (+) or
    below (−) the
    spine of the ischium measured in cm

Reflexes

Reflexes are usually graded on a 0 to 4+ scale. The designations +, ++, +++, and ++++ should not be used.

4+   may indicate disease often associated with clonus
     very brisk, hyperactive
3+   brisker than average
     possibly but not necessarily indicative of disease
2+   average
     normal
1+   low normal
     somewhat diminished
0   may indicate neuropathy
     no response

Muscle strength[1]

0—No muscular contraction detected
1—A barely detectable flicker or trace of contraction
2—Active movement of the body part with gravity eliminated
3—Active movement against gravity
4—Active movement against gravity and some resistance
5—Active movement against full resistance without evident fatigue. This is normal muscle strength

Pulse[1]

0   completely absent
+1 markedly impaired (or 1+)
+2 modererately impaired (or 2+)
+3 slightly impaired (or 3+)
+4 normal (or 4+)

Gradation of intensity of heart murmurs[1]

1/6 or I/VI	may not be heard in all positions very faint, heard only after the listener has "tuned in"
2/6 or II/VI	quiet, but heard immediately upon placing the stethoscope on the chest
3/6 or III/VI	moderately loud
4/6 or IV/VI	loud
5/6 or V/VI	very loud, may be heard with a stethoscope partly off the chest (thrills are associated)
6/6 or VI/VI	may be heard with the stethoscope entirely off the chest (thrills are associated)

Tonsil Size

0   no tonsils
1   less than normal
2   normal
3   greater than normal
4   touching

Grades of Severity of Knee Arthritis *(arthroscopic)*

Grade 1: Early changes show *fissuring* (breaks) in the cartilage
Grade 2: More extensive full thickness breaks in the cartilage
Grade 3: Intermittent loss of cartilage with breaks
Grade 4: Exposed *subchondral* (below the cartilage) bone

Metric Prefixes and Symbols

Prefix	Symbol	
tera-	T	1,000,000,000,000 or (10^{12}) one trillion
giga-	G	1,000,000,000 or (10^{9}) one billion
mega-	M	1,000,000 or (10^{6}) one million
kilo-	k	1,000 or (10^{3}) one thousand
hecto-	h	100 or (10^{2}) one hundred
deka-	da	10 or (10^{1}) ten
deci-	d	0.1 or (10^{-1}) one-tenth
centi-	c	0.01 or (10^{-2}) one-hundredth
milli-	m	0.001 or (10^{-3}) one-thousandth
micro-	μ	0.000,001 or (10^{-6}) one-millionth
nano-	n	0.000,000,001 or (10^{-9}) one-billionth
pico-	p	0.000,000,000,000,001 or (10^{-12}) one-trillionth
femto-	f	0.000,000,000,000,001 or (10^{-15}) one-quadrillionth
atto-	a	0.000,000,000,000,000,001 or (10^{-18}) one-quintillionth

Kilograms/Pounds Conversions
To convert pounds to kilograms, divide by 2.2
To convert kilograms to pounds, multiply by 2.2

After carrying out a calculation, always make sure your answer is reasonable by checking with the table below.

kilograms	pounds
0.5	1.1
1	2.2
5	11
10	22
25	55
50	110
75	165
100	220

Fahrenheit/Centigrade Conversions
To convert Centigrade to Fahrenheit

$°F = 32$ plus ($9/5$ times $°C$)　　　or　　　$°F = 32$ plus (1.8 times $°C$)

To convert Fahrenheit to Centigrade

$°C = 5/9$ times ($°F$ minus 32)　　　or　　　$°C ≈ 0.556$ times ($°F$ minus 32)

After carrying out a calculation, always make sure your answer is reasonable by checking with the table below.

°Centigrade	°Fahrenheit
0	32
2	36
8	46
15	59
20	68
25	77
30	86
36	96.8
37	98.6
38	100.4
39	102.2
40	104
41	105.8
50	122
100	212

#

Apothecary symbols (Should never be used)

The symbols presented below are for informational use. The apothecary system should **not** be used. Only the metric system should be used. The methods of expressing the symbols, the meanings, and the equivalence are not the classic ones, nor are they precise, but reflect the usual intended meanings when used by some older physicians in writing prescription directions.

ℨ or ℨ ī   dram, teaspoonful, (5 mL)

ℨ ii   two drams, 2 tea-spoonfuls, (10 mL)

ℨ ss   half ounce, table-spoonful, (15 mL)

℥ or ℥ ī   ounce, (30 mL)

gr   grain (approximately 65 mg)

♏   minim (approximately 0.06 mL)

gtt   drop

Reference

1. Adopted from Bates, B., *Bates' Guide to Physical Examinations and History Taking,* 9th ed. Philadelphia: Lippincott Williams and Wilkins; 2007.

Chapter 9

Cross-Referenced List of Generic and Brand Drug Names

Listed below is a cross-referenced index of generic and brand drug names. Generic names begin with a lower case letter while brand names begin with a capital letter. This partial list consists of frequently prescribed drugs, new drugs, and recently discontinued drugs.

In the web version of this book (see page vii), when the drug name is clicked, you are connected to its Wikipedia monograph. The web version is updated weekly.

The meanings of abbreviated and coded drug names can be found in Chapter 6 (Lettered Abbreviations and Acronyms).

This listing is intended to allow readers to reference generic and trade drug names. Since products are added and taken off the market daily, this listing can not be relied on for accuracy of availability. The best reference for checking on availability is the web version of Drug Facts and Comparisons[1] as it has a complete and current listing for drugs available as well as those no longer available.

Complete indices of United States drug names can be found in current editions of Drug Facts and Comparisons[1]. A complete list of world-wide names may be found in Martindales.[2] These and other references should be used to determine the equivalence of products, strengths, and dosage forms. Although several products may be listed under one generic name they may differ in strength, dosage form, or concentration available, as is the case with estradiol transdermal (Climara, Estraderm, and Vivelle).

When a product is often prescribed and/or labeled generically, the generic name is shown in italics. Some products are marketed without a brand name, as in the case of thioguanine. In such cases only the generic name is listed.

The following abbreviations are used in this listing:

EC	enteric coated	SR	sustained release tablets or capsules, and other designations for extended release dosage forms such as CR, LX, SA, LA, CC, XR, SR, CD, XT, etc.
HCl	hydrochloride		
IM	intramuscular	susp	suspension
IV	intravenous	(W)	withdrawn or discontinued from US market
inj	injection	(WA)	withdrawn or discontinued from U.S. Market but available under it's generic name and/or another brand name from another manufacturer(s)
oint	ointment		
ophth	ophthalmic		
soln	solution		

A

abacavir sulfate	Ziagen	abciximab	ReoPro
abarelix	Plenaxis	Abelcet	amphotericin B
abatacept	Orencia		lipid complex
Abbokinase (W)	urokinase (W)	Abilify	aripiprazole

Ablavar	gadofosveset trisodium inj	Actos	pioglitazone HCl
Abraxane	paclitaxel, albumin-bound inj	Acular	ketorolac tromethamine ophth
abobotulinumtoxin A inj	Dysport	*acyclovir*	Zovirax
ACAM 2000 (W)	smallpox (vaccinia) (W)	Adacel	*diphtheria, tetanus, and acellular pertussis (TdaP) vaccine (adult type)*
acamprosate calcium	Campral		
acarbose	Precose	Adalat CC	*nifedipine SR*
Accolate	zafirlukast	adalimumab	Humira
AccuNeb	albuterol inhalation soln	adapalene	Differin
Accupril	*quinapril HCl*	Adapin (WA)	*doxepin HCl*
Accuretic	*quinapril; hydrochlorothiazide*	Adderall	amphetamine; dextroamphet-
Accutane (W)	isotretinoin (W)		amine mixed salts
Accuzyme	papain; urea oint	adefovir	Hepsera
acebutolol HCl	Sectral	dipivoxil	Preveon
Aceon	perindopril erbumine	Adenocard	adenosine
acetaminophen	paracetamol	adenosine	Adenocard
	Tylenol	Adrenalin	epinephrine
acetaminophen 300 mg with Codeine Phosphate (15, 30, and 60 mg)	Phenaphen with Codeine (#2, 3, and 4) (WA)	Adriamycin	*doxorubicin HCl*
		Advair Diskus	fluticasone propionate; salmeterol inhalation powder
	Tylenol with Codeine (#2, 3, and 4)	Advicor	lovastatin; niacin
acetazolamide	Diamox	Advil	*ibuprofen*
acetohexamide (W)	Dymelor (W)	AeroBid	flunisolide
		Afluria	influenza vaccine
acetohydroxamic acid	Lithostat	Afrin nasal spray	*oxymetazoline HCl*
		agalsidase beta	Fabrazyme
acetylcholine ophth	Miochol E	Agenerase (W)	amprenavir (W)
		Aggrastat	tirofiban HCl
acetylcysteine	Mucomyst	Aggrenox	aspirin; extended-release dipyridamole
Achromycin (WA)	*tetracycline HCl*		
		Agriflu	influenza virus vaccine type A, susp inj
Aciphex	rabeprazole sodium		
acitretin	Soriatane	Agrylin (WA)	*anagrelide HCl*
Acora	argatroban	Akineton (W)	biperiden (W)
Actemra	tocilizumab inj	Alamast	pemirolast potassium ophth soln
Acthar (WA)	corticotropin		
ActHIB/Tripedia	Haemophilus b conjugate vaccine reconstituted with diphtheria and tetanus toxoids and acellular pertussis vaccine adsorbed	alatrofloxacin mesylate IV (W)	Trovan inj (W)
		albendazole	Albenza
		Albenza	albendazole
		albumin human	Albuminar
			Albutein
Acthrel	corticorellin ovine triflutate		Buminate
			Plasbumin
Actifed	*triprolidine HCl; pseudo-ephedrine HCl*	albumin (human), sonicated	Albunex
Actigall	*ursodiol*	Albuminar	*albumin human*
Actimmune	interferon gamma 1-b	Albunex	albumin (human),
Actiq	*fentanyl oral transmucosal*		sonicated
Activase	alteplase, recombinant	Albutein	*albumin human*
Activella (WA)	norethindrone acetate; estradiol	*albuterol*	AccuNeb
			Proventil
Actonel	risedronate sodium		

	salbutamol	Altabax	retapamulin oint
	Ventolin	Altace	*ramipril*
albuterol SR	Proventil Repetabs	alteplase,	Activase
	Volmax	recombinant	
albuterol sulfate	Proventil HFA	alteplase (for	Cathflo Activase
inhalation		catheter	
aerosol		occlusions)	
alcaftadine	Lastacaft	altretamine	Hexalen
Aldactazide	*spironolactone;*	aluminum	Domeboro
	hydrochlorothiazide	acetate	
Aldactone	*spironolactone*	aluminum	Basaljel (W)
Aldara	imiquimod cream	carbonate (W)	
aldesleukin	Proleukin	aluminum	Amphojel
Aldomet	*methyldopa*	hydroxide	
Aldoril	*methyldopa;*	*aluminum*	Maalox Liquid
	hydrochlorothiazide	*hydroxide;*	
Aldurazyme	laronidase	*magnesium*	
alefacept	Amevive	*hydroxide*	
alemtuzumab	Campath	Alupent	metaproterenol sulfate
alendronate	Fosamax	Alustra (W)	hydroquinone topical susp
sodium			(W)
Alesse	*levonorgestrel; ethinyl*	Alvesco	ciclesonide inhalation
	estradiol	alvimopan	Entereg
Alfenta	alfentanil HCl	*amantadine HCl*	Symmetrel
alfentanil HCl	Alfenta	Amaryl	*glimepiride*
alfuzosin	UroXatral	Ambien	*zolpidem tartrate*
alglucerase	Ceredase	AmBisome	liposomal amphotericin B
alglucosidase	Myozyme	ambrisentan	Letairis
alfa		amcinonide (W)	Cyclocort (W)
Alimta	pemetrexed disodium	Amerge	naratriptan HCl
aliskiren	Tekturna	Amevive	alefacept
hemifumarate		Amicar	*aminocaproic acid*
alitretinoin	Panretin	Amidate	*etomidate*
Allegra	*fexofenadine HCl*	amifostine	Ethyol
Alinia	nitazoxanide	*amikacin sulfate*	Amikin
Alkeran	melphalan	Amikin	*amikacin sulfate*
allopurinol	Zyloprim	*amiloride HCl*	Midamor
almotriptan	Axert	*amiloride; hydro-*	Moduretic
malate		*chlorothiazide*	
Alocril	nedocromil ophth soln	*amino acid inj*	Aminosyn
Alomide	lodoxamide tromethamine		Travasol
	ophth soln		TrophAmine
Alora	*estradiol transdermal*	amino acid with	Clinimix E (W)
alosetron	Lotronex	electrolytes in	
Aloxi	palonosetron HCl	dextrose with	
Alphagan (W)	brimonidine tartrate ophth	calcium inj	
	(W)	(various con-	
alpha₁-proteinase	Prolastin	centrations) (W)	
inhibitor		*aminocaproic*	Amicar
(human)		*acid*	
alprazolam	Xanax	aminocaproic	Caprogel
alprostadil	Caverject	acid gel	
	Edex	*aminogluteth-*	*aminoglutethimide*
	Prostin VR	*imide*	
alprostadil	Muse	aminolevulinic	Levulan Kerastick
urethral		acid HCl	
suppository		topical soln	
Alrex	loteprednol etabonate	*aminophylline*	*aminophylline*
	ophth susp		

aminosalicylic acid	Paser	Ampyra	dalfampridine
Aminosyn	*amino acid inj*	amrinone (former name)	inamrinone (new name)
amiodarone HCl	Cordarone		
Amitiza	lubiprostone	Amrix	*cyclobenzaprine SR*
amitriptyline HCl	*amitriptyline HCl*	amsacrine	Amsidyl
AmLactin	ammonium lactate lotion	Amsidyl	amsacrine
amlexanox oral paste	Aphthasol	Amvisc	sodium hyaluronate
		Amytal	amobarbital sodium inj
amlodipine besylate	Norvasc	Anadrol-50	oxymetholone
		Anafranil	*clomipramine HCl*
amlodipine besylate; atorvastatin calcium	Caduet	*anagrelide HCl*	Agrylin (WA)
		anakinra	Kineret
		Anaprox	*naproxen sodium*
		anastrozole	Arimidex
amlodipine besylate; benazepril HCl	Lotrel	Anbesol	benzocaine
		Ancef (WA)	*cefazolin sodium*
		Ancobon	flucytosine
		Androderm	*testosterone transdermal system*
amlodipine; valsartan	Exforge		
		AndroGel	testosterone gel
ammonium lactate lotion	AmLactin	Androgel-DHT	dihydrotestosterone transdermal
amobarbital sodium inj	Amytal	Anectine	*succinylcholine chloride*
		Anexsia	*hydrocodone bitartrate; acetaminophen*
amoxapine	*amoxapine*		
amoxicillin	Amoxil	Angiomax	bivalirudin
	Trimox	anidulafungin IV	Eraxis
	Wymox	Ansaid	*flurbiprofen*
amoxicillin; clavulanic acid	Augmentin	Antabuse	disulfiram
		Antagon	ganirelix acetate
amoxicillin; clavulanate potassium SR	Augmentin XR	antihemophilic factor (recombinant)	Kogenate ReFacto
		Antilirium	physostigmine salicylate
Amoxil	amoxicillin	antipyrine otic (W)	Auralgan (W)
amphetamine resins (W)	Biphetamine (W)	antithrombin, recombinant inj	Atryn
amphetamine; dextroamphet- amine mixed salts	Adderall	antithrombin III (human)	Thrombate III
		antithymocyte globulin, (rabbit)	Thymoglobulin
Amphojel (WA)	*aluminum hydroxide*	Antivert	*meclizine*
Amphotec	amphotericin B cholesteryl sulfate	Antizol	fomepizole
		Anturane (W)	sulfinpyrazone (W)
amphotericin B (W)	Fungizone (W)	Anzemet	dolasetron mesylate
		Aphthasol	amlexanox oral paste
amphotericin B cholesteryl sulfate	Amphotec	Apidra	insulin glulisine [rDNA origin]
		A.P.L. (WA)	*chorionic gonadotropin*
amphotericin B lipid complex	Abelcet	apligraf (W)	Graftskin (W)
ampicillin	Principen (WA)	Aplisol	tuberculin skin test
ampicillin sodium; sulbactam sodium	Unasyn	Apokyn	apomorphine HCl inj
		apomorphine HCl inj	Apokyn
amprenavir (W)	Agenerase (W)	Aposyn (W)	exisulind (W)

aprepitant — Emend capsules
Apresazide (W) — hydralazine HCl; hydrochloro-thiazide (W)
Apresoline (WA) — *hydralazine HCl*
aprotinin — Trasylol
Aptivus — tipranavir
AquaMEPHY-TON (WA) — *phytonadione*
Aralen — *chloroquine phosphate*
Aramine — metaraminol bitartrate
Aranesp — darbepoetin alfa
Arava — leflunomide
arbutamine HCl (W) — GenEsa (W)
Arcalyst — rilonacept
arcitumomab — CEA-Scan
ardeparin sodium (W) — Normiflo (W)
Arduan (W) — pipecuronium bromide (W)
Aredia — *pamidronate disodium*
Arestin — minocycline HCl dental microspheres
Arfonad (W) — trimethaphan camsylate (W)
argatroban — argatroban
arginine HCl — R-Gene
Aricept — donepezil HCl
Aridol — mannitol inhalation powder
Arimidex — *anastrozole*
aripiprazole — Abilify
Aristocort — triamcinolone
Arixtra — fondaparinux sodium
armodafinil — Nuvigil
Aromasin — exemestane
Arranon — nelarabine
arsenic trioxide — Trisenox
Artane (WA) — *trihexyphenidyl HCl*
artemether/lumafentrine combination — Coartem
Arthrotec — diclofenac; misoprostol
articaine; epinephrine — Septocaine
Artiss — fibrin sealant, human, topical
Arzerra — ofatumumab
Asacol — mesalamine
asenapine maleate — Saphris
Asendin (WA) — *amoxapine*
Aslera (W) — prasterone (W)
asparaginase — Elspar
aspirin 325 mg with codeine phosphate (30 and 60 mg) — Empirin with codeine #3 and #4

aspirin buffered — Bufferin
aspirin EC — Ecotrin
aspirin; extended-release dipyridamole — Aggrenox
Astelin — azelastine HCl nasal spray
astemizole (W) — Hismanal (W)
Atacand — candesartan cilexetil
Atarax (WA) — *hydroxyzine HCl*
atazanavir (W) sulfate — Reyataz (W)
atenolol — Tenormin
atenolol; chlorthalidone — Tenoretic
Atgam — lymphocyte imimmune globulin
Atacand HCT — candesartan cilexetil; hydrochlorothiazide
atazanavir (W) — Revetaz (W)
Ativan — *lorazepam*
Atomoxetine HCl — Strattera
atorvastatin calcium — Lipitor
atovaquone — Mepron
atovaquone; proguanil HCl — Malarone
atracurium besylate — Tracrium
Atridox — doxycycline hyclate gel
Atripla — efavirenz, emtricitabine, and tenofovir
Atromid-S (W) — clofibrate (W)
atropine sulfate tablets — Sal-Tropine
Atrovent — *ipratropium bromide*
Atryn — antithrombin, recombinant inj
Augmentin — *amoxicillin; clavulanic acid*
Augmentin XR — *amoxicillin; clavulanate potassium SR*
Auralgan (W) — antipyrine otic (W)
auranofin — Ridaura
Aurolate — gold sodium thiomalate
aurothioglucose (W) — Solganal (W)
Avalide — irbesartan; hydro-chlorothiazide
Avandamet — rosiglitazone maleate; metformin HCl
Avandia — Rosiglitazone maleate
Avanir (W) — docosanol cream (W)
Avapro — irbesartan
Avastin — bevacizumab
Avelox — moxifloxacin HCl
Aventyl — *nortriptyline HCl*
Avinza — *morphine sulfate tab SR*

Avita	*tretinoin cream 0.025%*
Avitene	collagen hemostat
Avodart	dutasteride
Avonex	interferon beta-la
Axert	almotriptan malate
Axid	*nizatidine*
azacitidine	Vidaza
Azactam	*aztreonam*
AzaSite	azithromycin ophth soln
azatadine maleate	Optimine
azathioprine	Imuran
azelaic acid cream	Azelex
	Finevin
azelastine HCl nasal spray	Astelin
azelastine HCl ophth soln	Optivar
Azelex	azelaic acid cream
Azilect	rasagiline mesylate
azithromycin	Zithromax
azithromycin ophth soln	AzaSite
Azmacort	triamcinolone acetonide aerosol
Azopt	brinzolamide ophth susp
aztreonam	Azactam
Azulfidine	*sulfasalazine*

B

Baciguent (W)	*bacitracin ointment*
baclofen	Lioresal
Bactrim	*sulfamethoxazole; trimeth-oprim*
Bactroban	mupirocin nasal ointment
BAL in Oil	dimercaprol
Banzel	rufinamide
Baraclude	entecavir
Basaljel (W)	aluminum carbonate (W)
balsalazide disodium	Colazal
basiliximab	Simulect
Baycol (W)	cerivastatin sodium (W)
BCG intravesical	Pacis TheraCys TICE BCG
becaplermin gel	Regranex
beclomethasone dipropionate	Beclovent (W) Beconase AQ Nasal Qvar Vancenase (W) Vancenase AQ Nasal (W) Vanceril (W)
Beclovent (WA)	*beclomethasone dipropionate*

Beconase AQ Nasal	*beclomethasone dipropionate*
belladonna alkaloids; phenobarbital	Donnatal (W)
Bellergal-S (W)	phenobarbital; ergotamine; belladonna (W)
Benadryl	*diphenhydramine HCl*
benazepril HCl	Lotensin
bendamustine HCl inj	Treanda
BeneFix	factor IX, (recombinant)
Benemid (WA)	*probenecid*
Benicar	olmesartan medoxomil
Benicar HCT	olmesartan medoxomil; hydrochlorothiazide
bentoquatam	IvyBlock
Bentyl	*dicyclomine HCl*
Benzamycin	erythromycin; benzoyl peroxide topical gel
benzocaine	Anbesol Hurricaine Orabase Orajel
benzocaine; tetracaine HCl	Cetacaine
benztropine mesylate	Cogentin
benzyl alcohol lotion	Ulesfia
bepotastine besilate ophth soln	Bepreve
Bepreve	bepotastine besilate ophth soln
bepridil (W)	Vascor (W)
beractant	Survanta
Berroca	*vitamin B complex; folic acid; vitamin C*
besifloxacin HCl ophth soln	Besivance
Besivance	besifloxacin HCL ophth soln
Betadine	povidone iodine
17β-estradiol; norgestimate	Ortho-Prefest
Betagan	levobunolol HCl
betaine anhydrous	Cystadane
betamethasone	Celestone
betamethasone dipropionate	Diprosone (WA)
betamethasone; clotrimazole cream	Lotrisone
betamethasone valerate (foam)	Luxiq
Betapace	*sotalol*

Betaseron — interferon beta-1b

betaxolol — Kerlone

betaxolol HCl ophth soln — Betoptic

betaxolol HCl ophth susp — Betoptic S

betaxolol HCl; pilocarpine HCl ophth soln (W) — Betoptic Pilo (W)

bethanechol chloride — Urecholine

Betoptic — betaxolol HCl ophth soln

Betoptic Pilo (W) — betaxolol HCl; pilocarpine HCl, ophth soln (W)

Betoptic S — betaxolol HCl ophth suspension

bevacizumab — Avastin

bexarotene gel — Targretin

Bextra (W) — valdecoxib (W)

Bexxar — tositumomab and I-131 tositumomab

Biaxin — *clarithromycin*

Biaxin XL — *clarithromycin SR*

bicalutamide — Casodex

Bicillin C-R — penicillin G benzathine; penicillin G procaine (for IM use only)

Bicillin L-A — penicillin G benzathine (for IM use only)

Bicitra (WA) — *sodium citrate; citric acid*

BiCNU — carmustine

BiDil — isosorbide dinitrate; hydralazine

Bilopaque (W) — tyropanoate sodium (W)

bimatoprost ophth soln (W) — Lumigan (W)

biperiden (W) — Akineton (W)

Biphetamine (W) — amphetamine resins (W)

bisacodyl — Dulcolax

bismuth subsalicylate; metronidazole; tetracycline HCl — Helidac

bisoprolol fumarate; hydrochlorothiazide — Ziac

bitolterol mesylate (W) — Tornalate (W)

bivalirudin — Angiomax

Blocadren — *timolol maleate*

Boniva — ibandronate

bortezomib — Velcade

bosentan — Tracleer

B & O Supprettes — opium; belladonna suppositories

Botox — botulinum toxin type A

botulinum toxin type A — Botox

botulinum toxin type B — Myobloc

Bravelle — urofollitropin

Brethaire — terbutaline sulfate aerosol

Brethine — *terbutaline sulfate tablets and inj*

bretylium tosylate (W) — Bretylol (W)

Bretylol (W) — bretylium tosylate (W)

Brevibloc — esmolol HCl

Brevital Sodium — methohexital sodium

Bricanyl (WA) — *terbutaline sulfate tablets and inj*

brimonidine tartrate ophth — Alphagan

brinzolamide ophth suspension — Azopt

bromfenac ophth soln — Xibrom

bromocriptine mesylate — Parlodel

brompheniramine maleate — *brompheniramine maleate*

brompheniramine maleate; phenylpropanolamime — Dimetapp Extentabs (WA)

Bronkometer (WA) — *isoetharine HCl aerosol*

Bronkosol (WA) — *isoetharine HCl soln*

Bucladin-S (W) — buclizine HCl (W)

buclizine HCl (W) — Bucladin-S (W)

budesonide capsule SR — Entocort EC

budesonide inhalation powder (W) — Pulmicort Turbuhaler (W)

budesonide nasal inhaler — Rhinocort

Bufferin — *aspirin buffered*

bumetanide — Bumex

Bumex — bumetanide

Buminate — albumin human

Buphenyl — phenylbutyrate sodium

bupivacaine HCl — Marcaine HCl

buprenorphine HCl — Subutex

buprenorphine HCl; naloxone HCl — Suboxone

bupropion HCl — Wellbutrin

bupropion HCl SR — Wellbutrin SR / Zyban

BuSpar — *buspirone HCl*

buspirone HCl — BuSpar

busulfan — Myleran

busulfan inj — Busulfex

Busulfex — busulfan inj

B
℞

butabarbital sodium	Butisol
butalbital; acetaminophen; caffeine	Fioricet
butalbital; aspirin; caffeine	Fiorinal
butenafine HCl	Mentax
Butisol	*butabarbital sodium*
butoconazole nitrate vaginal cream	Gynazole
butorphanol tartrate inj	Stadol
butorphanol tartrate nasal spray	Stadol NS
Byetta	exenatide inj

C

cabazitaxel inj	Jevtana
cabergoline	Dostinex (WA)
Ca-DTPA	calcium trisodium (trisodium calcium diethylenetriamine-pentaacetate)
Caduet	amlodipine besylate; atorvastatin calcium
Cafcit	*caffeine citrate inj*
Cafergot	ergotaminetartrate; caffeine
caffeine citrate inj	Cafcit
Calan SR	*verapamil HCl SR*
Calciferol	*ergocalciferol*
Calcimar	calcitonin
calcipotriene cream	Dovonex
calcitonin	Calcimar
calcitonin-salmon	Miacalcin
calcitriol	Rocaltrol
calcium carbonate	Os-Cal 500 Tums
calcium carbonate; vitamin D and K chewable	Viactiv
calcium trisodium (trisodium calcium diethylenetri-aminepenta-acetate)	Ca-DTPA

calfactant intratracheal susp	Infasurf
Campath	alemtuzumab
camphorated tincture of opium	paregoric
Campral	acamprosate calcium
Camptosar	*irinotecan HCl*
canakinumab inj	Ilaris
candesartan cilexetil	Atacand
candesartan cilexetil; hydrochlorothi-azide	Atacand HCT
Cancidas	caspofungin acetate
Capastat Sulfate	capreomycin sulfate
capecitabine	Xeloda
Capital w/ Codeine Suspension	codeine phosphate; acetaminophen suspension
Capitrol (W)	chloroxine (W)
Capoten	*captopril*
capreomycin sulfate	Capastat Sulfate
Caprogel	aminocaproic acid gel
capromab pendetide	ProstaScint
captopril	Capoten
Carac	fluorouracil cream
Carafate	sucralfate
carbachol (W)	Isopto Carbachol (W)
Carbaglu	carglumic acid
carbamazepine	Tegretol
carbamazepine SR	Carbatrol Tegretol-XR
carbamide peroxide otic	Debrox
Carbatrol	carbamazepine SR
carbenicillin (W)	Geocillin (W)
Carbex (WA)	*selegiline*
Carbocaine	*mepivacaine HCl*
carboplatin	*carboplatin*
Cardene	*nicardipine HCl*
Cardiolite	technetium Tc99m sestamibi
Cardiotec	technetium Tc-99m teboroxime kit
Cardizem	*diltiazem HCl*
Cardizem CD	*diltiazem HCl SR*
Cardura	*doxazosin mesylate*
carglumic acid	Carbaglu
carisoprodol	Soma
carmustine	BiCNU

carmustine implantable wafer — Gliadel
Carnitor — *levocarnitine*
Cartia XR (WA) — *diltiazem HCl SR*
carvedilol — Coreg
Casodex — *bicalutamide*
caspofungin acetate — Cancidas
Cataflam — *diclofenac potassium*
Catapres — *clonidine HCl*
Cathflo Activase — alteplase (for catheter occlusions)
Caverject — alprostadil
CEA-SCAN — arcitumomab
Ceclor (WA) — *cefaclor*
Cedax — ceftibuten
CeeNu — lomustine
cefaclor — Ceclor (WA)
cefadroxil — Duricef (WA)
Cefadyl (WA) — *cephapirin sodium*
cefamandole nafate (W) — Mandol (W)
cefazolin sodium — *cefazolin sodium*
cefdinir — Omnicef
cefditoren pivoxil — Spectracef
cefepime HCl — Maxipime
cefixime — Suprax
Cefizox — ceftizoxime sodium
Cefobid (W) — cefoperazone sodium (W)
cefonicid sodium (W) — Monocid (W)
cefoperazone sodium (W) — Cefobid (W)
Cefotan (WA) — *cefotetan*
cefotaxime sodium — Claforan
cefotetan — cefotetan
cefoxitin sodium — Mefoxin (WA)
cefpodoxime proxetil — Vantin
cefprozil — Cefzil (WA)
ceftazidime — Ceptaz
Fortaz
Tazicef
Tazidime (WA)
ceftibuten — Cedax
Ceftin — *cefuroxime axetil*
ceftizoxime sodium — Cefizox
ceftriaxone sodium — Rocephin
cefuroxime axetil — Ceftin

cefuroxime sodium — Kefurox (W)
Zinacef
Cefzil — *cefprozil*
Celebrex — celecoxib
celecoxib — Celebrex
Celestone — betamethasone
Celexa — *citalopram hydrobromide*
CellCept — *mycophenolate mofetil*
Cenestin — synthetic conjugated estrogens, A
Centrum — vitamins; minerals
cephalexin — *cephalexin HCl*
Keflex
cephalothin sodium (W) — Keflin (W)
cephapirin sodium (W) — Cefadyl (W)
cephradine (W) — Velosef (W)
Cephulac — lactulose
Ceprotin — protein C concentrate (human)
Ceptaz — ceftazidime
Cerebyx — fosphenytoin sodium
Ceredase — alglucerase
Cerezyme — imiglucerase
cerivastatin sodium (W) — Baycol (W)
Cernevit-12 — multivitamins for infusion
certolizumab pegol — Cimzia
Cerubidine — daunorubicin HCl
Cervarlx — human papillomavirus bivalent vaccine, recombinant, susp inj
Cervidil — dinoprostone vaginal insert
Cesamet — nabilone
Cl esterase inhibitor vaccine — Cinryze
Cetacaine — benzocaine; tetracaine HCl
cetirizine HCl — Zyrtec
cetirizine HCL; pseudoephedrine HCl SR — Zyrtec-D
cetrorelix — Cetrotide
Cetrotide — cetrorelix
cetuximab — Erbitux
cevimeline HCl — Evoxac
Chantix — varenicline
Chenodal — chenodiol
chenodiol — Chenodal
Chirocaine (W) — levobupivacaine (W)
chloral hydrate — *chloral hydrate*
chlorambucil — Leukeran
chloramphenicol sodium succinate — Chloromycetin inj (WA)

C
R̶

chloramphenicol ophth (W)	Chloroptic ophth (W)
chlordiazepoxide HCl	Librium
chlordiazepoxide HCl; amitriptyline HCl	Limbitrol
chlorhexidine gluconate	Hibiclens
chlorhexidine gluconate mouth rinse	Peridex
Chloromycetin (WA)	*chloramphenicol sodium succinate*
chloroprocaine HCl	Nesacaine
Chloroptic ophth (W)	chloramphenicol ophth (W)
chloroquine phosphate	Aralen
chlorothiazide	Diuril
chloroxine (W)	Capitrol (W)
chlorpheniramine maleate	Chlor-Trimeton
chlorpheniramine maleate SR	*chlorpheniramine maleate SR*
chlorpromazine	*chlorpromazine*
chlorpropamide	Diabinese
chlorthalidone	Hygroton
chlorthalidone; reserpine (W)	Regroton (W)
Chlor-Trimeton	*chlorpheniramine maleate*
chlorzoxazone 250 mg	Paraflex
chlorzoxazone 500 mg	Parafon Forte DSC
Cholebrine	iocetamic acid
Choledyl (W)	oxtriphylline (W)
cholestyramine (W)	Questran (W)
choline chloride inj	Intrachol
choline (W) magnesium trisalicylate	Trilisate (W)
Choloxin (W)	dextrothyroxine sodium (W)
chorionic gonadotropin	*chorionic gonadotropin*
choriogona-dotropin alfa	Ovidrel
Chronulac	lactulose
Chymodiactin	chymopapain
chymopapain	Chymodiactin
Cialis	tadalafil
Cibalith-S	lithium citrate
ciclesonide inhalation	Alvesco

ciclesonide nasal susp	Omnaris
ciclopirox cream and lotion	Loprox
ciclopirox soln	Penlac Nail Lacquer
cidofovir	Vistide
cilostazol	Pletal
Ciloxan	*ciprofloxacin ophth soln*
cimetidine HCl	Tagamet
Cimzia	certolizumab pegol
cinacalcet HCl	Sensipar
Cinryze	C1 esterase inhibitor vaccine
Cipro	*ciprofloxacin HCl*
ciprofloxacin HCl	Cipro
ciprofloxacin; hydrocortisone otic	Cipro HC Otic
ciprofloxacin ophth soln	Ciloxan
Cipro HC Otic	ciprofloxacin; hydrocortisone otic
cisapride (W)	Propulsid (W)
cisatracurium besylate	Nimbex
cisplatin	*cisplatin*
citalopram hydrobromide	Celexa
cladribine	Leustatin
Claforan	*cefotaxime sodium*
Clarinex	desloratadine
clarithromycin	Biaxin
clarithromycin SR	Biaxin XL
Claritin	*loratadine*
Claritin D	*loratadine; pseudoephed-rine sulfate*
clemastine fumarate	Tavist
Cleocin	clindamycin HCl
clevidipine butyrate	Cleviprex
Cleviprex	clevidipine butyrate
clidinium (W) bromide	Quarzan (W)
clidinium; chlordiaze-poxide	Librax
Climara	*estradiol transdermal*
clindamycin; benzoyl peroxide gel	BenzaClin
clindamycin HCl	Cleocin
clindamycin phosphate pledgets	Clindets
Clindets	clindamycin phosphate pledgets

Clinimix E (W)	amino acid with electrolytes in dextrose with calcium inj (various concentrations) (W)	colesevelam HCl	Welchol
		Colestid	colestipol HCl
		colestipol HCl	Colestid
		colistimethate sodium	Coly-Mycin M (WA)
Clinoril	*sulindac*	colistin sulfate; hydrocortisone, and neomycin otic soln	Coly-Mycin S
clioquinol (W)	Vioform (W)		
clobetasol foam	Olux		
clobetasol propionate gel (W)	Clobevate (W)		
		collagense clostridium histolyticum inj	Xiaflex
Clobevate (W)	clobetasol propionate gel (W)		
		collagen hemostat	Avitene
clofarabine	Clolar		
clofibrate (W)	Atromid-S (W)	collagenase	Santyl
Clolar	clofarabine	Collyrium	tetrahydrozoline HCl ophth
Clomid	*clomiphene citrate*		
clomiphene citrate	Clomid	Colomed	short chain fatty acids enema
clomipramine HCl	Anafranil	Coly-Mycin M (WA)	*colistimethate sodium*
clonazepam	Klonopin	Coly-Mycin S	colistin sulfate; hydrocortisone, and neomycin otic soln
clonidine HCl	Catapres		
clonidine HCl inj	Duraclon		
clopidogrel bisulfate	Plavix	CoLyte	*polyethylene glycol-electrolyte soln*
clorazepate dipotassium	Tranxene	CombiPatch	norethindrone acetate; estradiol transdermal
Clorpactin WCS-90	oxychlorosene sodium	Combivent	*ipratropium bromide; albuterol sulfate*
clotrimazole	Gyne-Lotrimin Lotrimin Mycelex	Combivir	lamivudine; zidovudine
		Combunox	oxycodone HCl, ibuprofen
		Compazine (WA)	*prochlorperazine*
clozapine	Clozaril	Comtan	entacapone
Clozaril	*clozapine*	Comvax	*Haemophilus b* conjugate; Hepatitis B vaccine
coagulation factor IX (recombinant)	BeneFix		
		Concerta	*methylphenidate HCl SR*
coagulation factor VII a (recombinant)	NovoSeven	Condylox	*podofilox gel*
		conivaptan HCl	Vaprisol
		Copaxone	glatiramer acetate
coal tar product	Zetar	Cordarone	*amiodarone HCl*
Coartem	artemether/lumafentrine combination	Coreg	carvedilol
		Corgard (WA)	*nadolol*
codeine phosphate; acetaminophen suspension	Capital w/ Codeine Suspension	Corlopam	fenoldopam mesylate
		Cortef	*hydrocortisone*
		corticorellin ovine triflutate	Acthrel
coenzyme Q10	UbiQGel		
Cogentin	*benztropine mesylate*	corticotropin	Acthar (WA)
Cognex (W)	tacrine HCl (W)	cortisone acetate	Cortone Acetate
Colace	*docusate sodium*	Cortone Acetate	cortisone acetate
Colazal	*balsalazide disodium*	Cortrosyn	cosyntropin
ColBENEMID (W)	*probenecid; colchicine*	Corvert	ibutilide fumarate
		Cosmegen	dactinomycin
colchicine tablets	Colcrys	Cosopt	*dorzolamide HCl; timolol maleate ophth soln*
colchinine inj (W)	*colchicine inj (W)*		
Colcrys	colchicine tablets	cosyntropin	Cortrosyn
		Cotazym (WA)	*pancrelipase*
		Cotazym-S (W)	*pancrelipase EC*

Cotrim	sulfamethoxazole; trimethoprim
co-trimoxazole	*Bactrim*
	Cotrim
	Septra
	sulfamethoxazole; trimethoprim
Coumadin	*warfarin sodium*
Covera HS	*verapamil HCl SR bedtime formulation*
Cozaar	*losartan potassium*
Creon	pancrelipase
Crestor	rosuvastatin calcium
Crinone	progesterone gel
Crixivan	indinavir
CroFab	crotalidae polyvalent immune fab (ovine)
cromolyn sodium	Gastrocrom
	Nasalcrom
	Opticrom
crotalidae polyvalent immune fab (ovine)	CroFab
crotamiton	Eurax
Cubicin	daptomycin
Cuprimine	penicillamine
Curosurf	poractant alpha intratracheal susp
Cutivate	fluticasone propionate cream & ointment
Cuvposa	glycopyrrolate
cyanocobalamin nasal gel	Nascobal
cyclobenzaprine HCl	Flexeril
cyclobenzaprine SR	Amrix
Cyclocort (W)	amcinonide (W)
Cyclogyl	cyclopentolate HCl
cyclopentolate HCl	Cyclogyl
cyclophospha-mide	Cytoxan (WA)
	Neosar (WA)
cycloserine	Seromycin
cyclosporine	Sandimmune
cyclosporine capsules (modified) and oral soln	Neoral
cyclosporine capsules, (modified)	Gengraf
cyclosporine ophth emulsion	Restasis
Cycrin (WA)	*medroxyprogesterone acetate*

Cylert (W)	pemoline (W)
Cymbalta	duloxetine HCl
Cypher stent	sirolimus-eluting stent
cyproheptadine HCl	*cyproheptadine HCl*
Cystadane	betaine anhydrous
Cytadren (W)	*aminoglutethimide*
cytarabine	*cytarabine*
cytarabine, liposomal inj	DepoCyt
Cytomel	*liothyronine sodium*
Cytosar-U (WA)	*cytarabine*
Cytotec	*misoprostol*
Cytovene	*ganciclovir*
Cytoxan (WA)	*cyclophosphamide*

D

dabigatran	Pradaxa
dacarbazine	DTIC-Dome (WA)
daclizumab (W)	Zenapax (W)
Dacogen	decitabine inj
dactinomycin	Cosmegen
dalfampridine	Ampyra
Dalmane (WA)	*flurazepam HCl*
dalteparin sodium	Fragmin
danaparoid sodium	Orgaran
danazol	Danocrine (WA)
Danocrine (WA)	*danazol*
Dantrium	dantrolene sodium
dantrolene sodium	Dantrium
dapsone	dapsone
daptomycin	Cubicin
Daranide (W)	dichlorphenamide (W)
Daraprim	pyrimethamine
darbepoetin alfa	Aranesp
darifenacin	Enablex
darunavir	Prezista
Darvocet-N 100 (W)	*propoxyphene napsylate; acetaminophen (W)*
Darvon (W)	*propoxyphene HCl (W)*
Darvon Compound 65 (W)	*propoxyphene HCl; aspirin; caffeine (W)*
dasatinib	Sprycel
daunorubicin citrate liposomal	DaunoXome
daunorubicin HCl	Cerubidine
DaunoXome	daunorubicin citrate liposomal
Daypro	oxaprozin

DDAVP	desmopressin acetate	desonide	Tridesilon
Debrox	carbamide peroxide otic	desoximetasone	Topicort
Decadron (WA)	dexamethasone	Desoxyn	methamphetamine HCl
Deca-Durabolin (W)	nandrolone decanoate (W)	desvenlafaxine succinate	Pristiq
decitabine inj	Dacogen	Desyrel (WA)	trazodone HCl
Declomycin	demeclocycline HCl	Detrol	tolterodine tartrate
deferasirox	Exjade	Detrol LA	tolterodine tartrate (SR)
deferoxamine mesylate	Desferal	dexamethasone	Decadron (WA) Hexadrol (WA)
degarelix inj	Firmagon	dexamethasone-eluting stent	Dexamet stent
delavirdine mesylate	Rescriptor		
Delestrogen	estradiol valerate	Dexamet stent	dexamethasone-eluting stent
Deltasone (WA)	prednisone		
Demadex	torsemide	dexchlorphenir-	dexchlorpheniramine
demecarium bromide (W)	Humorsol (W)	amine maleate SR	maleate SR
demeclocycline HCl	Declomycin	Dexedrine (WA)	dextroamphetamine sulfate
		dexfenfluramine HCl (W)	Redux (W)
Demerol	meperidine HCl		
Demser	metyrosine	Dexferrum	iron dextran inj
Demulen (WA)	ethynodiol diacetate; ethinyl estradiol	dexiansoprazole	Kapidex
		dexmedetomidine HCl inj	Precedex
Denavir	penciclovir cream		
denileukin diftitox	Ontak	dexmethyl- phenidate HCl	Focalin
Depacon	valproate sodium inj		
Depakene	valproic acid	dexrazoxane	Zinecard
Depakote	divalproex sodium	dextro-	dextroamphetamine sulfate
Depakote ER	divalproex sodium SR	amphetamine sulfate	
DepoCyt	cytarabine, liposomal inj		
DepoDur	morphine sulfate extended-release liposome inj	dextrothyroxine sodium (W)	Choloxin (W)
		D.H.E. 45	dihydroergotamine mesylate inj
Depo-Medrol	methylprednisolone acetate SR	DiaBeta	glyburide
		Diabinese	chlorpropamide
Depo-Provera	medroxyprogesterone acetate SR	Diamox	acetazolamide
		Diapid (W)	lypressin (W)
Depo- Testosterone	testosterone cypionate SR	Diastat	diazepam rectal gel
		diazepam	Valium
Desferal	deferoxamine mesylate	diazepam emulsified inj	Dizac
desflurane	Suprane		
desipramine HCl	Norpramin	diazepam rectal gel	Diastat
Desirudin	iprivask		
desloratadine	Clarinex	diazoxide	Hyperstat
desmopressin acetate	DDAVP	Dibenzyline	phenoxybenzamine HCl
		dibucaine	Nupercainal
Desogen	desogestrel; ethinyl estradiol	dichlorphena- mide (W)	Daranide (W)
desogestrel; ethinyl estradiol	Desogen Ortho-Cept	diclofenac gel	Solaraze
		diclofenac potassium	Cataflam
desogestrel and ethinyl estradiol; ethinyl estradiol	Mircette	diclofenac sodium	Voltaren
		diclofenac sodium; misoprostol	Arthrotec

diclofenac sodium SR	Voltaren-XR	diphenoxylate HCl; atropine sulfate	Lomotil
dicloxacillin sodium	dicloxacillin sodium	diphtheria and tetanus toxoids and acellular pertussis adsorbed and inactivated poliovirus vaccine	Kinrix
dicyclomine HCl	Bentyl		
didanosine	Videx		
didanosine SR	Videx EC		
Didronel	etidronate disodium		
diethylcarbama-zine citrate	Hetrazan		
diethylpropion HCl	diethylpropion HCl	diphtheria and tetanus toxoids and acellular pertussis adsorbed inactivated poliovirus and Haemophilus b conjugate	Pentacel
Differin	adapalene		
diflorasone diacetate	Florone		
Diflucan	fluconazole		
diflunisal	diflunisal		
difluprednate ophth emulsion	Durezol	diphtheria, tetanus, and acellular pertussis (TdaP) vaccine (adult type)	Adacel
Digibind	digoxin immune fab		
digoxin	Lanoxin		
digoxin capsules (W)	Lanoxicaps (W)		
digoxin immune fab	Digibind	dipivefrin	Propine
		Diprivan	propofol
dihydroergota-mine mesylate inj	D.H.E. 45	Diprosone (WA)	betamethasone dipropionate
		dipyridamole	Persantine
dihydroergota-mine mesylate nasal spray	Migranol	dirithromycin (W)	Dynabac (W)
		Disalcid	salsalate
		disopyramide phosphate	Norpace
dihydrotestoster-one transdermal	Androge12DHT	disulfiram	Antabuse
		Ditropan	oxybutynin chloride
Dilacor XR	diltiazem HCl SR	Diulo (WA)	metolazone
Dilantin	phenytoin	Diuril	chlorothiazide
Dilaudid	hydromorphone HCl	divalproex sodium	Depakote
diltiazem HCl	Cardizem		
diltiazem HCl SR	Cardizem CD	divalproex sodium SR	Depakote ER
	Cartia XR (WA)		
	Dilacor XR	Dizac	diazepam emulsified inj
	Tiazac	dobutamine HCl	Dobutrex
diltiazem maleate SR	Tiamate	Dobutrex (WA)	dobutamine HCl
		docetaxel	Taxotere
dimenhydrinate	Dramamine	docosanol cream (W)	Avanir (W)
dimercaprol	BAL in Oil		
Dimetane (WA)	brompheniramine maleate	docusate sodium	Colace
dinoprostone gel	Prepidil	docusate sodium; casanthranol	Peri-Colace
dinoprostone vaginal insert	Cervidil		
		dofetilide	Tikosyn
dinoprostone vaginal suppositories	Prostin E2	dolasetron mesylate	Anzemet
		Dolobid (WA)	diflunisal
Diovan	valsartan	Dolophine	methadone HCl
Diovan HCT	valsartan; hydrochloro-thiazide	Domeboro	aluminum acetate
		donepezil HCl	Aricept
Dipentum	olsalazine sodium	Donnatal (W)	belladonna alkaloids; phenobarbital
diphenhydramine HCl	Benadryl		
		dopamine HCl	Intropin (WA)

Dopar (W) — levodopa (W)
Dopram — doxapram HCl
Doribax — doripenem
doripenem — Doribax
dornase alpha — Pulmozyme
Doryx — *doxycycline hyclate SR*
dorzolamide HCI — Trusopt
dorzolamide HCl; timolol maleate ophth soln — Cosopt
Dostinex (WA) — *cabergoline*
Dovonex — calcipotriene cream
doxacurium chloride (W) — Nuromax (W)
doxapram HCl — Dopram
doxazosin mesylate — Cardura
doxepin HCl — *doxepin HCl* / Sinequan
doxepin HCl cream — Prudoxin
doxercalciferol — Hectorol
Doxil — doxorubicin, liposomal
doxorubicin HCl — Adriamycin / Rubex (WA)
doxorubicin, liposomal — Doxil
doxycycline hyclate — Vibramycin
doxycycline hyclate 20 mg tab & cap — Periostat
doxycycline hyclate gel — Atridox
doxycycline hyclate SR — Doryx
Dramamine — *dimenhydrinate*
Drisdol — *ergocalciferol*
Dristan Long Lasting — *oxymetazoline HCl*
Drixoral Syrup — pseudoephedrine HCl; bromphiramine maleate
dronabinol — Marinol
dronedarone — Multaq
droperidol — Inapsine (WA)
drospirenone; ethinyl estradiol — Yasmin
drotrecogin alfa — Xigris
Droxia — *hydroxyurea*
DTIC-Dome (WA) — *dacarbazine*
Dulcolax — *bisacodyl*
duloxetine HCl — Cymbalta
Durabolin (W) — nandrolone phenpropionate (W)

Duraclon — clonidine HCl epidural inj
Duragesic — *fentanyl transdermal*
Durezol — difluprednate ophth emulsion
Duramorph — morphine sulfate inj
Duranest (W) — etidocaine HCl (W)
Duricef (WA) — *cefadroxil*
dutasteride — Avodart
Dyazide — *triamterene 37.5 mg; hydrochlorothiazide 25 mg*
Dymelor (W) — acetohexamide (W)
Dynabac (W) — dirithromycin (W)
DynaCirc — *isradipine*
Dynapen (WA) — *dicloxacillin sodium*
dyphylline — Lufyllin
Dyrenium — triamterene
Dysport — abobotulinumtoxin A inj

E

EchoGen — perflenapent emulsion
echothiophate iodide (W) — Phospholine Iodide (W)
Ecotrin — *aspirin EC*
eculizumab — Soliris
Edecrin — ethacrynic acid
edetate disodium — Endrate
Edex — alprostadil inj
edrophonium chloride — Tensilon (WA)
E.E.S. 400 — erythromycin ethylsuccinate
efalizumab (W) — Raptiva (W)
efaproxiral — Efaproxyn
Efaproxyn — efaproxiral
efavirenz — Sustiva
efavirenz, emtricitabine, and tenofovir — Atripla
Effexor — *venlafaxine HCl*
Effexor XR — *venlafaxine HCl SR*
Effient — prasugrel
eflornithine HCl cream — Vaniqa
Efudex (WA) — fluorouracil cream; soln
Elaprase — idursulfase
Elavil (WA) — *amitriptyline HCl*
Eldepryl — selegiline HCl
Eldisine (W) — vindesine sulfate (W)
Elestat — epinastine
eletriptan hydrobromide — Relpax
Elidel — pimecrolimus cream
Eligard — *leuprolide acetate*

Elitek	rasburicase
Elixophyllin	theophylline
Ellence	*epirubicin HCl*
Elmiron	pentosan polysulfate sodium
Elocon	mometasone furoate topical
Eloxatin	oxaliplatin
Elspar	asparaginase
eltrombopag	Promacta
Emadine	emedastine difumarate opthth soln
Embeda	morphine sulfate and naltrexone HCl SR
Emcyt	estramustine phosphate sodium
emedastine difumarate opthth soln	Emadine
Emend capsule	aprepitant
Emend inj	fosaprepitant
EMLA Cream	*lidocaine; prilocaine cream*
Empirin with codeine #3 and #4	*aspirin 325 mg with codeine phosphate (30 and 60 mg)*
emtricitabine	Emtriva
emtricitabine, efavirenz, and tenofovir	Atripla
emtricitabine; tenofovir disoproxil	Truvada
Emtriva	emtricitabine
E-Mycin (WA)	*erythromycin*
Enablex	darifenacin
enalapril maleate	Vasotec
enalapril maleate; diltiazem malate (W)	Teczem (W)
enalapril maleate; felodipine SR (W)	Lexxel (W)
enalapril maleate; hydro-chlorothiazide	Vaseretic
Enbrel	etanercept
encainide HCl (W)	Enkaid (W)
Endep	amitriptyline HCl
Endocet	oxycodone HCl; acetaminophen
Endrate	edetate disodium
Enduron	*methyclothiazide*
enflurane	Ethrane
enfuvirtide	Fuzeon

Engerix-B	*hepatitis B vaccine*
Enkaid (W)	encainide HCl (W)
enoxaparin sodium	Lovenox
entacapone	Comtan
entecavir	Baraclude
Entereg	alvimopan
Entex LA	phenylpropanolamine HCl; guaifenesin SR
Entocort EC	budesonide capsule SR
Eovist	gadoxetate disodium inj
epinastine	Elestat
epinephrine	Adrenalin
epinephrine racemic (W)	Vaponefrin (W)
epirubicin HCl	Ellence
Epivir	lamivudine
Epivir HBV	lamivudine
eplerenone	Inspra
epoetin alfa	Epogen Procrit
Epogen	epoetin alfa
epoprostenol sodium	Flolan
eprosartan mesylate	Teveten
eprosartan mesylate; hydrochloro-thiazide	Teveten HCT
eptifibatide	Integrilin
Epzicom	lamivudine; abacavir sulfate
Equanil (WA)	*meprobamate*
Eraxis	anidulafungin IV
Erbitux	cetuximab
Ergamisol (W)	levamisole HCl (W)
ergocalciferol	Calciferol Drisdol
ergoloid mesylates	Hydergine
ergotamine tartrate; caffeine	Cafergot
ergotamine tartrate	Ergostat
Ergotrate	ergonovine maleate
erlotinib	Tarceva
Ertaczo	sertaconazole
ertapenem sodium	Invanz
Ery-Tab	erythromycin EC
Erythrocin Stearate	erythromycin stearate
erythromycin	*erythromycin*
erythromycin base coated particles	PCE Dispertab

erythromycin; benzoyl peroxide topical gel — Benzamycin

erythromycin EC — Ery-Tab

erythromycin estolate (W) — Ilosone (W)

erythromycin ethylsuccinate — E.E.S. 400

erythromycin ethylsuccinate; sulfisoxazole — Pediazole (WA)

erythromycin stearate — Erythrocin Stearate

escallantide inj — Kalbitor

escitalopram oxalate — Lexapro

Esclim — *estradiol transdermal*

Eserine Sulfate — physostigmine ophth ointment

Esidrix (WA) — hydrochlorothiazide

Esimil (W) — guanethidine monosulfate; hydrochlorothiazide (W)

Eskalith (WA) — *lithium carbonate*

esmolol HCl — Brevibloc

esomeprazole magnesium — Nexium

estazolam — *estazolam*

Estinyl (WA) — *ethinyl estradiol*

Estrace — *estradiol*

Estraderm — *estradiol transdermal*

estradiol — Estrace

estradiol hemihydrate vaginal tab — Vagifem

estradiol transdermal — Alora
Climara
Esclim
Estraderm
FemPatch (WA)
Menostar
Vivelle

estradiol vaginal ring — Estring

estradiol valerate — Delestrogen

estramustine phosphate sodium — Emcyt

Estratest — estrogens, esterified; methyltestosterone

Estratest H.S. — estrogens, esterified; methyltestosterone, half strength

Estring — estradiol vaginal ring

estrogens, conjugated — Premarin

estrogens conjugate, A synthetic — Cenestin

estrogens, conjugated; medroxyprogesterone acetate — Premphase
Prempro

estrogens, esterified; methyltestosterone — Estratest

estrogens, esterified methyltestosterone, half strength — Estratest H.S.

estropipate — Ogen

Estrostep — norethindrone acetate; ethinyl estradiol

eszopiclone — Lunesta

etanercept — Enbrel

ethacrynic acid — Edecrin

ethambutol HCl — Myambutol

ethchlorvynol (W) — Placidyl (W)

Ethezyme — papain; urea oint

ethinyl estradiol — Estinyl (WA)

ethinyl estradiol; levonorgestrel (91 day cycle) — Seasonale

ethionamide — Trecator-SC

Ethmozine — moricizine

ethosuximide — Zarontin

Ethrane — enflurane

ethyl chloride — *ethyl chloride*

ethynodiol diacetate; ethinyl estradiol — Demulen

Ethyol — amifostine

etidocaine HCl (W) — Duranest (W)

etidronate disodium — Didronel

etodolac — *etodolac*

etodolac SR — *etodolac SR*

etomidate — Amidate

etonogestrel; ethinyl estradiol vagina ring — NuvaRing

etonogestrel implant — Implanon

Etopophos — etoposide phosphate diethanolate

etoposide — VePesid

etoposide phosphate diethanolate — Etopophos

Etrafon	*perphenazine;*
	amitriptyline HCl
etravirine	Intelence
Eulexin (WA)	*flutamide*
Eurax	crotamiton
Euthroid (WA)	liotrix
Eutonyl	pargyline HCl
everolimus-eluting coronary stent system	Xience V
everolimus-eluting coronary stent system	Promus
Evista	raloxifene HCl
Evithrom	thrombin, topical (human)
Evoxac	cevimeline HCl
Exelon	*rivastigmine tartrate*
exemestane	Aromasin
exenatide inj	Byetta
Exforge	amlodipine; valsartan
exisulind (W)	Aposyn (W)
Exjade	deferasirox
Ex-Lax	*sennosides*
Extavia	interferon beta-1b
Extraneal	icodextrin 7.5% with electrolyte peritoneal dialysis soln
ezetimibe	Zetia
ezetimibe; simvastatin	Vytorin

F

Fabrazyme	agalsidase beta
Factive	gemifloxacin mesylate
factor IX, concentrate	BeneFix
Factrel (W)	gonadorelin HCl (W)
famciclovir	Famvir
famotidine	Pepcid
famotidine, oral disintegrating tablet	Pepcid RPD
Famvir	*famciclovir*
Fanapt	iloperidone
Fansidar (W)	sulfadoxine; pyrimethamine (W)
Fareston	toremifene citrate
Faslodex	fulvestrant
Fastin	*phentermine HCl*
fat emulsion	*Intralipid*
	Liposyn II and III
febuxostat	Uloric
felbamate	Felbatol
Felbatol	felbamate

Feldene	*piroxicam*
felodipine	Plendil
Femara	Ietrozole
Femhrt	norethindrone acetate; ethinyl estradiol
FemPatch (WA)	*estradiol transdermal*
fenfluramine HCl (W)	Pondimin (W)
fenofibrate	Tricor
fenofibric acid	TriLipix
fenoldopam mesylate	Corlopam
fenoprofen calcium	Nalfon
fentanyl citrate	Sublimaze
fentanyl citrate; droperidol (W)	Innovar (W)
fentanyl iontophoretic transdermal system	Ionsys
Fentanyl Oralet (WA)	*fentanyl transmucosal*
fentanyl transdermal	Duragesic
fentanyl transmucosal	Actiq
	Fentanyl Oralet (WA)
Feosol	*ferrous sulfate*
Feraheme	ferumoxytol inj
Fer-In-Sol	*ferrous sulfate*
Fergon	*ferrous gluconate*
Feridex	ferumoxide HCl
Ferrlecit	sodium ferric gluconate complex in sucrose inj
ferrous gluconate	Fergon
ferrous sulfate	Feosol
	Fer-In-Sol
ferrous sulfate SR	SlowFe
Fertinex	urofollitropin for inj
ferumoxetil oral suspension (W)	Gastromark (W)
ferumoxide HCl	Feridex
ferumoxytol inj	Feraheme
fesoterodine fumarate	Toviaz
fexofenadine HCl	Allegra
fibrin sealant, human, topical	Artiss
fibrinogen concentrate, human inj	Riastap
filgrastim	Neupogen
finasteride	Propecia 1 mg tablet
	Proscar 5 mg tablet
Finevin	azelaic cream
fingolimod	Gilenya

Fioricet	butalbital; acetaminophen; caffeine	flurbiprofen	Ansaid
		flutamide	Eulexin (WA)
		fluticasone propionate spray	Flonase
Fiorinal	butalbital; aspirin; caffeine		Flovent (WA)
Firmagon	degarelix inj	fluticasone propionate cream & ointment	Cutivate
Flagyl	metronidazole		
Flagyl ER	metronidazole SR		
flavocoxid	Limbrel		
flavoxate HCl	Urispas	fluticasone propionate; salmeterol inhalation powder	Advair Diskus
Flaxedil (W)	gallamine triethiodide (W)		
flecainide acetate	Tambocor		
Flexeril	cyclobenzaprine HCl		
Flolan	epoprostenol sodium		
Flomax	tamsulosin HCl	fluvastatin sodium	Lescol
Flonase	fluticasone propionate spray		
		fluvoxamine maleate SR	Luvox CR
Florinef (WA)	fludrocortisone acetate		
Florone	diflorasone diacetate	FML	fluorometholone
Floropryl (W)	isoflurophate (W)	Focalin	dexmethylphenidate HCl
Florotag (W)	synopinine (W)	Folex PFS (WA)	methotrexate inj
Flovent (WA)	fluticasone propionate spray	folic acid	Folvite
		Follistim	follitropin beta
Floxin	ofloxacin	follitropin alfa	Gonal-F
Floxin Otic	ofloxacin otic soln	follitropin beta	Follistim
floxuridine	FUDR	Folotyn	pralatrexate inj
fluconazole	Diflucan	Folvite	folic acid
flucytosine	Ancobon	fomepizole	Antizol
Fludara	fludarabine phosphate	fomivirsen sodium inj (W)	Vitravene (W)
fludarabine phosphate	Fludara		
fludrocortisone acetate	Florinef (WA)	fondaparinux sodium	Arixtra
		Foradil	formoterol fumarate
Flumadine	rimantadine	Forane	isoflurane
flumazenil	Romazicon	formoterol fumarate	Foradil
flunisolide	Aero Bid		
fluocinolone acetonide	Synalar (WA)	Fortaz	ceftazidime
		Forteo	teriparatide
fluocinonide	Lidex (WA)	Fortovase (W)	saquinavir soft gel capsule (W)
Fluor-I-Strip	fluorescein sodium strips		
fluorescein sodium soln	Fluorescite	Fosamax	alendronate sodium
		fosamprenavir calcium	Lexiva
fluorescein sodium strips	Fluor-I-Strip		
		fosaprepitant	Emend inj
Fluorescite	fluorescein sodium soln	foscarnet (W)	Foscavir (W)
fluorometholone	FML	Foscavir (W)	foscarnet (W)
Fluoroplex	fluorouracil cream; soln	fosfomycin tromethamine	Monurol
fluorouracil cream	Carac		
fluorouracil inj	fluorouracil inj	fosinopril sodium	Monopril
fluorouracil cream; soln	Efudex (WA) Fluoroplex	fosphenytoin sodium	Cerebyx
Fluothane (W)	halothane (W)	fospropofol disodium inj	Lusedra
fluoxetine HCl	Prozac Sarafem		
fluoxymesterone (W)	Halotestin (W)	Fosrenol	lanthanum carbonate
		Fragmin	dalteparin sodium
fluphenazine HCl	fluphenazine HCl	Frova	frovatriptan succinate
flurazepam HCl	flurazepam HCl		

F
Rx

frovatriptan succinate	Frova
FUDR	*floxuridine*
fulvestrant	Faslodex
Fulvicin P/G (WA)	*griseofulvin*
Fungizone (W)	amphotericin B (W)
Furacin (W)	nitrofurazone (W)
furosemide	Lasix
Fusilev	levoleucovorin for inj
Fuzeon	enfuvirtide

G

gabapentin	Neurontin
Gabitril	tiagabine HCl
gadobenate dimeglumine	MultiHance
gadofosveset trisodium inj	Ablavar Vasovist
gadopentetate dimeglumine	Magnevist
gadoteridol	ProHance
gadoversetamide	OptiMark
gadoxetate disodium inj	Eovist
galantamine HBr	Razadyne (formerly called Reminyl)
gallamine triethiodide (W)	Flaxedil (W)
gallium nitrate	Ganite
galsulfase	Naglazyme
Galzin	zinc acetate
Gamimune N	*immune globulin intravenous*
Gammagard S/D	*immune globulin intravenous*
Gammaplex	immune globulin, IV, human inj
ganciclovir	Cytovene
ganciclovir ophthalmic implant (W)	Vitrasert (W)
ganirelix acetate	Antagon
Ganite	gallium nitrate
Gantanol (W)	sulfamethoxazole (W)
Garamycin	*gentamicin sulfate*
Gardasil	quadrivalent human papillomavirus (types 6, 11, 16, 18) recombinant vaccine
Gastrocrom	cromolyn sodium
Gastromark (W)	ferumoxetil oral suspension (W)
gatifloxacin (W)	Tequin (W)

gatifloxacin ophth soln	Zymar
gefitinib	Iressa
gemcitabine HCl	Gemzar
gemfibrozil	*gemfibrozil*
gemifloxacin mesylate	Factive
gemtuzumab ozogamicin	Mylotarg
Gemzar	gemcitabine HCl
GenEsa (W)	arbutamine HCl (W)
Gengraf	*cyclosporine capsules, (modified)*
Genotropin	*somatropin for inj*
gentamicin sulfate	Garamycin
Geocillin (W)	carbenicillin (W)
Geodon	ziprasidone HCl
Geref	sermorelin acetate
Gilenya	fingolimod
glatiramer acetate	Copaxone
Gleevec	imatinib mesylate
Gliadel	carmustine implantable wafer
glimepiride	Amaryl
glipizide	Glucotrol
glipizide SR	Glucotrol XL
glipizide; metformin	Metaglip
GlucaGen	glucagon (rDNA origin)
glucagon	glucagon
glucagon (rDNA origin)	GlucaGen
Glucophage	*metformin HCl*
Glucophage XR	*metformin HCl SR*
Glucotrol	*glipizide*
Glucotrol XL	*glipizide SR*
Glucovance	*glyburide; metformin HCl*
glyburide	DiaBeta Micronase
glyburide; metformin HCl	Glucovance
glyburide micronized	Glynase
glycerin ophth soln	Ophthalgan
glycopyrrolate	Cuvposa Robinul
Glynase	*glyburide micronized*
Glyset	miglitol
gold sodium thiomalate	Aurolate Myochrysine
golimumab	Simponi
GoLYTELY	*polyethylene glycol-electrolyte soln*

gonadorelin HCl (W)	Factrel (W)
Gonal-F	follitropin alfa
goserelin acetate implant	Zoladex
graftskin (W)	Apligraf (W)
granisetron HCl	Kytril
grepafloxacin HCl (W)	Raxar (W)
Grifulvin V	griseofulvin microsize
griseofulvin microsize	Grifulvin V (WA)
guanfacine	Intuniv
guaifenesin	Organidin NR Robitussin
guaifenesin; codeine phosphate	Robitussin A-C Tussi-Organidin NR
guaifenesin; dextromethor- phan	Robitussin-DM
guanabenz acetate	Wytensin (WA)
guanadrel sulfate (W)	Hylorel (W)
guanethidine monosulfate (W)	Ismelin (W)
guanethidine monosulfate; hydrochlorothi- azide (W)	Esimil (W)
guanfacine HCl	Tenex
Gynazole	butoconazole nitrate vaginal cream
Gyne-Lotrimin	clotrimazole

H

Habitrol	nicotine transdermal system
Haemophilus b conjugate vaccine reconstituted with diphtheria and tetanus toxoids and acellular pertussis vaccine adsorbed	ActHIB/Tripedia
haemophilus b conjugate vaccine inj	Hiberix

Haemophilus b conjugate; Hepatitis B vaccine	Comvax
halcinonide	Halog
Halcion	*triazolam*
Haldol	*haloperidol*
Halfan	halofantrine HCl
halofantrine HCl	Halfan
Halog	halcinonide
haloperidol	Haldol
haloprogin (W)	Halotex (W)
Halotestin (W)	fluoxymesterone (W)
Halotex (W)	haloprogin (W)
halothane (W)	Fluothane (W)
Havrix	*hepatitis A vaccine, inactivated*
Healon	*sodium hyaluronate*
Hectorol	doxercalciferol
Helidac	bismuth subsalicylate; metronidazole; tetracycline HCl
heparin sodium	*heparin sodium*
hepatitis A inactivated; hepatitis B (recombinant) vaccine	Twinrix
hepatitis A vaccine, inactivated	Havrix Vaqta
hepatitis B immune globulin (human)	NABI-HB
hepatitis B vaccine	Engerix-B Recombivax HB
Hepsera	adefovir dipivoxil
Herceptin	trastuzumab
Herplex (W)	idoxuridine (W)
Hespan	*hetastarch*
hetastarch	Hespan
hetastarch in lactated electrolyte inj (W)	Hextend (W)
Hetrazan	diethylcarbamazine citrate
Hexadrol (WA)	*dexamethasone*
Hexalen	altretamine
Hextend (W)	hetastarch in lactated electrolyte inj (W)
Hiberix	haemophilus b conjugate vaccine inj
Hibiclens	*chlorhexidine gluconate*
Hiprex	*methenamine hippurate*
Hismanal (W)	astemizole (W)
Hivid (W)	zalcitabine (W)
homatropine hydrobromide ophth	Isopto Homatropine

H
R

Humalog	insulin, lispro (human)
Humalog Mix75/25	insulin lispro protamine susp 75%; insulin lispro inj 25% [rDNA origin]
human papilloma-virus bivalent vaccine, recombinant, susp inj	Cervarlx
Humatin	paromomycin sulfate
Humatrope	somatropin
Humira	adalimumab
Humorsol (W)	demecarium bromide (W)
Humulin 70/30	isophane insulin suspension 70%, insulin inj 30% (human)
Humulin L (W)	insulin zinc suspension (Lente) (human) (W)
Humulin N	isophane insulin suspension (NPH) (human)
Humulin R	insulin inj (human)
Humulin U Ultralente (W)	insulin zinc suspension, extended, (human) (W)
Hurricane	benzocaine
Hyalgan	sodium hyaluronate
hyaluronidase	Wydase
Hycamtin	topotecan HCl
Hydergine	ergoloid mesylates
hydralazine HCl	Apresoline (WA)
hydralazine HCl; hydrochloroth-iazide (W)	Apresazide (W)
hydralazine; hydrochloroth-iazide; reserpine (W)	Ser-Ap-Es (W)
Hydrea	*hydroxyurea*
hydrochloroth-iazide	Esidrix (WA) HydroDIURIL Microzide Oretic (WA)
hydrocodone bitartrate; acetaminophen	Anexsia 5/500 Anexsia 7.5/650 Lorcet 10/650 Lorcet-HD (5/500) Lorcet plus (7.5/650) Lortab 2.5/500; 5/500; 7.5/500; 10/500 Norco Vicodin Vicodin ES Zydone 5/400, 7.5/400, 10/400

hydrocodone bitartrate 7.5 mg; ibuprofen 200 mg	Vicoprofen
hydrocodone polistirex; chlorphenira-mine	Tussionex
hydrocortisone	Cortef Hydrocortone
hydrocortisone buteprate cream	Pandel
hydrocortisone sodium succinate	Solu-Cortef
hydrocortisone HydroDIURIL	*hydrocortisone* *hydrochlorothiazide*
hydroflumethia-zide (W)	Saluron (W)
hydromorphone HCl	Dilaudid
hydromorphone HCl SR	*hydromorphone HCl SR*
Hydromox (W)	quinethazone (W)
hydroquinone topical susp (W)	Alustra (W)
hydroquinone; tretinoin; fluocinolone cream	Tri-Luma
hydroxychloro-quine sulfate	Plaquenil
hydroxyurea	Droxia Hydrea
hydroxyzine HCl	Atarax (WA)
hydroxyzine pamoate	Vistaril
Hygroton	*chlorthalidone*
hylan G-F 20	Synvisc
Hylorel (W)	guanadrel sulfate (W)
hyoscyamine sulfate orally disintegrating tab	NuLev
hyoscyamine sulfate SR	Cystospaz-M (WA) Levbid
Hyperab (W)	rabies immune globulin, human
Hyperstat (WA)	*diazoxide*
Hyper-Tet (W)	tetanus immune globulin (human) (W)
Hytrin	*terazosin HCl*
Hyzaar	*losartan potassium; hydrochlorothiazide*

H
R̸

I

ibandronate	Boniva
ibritumomab tiuxetan	Zevalin
ibuprofen	Advil
	Motrin
ibutilide fumarate	Corvert
icodextrin 7.5% with electrolyte peritoneal dialysis soln	Extraneal
Idamycin	*idarubicin*
idarubicin	Idamycin
idoxuridine (W)	Herplex (W)
idursulfase	Elaprase
IFEX	ifosfamide
ifosfamide	IFEX
Ilaris	canakinumab inj
iloperidone	Fanapt
iloprost	Ventavis
Ilosone (W)	erythromycin estolate (W)
Imagent GI	perflubron
imatinib mesylate	Gleevec
imciromab pentetate	Myoscint
Imdur	*isosorbide mononitrate SR*
imiglucerase	Cerezyme
imipenem-cilastatin sodium	Primaxin
imipramine HCl	Tofranil
imiquimod cream	Aldara
Imitrex	*sumatriptan*
immune globulin intravenous	Gamimune N
	Gammagard S/D
immune globulin, IV, human inj	Gammaplex
Imodium	*loperamide HCl*
Imogam	rabies immune globulin, human
Implanon	etonogestrel implant
Imuran	*azathioprine*
inamrinone lactate	*inamrinone lactate*
Inapsine (WA)	*droperidol*
incobotulinumtoixin A	Xeomin
indapamide	Lozol
Inderal (WA)	*propranolol HCl*
Inderide (WA)	*propranolol HCl; hydrochlorothiazide*
indinavir	Crixivan

indium In-111 pentetreotide	OctreoScan
Indocin	*indomethacin*
indomethacin	Indocin
Infasurf	calfactant intratracheal susp
INFeD	*iron dextran inj*
Infergen	interferon alfacon-1
infliximab	Remicade
influenza vaccine	Afluria
influenza virus vaccine type A, susp inj	Agriflu
Innohep	tinzaparin sodium
Innovar (W)	fentanyl citrate; droperidol (W)
Inocor (WA)	*inamrinone lactate*
INOmax	nitric oxide for inhalation
Inspra	eplerenone
insulin aspart (rDNA origin)	NovoLog
insulin detemir [rDNA origin]	Levemir
insulin glargine (rDNA origin)	Lantus
insulin glulisine [rDNA origin]	Apidra
insulin inj (human)	Humulin R
	Novolin R
	Velosulin Human
insulin lispro (human)	Humalog
insulin lispro protamine susp 75%; insulin lispro inj 25% [rDNA origin]	Humalog Mix75/25
insulin zinc suspension (Lente) (human) (W)	Humulin L (W)
	Novolin L (W)
insulin zinc suspension, extended (beef)	Ultralente U
insulin zinc suspension, extended, (human)	Humulin U Ultralente
Integrilin	eptifibatide
Intelence	etravirine
interferon alfa-2a (W)	Roferon-A (W)
interferon alfa-2b	Intron A
interferon alfa-n¹ lymphoblastoid	Wellferon

interferon alfa-n3   Alferon
  (human
  leukocyte
  derived)

interferon alfa-n3 (human leukocyte derived)	Alferon
interferon alfacon-1	Infergen
interferon beta-la	Avonex
	Rebif
interferon beta-1b	Betaseron
	Extavia
interferon gamma 1-b	Actimmune
Intrachol	choline chloride inj
Intralipid	*fat emulsion*
Intron A	interferon alfa-2b
Intropin (WA)	*dopamine HCl*
Intuniv	guanfacine
Invanz	ertapenem sodium
Invega	paliperidone
Inversine (W)	mecamylamine HCl (W)
Invirase	saquinavir mesylate
iocetamic acid	Cholebrine
iodamide meglumine	Renovue 65
iodixanol	Visipaque
iohexol	Omnipaque
Ionamin	phentermine resin
Ionsys	fentanyl iontophoretic transdermal system
iopamidol	Isovue
iopanoic acid (W)	Telepaque (W)
iopromide	Ultravist
iotrolan	Osmovist
ioversol	Optiray
ioxilan (W)	Oxilan (W)
Iplex	mecasermin rinfabate
Ipol	poliovirus vaccine inactivated
ipratropium bromide	Atrovent
ipratropium bromide; albuterol sulfate	Combivent
iprivask	Desirudin
irbesartan	Avapro
irbesartan; hydrochlorothiazide	Avalide
Iressa	gefitinib
irinotecan HCl	Camptosar
iron dextran inj	INFeD
	Dexferrum
iron sucrose inj	Venofer
Isentress	raltegravir
Ismelin (W)	guanethidine monosulfate (W)
ISMO	*isosorbide mononitrate*
isocarboxazid	Marplan

isoetharine HCl aerosol	*isoetharine HCl aerosol*
isoetharine HCl soln	*isoetharine HCl soln*
isoflurane	Forane
isoflurophate (W)	Floropryl (W)
isoniazid	Nydrazid
isoniazid; rifampin	Rifamate
isophane insulin suspension (NPH) (human)	Humulin N
	Novolin N
isophane insulin suspension (NPH) 70%, insulin inj 30% (human)	Humulin 70/30
	Novolin 70/30
isoproterenol HCl	Isuprel
Isoptin	*verapamil HCl*
Isopto Carbachol	carbachol ophth
Isopto Carpine	pilocarpine HCl ophth
Isopto Homatropine	homatropine hydrobromide ophth
Isopto Hyoscine	scopolamine hydrobromide ophth
Isordil (WA)	*isosorbide dinitrate*
isosorbide dinitrate	Isordil (WA)
isosorbide dinitrate; hydralazine	BiDil
isosorbide mononitrate	ISMO
isosorbide mononitrate SR	Imdur
isotretinoin (W)	Accutane (W)
Isovue	iopamidol
isoxsuprine HCl	Vasodilan
isradipine	DynaCirc
Istodax	romidepsin inj
Isuprel	isoproterenol HCl
itraconazole	Sporanox
ivermectin	Stromectol
IvyBlock	bentoquatam
ixabepilone	Ixempra
Ixempra	ixabepilone
Ixiaro	Japanese encephalitis vaccine, inactivated adsorbed susp inj

J

Januvia	sitagliptin

Japanese encephalitis vaccine, inactivated adsorbed susp inj	Ixiaro
Jevtana	cabazitaxel inj

K

Kadian	*morphine sulfate SR*
Kalbitor	escallantide inj
Kaletra	lopinavir; ritonavir
kanamycin sulfate	Kantrex
Kantrex	*kanamycin sulfate*
Kaon	*potassium gluconate*
Kaon-Cl	*potassium chloride SR*
Kapidex	dexiansoprazole
Kayexalate	*polystyrene sulfonate sodium*
K-Dur	*potassium chloride SR*
Keflex	*cephalexin*
Keflin	*cephalothin sodium*
Keftab (WA)	*cephalexin HCl*
Kefurox (W)	*cefuroxime sodium*
Kefzol (WA)	*cefazolin sodium*
Kemadrin (W)	procyclidine HCl (W)
Kenalog	*triamcinolone acetonide*
Kepivance	palifermin
Keppra	*levetiracetam*
Kerlone	*betaxolol*
Ketalar	*ketamine HCl*
ketamine HCL	Ketalar
Ketek	telithromycin
ketoconazole	Nizoral
ketoprofen	Orudis (WA)
ketoprofen SR	Oruvail (WA)
ketorolac tromethamine	Toradol
ketorolac tromethamine ophth	Acular
ketotifen fumarate ophth soln	Zaditor
Kineret	anakinra
Kinrix	diphtheria and tetanus toxoids and acellular pertussis adsorbed and inactivated poliovirus vaccine
Klaron	sodium sulfacetamide lotion
Klonopin	*clonazepam*
Klor-Con 10	*potassium chloride SR*

K-Lyte	*potassium bicarbonate; potassium citrate effervescent*
K-Lyte/Cl	*potassium chloride potassium bicarbonate effervescent*
Kogenate	antihemophilic factor (recombinant)
Kolyum	*potassium chloride; potassium gluconate*
Konsyl-D	*psyllium*
Kuvan	sapropterin dihydrochloride
Kwell (WA)	*lindane*
Kytril	*granisetron HCl*

L

labetalol HCl	Normodyne Trandate
Lac-Hydrin	lactic acid; ammonium lactate lotion
lacosamide	Vimpat
lactic acid; ammonium lactate lotion	Lac-Hydrin
lactulose	Cephulac Chronulac
Lamictal	*lamotrigine*
Lamisil	*terbinafine HCl*
lamivudine	Epivir Epivir HBV
lamivudine; abacavir sulfate	Epzicom
lamivudine; zidovudine	Combivir
lamivudine; zidovudine; abacavir sulfate	Trizivir
lamotrigine	Lamictal
Lanoxicaps (W)	digoxin capsules (W)
Lanoxin	*digoxin*
lanreotide	Somatuline
lansoprazole	Prevacid
lansoprazole; amoxicillin; clarithromycin	Prevpac
lanthanum carbonate	Fosrenol
Lantus	insulin glargine (rDNA origin)
lapatinib	Tykerb
Lariam	mefloquine HCl

Larodopa (W)	levodopa (W)
laronidase	Aldurazyme
Lastacaft	alcaftadine
Lasix	furosemide
latanoprost	Xalatan
leflunomide	Arava
lenalidomide	Revlimid
lepirudin	Refludan
Lescol	fluvastatin sodium
Letairis	ambrisentan
letrozole	Femara
leucovorin calcium	Wellcovorin (WA)
Leukeran	chlorambucil
Leukine	sargramostim
leuprolide acetate	Eligard Lupron
leuprolide acetate implant	Viadur (WA)
Leustatin	cladribine
levalbuterol HCl inhalation soln	Xopenex
levamisole HCl (W)	Ergamisol (W)
Levaquin	levofloxacin
Levbid	*hyoscyamine sulfate SR*
Levemir	insulin detemir [rDNA origin]
levetiracetam	Keppra
Levitra	vardenafil HCl
Levlite	*levonorgestrel; ethinyl estradiol*
levobupivacaine	Chirocaine
levocabastine HCl ophth susp (W)	Livostin (W)
levocetirizine	Xylzal
Levo-Dromoran	levorphanol tartrate
levobunolol HCl	Betagan
levocarnitine	Carnitor
levodopa (W)	Dopar (W) Larodopa (W)
levodopa; carbidopa	Parcopa Sinemet
levodopa; carbidopa SR	Sinemet CR
levodopa, carbidopa, and entacapone	Stalevo
levofloxacin	Levaquin
levofloxacin ophth soln	Quixin
levoleucovorin for inj	Fusilev
levomethadyl acetate HCl (W)	Orlaam (W)
levonorgestrel	Plan B
levonorgestrel; ethinyl estradiol	Alesse Levlite Nordette Preven Emergency Contraceptive Kit Tri-Levlen Triphasil
levonorgestrel implant (W)	Norplant (W)
levonorgestrel-releasing intrauterine system	Mirena
Levophed	*norepinephrine bitartrate*
levorphanol tartrate	Levo-Dromoran
levothyroxine sodium	Levoxyl Synthroid
Levoxyl	*levothyroxine sodium*
Levulan Kerastick	aminolevulinic acid HCl topical soln
Lexapro	escitalopram oxalate
Lexiscan	regadenoson inj
Lexiva	fosamprenavir calcium
Lexxel	enalapril maleate; felodipine SR
Lialda	mesalamine multimatrix tablets
Librax	*clidinium; chlordiazepoxide*
Librium	*chlordiazepoxide HCl*
Lidex (WA)	*fluocinonide*
lidocaine HCl	Xylocaine HCl
lidocaine patch	Lidoderm
lidocaine; prilocaine cream	EMLA Cream
Lidoderm	lidocaine patch
Limbitrol	*chlordiazepoxide HCl; amitriptyline HCl*
Limbrel	flavocoxid
Lincocin	lincomycin HCl
lincomycin HCl	Lincocin
lindane	*lindane*
linezolid	Zyvox
Lioresal	*baclofen*
liothyronine sodium	Cytomel
liothyronine sodium inj	Triostat
liotrix	Thyrolar
Lipitor	atorvastatin calcium
liposomal amphotericin B	AmBisome
Liposyn II and III	*fat emulsion*

lisdexamfetamine dimesylate	Vyvanse
lisinopril	Prinivil Zestril
lisinopril; hydrochloro-thiazide	Zestoretic
lithium carbonate	*lithium carbonate*
lithium citrate	*lithium citrate*
Lithobid	*lithium carbonate*
Lithostat	*acetohydroxamic acid*
Livalo	pitavastatin calcium
Livostin (W)	levocabastine HCl ophth susp (W)
Lodine (WA)	*etodolac*
Lodine XL (WA)	*etodolac SR*
lodoxamide tromethamine ophth soln	Alomide
Loestrin	norethindrone acetate; ethinyl estradiol
lomefloxacin (W)	Maxaquin (W)
Lomotil	*diphenoxylate HCl; atropine sulfate*
lomustine	CeeNu
Loniten (WA)	*minoxidil tablets*
Lo/Ovral	norgestrel; ethinyl estradiol
loperamide HCl	Imodium
Lopid	*gemfibrozil*
lopinavir; ritonavir	Kaletra
Lopressor	*metoprolol tartrate*
Loprox	ciclopirox cream and lotion
loratadine	Claritin
loratadine; pseudoephe-drine sulfate	Claritin D
lorazepam	Ativan
Lorcet (various combinations)	*hydrocodone bitartrate; acetaminophen*
Lortab (various combinations)	*hydrocodone bitartrate; acetaminophen*
losartan potassium	Cozaar
losartan potassium; hydrochlorothi-azide	Hyzaar
Lotemax	loteprednol etabonate ophth susp
Lotensin	*benazepril HCl*
loteprednol	Alrex
etabonate ophth susp	Lotemax
Lotrel	*amlodipine besylate; benazepril HCl*
Lotrimin	clotrimazole
Lotrisone	betamethasone; clotrimazole cream
Lotronex (W)	alosetron (W)
lovastatin	Mevacor
lovastatin; niacin	Advicor
Lovaza	omega-3-acid ethyl esters
Lovenox	*enoxaparin sodium*
loxapine succinate	Loxitane
Loxitane	*loxapine succinate*
Lozol (WA)	*indapamide*
lubiprostone	Amitiza
Lucentis	ranibizumab inj
Ludiomil (WA)	*maprotiline HCl*
Lufyllin	dyphylline
LumenHance	manganese chloride
Lunelle (W)	medroxyprogesterone acetate; estradiol cypionate inj (W)
Lunesta	eszopiclone
Lupron	leuprolide acetate
Lusedra	fospropofol disodium inj
lutropin alfa	Luveris
Luveris	lutropin alfa
Luvox CR	*fluvoxamine maleate SR*
Luxiq	betamethasone valerate (foam)
Lyrica	pregabalin
Lyme disease vaccine (W)	LYMErix (W)
LYMErix (W)	Lyme disease vaccine (W)
lymphocyte immune globulin	Atgam
lypressin (W)	Diapid (W)
Lysodren	mitotane

M

Maalox liquid	*aluminum hydroxide; magnesium hydroxide*
Macrobid	*nitrofurantoin macrocrystals and monohydrate*
Macrodantin	*nitrofurantoin macrocrystals*
Macugen	pegaptanib
magaldrate	Riopan (WA)
manganese chloride	LumenHance

M
Rx

Magnacet	oxycodone; acetaminophen
magnesium chloride SR	Slow-Mag
magnesium oxide	MAG-OX 400
magnesium sulfate	*magnesium sulfate*
Magnevist	gadopentetate dimeglumine
MAG-OX 400	magnesium oxide
Malarone	atovaquone; proguanil HCl
Mandol (W)	cefamandole nafate (W)
mangafodipir trisodium	Teslascan
mannitol inhalation powder	Aridol
maprotiline HCl	*maprotiline HCl*
maraviroc	Selzentry
Marcaine HCl	*bupivacaine HCl*
Marinol	*dronabinol*
Marplan	isocarboxazid
Matulane	procarbazine HCl
Mavik	*trandolapril*
Maxalt	rizatriptan benzoate
Maxalt-MLT	rizatriptan oral disintegrating tablet
Maxaquin (W)	lomefloxacin (W)
Maxipime	*cefepime HCl*
Maxzide	*triamterene 75 mg; hydro-chlorothiazide 50 mg*
Maxzide-25MG	*triamterene 37.5 mg; hydro-chlorothiazide 25 mg*
mazindol	Sanorex
measles, mumps, rubella vaccines, combined	M-M-R II
Mebaral	*mephobarbital*
mebendazole	Vermox
mecamylamine HCl (W)	Inversine (W)
mecasermin rinfabate	Iplex
mechlorethamine HCl	Mustargen
Meclan (W)	meclocycline sulfosalicylate (W)
meclizine	Antivert
meclocycline sulfosalicylate (W)	Meclan (W)
meclofenamate sodium	*meclofenamate sodium*
Meclomen (W)	*meclofenamate sodium*
Medrol	*methylprednisolone*
medroxyproges-terone acetate	Cycrin (W) Provera
medroxyproges-terone acetate; estradiol cypionate inj (W)	Lunelle (W)
medroxyproges-terone acetate SR	Depo-Provera
mefenamic acid	Ponstel
mefloquine HCl	Lariam
Mefoxin (WA)	*cefoxitin sodium*
Megace	*megestrol acetate*
megestrol acetate	Megace
Mellaril (WA)	*thioridazine HCl*
meloxicam	Mobic
melphalan	Alkeran
memantine HCl	Namenda
Menactra	meningococcal vaccine
menadiol sodium diphosphate (W)	Synkayvite (W)
meningococcal (groups A, C, Y, and W-135) oligosaccharide diphtheria CRM197 conjugate vaccine	Menveo
meningococcal vaccine	Menactra Menomune
Menomune	meningococcal vaccine
Menostar	*estradiol transdermal system*
menotropins	Pergonal (WA) Repronex
Mentax	butenafine HCl
Menveo	meningococcal (groups A, C, Y, and W-135) oligosaccharide diphtheria CRM 197 conjugate vaccine
meperidine HCl	Demerol
mephentermine sulfate (W)	Wyamine (W)
mephenytoin (W)	Mesantoin (W)
mephobarbital	Mebaral
Mephyton	phytonadione
mepivacaine HCl	Carbocaine
meprobamate	Equanil (WA) Miltown
Mepron	atovaquone
mequinol; tretinoin	Solage
mercaptopurine	Purinethol
Meridia (W)	sibutramine HCl monohydrate (W)
meropenem	Merrem

Merrem	meropenem
Meruvax II	rubella virus vaccine live attenuated
mesalamine	Asacol
	Rowasa
mesalamine multimatrix tablets	Lialda
Mesantoin (W)	mephenytoin (W)
mesna	Mesnex
Mesnex	mesna
mesoridazine (W)	Serentil (W)
Mestinon	pyridostigmine bromide
Metadate ER	*methylphenidate HCl SR*
Metaglip	*glipizide; metformin*
Metamucil	*psyllium*
Metaprel	metaproterenol sulfate
metaproterenol sulfate	Alupent (WA)
	Metaprel
metaraminol bitartrate	Aramine
Metaret	suramin
Metastron	strontium-89 chloride inj
metformin HCl	Glucophage
metformin HCl SR	Glucophage XR
methadone HCl	Dolophine
methamphetamine HCl	Desoxyn
methazolamide	Neptazane
methenamine combination	Urised (WA)
methenamine hippurate	Hiprex
Methergine	*methylergonovine maleate*
methicillin sodium (W)	Staphcillin (W)
methimazole	Tapazole
methocarbamol	Robaxin
methohexital sodium	Brevital Sodium
methotrexate	Rheumatrex
	Trexall
methotrexate, sodium preservative-free inj	Folex PFS (WA)
methoxamine HCl (W)	Vasoxyl (W)
methoxsalen	Oxsoralen
methoxsalen extracorporeal administration	Uvadex
methoxy polyethylene glycol-epoetin beta	Mircera

methscopolamine bromide	Pamine
methyclothiazide	Enduron
methyldopa	Aldomet
methyldopa; hydrochlorothiazide	Aldoril
methylergonovine maleate	Methergine (WA)
Methylin	*methylphenidate HCl*
Methylin ER	*methylphenidate HCl SR*
methylnaltrexone bromide inj	Relistor
methylphenidate HCl	Methylin
	Ritalin
methylphenidate SR	Concerta
	Metadate ER
	Methylin ER
	Ritalin SR
methylprednisolone	Medrol
methylprednisolone acetate SR inj	Depo-Medrol
methylprednisolone sodium succinate inj	Solu-Medrol
methyltestosterone	*methyltestosterone*
methysergide maleate (W)	Sansert (W)
Meticorten (WA)	*prednisone*
metoclopramide HCl	Reglan
metolazone	Zaroxolyn
Metopirone	metyrapone
metoprolol succinate SR	Toprol XL
metoprolol tartrate	Lopressor
MetroGel-Vaginal	*metronidazole vaginal gel*
metronidazole	Flagyl
metronidazole SR	Flagyl ER
metronidazole vaginal gel	MetroGel-Vaginal
metyrapone	Metopirone
metyrosine	Demser
Mevacor	*lovastatin*
Mexate (WA)	*methotrexate*
mexiletine HCl	Mexitil
Mexitil	mexiletine HCl
Mezlin (W)	mezlocillin (W)
mezlocillin (W)	Mezlin (W)
Miacalcin	calcitonin-salmon
mibefradil dihydrochloride (W)	Posicor (W)

micafungin sodium	Mycamine
Micardis	telmisartan
Micro K	*potassium chloride SR*
miconazole nitrate	Monistat
Micronase	*glyburide*
Micronor	*norethindrone*
Microzide	*hydrochlorothiazide*
Midamor	*amiloride HCl*
midazolam HCl	*midazolam HCl*
midodrine HCl	ProAmatine
Mifeprex	mifepristone
mifepristone	Mifeprex
miglitol	Glyset
miglustat	Zavesca
Migranol	dihydroergotamine mesylate nasal spray
milnacipran	Savella
milrinone lactate	Primacor
Miltown	*meprobamate*
Minipress	*prazosin HCl*
Minocin	*minocycline HCl*
minocycline HCl	Minocin
minocycline HCl dental microspheres	Arestin
minoxidil tablets	Loniten (WA)
minoxidil topical	Rogaine
Mintezol (W)	thiabendazole (W)
Miochol E	acetylcholine ophth
MiraLax	polyethylene glycol 3350 powder
Mirapex	pramipexole dihydrochloride
Mircera	methoxy polyethylene glycol-epoetin beta
Mircette	desogestrel; ethinyl estradiol and ethinyl estradiol
Mirena	levonorgestrel-releasing intrauterine system
mirtazapine	Remeron
misoprostol	Cytotec
Mithracin (W)	plicamycin (W)
mitomycin	Mutamycin
mitotane	Lysodren
mitoxantrone HCl	Novantrone
Mivacron (W)	mivacurium chloride (W)
mivacurium chloride (W)	Mivacron (W)
M-M-R II	measles, mumps, rubella vaccines, combined
Moban (W)	molindone HCl (W)
Mobic	*meloxicam*
modafinil	Provigil
Moduretic	*amiloride HCl; hydrochlorothiazide*
moexipril HCl	Univasc
moexipril HCl; hydrochlorothiazide	Uniretic
molindone HCl (W)	Moban (W)
mometasone furoate topical	Elocon
Mometasone furoate monohydrate nasal spray	Nasonex
Monistat	*miconazole nitrate*
Monocid (W)	cefonicid sodium (W)
Monopril	*fosinopril sodium*
montelukast sodium	Singulair
Monurol	fosfomycin tromethamine
moricizine	Ethmozine
morphine sulfate	Roxanol
morphine sulfate extended-release liposome inj	DepoDur
morphine sulfate, immediate release concentrated oral soln	Roxanol-T
morphine sulfate inj	Duramorph
morphine sulfate SR	Avinza Kadian MS Contin Oramorph SR Roxanol SR
morphine sulfate and naltrexone HCl SR	Embeda
Motrin	ibuprofen
moxifloxacin HCl	Avelox
Mozobil	plerixafor inj
MS Contin	*morphine sulfate SR*
Mucomyst	*acetylcysteine*
Multaq	dronedarone
MultiHance	gadobenate dimeglumine
multivitamins for infusion	Cernevit-12 Multi-12 (vial 1 and vial 2)
mupirocin nasal ointment	Bactroban
muromonab-CD3	Orthoclone OKT3
Muse	alprostadil urethral suppository
Mustargen	mechlorethamine HCl
Mutamycin	mitomycin
M.V.I.-12	*vitamin, multiple inj*
Myambutol	ethambutol HCl

M
R̥

Mycamine	micafungin sodium
Mycelex (WA)	*clotrimazole*
Mycifradin Sulfate	neomycin sulfate oral soln
Myciguent (W)	neomycin sulfate ointment and cream (W)
Mycolog-II Cream	*nystatin; triamcinolone cream*
mycophenolate mofetil	CellCept
mycophenolic acid	Myfortic
Mycostatin (WA)	*nystatin*
Mydriacyl	*tropicamide*
Myfortic	mycophenolic acid
Mykrox	metolazone
Myleran	busulfan
Mylicon	*simethicone*
Mylotarg	gemtuzumab ozogamicin
Myobloc	botulinum toxin type B
Myochrysine	gold sodium thiomalate
Myoscint	imciromab pentetate
Myozyme	alglucosidase alfa
Mysoline	*primidone*

N

NABI-HB	hepatitis B immune globulin (human)
nabilone	Cesamet
nabumetone	Relafen
nadolol	*nadolol*
Nafcil (W)	*nafcillin sodium*
nafcillin sodium	Nafcil (W) Unipen (W)
Naglazyme	galsulfase
nalbuphine HCl	Nubain
Nalfon	*fenoprofen calcium*
nalidixic acid (W)	NegGram (W)
nalmefene HCl (W)	Revex (W)
naloxone HCl	Narcan (WA)
naltrexone	ReVia
Namenda	memantine HCl
nandrolone phenpropionate (W)	Durabolin (W)
nandrolone decanoate (W)	Deca-Durabolin (W)
naphazoline ophth soln	Vasocon
Naprelan	*naproxen sodium SR*
Naprosyn	*naproxen*
naproxen	Naprosyn
naproxen sodium	Anaprox

naproxen sodium SR	Naprelan
naratriptan HCl	Amerge
Narcan (WA)	*naloxone HCl*
Nardil	phenelzine sulfate
Naropin	ropivacaine HCl
Nasacort AQ	triamcinolone acetonide nasal inhaler
Nasalcrom	cromolyn sodium
Nascobal	cyanocobalamin nasal gel
Nasonex	Mometasone furoate monohydrate nasal spray
natalizumab (W)	Tysabri (W)
nateglinide	Starlix
Natrecor	nesiritide
Navane	*thiothixene*
Navelbine	*vinorelbine tartrate*
Nebcin (WA)	*tobramycin sulfate*
nebivolol	Bystolic
NebuPent	pentamidine isethionate aerosol
nedocromil inhalation	Tilade
nedocromil ophth soln	Alocril
nefazodone HCl (W)	Serzone (W)
NegGram (W)	nalidixic acid (W)
nelarabine	Arranon
nelfinavir mesylate	Viracept
Nembutal	pentobarbital sodium inj
Neo-Synephrine	phenylephrine HCl inj
neomycin sulfate ointment and cream (W)	Myciguent (W)
neomycin sulfate oral soln	Mycifradin Sulfate
Neoral	*cyclosporine capsules (modified) and oral soln*
Neosar (WA)	*cyclophosphamide*
Neosporin Cream	*polymyxin; neomycin*
Neosporin Ointment	*polymyxin; neomycin; bacitracin*
Neosporin ophth Ointment	*polymyxin; neomycin; bacitracin*
Neosporin ophth soln	*polymyxin; neomycin*
neostigmine methylsulfate	Prostigmin
nepafenac	Nevanac
Neptazane	*methazolamide*
Nesacaine	*chloroprocaine HCl*
nesiritide	Natrecor
netilmicin sulfate (W)	Netromycin (W)

N
R

Normiflo (W)	ardeparin sodium (W)	ofatumumab	Arzerra
Normodyne	*labetalol HCl*	*ofloxacin*	Floxin
Noroxin	norfloxacin	*ofloxacin otic*	Floxin Otic
Norpace	*disopyramide phosphate*	soln	
Norplant (W)	levonorgestrel implant (W)	Ogen	*estropipate*
		olanzapine	Zyprexa
Norpramin	*desipramine HCl*	olanzapine;	Symbyaz
nortriptyline HCl	Aventyl	fluoxetine	
	Pamelor	olmesartan	Benicar
Norvasc	*amlodipine besylate*	medoxomil	
Norvir	ritonavir	olmesartan	Benicar HCT
Novantrone	*mitoxantrone HCl*	medoxomil;	
Novocain HCl	*procaine HCl*	hydrochloro-	
Novolin 70/30	isophane insulin	thiazide	
	suspension (NPH) 70%,	olopatadine HCl	Patanol
	insulin inj 30%	ophth soln	
	(human)	olsalazine	Dipentum
Novolin N	isophane insulin	sodium	
	suspension (NPH)	Olux	clobetasol foam
	(human)	Omacor (name	omega-3-acid ethyl esters
Novolin R	insulin inj (human)	changed to	
NovoLog	insulin aspart (rDNA	Lovaza)	
	origin)	omalizumab	Xolair
NovoSeven	coagulation factor VII a	omega-3-acid	Lovaza (formerly called
	(recombinant)	ethyl ester	Omacor)
Noxafil	posaconazole	*omeprazole*	Prilosec
Nplate	romiplostim inj	Omnaris	ciclesonide nasal susp
Nubain	nalbuphine HCl	Omnicef	*cefdinir*
Nucynta	tapentadol	Omnipaque	iohexol
NuLev	hyoscyamine sulfate	Oncaspar	pegaspargase
	orally disintegrating tab	OncoScint	satumomab pendetide
Numorphan	oxymorphone HCl	Oncovin	*vincristine sulfate*
Nupercainal	*dibucaine*	*ondansetron*	Zofran
Nuromax (W)	doxacurium chloride (W)	*ondansetron*	Zofran ODT
Nuprin (WA)	*ibuprofen*	orally	
Nutropin	somatropin for inj	disintegrating	
Nutropin AQ	somatropin inj	tab	
NuvaRing	etonogestrel; ethinyl	Onglyza	saxagliptin
	estradiol vagina ring	Ontak	denileukin diftitox
Nuvigil	armodafinil	Onxol	*paclitaxel inj*
Nydrazid	*isoniazid*	Opana	oxymorphone HCl
nystatin	Mycostatin (WA)	Opana ER	oxymorphone HCl
nystatin topical	Nystop		extended
powder			release tablets
nystatin;	Mycolog-II Cream	Ophthaine (WA)	*proparacaine*
triamcinolone		Ophthalgan	glycerin ophth soln
cream		Ophthetic	proparacaine HCl
Nystop	*nystatin topical powder*	opium;	B & O
		belladonna	Supprettes
		suppositories	
O		oprelvekin	Neumega
		Opticrom	cromolyn sodium
		OptiMark	gadoversetamide
OctreoScan	indium In-111	Optimine	azatadine maleate
	pentetreotide	Optiray	ioversol
octreotide acetate	Sandostatin	Optivar	azelastine HCl ophth soln
octreotide acetate	Sandostatin LAR	Orabase	benzocaine
susp for inj	Depot	Orajel	benzocaine

O
R

Oramorph SR	morphine sulfate SR	*oxtriphylline*	*oxtriphylline*
Orap	pimozide	oxybate sodium	Xyrem
OraVerse	phentolamine mesylate inj	*oxybutynin*	Ditropan
Orencia	abatacept	*chloride*	
Oretic (WA)	*hydrochlorothiazide*	oxychlorosene	Clorpactin
Orfadin	nitisinone	sodium	WCS-90
Organidin NR	*guaifenesin*	*oxycodone HCl*	Percolone (WA)
Orgaran	danaparoid sodium		Roxicodone
Orinase (WA)	*tolbutamide*	*oxycodone HCl*	OxyContin
Orlaam (W)	levomethadyl acetate	*SR*	
	HCl (W)	*oxycodone HCl;*	Percocet 5/325;
orlistat	Xenical	*acetaminophen*	7.5/500; 10/650
Ornade	phenylpropanol-		Endocet
Spansules (W)	amine HCl;		Magnacet
	chlorphenir-amine		Roxicet
	maleate SR (W)	*oxycodone HCl;*	Percodan
orphenadrine	Norflex	*aspirin*	
citrate		oxycodone HCl;	Combunox
orphenadrine	Norgesic (W)	ibuprofen	
citrate; aspirin;		OxyContin	*oxycodone HCl SR*
caffeine (W)		*oxymetazoline*	Afrin nasal spray
Ortho-Cept	desogestrel; ethinyl	*HCl*	Dristan Long Lasting
	estradiol	oxymetholone	Anadrol-50
Orthoclone	muromonab-CD3	oxymorphone	Numorphan
OKT3		HCl	Opana tablets
Ortho Evra	norelgestromin; ethinyl	oxymorphone HCl	Opana ER
	estradiol transdermal	extended release	
	system	tablets	
Ortho-Novum	norethindrone; ethinyl	*oxytocin*	Pitocin
(products)	estradiol (or mestranol)		
Ortho-Prefest	17β-estradiol;		
	norgestimate		
Ortho Tri-Cyclen	norgestimate; ethinyl		**P**
	estradiol (combinations)		
Orudis (WA)	*ketoprofen*		
Oruvail (WA)	*ketoprofen SR*	Pacis	BCG intravesical
Os-Cal 500	*calcium carbonate*	*paclitaxel*	Onxol
oseltamivir	Tamiflu		Taxol
phosphate		paclitaxel,	Abraxane
Osmovist	iotrolan	albumin-bound	
Otrivin	xylometazoline	inj	
Ovidrel	choriogonadotropin alfa	paclitaxel-eluting	Taxus
ovine	Vitrase (W)	stent	
hyaluronidase		palifermin	Kepivance
(W)		paliperidone	Invega
Ovral	norgestrel; ethinyl	palivizumab	Synagis
	estradiol	Palladone XL	hydromorphone HCl SR
oxaliplatin	Eloxatin	palonosetron	Aloxi
Oxandrin	oxandrolone	HCl	
oxandrolone	Oxandrin	Pamelor	*nortriptyline HCl*
oxaprozin	Daypro	*pamidronate*	Aredia
oxazepam	Serax (WA)	*disodium*	
oxcarbazepine	Trileptal	Pamine	*methscopolamine bromide*
oxiconazole	Oxistat		Creon
nitrate cream		*pancrelipase EC*	*pancrelipase EC*
Oxilan (W)	ioxilan (W)		Pancrease
Oxistat	oxiconazole nitrate cream	*pancuronium*	Pavulon (WA)
Oxsoralen	methoxsalen	*bromide*	

O
Rx

Pandel	hydrocortisone buteprate cream
Panretin	alitretinoin
panitumumab	Vectibix
pantoprazole	Protonix
papain; urea oint	Accuzyme
	Ethezyme
papaverine HCl SR (W)	Pavabid (W)
papillomavirus quadrivalent human (types 6, 11, 16, 18) recombinant vaccine	Gardasil
paracetamol	*acetaminophen*
Paradione (W)	paramethadione (W)
Paraflex	*chlorzoxazone 250 mg*
Parafon Forte DSC	*chlorzoxazone 500 mg*
paramethadione (W)	Paradione (W)
Paraplatin (WA)	*carboplatin*
Parathar	teriparatide acetate
Parcopa	*levodopa; carbidopa*
paregoric	*camphorated tincture of opium*
pargyline HCl	Eutonyl
paricalcitol	Zemplar
Parlodel	*bromocriptine mesylate*
Parnate	*tranylcypromine sulfate*
paromomycin sulfate	Humatin
paroxetine HCl	Paxil
Paser	aminosalicylic acid
Patanol	olopatadine HCl ophth soln
Pavabid (W)	papaverine HCl SR (W)
Pavulon (WA)	*pancuronium bromide*
Paxil	*paroxetine HCl*
pazopanib	Votrient
PBZ (W)	tripelennamine HCl (W)
PCE Dispertab	erythromycin base coated particles
Pediazole (WA)	*erythromycin ethylsuccinate; sulfisoxazole*
pegaptanib	Macugen
pegaspargase	Oncaspar
Pegasys	peginterferon alfa-2a
pegfilgrastim	Neulasta
peginterferon alfa-2a	Pegasys
peginterferon alfa-2b (recombinant)	PEG-Intron
PEG-Intron	peginterferon alfa-2b (recombinant)

pegvisomant	Somavert
pemetrexed disodium	Alimta
pemirolast potassium ophth soln	Alamast
pemoline (W)	Cylert (W)
penicillamine	Cuprimine
penciclovir cream	Denavir
penicillin G benzathine	Bicillin L-A (for IM use only)
	Permapen (for IM use only)
penicillin G benzathine; penicillin G procaine	Bicillin C-R (for IM use only)
penicillin G procaine	Wycillin (for IM use only)
penicillin V potassium	*penicillin V potassium*
Penlac Nail Lacquer	ciclopirox soln
Pentacel	diphtheria and tetanus toxoids and acellular pertussis adsorbed, inactivated poliovirus and Haemophilus b conjugate
pentaerythritol tetranitrate (W)	Peritrate (W)
pentagastrin (W)	Peptavlon (W)
Pentam 300	pentamidine isethionate inj
pentamidine isethionate aerosol	NebuPent
pentamidine isethionate inj	Pentam 300
Pentaspan	pentastarch
pentastarch	Pentaspan
pentazocine HCl inj	Talwin
pentazocine HCl; naloxone HCl	Talwin Nx
pentetate zinc trisodium (tri-sodium zinc diethylenetri-aminepentaacetate)	Zn-DTPA
pentobarbital sodium inj	Nembutal
pentosan polysulfate sodium	Elmiron
pentostatin inj	Nipent
Pentothal	thiopental sodium inj

P
Rx

pentoxifylline	Trental	phentolamine	OraVerse
Pen Vee K (WA)	*penicillin V potassium*	mesylate	Regitine (WA)
Pepcid	*famotidine*	phenylbutyrate	Buphenyl
Pepcid RPD	*famotidine, oral*	sodium	
	disintegrating tablet	phenylephrine	Neo-Synephrine
Peptavlon (W)	pentagastrin (W)	HCl inj	
Percocet 5/325;	*oxycodone HCl;*	phenylpropanol-	Entex LA
7.5/500; 10/650	*acetaminophen*	amine HCl;	
Percodan	*oxycodone HCl; aspirin*	guaifenesin SR	
Percolone (WA)	*oxycodone HCl*	Phenytek	*phenytoin sodium*
perflenapent	EchoGen		*extended*
emulsion		*phenytoin*	Dilantin
perflubron	Imagent GI	*phenytoin*	Phenytek
Pergonal (WA)	*menotropins*	*sodium*	
Periactin (WA)	*cyproheptadine HCl*	*extended*	
Peri-Colace	docusate sodium; senna	Phospholine	echothiophate
	concentrate	Iodide (W)	iodide (W)
Peridex	chlorhexidine gluconate	Photofrin	porfimer sodium
	mouth rinse	physostigmine	Eserine Sulfate
perindopril	Aceon	ophth ointment	
erbumine		physostigmine	Antilirium
Periostat	*doxycycline hyclate*	salicylate	
	20 mg tab & cap	phytonadione	Mephyton
Peritrate (W)	pentaerythritol	pilocarpine HCl	Isopto Carpine
	tetranitrate (W)	ophth	
Permapen	penicillin G benzanthine	pilocarpine HCl	Salagen
	(for IM use only)	tablet	
permethrin	Nix	pimecrolimus	Elidel
Permitil (WA)	*fluphenazine HCl*	cream	
perphenazine	*perphenazine*	pimozide	Orap
perphenazine;	Etrafon	*pindolol*	Visken
amitriptyline	Triavil (WA)	pioglitazone HCl	Actos
HCl		pipecuronium	Arduan (W)
Persantine	*dipyridamole*	bromide (W)	
petrolatum,	Vaseline	*piperacillin*	Pipracil (WA)
white		*sodium*	
Phenaphen with	*acetaminophen*	piperacillin	Zosyn
Codeine (#2,	*300 mg with*	sodium;	
3, and 4) (WA)	*Codeine*	tazobactam	
	Phosphate (15, 30, and	sodium	
	60 mg)	Pipracil (WA)	*piperacillin sodium*
phenazopyridine	Pyridium	*piroxicam*	Feldene
HCl		pitavastatin	Livalo
phendimetrazine	Plegine	calcium	
tartrate		Pitocin	*oxytocin*
phenelzine	Nardil	Pitressin	*vasopressin*
sulfate		Placidyl (W)	ethchlorvynol (W)
Phenergan	*promethazine HCl*	Plan B	levonorgestrel
phenobarbital	*phenobarbital*	Plaquenil	*hydroxychloroquine*
phenobarbital,	Bellergal-S (W)		*sulfate*
ergotamine;		Plasbumin	*albumin human*
belladonna (W)		*plasma protein*	Plasma-Plex (WA)
phenoxybenza-	Dibenzyline	*fraction*	Plasmanate
mine HCl			Plasmatein (WA)
phentermine	Fastin		Protenate
HCl		Plasma-Plex (WA)	*plasma protein fraction*
phentermine	Ionamin	Plasmanate	*plasma protein fraction*
resin		Plasmatein	*plasma protein fraction*

Platinol AQ (WA)	*cisplatin*	poractant alpha intratracheal susp	Curosurf
Plavix	clopidogrel bisulfate		
Plegine	phendimetrazine tartrate		
Plenaxis	abarelix	porfimer sodium	Photofrin
Plendil	*felodipine*		
plerixafor inj	Mozobil	posaconazole	Noxafil
Pletal	cilostazol	Posicor (W)	mibefradil dihydrochloride (W)
Plexion	sulfacetamide sodium and sulfur lotion		
		potassium bicarbonate; potassium citrate effervescent	K-Lyte
plicamycin (W)	Mithracin (W)		
pneumococcal vaccine	Pneumovax		
pneumococcal 7-valent conjugate vaccine	Prevnar 7	*potassium chloride; potassium bicarbonate effervescent*	K-Lyte/Cl
pneumococcal 13-valent conjugate vaccine	Prevnar 13	*potassium chloride SR*	Kaon-Cl K-Dur Klor-Con 10 Slow-K (WA) Micro K
Pneumovax	pneumococcal vaccine		
podofilox gel	Condylox		
Polaramine Repetabs (WA)	*dexchlorpheniramine-maleate SR*	*potassium chloride; potassium gluconate*	Kolyum
poliovirus vaccine inactivated	Ipol		
polyethylene glycolelectro-lyte soln	CoLyte GoLYTELY	potassium citrate tab	Urocit-K
		potassium gluconate	Kaon
polyethylene glycol 3350 powder	MiraLax	povidone iodine	Betadine
		Pradaxa	dabigatran
poly-l-lactic acid	Sculptra	pralatrexate inj	Folotyn
polymyxin B sulfate inj	*polymyxin B sulfate inj*	pralidoxime chloride	Protopam
polymyxin B sulfate; trimethoprim ophth soln	Polytrim	pramipexole dihydrochloride	Mirapex
		pramlintide acetate	Symlin
polymyxin; neomycin	Neosporin Cream Neosporin ophth soln	pramoxine HCl	Tronothane HCl
		Prandin	repaglinide
polymyxin; neomycin; bacitracin	Neosporin Ointment Neosporin ophth Ointment	prasterone (W)	Aslera (W)
		prasugrel	Effient
		Pravachol	*pravastatin sodium*
polystyrene sulfonate sodium	Kayexalate	*pravastatin sodium*	Pravachol
		prazosin HCl	Minipress
polythiazide (W)	Renese (W)	Precedex	dexmedetomidine HCl inj
Polytrim	polymyxin B sulfate; trimethoprim ophth soln	Precose	acarbose
		prednisolone syrup	Prelone
Pondimin (W)	fenfluramine HCl (W)	*prednisone*	*prednisone*
		pregabalin	Lyrica
Ponstel	mefenamic acid	Prelone	*prednisolone syrup*
Pontocaine	*tetracaine HCl*	Premarin	estrogens, conjugated

Premphase	estrogens,
Prempro	conjugated;
	medroxyprogesterone
	acetate
Prepidil	dinoprostone gel
Preven	levonorgestrel;
Emergency	ethinyl
Contraceptive	estradiol
Kit	
Prevacid	*lansoprazole*
Prevnar 7	pneumococcal 7-valent
	conjugate vaccine
Prevnar 13	pneumococcal 3-valent
	conjugate vaccine
Preveon	adefovir dipivoxil
Prevpac	lansoprazole; amoxicillin;
	clarithromycin
Prezista	darunavir
Prialt	ziconotide
Priftin	rifapentine
Prilosec	*omeprazole*
Primacor	milrinone lactate
Primaxin	imipenemcilastatin sodium
primidone	Mysoline
Primsol (W)	trimethoprim (W)
Principen (WA)	*ampicillin*
Prinivil	*lisinopril*
Priscoline (W)	tolazoline (W)
Pristiq	desvenlafaxine succinate
ProAmatine	*midodrine HCl*
Pro-Banthine (WA)	*propantheline bromide*
probenecid	*probenecid*
probenecid;	ColBENEMID
colchicine	(WA)
procaine HCl	Novocain HCl
procarbazine	Matulane
HCl	
Procardia	*nifedipine*
Procardia XL	*nifedipine SR*
Prochieve	progesterone gel
prochlorperazine	Compazine (WA)
Procrit	epoetin alfa
procyclidine HCl	Kemadrin (W)
(W)	
progesterone gel	Crinone
	Prochieve
progesterone	Prometrium
micronized	
Prograf	*tacrolimus*
ProHance	gadoteridol
ProHIBiT	haemophilus b vaccine
Prokine (WA)	sargramostim
Prolastin	alpha$_1$-proteinase inhibitor
	(human)
Proleukin	aldesleukin
Prolixin (WA)	*fluphenazine HCl*
Proloid (W)	thyroglobulin (W)
Promacta	eltrombopag

promethazine HCl	Phenergan
Prometrium	progesterone micronized
Promus	everolimus-eluting
	coronary stent system
Propacet-100	propoxyphene napsylate;
	acetaminophen
propafenone HCl	Rythmol
propantheline	Pro-Banthine
bromide	
proparacaine	Ophthaine (WA)
HCl	Ophthetic
Propecia	finasteride tablets 1 mg
Propine	dipivefrin
propofol	Diprivan
propoxyphene	Darvon (W)
HCl (W)	
propoxyphene	*propoxyphene HCl;*
HCl;	*acetaminophen* (W)
acetaminophen	
(W)	
propoxyphene	Darvon
HCl; aspirin;	Compound 65 (W)
caffeine (W)	
propoxyphene	Darvocet-N 100
napsylate;	Propacet-100 (W)
acetaminophen	
(W)	
propranolol HCl	Inderal (WA)
propranolol HCl;	Inderide (WA)
hydrochlorothi-	
azide	
Propulsid (W)	cisapride (W)
Proscar	*finasteride tablets 5 mg*
ProSom (WA)	*estazolam*
ProstaScint	capromab pendetide
Prostep	*nicotine transdermal*
	system
Prostigmin	*neostigmine methylsulfate*
Prostin E$_2$	dinoprostone vaginal
	suppositories
Prostin VR	alprostadil
protamine sulfate	*protamine sulfate*
protein C	Ceprotin
concentrate	
(human)	
Protenate	plasma protein fraction
Protonix	*pantoprazole*
Protopam	pralidoxime chloride
Protopic	tacrolimus oint
protriptyline HCl	*protriptyline HCl*
Protropin	somatrem
Protropin II	*somatropin for inj*
Proventil	*albuterol*
Proventil HFA	*albuterol sulfate*
	inhalation aerosol
Proventil	*albuterol SR*
Repetabs	

Provera	*medroxyproges-terone acetate*
Provigil	modafinil
Prozac	*fluoxetine HCl*
Prudoxin	doxepin HCl cream
Prussian blue	Radiogardase
pseudoephedrine HCl	Sudafed
pseudoephedrine HCl; bromphiramine maleate	Drixoral Syrup
psyllium	Konsyl-D Metamucil
Pulmicort Turbuhaler (W)	budesonide inhalation powder (W)
Pulmozyme	dornase alfa
Purinethol	*mercaptopurine*
Pyridium	*phenazopyridine HCl*
pyridostigmine bromide	Mestinon
pyrimethamine	Daraprim
pyrimethamine; sulfadoxine	Fansidar

Q

Quadramet	samarium SM 153 lexidronam
Qualaquin	quinine sulfate
Quarzan (W)	clidinium bromide (W)
Questran (W)	cholestyramine (W)
quetiapine fumerate	Seroquel
Quinaglute (WA)	*quinidine gluconate SR*
quinapril HCl	Accupril
quinapril; hydrochloro-thiazide	Accuretic
quinethazone (W)	Hydromox (W)
Quinidex Extentabs (WA)	*quinidine sulfate SR*
quinidine gluconate SR	*quinidine gluconate SR*
quinidine sulfate	*quinidine sulfate*
quinidine sulfate SR	Quinidex Extentabs (WA)
quinine sulfate	Qualaquin
quinupristin; dalfopristin	Synercid
Quixin	levofloxacin ophth soln
Qvar	beclomethasone diproprionate inhalation aerosol

R

RabAvert	rabies vaccine for human use
rabeprazole sodium	Aciphex
rabies immune globulin, human	Hyperab (W) Imogam
rabies vaccine for human use	RabAvert
Radiogardase	Prussian blue
raloxifene HCl	Evista
raltegravir	Isentress
ramelteon	Rozerem
ramipril	Altace
Ranexa	ranolazine
ranibizumab inj	Lucentis
ranitidine bismuth citrate (W)	Tritec (W)
ranitidine HCl	Zantac
ranolazine	Ranexa
rapacuronium bromide (W)	Raplon (W)
Rapaflo	silodosin
Rapamune	sirolimus
Raplon (W)	rapacuronium bromide (W)
Raptiva (W)	efalizumab (W)
rasagiline mesylate	Azilect
rasburicase	Elitek
rattlesnake anti-venom	CroFab
Raxar (W)	grepafloxacin HCl (W)
Razadyne	*galanthamine HBr*
Rebetol	*ribavirin*
Rebetron (W)	ribavirin; interferon alfa-2b (W)
Rebif	interferon beta-1a
reboxetine mesylate	Vestra
Reclast intravenous infusion	zoledronic acid inj
Recombivax HB	*hepatitis B vaccine*
Recothrom	thrombin, topical (recombinant)
Redux (W)	dexfenfluramine HCl (W)
Refacto	antihemophilic factor (recombinant)
Refludan	lepirudin
regadenoson inj	Lexiscan
Regitine (WA)	*phentolamine mesylate*
Reglan	*metoclopramide HCl*
Regranex	becaplermin gel

R
R℞

Regroton (W)	chlorthalidone; reserpine (W)
Relafen	nabumetone
Relenza	zanamivir for inhalation
Relistor	methylnaltrexone bromide inj
Relpax	eletriptan hydrobromide
Remeron	*mirtazapine*
Remicade	infliximab
remifentanil HCl	Ultiva
Reminyl	name changed to Razadyne
Remodulin	treprostinil sodium
Renagel (W)	sevelamer HCl (W)
Renese (W)	polythiazide (W)
Renova	*tretinion topical*
Renovue 65	iodamide meglumine
ReoPro	abciximab
repaglinide	Prandin
Repronex	*menotropins*
Requip	*ropinirole HCl*
Rescriptor	delavirdine mesylate
Rescula (W)	unoprostone isopropyl ophth soln (W)
reserpine	Serpasil (WA)
RespiGam	respiratory syncytial virus immune globulin intravenous (human)
respiratory syncytial virus immune globulin intravenous (human)	RespiGam
Restasis	cyclosporine ophth emulsion
Restoril	*temazepam*
retapamulin oint	Altabax
Retavase	reteplase
reteplase	Retavase
Retin-A	*tretinoin topical*
Retin-A Micro	*tretinoin gel*
Retrovir	*zidovudine*
Revex (W)	nalmefene HCl (W)
ReVia	*naltrexone*
Revlimid	lenalidomide
Reyataz (W)	atazanavir sulfate (W)
Rezulin (W)	troglitazone (W)
R-Gene	arginine HCl
Rheumatrex	*methotrexate tablets*
Rhinocort	budesonide nasal inhaler
RH$_O$ (D) immune globulin	RhoGAM
RH$_O$ (D) immune globulin IV (human)	WinRho SD
RhoGAM	RH$_O$ (D) immune globulin

Riastap	fibrinogen concentrate, human inj
ribavirin	Rebetol
	Virazole
ribavirin; interferon alfa-2b	Rebetron
Ridaura	auranofin
Rifadin	*rifampin*
Rifamate	isoniazid; rifampin
rifampin	Rifadin
	Rimactane
rifapentine	Priftin
rifaximin	Xifaxan
rilonacept	Arcalyst
Rilutek	riluzole
riluzole	Rilutek
Rimactane	*rifampin*
rimantadine	Flumadine
rimexolone	Vexol
Riopan	magaldrate
risedronate sodium	Actonel
Risperdal	*risperidone*
risperidone	Risperdal
Ritalin	*methylphenidate HCl*
Ritalin SR	*methylphenidate SR*
ritodrine HCl (W)	Yutopar (W)
ritonavir	Norvir
Rituxan	rituximab
rituximab	Rituxan
rivastigmine tartrate	Exelon
rizatriptan benzoate	Maxalt
rizatriptan oral disintegrating tablet	Maxalt-MLT
Robaxin	*methocarbamol*
Robinul	*glycopyrrolate*
Robitussin	*guaifenesin*
Robitussin A-C	*guaifenesin; codeine phosphate*
Robitussin-DM	*guaifenesin; dextromethorphan*
Rocaltrol	calcitriol
Rocephin	*ceftriaxone sodium*
rofecoxib (W)	Vioxx (W)
Roferon-A (W)	interferon alfa-2a (W)
Rogaine	*minoxidil topical*
Romazicon	flumazenil
romidepsin inj	Istodax
romiplostim inj	Nplate
ropinirole HCl	Requip
ropivacaine HCl	Naropin
Rosiglitazone maleate	Avandia
rosiglitazone maleate; metformin HCl	Avandamet

rosuvastatin calcium	Crestor
Rotarix	rotavirus vaccine, live, oral
Rotashield (W)	rotavirus (W) vaccine, live, oral, tetravalent
rotavirus vaccine live, oral	Rotarix
rotavirus vaccine, live, oral, (W) tetravalent	Rotashield (W)
rotigotine transdermal system	Neupro
Rowasa	mesalamine
Roxanol	*morphine sulfate*
Roxanol SR	*morphine sulfate SR*
Roxanol-T	*morphine sulfate, immediate release concentrated oral soln*
Roxicet	*oxycodone HCl; acetaminophen*
Roxicodone	*oxycodone HCl*
Rozerem	ramelteon
rubella virus vaccine live attenuated	Meruvax II
Rubex (WA)	*doxorubicin HCl*
rufinamide	Banzel
Rythmol	*propafenone HCl*

S

Sabril	vigabatrin
sacrosidase	Sucraid
Saizen	*somatropin*
Salagen	*pilocarpine HCl tablet*
salbutamol sulfate	*albuterol sulfate*
salmeterol xinafoate	Serevent
salmeterol xinafoate inhalation powder	Serevent Diskus
salsalate	Disalcid
Sal-Tropine	atropine sulfate tablets
Saluron (W)	hydroflumethiazide (W)
samarium SM 153 lexidronam	Quadramet
Samsca	tolvaptan oral
Sanctura	trospium chloride
Sandimmune	*cyclosporine*

Sandoglobulin (WA)	*immune globulin intravenous*
Sandostatin	*octreotide acetate*
Sandostatin LAR Depot	octreotide acetate susp for inj
Sanorex	mazindol
Sansert (W)	methysergide maleate (W)
Santyl	collagenase
Saphris	asenapine maleate
sapropterin dihydrochloride	Kuvan
saquinavir mesylate	Invirase
saquinavir soft gel capsule (W)	Fortovase (W)
Sarafem	*fluoxetine*
sargramostim	Leukine
	Prokine (WA)
satumomab pendetide	OncoScint
Savella	milnacipran
saxagliptin	Onglyza
Sclerosol	talc, sterile aerosol
Scopace	scopolamine hydrobromide, soluble tab
scopolamine hydrobromide ophth	Isopto Hyoscine
scopolamine hydrobromide, soluble tab	Scopace
scopolamine transdermal	Transderm Scop
Sculptra	poly-l-lactic acid
Seasonale	ethinyl estradiol; levonorgestrel (91 day cycle)
Sectral	*acebutolol HCl*
Seldane (W)	terfenadine (W)
Seldane D (W)	terfenadine; pseudoephedrine HCl (W)
selegiline HCl	Carbex (WA) Eldepryl
selenium sulfide	Selsun Blue
Selsun Blue	*selenium sulfide*
Selzentry	maraviroc
Sensipar	cinacalcet
sennosides	Ex Lax
sennosides	Senokot
sennosides; docusate sodium	Senokot-S
Senokot	*senna concentrates*
Senokot-S	*sennosides; docusate sodium*
Sensipar	cinacalcet HCl
Septocaine	articaine; epinephrine

S
℞

Septra	sulfamethoxazoletrimeth-oprim	sodium ferric gluconate complex in sucrose inj	Ferrlecit
Ser-Ap-Es (W)	hydralazine; hydrochloro-thiazide; reserpine (W)		
		sodium hyaluronate	Amvisc Healon Hyalgan
Serax (WA)	oxazepam		
Serentil (W)	mesoridazine (W)	sodium oxybate	Xyrem
Serevent	salmeterol xinafoate	sodium phenylbutyrate	Buphenyl
Serevent Diskus	salmeterol xinafoate inhalation powder		
		sodium phosphate tab	Visicol
Serlect	sertindole		
sermorelin acetate	Geref	sodium sulfacetamide lotion	Klaron
Seromycin	cycloserine		
Seroquel	quetiapine fumerate	sodium tetradecyl sulfate	Sotradecol
Serostim	somatropin (rDNA origin) for inj		
		Solage	mequinol; tretinoin
Serpasil (WA)	reserpine		
sertaconazole	Ertaczo	Solaraze	diclofenac gel
sertindole	Serlect	Solganal (W)	aurothioglucose (W)
sertraline HCl	Zoloft	solifenacin succinate	Vesicare
Serzone (W)	nefazodone HCl (W)		
sevelamer HCl (W) (W)	Renagel (W)	Soliris	eculizumab
		Solu-Cortef	hydrocortisone sodium succinate
sevoflurane	Ultane		
short chain fatty acids enema	Colomed	Solu-Medrol	methylprednisolone sodium succinate
sibutramine HCl monohydrate	Meridia	Soma	carisoprodol
		Somatuline	lanreotide
sildenafil citrate	Viagra	somatrem	Protropin
silodosin	Rapaflo	somatropin for inj	Genotropin Humatrope Norditropin Nutropin Protropin II Saizen
Silvadene	silver sulfadiazine		
silver sulfadiazine	Silvadene		
simethicone	Mylicon		
Simponi	golimumab		
Simulect	basiliximab		
simvastatin	Zocor		
sinecatechins oint	Veregen	somatropin inj	Nutropin AQ
Sinemet	levodopa; carbidopa	somatropin (rDNA origin) for inj	Serostim
Sinemet CR	levodopa; carbidopa SR		
Sinequan (WA)	doxepin HCl		
Singulair	montelukast sodium	Somavert	pegvisomant
sirolimus	Rapamune	Sonata	zaleplon
sirolimus-eluting stent	Cypher stent	sorafenib tosylate	Nexavar
		Soriatane	acitretin
sitagliptin	Januvia	sotalol	Betapace
Skelid	tiludronate disodium	Sotradecol	sodium tetradecyl sulfate
Slo-bid	theophylline SR	sparfloxacin (W)	Zagam (W)
Slo-Phyllin	theophylline	stavudine	Zerit
Slow Fe	ferrous sulfate SR	spectinomycin HCl (W)	Trobicin (W)
Slow-K (WA)	potassium chloride SR		
Slow-Mag	magnesium chloride SR	Spectracef	cefditoren pivoxil
smallpox (vaccinia) (W)	ACAM 2000 (W)	Spiriva HandiHaler	tiotropium bromide inhalation powder
sodium citrate; citric acid	Bicitra (WA)		
		spironolactone	Aldactone

S
R

spironolactone; hydrochloro- thiazide	Aldactazide
Sporanox	*itraconazole*
Sprycel	dasatinib
Stadol	butorphanol tartrate inj
Stadol NS (WA)	*butorphanol tartrate nasal spray*
Stalevo	levodopa; carbidopa; entacapone
stanozolol (W)	Winstrol (W)
Staphcillin (W)	methicillin sodium (W)
Starlix	nateglinide
stavudine SR	Zerit XR
Stelara	ustekinumab
Stelazine (WA)	*trifluoperazine HCl*
Strattera	Atomoxetine HCl
Streptase (W)	streptokinase (W)
streptokinase (W)	Streptase (W)
streptomycin sulfate	streptomycin sulfate
streptozocin	Zanosar
Striant	testosterone buccal
Stromectol	ivermectin
strontium-89 chloride inj	Metastron
Sublimaze	fentanyl citrate inj
Suboxone	buprenorphine HCl; naloxone HCl
Subutex	buprenorphine HCl
succinylcholine chloride	Anectine
Sucraid	sacrosidase
sucralfate	Carafate
Sudafed	pseudoephedrine HCl
Sufenta	sufentanil citrate
sufentanil citrate	Sufenta
Sulamyd sodium (WA)	*sulfacetamide sodium ophth*
Sular	*nisoldipine SR*
sulfacetamide sodium and sulfur lotion	Plexion
sulfacetamide sodium ophth	*sulfacetamide sodium ophth*
sulfadoxine; pyrimethamine (W)	Fansidar (W)
sulfamethoxazole (W)	Gantanol (W)
sulfamethoxazole- trimethoprim	Bactrim Cotrim co-trimoxazole Septra
sulfasalazine	Azulfidine
sulfinpyrazone (W)	Anturane (W)
sulindac	Clinoril

Sultrin (W)	triple sulfa vaginal cream (W)
sumatriptan	Imitrex
sumatriptan; naproxen sodium	Treximet
Sumycin (WA)	*tetracycline HCl*
sunitinib malate	Sutent
Suprane	desflurane
Suprax	cefixime
suramin	Metaret
Surmontil	*trimipramine maleate*
Survanta	beractant
Sustiva	Efavirenz
Sutent	sunitinib malate
Symbyax	olanzapine; fluoxetine
Symlin	pramlintide acetate
Symmetrel	*amantadine HCl*
Synagis	palivizumab
Synalar (WA)	*fluocinolone acetonide*
Synercid	quinupristin; dalfopristin
Synkayvite (W)	menadiol sodium diphosphate (W)
synopinine (W)	Florotag (W)
synthetic conjugated estrogens, A	Cenestin
Synthroid	*levothyroxine sodium*
Synvisc	hylan G-F 20

T

tacrine HCl (W)	Cognex (W)
tacrolimus	Prograf
tacrolimus oint	Protopic
tadalafil	Cialis
Tagamet	*cimetidine HCl*
talc, sterile aerosol	Sclerosol
Talwin	*pentazocine HCl*
Talwin Nx	*pentazocine HCl; naloxone HCl*
Tambocor	*flecainide acetate*
Tamiflu	oseltamivir phosphate
tamoxifen citrate	*tamoxifen citrate*
tamsulosin HCl	Flomax
Tapazole	*methimazole*
Tapentadol	tapentadol HCl tablets
tapentadol	Nucynta
tapentadol HCl tablets	Tapentadol
Tarceva	erlotinib
Targretin	bexarotene gel

Tarka	trandolapril; verapamil SR	terbutaline sulfate aerosol	Brethaire
tarzarotene gel	Tazorac		
Tasigna	nilotinib	terbutaline sulfate tablets and inj	Brethine Bricanyl
Tasmar	tolcapone		
tasosartan (W)	Verdia (W)		
Tavist	*clemastine fumarate*	*terconazole*	Terazol
Taxol	*paclitaxel*	terfenadine (W)	Seldane (W)
Taxotere	docetaxel	terfenadine; pseudoephed-rine HCl (W)	Seldane D (W)
Taxus	paclitaxel-eluting stent		
Tazicef	*ceftazidime*		
Tazidime (WA)	*ceftazidime*	teriparatide	Forteo
Tazorac	tarzarotene gel	teriparatide acetate	Parathar
technetium Tc-99m bicisate kit	Neurolite		
		Teslac (W)	testolactone (W)
		Teslascan	mangafodipir trisodium
technetium Tc-99m red blood cell kit	Ultratag	Testim	testosterone gel
		Testoderm (WA)	*testosterone transdermal*
		Testoderm TTS (WA)	*testosterone transdermal*
technetium Tc-99m	Cardiotec		
		testolactone (W)	Teslac (W)
technetium Tc99m sestamibi teboroxime kit	Cardiolite	testosterone buccal	Striant
		testosterone cypionate SR	DEPO-Testosterone
Teczem (W)	enalapril maleate; diltiazem malate (W)	testosterone gel	AndroGel Testim
tegaserod maleate (W)	Zelnorm (W)	*testosterone transdermal*	Androderm Testoderm (WA) Testoderm TTS (WA)
Tegretol	*carbamazepine*		
Tekturna	aliskiren hemifumarate	tetrabenazine	Xenazine
telavancin HCl	Vibativ	*tetracaine HCl*	Pontocaine
telbivudine	Tyzeka	*tetracycline HCl*	Achromycin (WA) Sumycin (WA)
Teldrin (WA)	*chlorpheniramine maleate SR*		
		tetrahydrozoline HCl ophth	Collyrium Visine Extra
Telepaque (W)	iopanoic acid (W)		
telithromycin	Ketek	Teveten	eprosartan mesylate
telmisartan	Micardis	Teveten HCT	eprosartan mesylate; hydrochlorothiazide
temazepam	Restoril		
Temodar	temozolomide	thalidomide	Thalomid
temozolomide	Temodar	Thalomid	thalidomide
temsirolimus	Torisel	Tham	tromethamine
tenecteplase	TNKase	Theo-Dur (WA)	*theophylline SR*
Tenex	*guanfacine HCl*	*theophylline*	Elixophyllin Slo-Phyllin
teniposide	Vumon		
tenofovir disoproxil fumarate	Viread	*theophylline SR*	Slo-bid Theo-Dur (WA) Uniphyl
tenofovir, efavirenz, and emtricitabine	Atripla	TheraCys	BCG intravesical
		Theragran	*vitamins*
		thiabendazole (W)	Mintezol (W)
Tenoretic	*atenolol; chlorthalidone*	thiethylperazine maleate (W)	Torecan (W)
Tenormin	*atenolol*		
Tensilon (WA)	*edrophonium chloride*	thioguanine	thioguanine
Tenuate	diethylpropion HCl	thiopental sodium inj	Pentothal
Tequin (W)	gatifloxacin (W)		
Terazol	*terconazole*	Thioplex	thiotepa
terazosin HCl	Hytrin	*thioridazine HCl*	Mellaril (WA)
terbinafine HCl	Lamisil	*thiotepa*	Thioplex (WA)

thiothixene | Navane
Thorazine (WA) | *chlorpromazine*
Thrombate III | antithrombin III (human)
thrombin, topical (human) | Evithrom
thrombin, topical (recombinant) | Recothrom
thymalfasin | Zadaxin
Thymitaq (W) | nolatrexed dihydrochloride (W)
Thymoglobulin | anti-thymocyte globulin, (rabbit)
thyroglobulin (W) | Proloid (W)
thyroid | *thyroid*
Thyrogen | thyrotropin alpha
Thyrolar | liotrix
thyrotropin (W) | Thytropar (W)
thyrotropin alpha | Thyrogen
Thytropar (W) | thyrotropin (W)
tiagabine HCl | Gabitril
Tiamate | *diltiazem maleate SR*
Tiazac | *diltiazem HCl SR*
Ticar (W) | ticarcillin disodium (W)
ticarcillin disodium (W) | Ticar (W)
ticarcillin; clavulanic acid | Timentin
TICE BCG | BCG intravesical
Ticlid (WA) | *ticlopidine*
ticlopidine | Ticlid (WA)
Tigan | *trimethobenzamide HCl*
tigecycline inj | Tygacil
Tikosyn | dofetilide
Tilade | nedocromil inhalation
tiludronate disodium | Skelid
Timentin | ticarcillin; clavulanic acid
timolol maleate ophth soln | Timoptic
timolol maleate ophth soln, gel forming | Timoptic-XE
timolol maleate | Blocadren
timolol maleate; dorzolamide HCl | Cosopt
Timoptic-XE | *timolol maleate ophth soln, gel forming*
Timoptic | *timolol maleate ophth soln*
Tinactin | tolnaftate
Tindamax | tinidazole
tinidazole | Tindamax
tinzaparin sodium | Innohep
TNKase | tenecteplase
tioconazole | Vagistat-1

tiotropium bromide inhalation powder | Spiriva HandiHaler
tipranavir | Aptivus
tirofiban HCl | Aggrastat
tizanidine HCl | Zanaflex
TOBI | tobramycin soln for inhalation
TobraDex | tobramycin; dexamethasone oint and susp
tobramycin sulfate inj | *tobramycin sulfate inj*
tobramycin sulfate ophth | Tobrex
tobramycin; dexamethasone oint and susp | TobraDex
tobramycin soln for inhalation | TOBI
Tobrex | tobramycin sulfate ophth
tocainide HCl | Tonocard
tocilizumab inj | Actemra
Tofranil | *imipramine HCl*
tolazamide | Tolinase
tolazoline (W) | Priscoline (W)
tolbutamide | Orinase (WA)
tolcapone | Tasmar
Tolectin | *tolmetin sodium*
Tolinase (WA) | *tolazamide*
tolmetin sodium | Tolectin
tolnaftate | Tinactin
tolterodine tartrate | Detrol
tolterodine tartrate (SR) | Detrol LA
tolvaptan Oral | Samsca
Tonocard | tocainide HCl
Topamax | *topiramate*
Topicort | desoximetasone
topiramate | Topamax
topotecan HCl | Hycamtin
Toprol XL | *metoprolol succinate SR*
Toradol | *ketorolac tromethamine*
Torecan | thiethylperazine maleate
toremifene citrate | Fareston
Torisel | temsirolimus
Tornalate (W) | bitolterol mesylate (W)
torsemide | Demadex
tositumomab and I-131 tositumomab | Bexxar
Totacillin-N | ampicillin sodium
Toviaz | fesoterodine fumarate
Tracleer | bosentan
Tracrium | atracurium besylate

T
R̶

tramadol; acetaminophen	Ultracet
tramadol HCl	Ultram
Trandate	*labetalol HCl*
trandolapril	Mavik
trandolapril; verapamil SR	Tarka
Transderm Scop	*scopolamine transdermal*
Transderm-Nitro	*nitroglycerin transdermal*
Tranxene	*clorazepate dipotassium*
tranylcypromine sulfate	Parnate
trastuzumab	Herceptin
Trasylol	aprotinin
Travasol	*amino acid inj*
Travatan	travoprost ophth soln
travoprost ophth soln	Travatan
trazodone HCl	*trazodone HCl*
Treanda	bendamustine HCl inj
Trecator-SC	ethionamide
Trelstar Depot	triptorelin pamoate
Trelstar LA	triptorelin pamoate (3 month inj)
Trental	*pentoxifylline*
treprostinil sodium	Remodulin
tretinoin cream 0.025%	Avita
tretinoin gel	Retin-A Micro
tretinion topical	Renova Retin-A
tretinoin capsules	Vesanoid (WA)
Trexall	*methotrexate tablets*
Treximet	sumatriptan; naproxen sodium
triamcinolone	Aristocort (W) Kenalog
triamcinolone acetonide aerosol	Azmacort
triamcinolone acetonide nasal inhaler	Nasacort AQ Tri-Nasal
triamcinolone acetonide ophth inj	Trivaris
triamterene	Dyrenium
triamterene 37.5 mg; hydro-chlorothiazide 25 mg	Maxzide -25MG Dyazide
triamterene 75 mg; hydro-chlorothiazide 50 mg	Maxzide
Triavil (WA)	*perphenazine; amitriptyline HCl*

triazolam	*Halcion*
Tricor	*fenofibrate*
Tri-Cyclen	norgestimate; ethinyl estradiol
Tridesilon	desonide
Tridil (WA)	*nitroglycerin inj*
Tridione (W)	trimethadione (W)
trifluoperazine HCl	*trifluoperazine HCl*
trifluridine	Viroptic
trihexyphenidyl HCl	*trihexyphenidyl HCl*
Trileptal	*oxcarbazepine*
Trilafon (WA)	*perphenazine*
Tri-Levlen	*levonorgestrel; ethinyl estradiol*
TriLipix	fenofibric acid
Trilisate (W)	choline magnesium trisalicylate (W)
Tri-Luma	hydroquinone; tretinoin; fluocinolone cream
trimethadione (W)	Tridione (W)
trimethaphan camsylate (W)	Arfonad (W)
trimethobenza-mide HCl	Tigan
trimethoprim (W)	Primsol (W)
trimetrexate glucuronate	Neutrexin
trimipramine maleate	Surmontil
Trimox	*amoxicillin*
Tri-Nasal (WA)	*triamcinolone acetonide nasal spray*
Triostat	liothyronine sodium inj
tripelennamine HCl (W)	PBZ (W)
Triphasil	*levonorgestrel; ethinyl estradiol*
triple sulfa vaginal cream (W)	Sultrin (W)
triprolidine HCl; pseudoephed-rine HCl	Actifed
triptorelin pamoate	Trelstar Depot
triptorelin pamoate (3 month inj)	Trelstar LA
Trisenox	arsenic trioxide
Tritec (W)	ranitidine bismuth citrate (W)
Trivaris	triamcinolone acetonide ophth inj
Tri-Vi-Flor	vitamins A, D, & C; fluoride
Trizivir	lamivudine; zidovudine; abacavir sulfate

Trobicin (W)   spectinomycin HCl (W)

troglitazone (W)   Rezulin (W)

tromethamine   Tham

Tronothane HCl   pramoxine HCl

TrophAmine   *amino acid inj*

Tropicacyl (WA)   *tropicamide*

tropicamide   Mydriacyl
     Tropicacyl

trospium   Sanctura
   chloride

trovafloxacin (W)   Trovan tablets (W)

Trovan tablet (W)   trovafloxacin mesylate
     (W)

Trovan inj (W)   alatrofloxacin mesylate IV
     (W)

Trusopt   dorzolamide HCl

Truvada   emtricitabine;
     tenofovir disoproxil

trypan blue   VisionBlue
   ophth soln

tuberculin skin   Aplisol
   test

tubocurarine   *tubocurarine*

Tucks   witch hazel pads

Tums   *calcium*
     carbonate

Tussi-Organidin   guaifenesin;
   NR   codeine
     phosphate

Tussionex   hydrocodone polistirex;
     chlorpheniramine

Twinrix   hepatitis A
     inactivated; hepatitis B
     (recombinant) vaccine

Tygacil   tigecycline inj

Tykerb   lapatinib

Tylenol   *acetaminophen*

Tylenol with   *acetaminophen*
   Codeine (#2,   *300 mg with*
   3, and 4)   *Codeine Phosphate (15,*
     30, and 60 mg)

Typhim Vi   typhoid Vi polysaccharide
     vaccine

typhoid Vi   Typhim Vi
   polysaccharide
   vaccine

tyropanoate   Bilopaque
   sodium

Tysabri   natalizumab

Tyzeka   telbivudine

U

UbiQGel   coenzyme Q10

Ulesfia   benzyl alcohol lotion

Ultane   *sevoflurane*

Ultiva   remifentanil HCl

Ultracet   *tramadol HCl;*
     acetaminophen

Ultralente U   insulin zinc suspension,
     extended (beef)

Ultram   *tramadol HCl*

Ultratag   technetium Tc-99m red
     blood cell kit

Ultravist   iopromide

Unasyn   *ampicillin sodium;*
     sulbactam sodium

Unipen (WA)   *nafcillin sodium*

Uniphyl   *theophylline SR*

Uniretic   *moexipril HCl;*
     hydrochlorothiazide

Univasc   *moexipril HCl*

Urecholine   *bethanechol chloride*

Urised (WA)   *methenamine combination*

Urispas   flavoxate HCl

urofollitropin   Bravelle

urofollitropin for   Fertinex
   inj

urokinase (W)   Abbokinase (W)

unoprostone   Rescula (W)
   isopropyl
   ophth soln (W)

UroXatral   alfuzosin

Uprima (WA)   *apomorphine HCl*

URSO   *ursodiol*

ursodiol   Actigall
     URSO

ustekinumab   Stelara

Uvadex   methoxsalen
     extracorporeal
     administration

V

Vagifem   estradiol hemihydrate
     vaginal tab

Vagistat-1   tioconazole

valacyclovir   Valtrex

Valcyte   valganciclovir

valdecoxib (W)   Bextra (W)

valganciclovir   Valcyte

Valium   *diazepam*

valproate sodium   Depacon
   inj

valproic acid   Depakene

valrubicin, (for   Valstar
   intravesical use)

valsartan   Diovan

valsartan;   Diovan HCT
   hydro-
   chlorothiazide

V
R̸

Valstar	valrubicin, (for intravesical use)
Valtrex	*valacyclovir*
Vancenase	beclomethasone dipropionate
Vancenase AQ Nasal (WA)	beclomethasone dipropionate
Vanceril (WA)	beclomethasone dipropionate
Vancocin	*vancomycin HCl*
vancomycin HCl	Vancocin
Vaniqa	eflornithine HCl cream
Vantin	cefpodoxime proxetil
Vaponefrin (W)	epinephrine racemic (W)
Vaprisol	conivaptan HCl
Vaqta	*hepatitis A vaccine, inactivated*
vardenafil HCl	Levitra
varicella virus vaccine	Varivax
varenicline	Chantix
Varivax	varicella virus vaccine
Vascor (W)	bepridil (W)
Vaseline	petrolatum, white
Vaseretic	*enalapril maleate; hydrochlorothiazide*
Vasocon	naphazoline ophth soln
Vasodilan	*isoxsuprine HCl*
vasopressin	Pitressin
Vasotec	*enalapril maleate*
Vasovist	gadofosveset trisodium inj
Vasoxyl (W)	methoxamine HCl (W)
Vectibix	panitumumab
vecuronium bromide	Norcuron
velaglucerase alfa inj	Vpriv
Velban	vinblastine sulfate
Velcade	bortezomib
Velosef (W)	cephradine (W)
Velosulin Human	insulin inj (human)
venlafaxine HCl	Effexor
venlafaxine HCl SR	Effexor XR
Venofer	*iron sucrose inj*
Ventavis	iloprost
Ventolin	albuterol
VePesid	*etoposide*
verapamil HCl	Isoptin
verapamil HCl SR	Calan SR Verelan
verapamil HCl SR bedtime formulation	Covera HS Verelan PM
Verdia (W)	tasosartan (W)
Veregen	sinecatechins oint
Verelan	*verapamil HCl SR*
Verelan PM	*verapamil HCl SR bedtime formulation*
Verluna (W)	nofetumomab (W)
Vermox	mebendazole
Versed (WA)	*midazolam HCl*
verteporfin inj	Visudyne
Vesanoid (WA)	*tretinoin capsules*
Vesicare	solifenacin succinate
Vestra	reboxetine mesylate
Vexol	rimexolone
Vfend	voriconazole
V-Flex plus PTX stent	paclitaxel-eluting stent
Viactiv	calcium carbonate; vitamin D and K chewable
Viadur (WA)	leuprolide acetate implant
Viagra	sildenafil citrate
Vibativ	telavancin HCl
Vibramycin	*doxycycline hyclate*
Vicodin	*hydrocodone bitartrate; acetaminophen*
Vicoprofen	*hydrocodone bitartrate 7.5 mg; ibuprofen 200 mg*
vidarabine monohydrate (W)	Vira-A (W)
Vidaza	azacitidine
Videx	didanosine
Videx EC	*didanosine SR*
vigabatrin	Sabril
Vimpat	lacosamide
vinblastine sulfate	Velban
vincristine sulfate	Oncovin
vindesine sulfate (W)	Eldisine (W)
vinorelbine tartrate	Navelbine
Vioform (W)	clioquinol (W)
Vioxx (W)	rofecoxib (W)
Vira-A (W)	vidarabine monohydrate (W)
Viracept	nelfinavir mesylate
Viramune	nevirapine
Virazole	ribavirin
Viread	tenofovir disoproxil fumarate
Viroptic	trifluridine
Visicol	sodium phosphate tab
Visine Extra	tetrahydrozoline HCl ophth
VisionBlue	trypan blue ophth soln
Visipaque	iodixanol
Visken	*pindolol*
Vistaril	*hydroxyzine pamoate*
Vistide	cidofovir
Visudyne	verteporfin inj
Vitrase	ovine hyaluronidase
Vitravene (W)	fomivirsen sodium inj (W)

V
Ŗ

Vivactil (WA)	*protriptyline HCl*
Vivelle	*estradiol transdermal system*
Volmax	albuterol SR
Voltaren	*diclofenac sodium*
Voltaren-XR	*diclofenac sodium SR*
voriconazole	Vfend
vorinostat	Zolinza
Votrient	pazopanib
Vpriv	velaglucerase alfa inj
Vumon	teniposide
Vytorin	ezetimibe; simvastatin
Vyvanse	lisdexamfetamine dimesylate

W

warfarin sodium	Coumadin
Welchol	colesevelam HCl
Wellbutrin	bupropion HCl
Wellbutrin SR	bupropion HCl SR
Wellcovorin (WA)	*leucovorin calcium*
Wellferon	interferon ALFA-n[1] lymphoblastoid
WinRho SD	RH_O (D) immune globulin IV (human)
Winstrol (W)	stanozolol (W)
witch hazel pads	Tucks
Wyamine (W)	mephentermine sulfate (W)
Wycillin (for IM use only)	penicillin G procaine (for IM use only)
Wydase (W)	hyaluronidase (W)
Wygesic (WA)	*propoxyphene HCl; acetaminophen*
Wymox (WA)	*amoxicillin*
Wytensin (WA)	*guanabenz acetate*

XYZ

Xalatan	latanoprost
Xanax	*alprazolam*
Xeloda	capecitabine
Xenazine	tetrabenazine
Xenical	orlistat
Xeomin	incobotulinumtoixin A
Xiaflex	collagenase clostridium histolyticum inj
Xibrom	bromfenac ophth soln
Xience V	everolimus-eluting coronary stent system

Xifaxan	rifaximin
Xigris	drotrecogin alfa
Xolair	omalizumab
Xopenex	*levalbuterol HCl inhalation soln*
Xylocaine HCl	*lidocaine HCl*
xylometazoline	Otrivin
Xylzal	levocetirizine
Xyrem	oxybate sodium
Yasmin	drospirenone; ethinyl estradiol
Yutopar (W)	ritodrine HCl (W)
Zadaxin	thymalfasin
Zaditor	ketotifen fumarate ophth soln
zafirlukast	Accolate
Zagam (W)	sparfloxacin (W)
zalcitabine (W)	Hivid (W)
zaleplon	Sonata
Zanaflex	*tizanidine HCl*
zanamivir for inhalation	Relenza
Zanosar	streptozocin
Zantac	*ranitidine HCl*
Zarontin	*ethosuximide*
Zaroxolyn	*metolazone*
Zavesca	miglustat
Zelnorm (W)	tegaserod maleate (W)
Zemplar	paricalcitol
Zenapax (W)	daclizumab (W)
Zerit XR	*stavudine SR*
Zestoretic	*lisinopril; hydrochloro-thiazide*
Zestril	*lisinopril*
Zetar	coal tar product
Zetia	ezetimibe
Zevalin	ibritumomab tiuxetan
Ziac	*bisoprolol fumarate; hydrochlorothiazide*
Ziagen	abacavir sulfate
ziconotide	Prialt
zidovudine	Retrovir
zidovudine; lamivudine	Combivir
zileuton	Zyflo
Zinacef	*cefuroxime sodium*
zinc acetate	Galzin
Zinecard	*dexrazoxane*
ziprasidone HCl	Geodon
Zithromax	*azithromycin*
Zn-DTPA	pentetate zinc trisodium (trisodium zinc diethylenetriamine-pentaacetate)
Zocor	*simvastatin*
Zofran	*ondansetron*
Zofran ODT	*ondansetron orally disintegrating tab*

Zoladex — goserelin acetate implant

zoledronic acid for inj — Zometa

zoledronic acid inj — Reclast intravenous infusion

Zolinza — vorinostat

zolmitriptan — Zomig

zolmitriptan orally disintegrating tablet — Zomig-ZMT

Zoloft — *sertraline HCl*

zolpidem tartrate — Ambien

Zometa — zoledronic acid for inj

Zomig — zolmitriptan

Zomig-ZMT — zolmitriptan orally disintegrating tablet

Zonegran — *zonisamide*

zonisamide — Zonegran

Zosyn — piperacillin sodium; tazobac tam sodium

Zovirax — *acyclovir*

Zyban — bupropion HCl SR

Zydone 5/400, 7.5/400, 10/400 — *hydrocodone bitartrate; acetaminophen*

Zyflo — zileuton

Zyloprim — *allopurinol*

Zymar — gatifloxacin opth soln

Zyprexa — olanzapine

Zyrtec — *cetirizine HCl*

Zyrtec-D — cetirizine HCl; pseudo-ephedrine HCl SR

Zyvox — linezolid

References

1. Facts and Comparisons. St. Louis, MO: Wolters Kluwer Health; Facts and Comparisons, Inc. (published monthly and online)

2. Sweetman SC. Ed. Martindale: 36th edition. The Pharmaceutical Press. London, 2009 (and online).

Chapter 10

Normal Adult Laboratory Values*

In the following tables, normal reference values for commonly requested laboratory tests are listed in traditional units and in SI units. The tables are a guideline only. Values are method dependent and "normal values" may vary between laboratories.

Blood, Plasma or Serum		
	Reference Value	
Determination	Conventional Units	SI Units
Ammonia (NH₃) − diffusion	20–120 mcg/dl	12–70 mcmol/L
Ammonia Nitrogen	15–45 mcg/dl	11–32 μmol/L
Amylase	35–118 IU/L	0.58–1.97 mckat/L
Anion Gap (Na⁺ − [Cl⁻ + HCO₃⁻]) (P)	7–16 mEq/L	7–16 mmol/L
Antinuclear antibodies	negative at 1:10 dilution of serum	negative at 1:10 dilution of serum
Antithrombin III (AT III)	80–120 units/dl	800–1200 units/L
Bicarbonate: Arterial Venous	21–28 mEq/L 22–29 mEq/L	21–28 mmol/L 22–29 mmol/L
Bilirubin: Conjugated (direct) Total	≤0.2 mg/dl 0.1–1 mg/dl	≤4 mcmol/L 2–18 mcmol/L
Calcitonin	<100 pg/mL	<100 pg/mL
Calcium: Total Ionized	8.6–10.3 mg/dl 4.4–5.1 mg/dl	2.2–2.74 mmol/L 1–1.3 mmol/L
Carbon dioxide content (plasma)	21–32 mmol/L	21–32 mmol/L
Carcinoembryonic antigen	<3 ng/mL	<3 mcg/L
Chloride	95–110 mEq/L	95–110 mmol/L
Coagulation screen: Bleeding time Prothrombin time Partial thromboplastin time (activated) Protein C Protein S	3–9.5 min 10–13 sec 22–37 sec 0.7–1.4 μ/mL 0.7–1.4 μ/mL	180–570 sec 10–13 sec 22–37 sec 700–1400 units/mL 700–1400 units/mL
Copper, total	70–160 mcg/dl	11–25 mcmol/L
Corticotropin (ACTH adrenocorticotropic hormone) − 0800 hr	<60 pg/mL	<13.2 pmol/L
Cortisol: 0800 hr 1800 hr 2000 hr	5–30 mcg/dl 2–15 mcg/dl ≤50% of 0800 hr	138–810 nmol/L 50–410 nmol/L ≤50% of 0800 hr
Creatine kinase: Female Male	20–170 IU/L 30–220 IU/L	0.33–2.83 mckat/L 0.5–3.67 mckat/L
Creatine kinase isoenzymes, MB fraction	0–12 IU/L	0–0.2 mckat/L
Creatinine	0.5–1.7 mg/dl	44–150 mcmol/L
Fibrinogen (coagulation factor I)	150–360 mg/dl	1.5–3.6 g/L

Blood, Plasma or Serum (Cont.)		
	Reference Value	
Determination	Conventional Units	SI Units
Follicle-stimulating hormone (FSH):		
Female	2–13 mIU/mL	2–13 IU/L
Midcycle	5–22 mIU/mL	5–22 IU/L
Male	1–8 mIU/mL	1–8 IU/L
Glucose, fasting	65–115 mg/dl	3.6–6.3 mmol/L
Glucose Tolerance Test (Oral)	mg/dL	mmol/L
	Normal	Normal
Fasting	70–105	3.9–5.8
60 min	120–170	6.7–9.4
90 min	100–140	5.6–7.8
120 min	70–120	3.9–6.7
	Diabetic	Diabetic
Fasting	>140	>7.8
60 min	≥200	≥11.1
90 min	≥200	≥11.1
120 min	≥140	≥7.8
(γ) − Glutamyltransferase (GGT):		
Male	9–50 units/L	9–50 units/L
Female	8–40 units/L	8–40 units/L
Haptoglobin	44–303 mg/dl	0.44–3.03 g/L
Hematologic tests:		
Fibrinogen	200–400 mg/dl	2–4 g/L
Hematocrit (Hct), female	36%–44.6%	0.36–0.446 fraction of 1
male	40.7%–50.3%	0.4–0.503 fraction of 1
Hemoglobin A$_{1C}$	5.3%–7.5% of total Hgb	0.053–0.075
Hemoglobin (Hb), female	12.1–15.3 g/dl	121–153 g/L
male	13.8–17.5 g/dl	138–175 g/L
Leukocyte count (WBC)	3800–9800/mcl	$3.8–9.8 \times 10^9$/L
Erythrocyte count (RBC), female	$3.5–5 \times 10^6$/mcl	$3.5–5 \times 10^{12}$/L
male	$4.3–5.9 \times 10^6$/mcl	$4.3–5.9 \times 10^{12}$/L
Mean corpuscular volume (MCV)	80–97.6 mcm^3	80–97.6 fl
Mean corpuscular hemoglobin (MCH)	27–33 pg/cell	1.66–2.09 fmol/cell
Mean corpuscular hemoglobin concentrate (MCHC)	33–36 g/dl	20.3–22 mmol/L
Erythrocyte sedimentation rate (sedrate, ESR)	≤30 mm/hr	≤30 mm/hr
Erythrocyte enzymes: Glucose-6-phosphate dehydrogenase (G-6-PD)	$250–5000$ units/10^6 cells	250–5000 mcunits/cell
Ferritin	10–383 ng/mL	23–862 pmol/L
Folic acid: normal	>3.1–12.4 ng/mL	7–28.1 nmol/L
Platelet count	$150–450 \times 10^3$/mcl	$150–450 \times 10^9$/L
Reticulocytes	0.5%–1.5% of erythrocytes	0.005–0.015
Vitamin B$_{12}$	223–1132 pg/mL	165–835 pmol/L
Iron: Female	30–160 mcg/dl	5.4–31.3 mcmol/L
Male	45–160 mcg/dl	8.1–31.3 mcmol/L
Iron binding capacity	220-420 mcg/dl	39.4–75.2 mcmol/L
Isocitrate Dehydrogenase	1.2–7 units/L	1.2–7 units/L
Isoenzymes		
Fraction 1	14%–26% of total	0.14–0.26 fraction of total
Fraction 2	29%–39% of total	0.29–0.39 fraction of total
Fraction 3	20%–26% of total	0.20–0.26 fraction of total
Fraction 4	8%–16% of total	0.08–0.16 fraction of total
Fraction 5	6%–16% of total	0.06–0.16 fraction of total
Lactate dehydrogenase	100–250 IU/L	1.67–4.17 mckat/L

Normal Adult Laboratory Values (Cont.) Blood*

	Blood, Plasma or Serum (Cont.)	
	Reference Value	
Determination	**Conventional Units**	**SI Units**
Lactic acid (lactate)	6–19 mg/dl	0.7–2.1 mmol/L
Lead	≤50 mcg/dl	≤2.41 mcmol/L
Lipase	10–150 units/L	10–150 units/L

Lipids:
  Total Cholesterol
    Desirable
    Borderline-high
    High
  LDL
    Desirable
    Borderline-high
    High
  HDL (low)
  Triglycerides
    Desirable
    Borderline-high
    High
    Very high
	
	<200 mg/dl
	200–239 mg/dl
	>239 mg/dl
	
	<130 mg/dl
	130–159 mg/dl
	>159 mg/dl
	<35 mg/dl
	
	<200 mg/dl
	200–400 mg/dl
	400–1000 mg/dl
	>1000 mg/dl
		
		<5.2 mmol/L
		<5.2–6.2 mmol/L
		>6.2 mmol/L
		
		<3.36 mmol/L
		3.36–4.11 mmol/L
		>4.11 mmol/L
		<0.91 mmol/L
		
		<2.26 mmol/L
		2.26–4.52 mmol/L
		4.52–11.3 mmol/L
		>11.3 mmol/L

Magnesium	1.3–2.2 mEq/L	0.65–1.1 mmol/L
Osmolality	280–300 mOsm/kg	280–300 mmol/kg
Oxygen saturation (arterial)	94%–100%	0.94–1 fraction of 1
PCO_2, arterial	35–45 mm Hg	4.7–6 kPa
pH, arterial	7.35–7.45	7.35–7.45
PO_2, arterial: Breathing room air[1] On 100% O_2	80–105 mm Hg >500 mm Hg	10.6–14 kPa
Phosphatase (acid), total at 37°C	0.13–0.63 IU/L	2.2–10.5 IU/L or 2.2–10.5 mckat/L
Phosphatase alkaline[2]	20–130 IU/L	20–130 IU/L or 0.33–2.17 mckat/L
Phosphorus, inorganic,[3] (phosphate)	2.5–5 mg/dl	0.8–1.6 mmol/L
Potassium	3.5–5 mEq/L	3.5–5 mmol/L

Progesterone
  Female
    Follicular phase
    Luteal phase
  Male
	
	0.1–1.5 ng/mL
	0.1–1.5 ng/mL
	2.5–28 ng/mL
	<0.5 ng/mL
		
		0.32–4.8 nmol/L
		0.32–4.8 nmol/L
		8–89 nmol/L
		<1.6 nmol/L

Prolactin	1.4–24.2 ng/mL	1.4–24.2 mcg/L

Prostate specific antigen
Protein: Total
    Albumin
    Globulin
	0–4 ng/mL
	6–8 g/dl
	3.6–5 g/dl
	2.3–3.5 g/dl
		0–4 ng/mL
		60–80 g/L
		36–50 g/L
		23–35 g/L

Rheumatoid factor	<60 IU/mL	<60 kIU/L
Sodium	135–147 mEq/L	135–147 mmol/L
Testosterone: Female Male	6–86 ng/dl 270–1070 ng/dl	0.21–3 mmol/L 9.3–37 nmol/L

[1]Age dependent
[2]Infants and adolescents up to 104 IU/L
[3]Infants in the first year up to 6 mg/dl

Normal Adult Laboratory Values (Cont.) Blood*

Blood, Plasma or Serum (Cont.)		
	Reference Value	
Determination	**Conventional Units**	**SI Units**
Thyroid Hormone Function Tests:		
Thyroid-stimulating hormone (TSH)	0.35–6.2 mcU/mL	0.35–6.2 mU/L
Thyroxine-binding globulin capacity	10–26 mcg/dl	100–260 mcg/L
Total triiodothyronine (T_3)	75–220 ng/dl	1.2–3.4 nmol/L
Total thyroxine by RIA (T_4)	4–11 mcg/dl	51–142 nmol/L
T_3 resin uptake	25%–38%	0.25–0.38 fraction of 1
Transaminase, AST (aspartate aminotransferase, SGOT)	11–47 IU/L	0.18–0.78 mckat/L
Transaminase, ALT (alanine aminotransferase, SGPT)	7–53 IU/L	0.12–0.88 mckat/L
Transferrin	220–400 mg/dL	2.20–4.00 g/L
Urea nitrogen (BUN)	8–25 mg/dl	2.9–8.9 mmol/L
Uric acid	3–8 mg/dl	179–476 mcmol/L
Vitamin A (retinol)	15–60 mcg/dl	0.52–2.09 mcmol/L
Zinc	50–150 mcg/dl	7.7–23 mcmol/L

Normal Laboratory Values—Urine

Urine		
	Reference Value	
Determination	**Conventional Units**	**SI Units**
Calcium[1]	50–250 mcg/day	1.25–6.25 mmol/day
Catecholamines: Epinephrine	<20 mcg/day	<109 nmol/day
Norepinephrine	<100 mcg/day	<590 nmol/day
Catecholamines, 24-hr	<110 mcg	<650 nmol
Copper[1]	15–60 mcg/day	0.24–0.95 mcmol/day
Creatinine: Child	8–22 mg/kg	71–195 μmol/kg
Adolescent	8–30 mg/kg	71–265 μmol/kg
Female	0.6–1.5 g/day	5.3–13.3 mmol/day
Male	0.8–1.8 g/day	7.1–15.9 mmol/day
pH	4.5–8	4.5–8
Phosphate[1]	0.9–1.3 g/day	29–42 mmol/day
Potassium[1]	25–100 mEq/day	25–100 mmol/day
Protein		
Total	1–14 mg/dL	10–140 mg/L
At rest	50–80 mg/day	50–80 mg/day
Protein, quantitative	<150 mg/day	<0.15 g/day
Sodium[1]	100–250 mEq/day	100–250 mmol/day
Specific Gravity, random	1.002–1.030	1.002–1.030
Uric Acid, 24-hr	250–750 mg	1.48–4.43 mmol

[1]Diet dependent

Normal Adult Laboratory Values—Drug Levels*

Drug Levels†			
		Reference Value	
	Drug Determination	Conventional Units	SI Units
Aminoglycosides	Amikacin		
	(trough)	1–8 mcg/mL	1.7–13.7 mcmol/L
	(peak)	20–30 mcg/mL	34–51 mcmol/L
	Gentamicin		
	(trough)	0.5–2 mcg/mL	1–4.2 mcmol/L
	(peak)	6–10 mcg/mL	12.5–20.9 mcmol/L
	Kanamycin		
	(trough)	5–10 mcg/mL	nd
	(peak)	20–25 mcg/mL	nd
	Netilmicin		
	(trough)	0.5–2 mcg/mL	nd
	(peak)	6–10 mcg/mL	nd
	Streptomycin		
	(trough)	<5 mcg/mL	nd
	(peak)	5–20 mcg/mL	nd
	Tobramycin		
	(trough)	0.5–2 mcg/mL	1.1–4.3 mcmol/L
	(peak)	5–20 mcg/mL	12.8–21.8 mcmol/L
Antiarrhythmics	Amiodarone	0.5–2.5 mcg/mL	1.5–4 mcmol/L
	Bretylium	0.5–1.5 mcg/mL	nd
	Digitoxin	9–25 mcg/L	11.8–32.8 nmol/L
	Digoxin	0.8–2 ng/mL	0.9–2.5 nmol/L
	Disopyramide	2–8 mcg/mL	6–18 mcmol/L
	Flecainide	0.2–1 mcg/mL	nd
	Lidocaine	1.5–6 mcg/mL	4.5–21.5 mcmol/L
	Mexiletine	0.5–2 mcg/mL	nd
	Procainamide	4–8 mcg/mL	17–34 mcmol/mL
	Propranolol	50–200 ng/mL	190–770 nmol/L
	Quinidine	2–6 mcg/mL	4.6–9.2 mcmol/L
	Tocainide	4–10 mcg/mL	nd
	Verapamil	0.08–0.3 mcg/mL	nd
Anti-convulsants	Carbamazepine	4–12 mcg/mL	17–51 mcmol/L
	Phenobarbital	10–40 mcg/mL	43–172 mcmol/L
	Phenytoin	10–20 mcg/mL	40–80 mcmol/L
	Primidone	4–12 mcg/mL	18–55 mcmol/L
	Valproic acid	40–100 mcg/mL	280–700 mcmol/L
Antidepressants	Amitriptyline	110–250 ng/mL[3]	500–900 nmol/L
	Amoxapine	200–500 ng/mL	nd
	Bupropion	25–100 ng/mL	nd
	Clomipramine	80–100 ng/mL	nd
	Desipramine	115–300 ng/mL	nd
	Doxepin	110–250 ng/mL[3]	nd
	Imipramine	225–350 ng/mL[3]	nd
	Maprotiline	200–300 ng/mL	nd
	Nortriptyline	50–150 ng/mL	nd
	Protriptyline	70–250 ng/mL	nd
	Trazodone	800–1600 ng/mL	nd
Antipsychotics	Chlorpromazine	50–300 ng/mL	150–950 nmol/L
	Fluphenazine	0.13–2.8 ng/mL	nd
	Haloperidol	5–20 ng/mL	nd
	Perphenazine	0.8–1.2 ng/mL	nd
	Thiothixene	2–57 ng/mL	nd

†The values given are generally accepted as desirable for treatment without toxicity for most patients. However, exceptions are not uncommon.
[1]24 hour trough values
[2]Toxic: 50–100 mg/dl (10.9–21.7 mmol/L)
[3]Parent drug plus N-desmethy7l metabolite
nd — No data available

L A B

Normal Adult Laboratory Values (Cont.) Drug Levels*

Drug Levels†

	Drug Determination	Reference Value: Conventional Units	Reference Value: SI Units
Miscellaneous	Amantadine	300 ng/mL	nd
	Amrinone	3.7 mcg/mL	nd
	Chloramphenicol	10–20 mcg/mL	31–62 mcmol/L
	Cyclosporine[1]	250–800 ng/mL (whole blood, RIA)	nd
		50–300 ng/mL (plasma, RIA)	nd
	Ethanol[2]	0 mg/dl	0 mmol/L
	Hydralazine	100 ng/mL	nd
	Lithium	0.6–1.2 mEq/L	0.6–1.2 mmol/L
	Salicylate	100–300 mg/L	724–2172 mcmol/L
	Sulfonamide	5–15 mg/dl	nd
	Terbutaline	0.5–4.1 ng/mL	nd
	Theophylline	10–20 mcg/mL	55–110 mcmol/L
	Vancomycin		
	(trough)	5–15 ng/mL	nd
	(peak)	20–40 mcg/mL	nd

†The values given are generally accepted as desirable for treatment without toxicity for most patients. However, exceptions are not uncommon.

[1]24 hour trough values

[2]Toxic: 50–100 mg/dl (10.9–21.7 mmol/L)

nd — No data available

#1 in its Field

Order Form and Prices for the 15th Edition of
Medical Abbreviations: 32,000 Conveniences at the
Expense of Communication and Safety
Authored by Neil M Davis
ISBN 978-0-931431-15-9

THE BOOK (prices shown include a 1-year single-user access license to the Internet version of the book which is updated with 20 new entries per week)

1–19 copies (book and Internet version)	$28.95 each plus S & H
20 or more copies (book and Internet version)	$20.25 each plus S & H

Shipping and handling charges to the 48 contiguous US states shown below

Number of books ordered	For the 48 contiguous US states
1	$7.00 + the price shown above
2	$9.00 + the price shown above
3–6	$12.00 + the price shown above
7–11	$15.00 + the price shown above
12–20	$19.00 + the price shown above
21–40	$36.00 + the price shown above
41 or more	$48.00 + the price shown above

For S & H costs to Hawaii, Alaska, Puerto Rico, or countries other than the USA, contact one of the sites shown below.
- Orders shipped to Pennsylvania, add 6% sales tax.
- No sales tax for other US states (subject to change)
- Purchase orders are accepted

1-YEAR SINGLE-USER ACCESS LICENSE TO THE INTERNET VERSION OF THE BOOK WHICH IS UPDATED WITH 20 NEW ENTRIES PER WEEK (no book, just the Internet version)

1-year, Single-User Access License (Internet version only—no book) For computers and/or WiFi-enabled devices	$19.95

- Orders from Pennsylvania, add 6% sales tax.
- No sales tax for other US states (subject to change)
- No S & H charges
- Credit Cards or other forms of prepayment only (secure web site)

PAYABLE BY–

Visa	MasterCard	Discover
American Exp.	Check	Money Order

ORDER FROM AND MAKE CHECK PAYABLE TO–

Neil M Davis Associates
2049 Stout Drive, B-3
Warminster PA 18974-3861

(continued)

Order and Price Information—continued

ORDERS MAY BE MAILED TO THE ADDRESS ON PREVIOUS PAGE OR

Phone 215 442 7430 or 888 333 1862
Fax 215 442 7432 or 888 333 4915
Secure Web site www.medabbrev.com
E-mail ev@neilmdavis.com

Where applicable, please have ready your credit card number, expiration date, security code number, phone number, and mailing address.

COUNTRIES OTHER THAN THE UNITED STATES

- Pay by credit card or in US dollars through corresponding US bank or an International Money Order in US currency.
- Prices shown on previous page
- To obtain shipping costs or provide shipping instructions call 215 442 7430, FAX 215 442 7432 or E-mail to ev@neilmdavis.com

Information Needed on Order Form

PLEASE PRINT OR TYPE

Name _____

Address _____

_____

City _____ State _____ Zip Code _____

Phone (____) _____

Attention (If Applicable) _____

Number of **books** ordered (**includes** a 1-year, single-user Internet access license) _____

Number of 1-year, single-user Internet access licenses (No book wanted) _____

PO # (If applicable) _____

Method of payment:

_____ Check or money order enclosed

_____ Visa _____ MasterCard

_____ Discover _____ American Express

Card Number _____

Exp. Date _____ Security Code _____

Cardholder's Name _____

Phone Number _____

Signature _____

CONCURRENT MULTI-USER ACCESS LICENSES TO THE INTERNET VERSION are available. The ability exists for you to add and control a list on abbreviations which are unique to your locale and/or organization, that would not normally appear in a national list. Hospitals and other healthcare facilities have the ability to add and control their own list of dangerous abbreviations which should not be used. To obtain a price list, a copy of the license agreement, and a 3-week free trial call 215 442 7430, FAX 215 442 7432 or E-mail ev@neilmdavis.com

iPhone®, iPad®, iPod®, iPod Touch®, DROID™, Windows Mobile, BlackBerry®, Palm, and other WiFi-enabled devices

The Internet version of the book which you receive can be accessed from any WiFi-enabled device. Add it to your home screen as an icon or bookmark it.

The Internet version is comprehensive and current as **20 new entries are added each week**. You can order the print addition of the book which comes with a 1-year, single-user access license to the Internet version or you can order the Internet version alone (see pricing and ordering information on the previous page)

Additions

Please forward additional meanings for these abbreviations, additional abbreviations and their meanings, or corrections to the author so that the Internet version, and book can be updated. Thank you. Dr. Neil M Davis, 2049 Stout Drive, B-3, Warminster, PA 18974. FAX 215 442 7432 or 888 333 4915. E-mail med@neilmdavis.com

Additions and Notes

(See the preface (page vii) for instructions on how to access to the Internet version of this book which is updated each week with about 20 new entries. Your suggestions are appreciated.)

Additions and Notes

(See the preface (page vii) for instructions on how to access to the Internet version of this book which is updated each week with about 20 new entries. Your suggestions are appreciated.)

Additions and Notes

(See the preface (page vii) for instructions on how to access to the Internet version of this book which is updated each week with about 20 new entries. Your suggestions are appreciated.)

dditions and Notes

(See the preface (page vii) for instructions on how to access to the Internet version of this book which is updated each week with about 20 new entries. Your suggestions are appreciated.)

www.medabbrev.com

- Have you used this Internet site?
- You are entitled to a no-cost, one-year, single-user access license.
- See page vii for activation instructions.

Features

- Contains the entire contents of this book
- At no extra cost, add it to your WiFi-enabled devices' home page as an icon, or bookmark it.
- Has a high-speed search engine to find—
  - the meaning(s) of an abbreviation
  - all the abbreviations that contain a particular word
  - trade and generic drug names
- Each week about 20 new entries are added.
- Click any word or drug name and be connected to the Wikipedia definition/monograph.
- You can renew your license each year, see page 417.